To the Dingly
Memorial Library
with best wishes
8/26/97 David H Goodel

From Tang Q

Percutaneous Balloon Valvuloplasty

Percutaneous Balloon Valvuloplasty

Edited by:
Tsung O. Cheng, M.D.
Professor of Medicine
Division of Cardiology
Department of Medicine
The George Washington University
School of Medicine and Health Sciences
Washington, D.C.

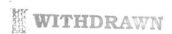
IGAKU-SHOIN New York · Tokyo

Published and distributed by

IGAKU-SHOIN Medical Publishers, Inc.
One Madison Avenue, New York, N.Y. 10010

IGAKU-SHOIN Ltd.,
5-24-3 Hongo, Bunkyo-ku, Tokyo

Library of Congress Cataloging-in-Publication Data

Percutaneous balloon valvuloplasty / edited by Tsung O. Cheng
    p.   cm.
    Includes bibliographical references and index.
    1. Percutaneous balloon valvuloplasty.   [1. Balloon Dilation.
  2. Heart Valve Diseases—surgery.]   I. Cheng, Tsung O.
  [DNLM: WG 260 P429]
  RD598.35.P37P48 1992
  617.4′12—dc20
  DNLM/DLC
  for Library of Congress   91-20887
                       CIP

ISBN: 0-89640-216-9 (New York)
ISBN: 4-260-14216-X (Tokyo)
Printed and bound in the U.S.A.

10 9 8 7 6 5 4 3 2 1

Dedication

To the memory of my father,
KIEN SUE CHENG
September 28, 1898–January 20, 1991

Foreword

This book on percutaneous techniques for relieving stenotic lesions of the heart and great vessels represents one aspect of the invasive treatment of heart disease. As is the case with most such techniques, there is the opportunity of providing enormous benefit to patients. Unfortunately, this beneficial potential is combined with the temptation for self-aggrandizement and divisiveness, which in some curious way is generated by the excitement of dramatically improving the well-being of another human being and is aggravated by the monetary advantages that can be accrued.

The development of a surgical intervention for mitral stenosis, probably begun in truth by Souttar in 1925, no doubt was not only an early but a very powerful stimulus to the development of the invasive treatment of heart disease in general. In fact, the development of cardiac surgery in the early 1950s consisted in considerable part of efforts to apply the techniques that had been successful in the treatment of mitral stenosis to adult calcific aortic stenosis — efforts that proved to be as unsuccessful as they had been successful when applied to mitral stenosis. In this same era, the other semilunar valve, the pulmonary valve, was the target of similar efforts. Pulmonary valvotomy, however, proved to be more successful than did aortic valvotomy, surely because the adverse effects of pulmonary valve incompetence were less evident. This early surgical experience appears to have been highly predictive of the current efforts to accomplish these goals percutaneously.

These developments of the late 1940s and early 1950s antedated the ready availability of methods for performing procedures on the cardiac valves, the coronary arteries, and the great arteries under direct vision by means of cardiopulmonary bypass. The actual procedures in that era, although surgical, manipulated narrowings in these structures from a distance, short as the distance may have been. It is only surprising that the interval has been so long between the development of those techniques, and those for manipulating narrowings in these structures from a greater distance, by percutaneous techniques.

This interval witnessed not only the further development of techniques for opening these narrowings under direct vision, but also the development of methods for replacing or bypassing the structures that were narrowed. Thus we need, and society must surely soon demand, appropriate and adequate comparisons of outcomes provided by these percutaneous techniques, not only with those accomplished surgically but also with those which can be achieved by replacing or bypassing the narrowed structures.

The table of contents of Professor Cheng's magnificent book gives evidence of the plethora of information that is available about the different outcomes that can be achieved by these percutaneous techniques. The table of contents also gives evidence of the paucity of information of the type which we and society really need: patient-specific studies comparing the outcomes after percutaneous techniques for opening narrowings in the cardiac valves, the coronary arteries, and great arteries with those after surgical techniques for accomplishing this and with those after the replacement or bypassing of these narrowings by surgical methods. This is said, not in criticism, but in anticipation of the stimulus to reaching this goal which Professor Cheng's book will provide.

The encyclopedic coverage of the results of percutaneous techniques provides an important basis, and thus a stimulus, for such further studies. It does not address the self-aggrandizement and divisiveness that have characterized the activities of many interventional cardiologists. Some have said that interventional cardiology, both pediatric and adult, has made the cardiologists much more like surgeons! Certain it is that true progress and true growth of knowledge in cardiac surgery have been impeded by these two tendencies, just as is, in my opinion at least, the case in interventional cardiology. I hope that the outstanding individuals who have contributed to this book will inspire others to lay aside the tendency to report "records of achievement" and instead to generate truly useful information which someday can be incorporated into appropriate comparisons and predictions. I also hope that the need to generate these comparisons and predictions — an activity which is surely best done when it is multidisciplinary — will again bring together to work in unison the noninterventional cardiologists, the interventional cardiologists, the cardiac surgeons, and others including biostatisticians. This spontaneous reunion can certainly be more productive than one forced upon us by society.

John W. Kirklin, M.D.
Professor of Surgery
Division of Cardiothoracic Surgery
Department of Surgery
The University of Alabama at Birmingham
Birmingham, Alabama
and
Editor-in-Chief
The Journal of Thoracic and Cardiovascular Surgery

Preface

Interventional cardiology has entered an exciting era with the advent of percutaneous balloon valvuloplasty following the successful application of percutaneous transluminal coronary angioplasty. It is now a well-established alternative to surgical treatment of many congenital and acquired valvular stenotic lesions. Many different approaches and techniques have been employed with various degrees of success. The purpose of this book is to put all these techniques into one reference text which summarizes their place and application for practicing physicians, cardiologists, cardiac surgeons, cardiovascular radiologists, and all others who are involved in caring for patients with stenotic cardiovascular diseases.

This volume was written by acknowledged experts in the field to describe the current status of percutaneous balloon valvuloplasty. It begins with a discussion of the pathology and pathophysiology of valvular stenosis. The methods for examining patients with valvular stenosis are then discussed. Clinical evaluation, electrocardiography, echocardiography, and magnetic resonance imaging are covered in depth before management of individual stenotic lesions and its results are addressed. There being no field where the interaction between cardiologists and cardiac surgeons is more vital, a special section on a surgeon's point of view is also included.

This is a constantly evolving field. What appears to be merely a conjectural possibility for the future may quickly become the present practical reality.

I would like to take this opportunity to thank all the individual authors from different parts of the world for their valuable contributions. I learned a great deal while editing this text. I am grateful to TORAY Industries (America), Cook Incorporated, Mansfield/Boston Scientific Corporation, and Datascope Corporation for their generous support in bearing a portion of the preparation costs for the text and the full cost of the color illustrations.

Tsung O. Cheng, M.D.

Contributors

Vivian M. Abascal, M.D.
Former Research Fellow in Medicine
Massachusetts General Hospital
Harvard Medical School
Boston, Massachusetts
and
Internal Medicine Resident
Medical Center of Central Massachusetts
Worchester, Massachusetts
  (*Echocardiographic Evaluation*)

Marcus Allen
Department of Medical Media
Indiana University Medical Center
Indianapolis, Indiana
  (*Stenotic Porcine Bioprosthetic Valves*)

Robert H. Anderson, B. Sc., M.D., F.R.C. Path.
Joseph Levy Professor of Pediatric Cardiac Morphology
National Heart and Lung Institute
London, United Kingdom
  (*Anatomy and Pathology of Valvular Stenosis*)

Anton E. Becker, M.D., F.A.C.C.
Professor of Pathology
Academic Medical Center
University of Amsterdam
Amsterdam, The Netherlands
  (*Anatomy and Pathology of Valvular Stenosis*)

Peter C. Block, M.D.
Associate Director
The St. Vincent's Heart Institute
Portland, Oregon
(*Acquired Mitral Stenosis: Double Balloon Catheter Technique*)

Chuan-Rong Chen, M.D.
Director, Cardiac Catheterization Laboratory
Vice Chairman, Department of Cardiology
Guangdong Cardiovascular Institute
Guangzhou, China
(*Mitral Stenosis: Inoue Balloon Catheter Technique*)

Chunguang Chen, M.D.
Director, Echocardiographic Laboratory
Department of Cardiology
University Hospital Hamburg
Hamburg, Germany
(*Echocardiographic Evaluation*)

Tsung O. Cheng, M.D.
Professor of Medicine
Division of Cardiology
Department of Medicine
The George Washington University School of Medicine and Health Sciences
Washington, D.C.
(*Preface; A History of Percutaneous Balloon Valvuloplasty; Mitral Stenosis: Inoue Balloon Catheter Technique; Concurrent Multivalve Balloon Valvuloplasty; Future Prospects.*)

Alain Cribier, M.D.
Professor of Medicine, Universite de Rouen
Associate Chief, Department of Cardiology
Hôpital Charles-Nicolle
Rouen, France
(*Acquired Aortic Stenosis*)

Daniel J. Diver, M.D.
Associate Director, Cardiac Catheterization Laboratory
Beth Israel Hospital
and
Assistant Professor of Medicine
Harvard Medical School
Boston, Massachusetts
(*Concurrent Balloon Valvuloplasty and Coronary Angioplasty*)

Frank Gavini, M.D.
Interventional Fellow
Cardiovascular Laboratory
White Memorial Medical Center
Los Angeles, California
(*Tricuspid Stenosis*)

Harry Goldberg, M.D.
Head Emeritus, Division of Cardiology

Director, Women's League for Medical Research
Cardiopulmonary and Renal Laboratories
Albert Einstein Medical Center
Philadelphia, Pennsylvania
and
Chairman Emeritus
Department of Cardiology
Deborah Heart and Lung Center
Browns Mills, New Jersey
and
Professor of Medicine
Temple University School of Medicine
Philadelphia, Pennsylvania
  (*Pathophysiology of Valvular Stenosis*)

Donald J. Hagler, M.D.
Professor of Pediatrics
Division of Pediatric Cardiology
Mayo Clinic
Rochester, New York
  (*Conduits and Conduit Valves*)

E. William Hancock, M.D.
Professor of Medicine (Cardiovascular Medicine)
Stanford University School of Medicine
Stanford, California
  (*Electrocardiographic Evaluation*)

Enrique Hernández, M.D.
Unidad de Cardiología
Hospital Ntra. Sra. del Pino
University of Las Palmas
Las Palmas, Spain
  (*Mitral Restenosis: The Cordoba-Las Palmas Experience*)

Jui-Sung Hung, M.D.
Professor of Medicine
Chang Gung Medical College
Taipei, Taiwan, ROC
  (*Mitral Stenosis: Inoue Balloon Catheter Technique; Mitral Stenosis
    With Left Atrial Thrombi: Inoue Balloon Catheter Technique.*)

Kanji Inoue, M.D.
Cardiovascular Surgeon
Department of Cardiac Surgery
Izinkai Takeda General Hospital
Kyoto, Japan
  (*Mitral Stenosis: Inoue Balloon Catheter Technique*)

Robert G. Johnson, M.D.
Assistant Professor of Surgery
Harvard Medical School
and

Cardiothoracic Surgeon
Beth Israel Hospital
Boston, Massachusetts
(*A Surgeon's Point of View*)

Dave Joseph, M.D.
Interventional Fellow
Cardiovascular Laboratory
White Memorial Medical Center
Los Angeles, California
(*Tricuspid Stenosis*)

Zuhdi Lababidi, M.D.
Professor and Director
Pediatric Cardiology
University of Missouri – Columbia
Columbia, Missouri
(*Congenital Obstruction of the Left Ventricular Outflow Tract*)

Eva Laraudogoitia, M.D.
Unidad de Cardiología
Hospital Ntra. Sra. del Pino
University of Las Palmas
Las Palmas, Spain
(*Mitral Restenosis: The Cordoba-Las Palmas Experience*)

Francis Y. K. Lau, M.D.
Professor of Medicine
Loma Linda University
and
White Memorial Medical Center
Los Angeles, California
(*Tricuspid Stenosis*)

Brice Letac, M.D.
Professor of Medicine, Universite de Rouen
Chief, Department of Cardiology
Hôpital Charles-Nicolle
Rouen, France
(*Acquired Aortic Stenosis*)

Vladir Maranhao, M.D.
Chairman, Department of Cardiology
Vice President, Medical Affairs
Deborah Heart and Lung Center
Browns Mills, New Jersey
and
Clinical Associate Professor of Medicine
University of Medicine and Dentistry of New Jersey –
  Robert Wood Johnson Medical School
New Brunswick, New Jersey
(*Pathophysiology of Valvular Stenosis*)

Charles McKay, M.D.
Associate Professor of Medicine
Division of Cardiology
University of Iowa
Iowa City, Iowa
(*Stenotic Porcine Bioprosthetic Valves*)

Alfonso Medina, M.D.
Unidad de Cardiología
Hospital Ntra. Sra. del Pino
University of Las Palmas
Las Palmas, Spain
(*Mitral Restenosis: The Cordoba-Las Palmas Experience*)

Francisco Melian, M.D.
Unidad de Cardiología
Hospital Ntra. Sra. del Pino
University of Las Palmas
Las Palmas, Spain
(*Mitral Restenosis: The Cordoba-Las Palmas Experience*)

Raad H. Mohiaddin, M.D., M.Sc.
Senior Research Fellow and Head of the Clinical Science Division
Magnetic Resonance Unit
Royal Brompton National Heart and Lung Hospital
and
The National Heart and Lung Institute
London, United Kingdom
(*Magnetic Resonance Assessment*)

Charles E. Mullins, M.D.
Professor of Clinical Pediatrics
Baylor College of Medicine
and
Medical Director, Cardiac Catheterization Laboratories
Texas Children's Hospital
Houston, Texas
(*Nonvalvular Lesions*)

Igor F. Palacios, M.D.
Director, Interventional Cardiology
Cardiac Catheterization Laboratories
Massachusetts General Hospital
and
Associate Professor of Medicine
Harvard Medical School
Boston, Massachusetts
(*Acquired Mitral Stenosis: Double Balloon Catheter Technique*)

Manuel Pan, M.D.
Servico de Cardiología
Hospital "Reina Sofía"

University of Córdoba
Córdoba, Spain
 (*Mitral Restenosis: The Cordoba-Las Palmas Experience*)

Djordje Pavlovic, M.D.
Servicio de Cardiología
Hospital "Reina Sofía"
University of Córdoba
Córdoba, Spain
 (*Mitral Restenosis: The Cordoba-Las Palmas Experience*)

Dudley J. Pennell, M.R.C.P.
Research Fellow
Magnetic Resonance Unit
Royal Brompton National Heart and Lung Hospital
and
The National Heart and Lung Institute
London, United Kingdom
 (*Magnetic Resonance Assessment*)

Joseph K. Perloff, M.D.
Streisand/American Heart Association
Professor of Medicine and Pediatrics
Division of Cardiology
UCLA School of Medicine
Los Angeles, California
 (*Clinical Evaluation*)

Richard M. Pomerantz, M.D.
Assistant Director
Cardiac Catheterization Laboratory
University of Rochester Medical Center
Rochester, New York
 (*Concurrent Balloon Valvuloplasty and Coronary Angioplasty*)

P. Syamasundar Rao, M.D.
Professor of Pediatrics
University of Wisconsin Medical School
and
Head, Division of Pediatric Cardiology
University of Wisconsin Children's Hospital
Madison, Wisconsin
 (*Pulmonic Stenosis*)

Albert P. Rocchini, M.D.
Ruben/Bentson Professor of Pediatrics
University of Minnesota
and
Director of Pediatric Cardiology
Variety Club Children's Hospital
Minneapolis, Minnesota
 (*Congenital Mitral Stenosis*)

Miguel Romero, M.D.
Servicio de Cardiología
Hospital "Reina Sofía"
University of Córdoba
Córdoba, Spain
(*Mitral Restenosis: The Cordoba-Las Palmas Experience*)

Carlos E. Ruiz, M.D.
Professor of Medicine
Loma Linda University
and
White Memorial Medical Center
Los Angeles, California
(*Tricuspid Stenosis*)

Robert D. Safian, M.D.
Director, Interventional Cardiology
Division of Cardiology
William Beaumont Hospital
Royal Oak, Michigan
(*Concurrent Balloon Valvuloplasty and Coronary Angioplasty*)

José Suárez de Lezo, M.D.
Servicio de Cardiología
Hospital "Reina Sofía"
University of Córdoba
Córdoba, Spain
(*Mitral Restenosis: The Cordoba-Las Palmas Experience*)

James Van Tassel, M.D.
Nasser, Smith and Pinkerton Cardiology, Inc.
Indianapolis, Indiana
(*Stenotic Porcine Bioprosthetic Valves*)

Bruce F. Waller, M.D.
Clinical Professor of Pathology and Medicine
Indiana University Medical Center
and
Director
Cardiovascular Pathology Registry
St. Vincent Hospital
and
Nasser, Smith and Pinkerton Cardiology, Inc.
Indianapolis, Indiana
(*Stenotic Porcine Bioprosthetic Valves*)

Ronald M. Weintraub, M.D.
Associate Professor of Surgery
Harvard Medical School
and
Chief, Division of Cardiothoracic Surgery
Beth Israel Hospital

Boston, Massachusetts
(*A Surgeon's Point of View*)

Sing San Yang, M.D.
Head, Cardiac Noninvasive Laboratory
Deborah Heart and Lung Center
Browns Mills, New Jersey
and
Clinical Assistant Professor of Medicine
University of Medicine and Dentistry of New Jersey—
    Robert Wood Johnson Medical School
New Brunswick, New Jersey
(*Pathophysiology of Valvular Stenosis*)

Lawrence A. Yeatman, M.D.
Clinical Professor of Medicine
Division of Cardiology
UCLA School of Medicine
Los Angeles, California
(*Clinical Evaluation*)

Contents

Percutaneous Balloon Valvuloplasty

CHAPTER 1

A History of Percutaneous Balloon Valvuloplasty

TSUNG O. CHENG

The birth of therapeutic balloon dilatation in the management of cardiovascular disease can be traced to the late Dr. William Rashkind (Fig. 1.1), who reported a balloon atrial septostomy in 1966. He should also be credited for introducing the percutaneous approach, because he and Miller[1] entitled their landmark paper the creation of an atrial septal defect "without thoracotomy." By sheer coincidence, a printing error in their original article transformed the word "magnified" to "magnificent" (Fig. 1.2). Little did they know then what a magnificent contribution they indeed made in therapeutic cardiac catheterization and the entire field of interventional cardiology, which has ballooned to such a magnitude a quarter of a century later.

In the field of therapeutic dilatation by catheterization Dotter and Judkins (Fig. 1.3)[2] actually anteceded Rashkind by 2 years. In 1964 they reported passing progressively larger vessel dilators and coaxially and sequentially across an area of stenosis to open atherosclerotic obstructions in the iliofemoral circulation. However, the dilatation catheters used were stiff and complication rate was high. It was not until 1978 that Grüntzig[3] (Fig. 1.4) reported developing a flexible balloon catheter miniaturized sufficiently to be applicable for percutaneous transluminal coronary angioplasty. Therapeutic balloon dilatation then began to be applied to stenotic heart valves.

CHRONOLOGY OF DEVELOPMENT

Pulmonic Stenosis

The first valve to be dilated by a balloon catheter was the pulmonic valve. Recognition of the potential usefulness of balloon dilatation in the treatment of congenital pulmonic stenosis was a natural consequence of the early surgical success with mechanical dilatation of the stenotic pulmonic valve by the Brock procedure.[4] In this operation, reported in 1961, a cutting valvotome was introduced through a small right ventriculotomy and advanced to the pulmonic valve where the congenitally fused commissures were incised. The commissural incisions were subsequently enlarged

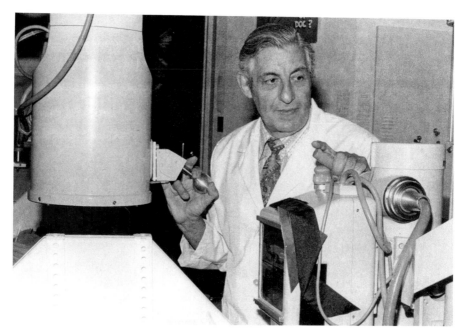

Figure 1.1 William J. Rashkind, M.D.

with a graded series of bougies, and the valvulotomy was then completed with a hinged dilator. This early success of the Brock procedure and its long-term postoperative result suggested that congenitally stenosed pulmonic valves might be opened simply by mechanical dilatation alone. Consequently, in 1979 Semb and associates[5] reported the successful use of a Berman angiographic balloon catheter in a critically ill 2-day-old boy with pulmonic stenosis and tricuspid regurgitation, reducing the systolic pressure gradient across the pulmonic valve from 20 to 6 mmHg.

In 1982, Kan and associates[6] reported the first case of percutaneous balloon valvuloplasty in treating an 8-year-old child with congenital pulmonic stenosis. After dilatation the systolic gradient across the pulmonic valve decreased from 48 to 14 mmHg, and the systolic ejection murmur also decreased in harshness and intensity. Serial electrocardiograms at 1 and 4 months after valvuloplasty showed a decrease in right ventricular hypertrophy; repeat cardiac catheterization at 4 months showed maintenance of a good result with a residual gradient of 20 mmHg at an unchanged cardiac output.

Congenital Aortic Stenosis

Lababidi[7] reported in 1983 the successful use of percutaneous balloon valvuloplasty in an 8-year-old boy with severe congenital aortic stenosis; the peak systolic gradient across the aortic valve was reduced from 85 to 28 mmHg and there was no aortic insufficiency at the end of the procedure.

Mitral Stenosis

As with balloon pulmonic valvuloplasty, early surgical experiences with the treatment of mitral stenosis paved the way for the subsequent use of a percutaneously introduced

Preliminary Communication

Creation of an Atrial Septal Defect Without Thoracotomy

A Palliative Approach to Complete Transposition of the Great Arteries

William J. Rashkind, MD, and William W. Miller, MD

Transposition of the great vessels (TGV) occurs in approximately 20% of children who die with congenital heart disease.[1] With rare exceptions, patients with this lesion die in the first 6 months of life (50% within the first month). Approximately 40% of patients with TGV have an otherwise normal heart. In recent years, various types of complete corrections for this lesion have been attempted. Mustard et al[2] has simplified these procedures and has reduced mortality to reasonable levels. Best results are obtained in children well beyond 6 months of age. Therefore, it is imperative to provide early palliation that is effective until the optimal age for complete correction and that does not interfere significantly with subsequent surgery. Creation of an interatrial communication seems the best available choice to suit these requirements. The Blalock-Hanlon technique,[3] or some modified version, is commonly used to remove a portion of the atrial septum surgically. The purpose of this report is to present a technique for producing an atrial septal defect without thoracotomy and without anesthesia, using a cardiac catheter introduced into a femoral vein.

Method and Material

The femoral vein is exposed as for routine cardiac catheterization in infancy. The device is a double-lumen cardiac catheter. One lumen continues the entire length of the catheter, the other ends in the balloon. It is passed via the femoral vein into the right atrium and is then manipulated through the foramen ovale into the left atrium. Location in the left atrium is verified by passing the catheter tip into a pulmonary vein, by sampling highly saturated blood, or by selective angiography. The balloon is inflated in the left atrium with 2 to 6 ml of dilute radiopaque solution. It is then withdrawn rapidly (one to two seconds) into the right atrium tearing the atrial septum. The balloon is then deflated rapidly (two to four seconds) and

From the Cardiovascular Laboratories, The Children's Hospital of Philadelphia.
Reprint requests to Children's Hospital of Philadelphia, 18th and Bainbridge Streets, Philadelphia 19146 (Dr. Rashkind).

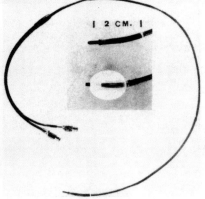

1. Illustration of the special balloon-tipped catheter (6.5 F). Insert shows the tip magnified in both deflated and inflated positions.

the procedure repeated until the filled balloon can be withdrawn from the left to the right atrium without resistance. Figure 1 illustrates the special catheter. The insert is a magnificent view of the catheter tip with the balloon deflated and inflated.

septal defects created by the technique described. The seventh served as a normal control. Five of the puppies have been sacrificed at intervals of one hour to two months after the procedure. The remaining puppy is being kept for one year of follow-up study. Figure 2 compares the atrial septal defect and the tricuspid valve in the animal sacrificed two months after septotomy.

Three infants with TGV, age 15 hours, 5 weeks, and 6 weeks, have been treated successfully with this technique. None of them showed ventricular or ductal shunting on angiography. They are now

---

Figure 1.2 Title page from the 1966 article by Rashkind and Miller[1] on balloon atrial septostomy in which a printing error transformed the word "magnified" into "magnificent." (From: Rashkind WJ, Miller WW: Creation of an atrial septal defect without thoracotomy. A palliative approach to complete transposition of the great arteries, *JAMA.* 196:991–992, 1966. With permission.)

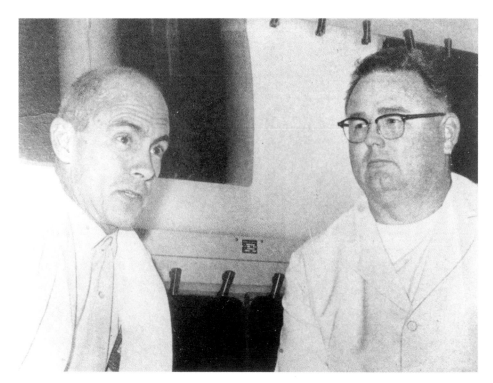

Figure 1.3 *Left,* Charles T. Dotter, M.D. *Right,* Melvin P. Judkins, M.D.

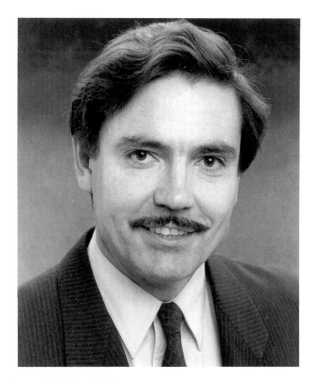

Figure 1.4 Andreas Grüntzig, M.D.

balloon catheter to produce mechanical dilatation of the stenotic mitral valve. As early as 1923, Cutler,[8] Souttar,[9] Bailey,[10] Harken,[11] and their associates reported on several various techniques of surgical mitral commissurotomy using finger fractures, transventricular dilators, and valvulotomes. These reports suggested that fused commissures in mitral stenosis could be separated with simple mechanical dilatation. Incidentally, these pioneering surgeons had to work against such skeptics and detractors as Carey Coombs and Thomas Lewis. Carey Coombs, commenting in 1924 on the previous year's report by Cutler and Levine, wrote that "the operation can *never* become a general method of treatment for a disease of which the mitral lesion is only one feature — to say nothing of the technical difficulties attending surgical approach to such a structure."[12] Sir Thomas Lewis, the "father of clinical science,"[13] wrote in 1943: "Although many symptoms may be complained of by the patients suffering from mitral stenosis, there are none that can be ascribed properly and usefully to this deformity of the valve."[14] Of course, Thomas Lewis' opinion proved wrong within a few years, as closed mitral commissurotomy by Bailey[10] and Harken[11] transformed the lives of thousands. On the basis of these surgical experiences and their brilliant results, successful use of a balloon catheter for opening a stenotic mitral valve might have been predicted. Equally important in the development of the technology for balloon mitral valvuloplasty was the introduction of Brockenbrough's transseptal left heart catheterization[15] and Rashkind's balloon atrial septostomy.[1] These two techniques are essential to the execution of percutaneous balloon mitral valvuloplasty.

Inoue[16] in 1984 reported the first clinical application of a balloon catheter in the nonoperative management of mitral stenosis. Inspired by Rashkind's work, Inoue actually began to design and develop a double-lumen coaxial balloon catheter in 1980 to create an atrial septal defect in children with transposition of the great arteries, tricuspid atresia, and other types of cyanotic congenital heart disease.[17] He also used the device to treat membranous obstruction of the hepatic portion of the inferior vena cava[16,18-20] and stenotic lesions in iliofemoral arteries.[21] The ability of the balloon to separate fused commissures of the mitral valve was then evaluated under direct vision as an auxiliary means of open mitral commissurotomy.[22] The first clinical application by Inoue of his balloon catheter, which took place on June 3, 1982, was for a 33-year-old male with severe rheumatic mitral stenosis.[23] The prototype balloon catheter used in the early stage of clinical trials had a large-profile balloon that required a cutdown for its insertion in the saphenous vein. Subsequent modifications in catheter designs enabled percutaneous introduction of the catheter through the femoral vein, and the procedure was named "percutaneous transvenous mitral commissurotomy."[18]

Several modifications of the transseptal approaches to percutaneous balloon mitral valvuloplasty have been introduced. Instead of the antegrade approach, a retrograde transarterial technique was introduced in 1986 by Babic and associates from Yugoslavia.[24] A balloon catheter was inserted percutaneously from the left femoral artery over a long guidewire which was introduced into the right femoral vein, advanced transseptally through the Brockenbrough catheter into the left atrium and left ventricle, and drawn out of the body through the left femoral artery using an intravascular retriever set. In comparison to the transvenous mitral commissurotomy technique of Inoue,[18] the advantages of the transarterial approach, according to Babic and associates,[24] are (1) easy placement of the balloon into the mitral valve orifice; (2) with both ends of the long guidewire under manual control outside the body, easy fixation of the balloon during inflation; (3) larger balloon catheters to be inflated with contrast material; (4) no danger of embolization in the event of balloon rupture; and (5) no danger of creating an iatrogenic atrial septal defect.

This retrograde approach of percutaneous balloon mitral valvuloplasty was further modified in 1987 by Buchler from Brazil,[25] who omitted the transseptal puncture altogether and used the retrograde transarterial approach exclusively in catheterizing the left atrium. He used the Sones catheter to enter the left atrium from the left ventricle. The chief advantage of the Buchler technique is total avoidance of a transseptal puncture with its associated risks and accompanying complication of an iatrogenic atrial septal defect. However, there are two major disadvantages, as pointed out by McKay.[26] The first concerns the retrograde crossing of the mitral valve with a guidewire; improper positioning of this guidewire through the mitral chordae could subsequently lead to improper positioning of a mitral valvuloplasty balloon catheter, thereby causing chordal rupture and massive mitral regurgitation. The second concern is the percutaneous arterial insertion of a large valvuloplasty balloon catheter with resultant damage to the femoral artery.

Acquired Aortic Stenosis

In contrast to experiences with the treatment of pulmonic stenosis and mitral stenosis, early reports on the surgical therapy of acquired aortic stenosis did not predict a favorable response to mechanical valvular dilatation.[27-29] However, Cribier and associates[30] in 1986 reported three elderly patients with calcific aortic stenosis who underwent successful percutaneous balloon aortic valvuloplasty. The procedure reduced the peak aortic systolic gradient from 75 to 33 mmHg and increased the calculated aortic valve area from 0.5 to 0.8 cm^2, with no significant increase in aortic regurgitation or emboli and with striking clinical improvement. Following the initial reports of successful balloon aortic valvuloplasty in elderly patients by Cribier[30] and McKay[31] and their associates, several larger series[32-35] have reported similar results.

Several modifications of the percutaneous retrograde balloon aortic valvuloplasty techniques have been described. An antegrade approach with positioning of the balloon catheter over a guidewire introduced transseptally from the femoral vein was described by Block and Palacios.[36] Use of a surgical cutdown to achieve femoral arterial access for balloon catheters has been described by Isner and associates.[37] Both of these techniques offered an alternative to reduce or avoid the vascular complications associated with percutaneous insertion of aortic valvuloplasty balloon catheters.

Finally, use of a double-balloon technique for performing percutaneous balloon aortic valvuloplasty was described by Dorros and associates.[38] Using a combined brachial and femoral arterial approach to insert two valvuloplasty catheters simultaneously, they achieved successful aortic valve dilatation in 10 patients with a reduction in peak systolic gradient across the aortic valve from 77.6 ± 28 to 27.8 ± 15 mmHg and an increase in calculated aortic valve area from 0.56 ± 0.3 to 1.03 ± 0.6 cm^2. This technique significantly reduced the "ping-pong-ball" effect hindering the seating of the single balloon catheter and yet achieved good hemodynamic results with a low vascular complication rate.

Tricuspid Stenosis

The last heart valve to undergo successful percutaneous balloon dilatation was the tricuspid valve. Al Zaibag[39] in 1987 first reported the use of a double-balloon technique in a 27-year-old woman with rheumatic tricuspid stenosis; the procedure increased tricuspid valve area and cardiac output, and brought about marked symptomatic improvement.

CATHETER DESIGNS

Several types of dilating balloon catheters have been introduced over the years. The most common type, and also the earliest in use, has a single cylindrical balloon mounted on a shaft. It is delivered to the stenotic valve either antegradely or retrogradely, over a guidewire. This type of catheter has the advantage of distributing wall stress equally around the circumference and folding to a relatively small profile in its collapsed state. However, it tends to obstruct blood flow completely during inflation. Also, there is a limitation in the diameter of the balloon which can be mounted on the catheter and in inflation pressure of the balloon, beyond which it may rupture. Balloons are designed to rupture longitudinally. If the rupture is transverse, as occurs occasionally, part of the balloon may be sheared off the shaft and could be a source of systemic embolism.[40] Rupture may also be circumferential,[41] which besides presenting a risk of embolization may increase the hazard of vascular injury during percutaneous removal of the balloon catheter.[42]

Catheters with two (bifoil) or three (trefoil) balloons mounted around a central shaft were designed to prevent obstructing the blood flow completely during inflation by allowing blood flow through the interballoon "commissures." However, their failure to distribute wall stress evenly and their tendency to kink and thereby prevent full deflation may engender untoward clinical consequences.

Using two balloon catheters at the same time overcomes the limitation in diameter and inflation pressure of a single balloon catheter. However, their larger profile is more apt to cause intravascular damage at the entry site or intracardiac damage during manipulation.

The Inoue balloon catheter used for mitral valvuloplasty contains a single rubber-nylon micromeshed balloon shaped like a peanut shell. Its differential compliance allows greater inflation of the more compliant segments on either side of the valve, thereby helping to secure the less compliant waist within the mitral orifice during balloon inflation. The Inoue balloon eliminates the need for a longer balloon previously employed to prevent the "trombone effect" associated with the shorter balloons developed originally for pulmonic valvuloplasty. The longer balloon is difficult to accommodate within a typically small cavity of the left ventricle in mitral stenosis and also predisposes to perforation of the left ventricular free wall. On the other hand the Inoue balloon, because of its design, always pulls itself away from the apex of the left ventricle toward the mitral valve and maintains its position at the mitral valve during inflation. Therefore the patient is not at risk for left ventricular perforation. The shorter inflation time at a lower inflation pressure with the Inoue balloon also minimizes interference with the systemic circulation. The Inoue rubber-nylon balloon is also stronger than the polyethylene balloon.

Refinements in equipment have enabled modern cardiologists, both adult and pediatric, to proceed in two directions. With small steerable balloons, they have been able to reach more distal branches of the pulmonary arteries.[43] With larger balloons they have been able to approach major vessels — eg, in treating coarctation of aorta[44] and membranous obstruction of inferior vena cava[19,20] and to dilate every native heart valve, prosthetic heart valves,[45] valve conduits,[46] and multiple valves at the same setting.[47,48]

Table 1.1 Milestones in Percutaneous Balloon Valvuloplasty

Year	Investigators	Disease	Procedure
1964	Dotter & Judkins[2]	Iliofemoral arteriosclerotic obstruction	Transluminal recanalization
1966	Rashkind & Miller[1]	Transposition of great arteries	Balloon atrial septostomy
1978	Grüntzig[3]	Coronary artery disease	Percutaneous transluminal angioplasty
1982	Kan et al[6]	Pulmonic stenosis	Percutaneous balloon valvuloplasty
1982	Singer et al[44]	Coarctation of the aorta	Transluminal balloon angioplasty
1983	Lock et al[43]	Hypoplastic or stenotic pulmonary artery branches	Balloon angioplasty
1983	Lababidi[7]	Congenital aortic stenosis	Balloon valvuloplasty
1984	Inoue et al[16]	Mitral stenosis	Transvenous mitral commissurotomy
1986	Cribier et al[30]	Acquired aortic stenosis	Percutaneous transluminal valvuloplasty
1986	Feit et al[45]	Stenosis of bioprosthetic tricuspid valve	Percutaneous valvuloplasty
1987	Al Zaibag et al[39]	Tricuspid stenosis	Percutaneous valvotomy
1987	Lloyd et al[46]	Obstructed valve conduits	Balloon valvuloplasty
1987	Kritzer et al[47]	Multivalve stenoses	Simultaneous valvotomies

CONCLUSIONS

Perspective

Balloon dilatation began nearly three decades ago as a last-ditch effort to salvage the ischemic leg of a patient with iliofemoral atherosclerosis by means of transluminal catheter recanalization.[2] Not long thereafter, balloon septostomy was used to increase systemic oxygen hemoglobin saturation in complete transposition of the great arteries by creation of an atrial septal defect.[1] These early efforts have evolved into a long list of successful transcatheter therapeutic procedures (Table 1.1) that will continue to grow. This text in its ensuing chapters focuses on the percutaneous techniques of balloon dilatation of stenotic heart valves, conduits, and blood vessels that are available today for treating patients with congenital and acquired cardiovascular diseases.

Nomenclature

A number of terms have been used in the English literature for balloon dilatation (or dilation) of stenotic valves. Some investigators[49] suggested that balloon valvotomy is a better term than balloon valvuloplasty because the latter "may be interpreted as a surgical procedure." The word valvotomy actually sounds more "surgical," being defined in *Webster's Third New International Dictionary* as "the operation of enlarging a narrowed heart valve by cutting through the mitral commissures to relieve the symptoms of mitral stenosis" and in *Dorland's Illustrated Medical Dictionary* as "incision of a valve such as a valve of the heart." Balloon valvuloplasty is certainly as appropriate a term for nonsurgical dilatation of a cardiac valve by means of a balloon as the term coronary angioplasty is for nonsurgical balloon dilatation of a stenosed coronary artery.[50]

The term "commissurotomy" was first used by Bailey[10] in 1949 when he described the original surgical operation of closed dilatation of the stenosed mitral valve. But the same operative procedure had been termed "valvuloplasty" by Harken[11] a year earlier. Harken believed valvuloplasty to be a better term than commissurotomy because the operation "corrected all components of mitral stenosis and not just commissural fusion."[51] Furthermore, depending on the etiology of the stenotic lesion and the pathology of the specific valve, balloon dilatation improves the valve area by several means other than separation of commissural fusion as in mitral stenosis, such as leaflet tearing in pulmonic stenosis;[52] anular, cuspal, and calcific nodular fracture and improved cuspal mobility in adult calcific aortic stenosis;[31] compression and fracture of the subaortic "membrane" in discrete subaortic stenosis;[53] or a combination of these mechanisms. The term valvuloplasty is therefore preferable to commissurotomy.

The use of "valvular" (and valvotomy, etc) instead of "valvar" (and valvotomy, etc), is entirely a matter of custom or habit. The British prefer "valvar" to valvular" because the adjective derived from "valve" should be "valvar" and the noun form of "valvular" would be "valvule," which means a little valve (Robert H. Anderson, personal communication, 12 November 1990). The Americans, however, always use "valvular," as in valvular heart disease, valvular stenosis, valvuloplasty, and so on. These terms used are in all the textbooks, journal articles, and *Cumulated Index Medicus.* I do not know how and when the custom of adding the "ul" to the word "valve" commenced, but old habits die hard. Therefore the term *percutaneous balloon valvuloplasty* will be used throughout this text.

REFERENCES

1. Rashkind WJ, Miller WW: Creation of an atrial septal defect without thoracotomy. A palliative approach to complete transposition of the great arteries. *JAMA.* 196:991–992, 1966.

2. Dotter CT, Judkins MP: Transluminal treatment of arteriosclerotic obstruction. Description of a new technic and a preliminary report of its application. *Circulation.* 30:654–670, 1964.

3. Grüntzig A: Transluminal dilatation of coronary artery stenosis. *Lancet.* 1:263, 1978.

4. Brock R: The surgical treatment of pulmonary stenosis. *Br Heart J.* 23:337–356, 1961.

5. Semb BKH, Tjönneland S, Stake G, et al: "Balloon valvulotomy" of congenital pulmonary valve stenosis with tricuspid valve insufficiency. *Cardiovasc Radiol.* 2:239–241, 1979.

6. Kan JS, White RI, Mitchell SE, et al: Percutaneous balloon valvuloplasty: a new method for treating congenital pulmonary valve stenosis. *N Engl J Med.* 307:540–542, 1982.

7. Lababidi Z: Aortic balloon valvuloplasty. *Am Heart J.* 106:751–752, 1983.

8. Cutler EC, Levine SA: Cardiotomy and valvulotomy for mitral stenosis. Experimental observations and clinical notes concerning an operated case with recovery. *Boston Med Surg J.* 188:1023–1027, 1923.

9. Souttar HS: The surgical treatment of mitral stenosis. *Br Heart J.* 2:603–606, 1925.

10. Bailey CP: The surgical treatment of mitral stenosis (mitral commissurotomy). *Dis Chest.* 15:377–393, 1949.

11. Harken DE, Ellis LB, Ware PF, et al: The surgical treatment of mitral stenosis, I: valvuloplasty. *N Engl J Med.* 239:801–809, 1948.

12. Coombs CF: *Rheumatic Heart Disease.* Marshall Hamilton Kent and Co, 1924. Reprint. Birmingham, Ala: Gryphon Editions, 1989, p 330.

13. Treasure T: Balloon dilatation of the aortic valve in adults: a surgeon's view. *Br Heart J.* 63:205–206, 1990.

14. Lewis T: *Diseases of the Heart.* 3rd ed. London: Macmillan, 1943, p 130.

15. Brockenbrough EC, Braunwald E: A new technic for left ventricular angiocardiography and transseptal left heart catheterization. *Am J Cardiol.* 6:1062–1064, 1960.

16. Inoue K, Owaki T, Nakamura T, et al: Clinical application of transvenous mitral commissurotomy by a new balloon catheter. *J Thorac Cardiovasc Surg.* 87:394–402, 1984.

17. Inoue K, Kitamura F, Chikusa H, et al: Atrial septostomy by a new balloon catheter. *Jpn Circ J.* 45:730–738, 1981.

18. Inoue K, Hung J-S: Percutaneous transvenous mitral commissurtomy (PTMC): the Far East experience. In: Topol EJ. *Textbook of Interventional Cardiology.* Philadelphia: WB Saunders Co, 1990, p 887.

19. Cheng TO: Membranotomy for Budd-Chiari syndrome. *Ann Thorac Surg.* 51:522–523, 1991.

20. Yang XL, Chen CR, Cheng TO: Nonoperative treatment of membranous obstruction of inferior vena cava by percutaneous balloon transluminal angioplasty. *Circulation* 84 (Supp II): II–27, 1991.

21. Inoue K: A new balloon catheter for percutaneous transluminal angioplasty. *AJR.* 144:1069–1071, 1985.

22. Inoue K, Nakamura T, Kitamura F, et al: Nonoperative mitral commissurotomy by a new balloon catheter. *Jpn Circ J.* 46:877, 1982.

23. Cheng TO: The Inoue balloon catheter. *Mayo Clin Proc.* 66; 761, 1991.

24. Babic UU, Pejcic P, Djurisic Z, et al: Percutaneous transarterial balloon valvuloplasty for mitral valve stenosis. *Am J Cardiol.* 57:1101–1104, 1986.

25. Buchler JR: Percutaneous balloon dilation of rheumatic mitral stenosis by the transarterial approach. *J Am Coll Cardiol.* 10:1366–1367, 1987.

26. McKay RG: Percutaneous balloon dilation of rheumatic mitral stenosis by the transarterial approach-reply. *J Am Coll Cardiol.* 10:1367, 1987.

27. Bailey CP, Glover RP, O'Neill TJE, et al: Experiences with the experimental surgical relief of aortic stenosis. *J Thorac Surg.* 20:516–540, 1950.

28. Brock RC: The arterial route to the aortic and pulmonary valves. The mitral route to the aortic valve. *Guy's Hosp Rep.* 99:236–246, 1950.

29. Bailey CP, Bolton HE, Jamison WL, et al: Commissurotomy for rheumatic aortic stenosis, I: surgery. *Circulation.* 9:23–31, 1954.

30. Cribier A, Savin T, Saoudi N, et al: Percutaneous transluminal valvuloplasty of acquired aortic stenosis in elderly patients: an alternative to valve replacement? *Lancet.* 1:63–67, 1986.

31. McKay RG, Safian RD, Lock JE, et al: Balloon dilatation of calcific aortic stenosis in elderly patients: postmortem, intraoperative, and percutaneous valvuloplasty studies. *Circulation.* 74:119–125, 1986.

32. Schneider JF, Wilson M, Gallant TE: Percutaneous balloon aortic valvuloplasty for aortic stenosis in elderly patients at high risk for surgery. *Ann Intern Med.* 106:696–699, 1987.

33. Safian RD, Berman AD, Diver DJ, et al: Balloon aortic valvuloplasty in 170 consecutive patients. *N Engl J Med.* 319:125–130, 1988.

34. Desnoyers MR, Isner JM, Pandian NG, et al: Clinical and noninvasive hemodynamic results after aortic balloon valvuloplasty for aortic stenosis. *Am J Cardiol.* 62:1078–1984, 1988.

35. Cribier A, Gerber LI, Letac B: Percutaneous balloon aortic valvuloplasty: the French experience. In: Topol EJ. *Textbook of Interventional Cardiology.* Philadelphia: WB Saunders Co, 1990, pp 849–867.

36. Block PC, Palacios IF: Aortic and mitral balloon valvuloplasty: the United States experience. In: Topol EJ. *Textbook of Interventional Cardiology.* Philadelphia: WB Saunders Co, 1990, pp 831–832.

37. Isner JM, Salem DN, Desnoyers MR, et al: Treatment of calcific aortic stenosis by balloon valvuloplasty. *Am J Cardiol.* 59:313–317, 1987.

38. Dorros G, Lewin RF, King JF, et al: Percutaneous transluminal valvuloplasty in calcific aortic stenosis: the double balloon technique. *Cathet Cardiovasc Diagn.* 13:151–156, 1987.

39. Al Zaibag M, Ribeiro P, Al Kasab S: Percutaneous balloon valvotomy in tricuspid stenosis. *Br Heart J.* 57:51–53, 1987.

40. Vahanian A, Michel P-L, Cormier B, et al: Mitral valvuloplasty: the French experience. In: Topol EJ. *Textbook of Interventional Cardiology.* Philadelphia, WB Saunders Co, 1990, pp 872–873.

41. Weinhaus L, Lababidi Z: Catheter rupture during balloon valvuloplasty. *Am Heart J.* 113:1035–1036, 1987.

42. Isner JM, and the Mansfield Scientific Aortic Valvuloplasty Registry Investigators: Acute catastrophic complications of balloon aortic valvuloplasty. *J Am Coll Cardiol.* 17: 1436–1444, 1991.

43. Lock JE, Castaneda–Zuniga WR, Fuhrman BP, et al: Balloon dilation angioplasty of hypoplastic and stenotic pulmonary arteries. *Circulation.* 67:962–967, 1983.

44. Singer MI, Rowen M, Dorsey TJ: Transluminal aortic balloon angioplasty for coarctation of the aorta in the newborn. *Am Heart J.* 103:131–132, 1982.

45. Feit F, Stecy PJ, Nachamie MS: Percutaneous balloon valvuloplasty for stenosis of a porcine bioprosthesis in the tricuspid valve position. *Am J Cardiol.* 58:363–364, 1986.

46. Lloyd TR, Marvin WJ, Mahoney LT, et al: Balloon dilation valvuloplasty of bioprosthetic valves in extracardiac conduits. *Am Heart J.* 114:268–274, 1987.

47. Kritzer GL, Block PC, Palacios I: Simultaneous percutaneous mitral and aortic balloon valvotomies in an elderly patient. *Am Heart J.* 114:420–423, 1987.

48. Cheng TO: Multivalve percutaneous balloon valvuloplasty. *Cathet Cardiovasc Diagn.* 16:109–112, 1989.

49. Ribeiro PA, Zaibag MA, Sawyer W: Nomenclature for the use of balloon catheters. *Am J Cardiol.* 63:262, 1989.

50. Cheng TO: Balloon valvuloplasty instead of balloon valvotomy. *Am J Cardiol.* 63:1540, 1990.

51. Harken DE: The emergence of cardiac surgery, I: personal recollections of the 1940s and 1950s. *J Thorac Cardiovasc Surg.* 98:805–813, 1989.

52. Hill JA, Lambert CR, Pepine CJ: Catheter balloon valvuloplasty. *Modern Concepts Cardiovasc Dis.* 60(1):1–6, 1991.

53. De Lezo JS, Pan M, Sancho M, et al: Percutaneous transluminal balloon dilatation for discrete subaortic stenosis. *Am J Cardiol.* 58:619–621, 1986.

CHAPTER **2**

Anatomy and Pathology of Valvular Stenosis

ROBERT H. ANDERSON
ANTON E. BECKER

The option of using the inflation of balloons, introduced on catheters, to dilate obstructive lesions within the heart has revolutionized the treatment of both congenital and acquired cardiac malformations. Fully to optimize the potential of these techniques, it is essential to choose carefully those obstructive lesions that are most suited to balloon dilatation, and to refer to alternative therapies, such as surgery, those cases deemed to be unsuitable for transcatheter treatment. Appropriate selection of patients with valvular disease demands a firm understanding of the pathologic processes producing stenosis. Knowledge of the pathology must, in turn, be founded on correct appreciation of normal valvular anatomy. Surprisingly, it is rare to find accounts that describe anatomy as we observe it. All too often, the descriptions to be found in standard textbooks are based on mythical conceptions, concerned most notably with the oft-described, yet rarely illustrated, "annulus" supporting the leaflets of the arterial valves. In this chapter, therefore, we illustrate the functional anatomy of the atrioventricular and arterial valves of the heart. We show how fundamental differences in morphology dictate the pathologic changes responsible for valvular stenosis, and how these different features must be taken into account if appropriate selection is to be made of those cases that are suitable for balloon dilatation. If we are adequately to describe these anatomopathologic features, it is essential that we start with a brief section defining our understanding of some of the potentially contentious words we will use in our chapter.

DEFINITION OF TERMS

The mere existence of a section of text devoted to definitions is often sufficient to deter some readers from proceeding further with their inquiries. In this respect, "definition" has the same effect as has "culture" on the man whose reaction was to release the safety catch of his Browning revolver ("Wenn ich Kultur höre . . . entsichere ich meinen Browning" — from the play *Schlageter* by Hanns Johst, although often inappropriately attributed to Herman Göring). We hope, therefore, that those who have not, at this stage, reached for their revolvers, will bear with us while we describe our understanding of several terms that are used inconsistently by current writers.

Leaflet: The segments of fibrous and collagenous tissue that make up the functional segments of the cardiac valves are here described as leaflets in both the arterial and atrioventricular valves. Often, these structures are described as cusps. Those who use the latter word display an ignorance of its meaning. A cusp is a point or elevation, and the word is used appropriately by dentists when describing the crowns of molar teeth.

Commissure: The junctions between adjacent leaflets are herein described as commissures. As such, the commissures extend from the peripheral attachments of the leaflets to the center of the valve when its leaflets are closed. In other words, the commissures have length when the valve is closed. This is an important point, since the pathologist and the anatomist often describe only the peripheral extent of these junctions as the commissure. It follows that, strictly speaking, a valve with only two leaflets, such as the mitral valve, has only one commissure between its leaflets (Fig 2.1, *upper*). Almost always, however, both ends of this line of apposition between the leaflets are described as commissures in posteromedial and anterolateral location. In defining a commissure in the way we suggest, problems arise concerning the nature of the so-called "scallops" of the mitral valve. In many hearts, these scallops fulfil our definition given above for a leaflet. Indeed, some have argued that the mitral valve is best considered as a structure with four leaflets.[1] We have to admit that, in many instances, the junctions between scallops also fulfill our chosen definition for a commissure. Yet, in other circumstances still other breaches appear within the skirt of leaflet tissue which do not approximate to the proposed quadrifoliate pattern (Fig. 2.1, *lower*). At present, this situation remains unresolved. We think most would still contend that the valve has only two leaflets. If this is the case, those leaflets must have a common zone of apposition (the commissure) with length as well as ends. In valves with three leaflets, this problem does not occur, and examination of an arterial valve from above illustrates convincingly the true nature of the commissure (Fig. 2.2). This debate does impinge again on the conventional definition of commissures in atrioventricular valves. It has become conventional to define the commissure in terms of its cordal support, demanding the presence of a fan-shaped cord atop a papillary muscle to justify the presence of a commissure.[2,3] We dislike this approach and, as discussed, prefer to define a commissure on its appearance as a line of apposition between adjacent leaflets, while recognizing the problems discussed above, as yet unsolved, which our approach raises in the case of the mitral valve.

Annulus: Although the definition of a commissure is perhaps the most important terminological problem, the nature of the valvular annulus is undoubtedly the most controversial. Surgeons talk all the time about "transannular" patches, whereas interventional cardiologists speak with equal frequency of measuring the valvular "annulus" so as to size their balloons. What do they mean? It is an anatomic fact that the leaflets of the atrioventricular valves are suspended in ringlike fashion around the atrioventricular junctions (Fig. 2.3). In the atrioventricular junction, therefore, it is appropriate to describe the valvular annulus, even though it is the exception rather than the rule to find a firm and well-structured collagenous cord supporting the leaflets throughout their circumference (see below). At the ventriculoarterial junctions, in contrast, it is not possible to find any annular structure supporting the attachment of the valvular leaflets.[4] The only ringlike construction is the area over

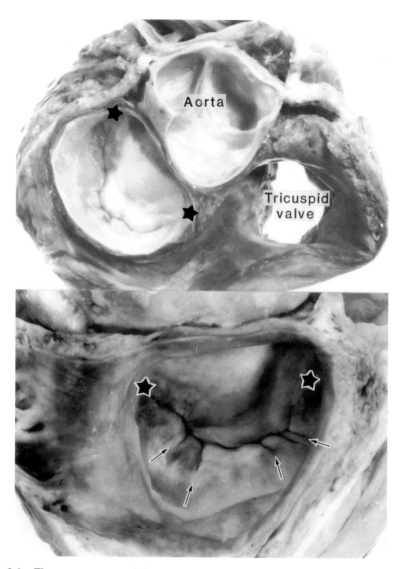

Figure 2.1 These views are of the mitral valve in closed position from above, after inflation of the left ventricle under pressure. The upper figure shows a solitary line of apposition (the commissure), with two ends (*stars*) between the aortic and mural leaflets of the valve. The lower valve, however, has several smaller lines of apposition between segments of leaflet (*arrows*). Are these junctions also to be considered as commissures? They would fit within our preferred definition, but it is unlikely that many would recognize them as commissures. The most appropriate definition of a commissure for the mitral valve has still to be agreed upon. Our approach is to consider the major line of apposition (*upper, lower,* between stars) as the commissure, with two ends (at the stars).

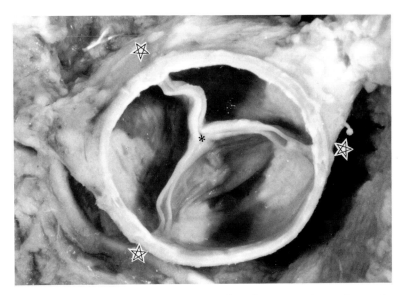

Figure 2.2 This view of an arterial valve in closed position from above shows that no problems exist in defining commissures in valves with three leaflets. The commissures are the lines of apposition extending from the periphery (*stars*) to the center (*asterisk*) of the valve.

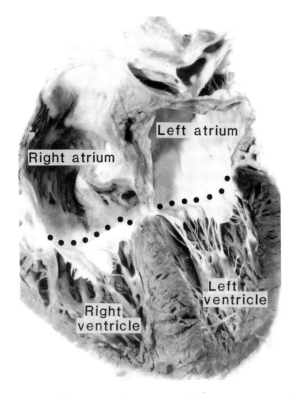

Figure 2.3 This view of the posterior aspect of the atrioventricular junctions, revealed by sectioning the heart in "four-chamber" projection, shows half of the annular attachments of the mitral and tricuspid valves (*dotted lines*).

15

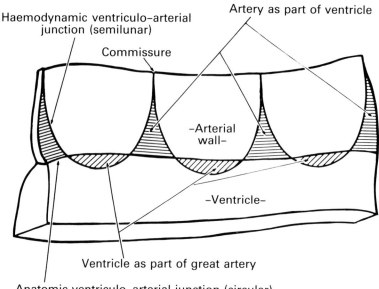

Figure 2.4 This diagram illustrates the mode of attachment of the leaflets of arterial valves, and the effect this has on the structure of the ventricular outflow tracts. There is no "annulus" supporting the valvar leaflets, which are attached in semilunar fashion.

which the wall of the arterial trunk (aorta or pulmonary trunk) is supported by the ventricular structures. The leaflets of the arterial valves are then attached in semilunar fashion, the locus of attachment (the hemodynamic ventriculoarterial junction) crossing the anatomic junction of arterial wall with ventricular mass (Fig. 2.4). The segments of ventricular outflow tracts within which the leaflets of the arterial valves are attached have considerable length. This point will be elaborated when considering the valvular anatomy in reference to balloon dilatation.

ANATOMY OF THE CARDIAC VALVES

In terms of overall structure, the heart can be considered in terms of a muscular pump driven by electricity. The function of this pump depends on the proper working of the valves at the atrioventricular and ventriculoarterial junctions. The morphology of these valves reflects the hemodynamic conditions under which they must work. Thus, the atrioventricular valves open during atrial systole and ventricular diastole, yet must close, and remain competent, against the full force of ventricular contraction (Fig. 2.5, *upper*). Hence, the atrioventricular valves are furnished with an extensive tension apparatus to ensure their competent closure and, more important, to prevent their eversion during ventricular systole. In contrast, the arterial valves are open during the high pressures of systole. They close while the ventricles are quiescent, and their structure reflects the fact that closure is effected by the hydrostatic pressure of the column of blood they support within the arterial systems (Fig. 2.5, *lower*). Overall, therefore, the structure of an arterial valve is simpler than that of an atrioventricular valve, although the valve should not be dismissed merely in terms of having leaflets. It

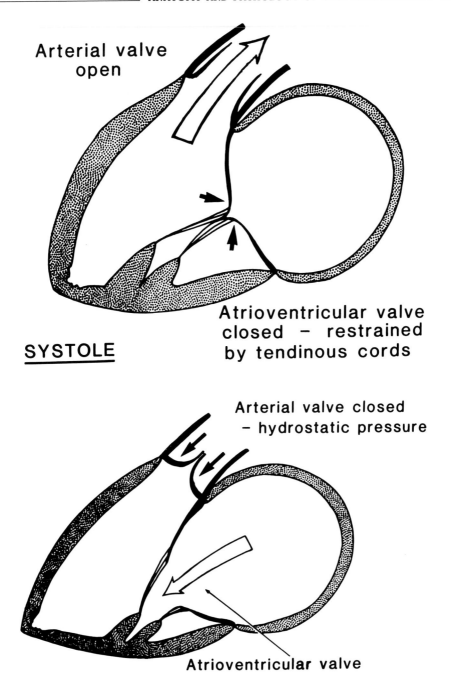

Figure 2.5 These diagrams show the mode of action of the valves and the anatomic arrangement to fit this function, in (*upper*) systole and (*lower*) diastole.

is the arrangement of these leaflets within and across the ventriculoarterial junction that is the key to correct function.

Anatomy of the Atrioventricular Valves

The atrioventricular valves are made up of a complex of atrial myocardium, annulus, leaflets, tension apparatus, and papillary muscles, the last supported in turn by the ventricular myocardium (Fig. 2.6). All these units must function appropriately and in concert if the valve is to work properly.[5] The basic arrangement is the same in both tricuspid and mitral valves but, from the perspective of balloon dilatation, almost all procedures are carried out on the mitral valve. We will concentrate our description on the mitral valve, therefore, emphasizing only those features of the tricuspid valve which differ from the basic pattern.

The leaflets of the mitral valve are suspended from the annulus, with atrial myocardium inserting within their uppermost part. A major feature of the mitral valve is that the annulus has scant relationship to the septal structures, largely being lifted away from the septum by the deep extension of the left ventricular outflow tract which extends toward the crux (Fig. 2.7). There is also a marked difference in the arrangement of the leaflets around the annulus. One leaflet, often termed the "anterior" leaflet, is a deep structure, but one which guards only one third of the overall junctional circumference. The other leaflet, usually termed "posterior," has much less depth, yet guards two thirds of the overall valvular circumference. As can be seen in Fig. 2.7, the valvular orifice has marked obliquity relative to the axis of the heart, and part of the "posterior" leaflet, when the heart is in its in situ position, is anterior to its counterpart. It is much more accurate anatomically to describe the "posterior" leaflet as mural, and, recognizing its relationship to the leaflets of the aortic valve, to describe the other leaflet as aortic (Fig. 2.8). The commissure between these leaflets is also

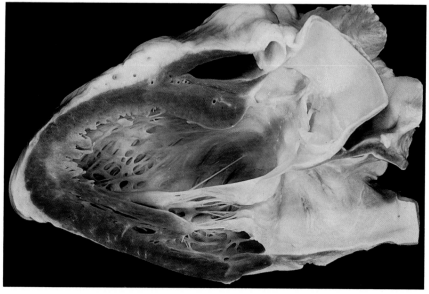

Figure 2.6 This cross-section in the long axis of the left ventricle shows the basic arrangement of the components of an atrioventricular valve.

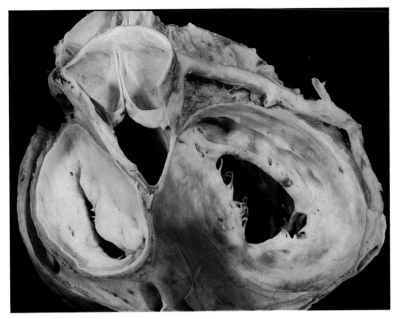

Figure 2.7 This dissection of a normal heart, viewed from above, is made by removing the noncoronary sinus of the aorta. It shows the deep extension of the left ventricular outlet which "lifts" the mitral valve away from the septum. Note the obliquity of the leaflets of the mitral valve.

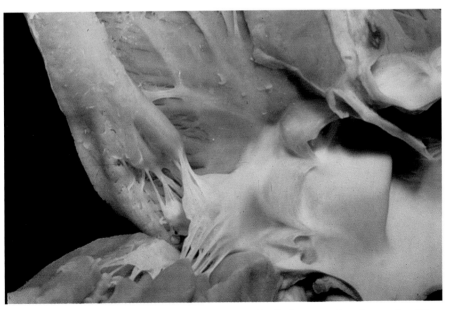

Figure 2.8 This view of the outflow tract of the left ventricle shows the fibrous continuity between the leaflets of the aortic and mitral valves. Note the so-called strut cords on the ventricular surface of the aortic leaflet of the mitral valve.

oblique (see Fig. 2.7) and extends in a posteromedial to an anterolateral direction. There are usually discrete segments within the mural leaflets, which some identify as leaflets in their own right.[1] As discussed, although there is much to commend this approach, it is still conventional to regard the scallops as subunits of the mural leaflet. The tension apparatus of the valve is composed of tendinous cords that tether the leaflets to the papillary muscles and to the ventricular wall. Most cords are attached to the characteristically paired papillary muscles. These muscles, like the ends of the commissure, are located posteromedially and anterolaterally within the left ventricle, being positioned at the points of maximal mechanical advantage relative to the valvular orifice (Fig. 2.9). The cords tethering the leaflets arise either from their free

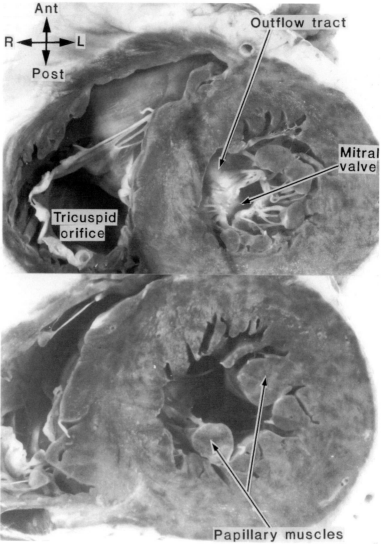

Figure 2.9 These sections in the short axis of the ventricular mass, viewed from beneath, show the oblique arrangement of the orifice of the mitral valves relative to the septum (*upper*) and show how the papillary muscles are positioned beneath the ends of the commissure (line of apposition) between the leaflets (*lower*).

edges or from their ventricular surfaces. Those arising from the free edges support all areas of both leaflets and connect adjacent edges to the papillary muscles. The cords supporting the apices of the ends of the commissure are particularly prominent, having a fan-shaped arrangement, but similar fan-shaped cords can be found between the scallops of the mural leaflet.[6] Prominent and thick cords arise from the ventricular surface of the aortic leaflet; these are known as the strut cords (Fig. 2.8). Other cords arise from the ventricular surface of the mural leaflet and insert directly to the ventricular wall; these are the basal cords.

The major differences in the tricuspid relative to the mitral valve are in the number of leaflets and the arrangements of the tension apparatus. As the name suggests, there are three leaflets in the tricuspid valve, and these are located in septal, anterosuperior, and inferior (or mural) positions (Fig. 2.10). The single most distinguishing feature of the tricuspid valve, however, is the attachment of the tendinous cords from the septal leaflet directly to the ventricular septum. The other leaflets are supported by small papillary muscles (for the inferior leaflet) and by the characteristic medial and anterior muscles (for the septal and anterosuperior leaflets).

The Arterial Valves

As with the atrioventricular valves, both arterial valves have the same basic morphologic arrangement, with the leaflets attached in semilunar fashion across the anatomic ventriculoarterial junction.[4] The locus of this attachment rises to the apices of the commissures and falls to the troughs of the leaflets (Fig. 2.11). Within this pattern, three important rings can be identified which might be candidates for the enigmatic "annulus." The most distal ring is at the level of the attachment of the apices of the commissures. This ring is particularly prominent in both the aorta and

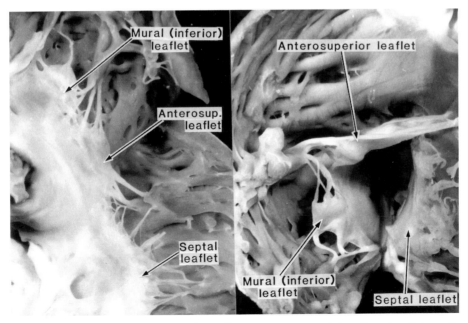

Figure 2.10 These photographs show the arrangement of the three leaflets of the tricuspid valve as seen from (*left*) the inlet and (*right*) the infundibular aspects.

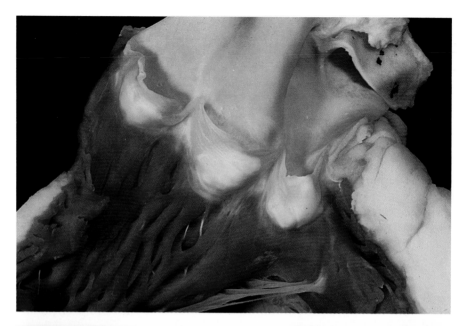

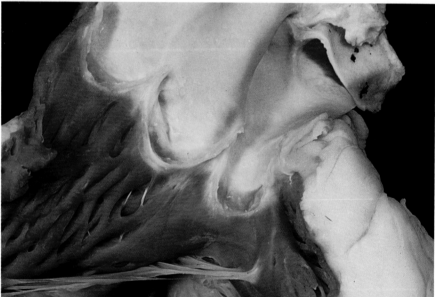

Figure 2.11 These photographs show the spread-open outflow tract of the right ventricle before (*upper*) and after (*lower*) removal of the leaflets of the pulmonary valve. They show how the valvular leaflets have a semilunar attachment, the only ringlike structure being the attachment of the wall of the pulmonary trunk to the infundibular musculature (see Fig. 2.4).

the pulmonary trunk. It forms the junction between the tubular wall of the arterial trunk and the expanded sinuses that house the leaflets of the valves during ventricular systole (Fig. 2.12). It is best described as the sinutubular junction (or bar). There is then a middle ring that is crossed by the attachments of the semilunar leaflets (Fig. 2.11 *lower*). This is the anatomic ventriculoarterial junction (Fig. 2.4). The third

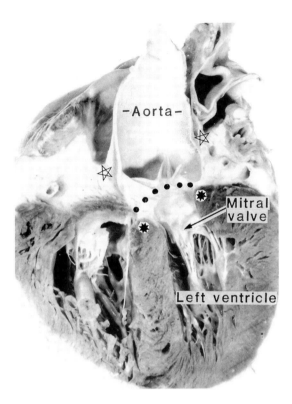

Figure 2.12 This "four-chamber" section through the aortic root shows how the leaflets of the aortic valve are attached across a segment of outflow tract with considerable length. Within this segment, there are three "rings"—the sinutubular junctions (*stars*), the junction of the aortic wall with the supporting ventricular structures (*dotted*), and the basal attachment of the semilunar leaflets (*asterisks*).

ring in the outflow tracts can then be constructed by joining the basal attachments of the troughs of the three leaflets, this ring marking the most proximal extent of the valvular apparatus within the ventricles (Fig. 2.11). None of these rings supports the entirety of attachment of the valvular leaflets which, unlike the atrioventricular valves, are attached in semilunar rather than annular fashion. It is the superior and inferior rings that are important in determining the anatomy of valvular stenosis, together with the narrowed orifice of the stenosed valve (see below). Both of these rings should be considered when measuring the diameter of the outlet, which has length across the area of the leaflets (Fig. 2.12). The semilunar pattern of attachment of the leaflets is also significant in that it incorporates three triangular areas of the arterial walls as extensions of the ventricular outflow tracts, while enclosing three crescents of the ventricle as part of the arterial sinuses (Fig. 2.4).

The fundamental differences between the aortic and pulmonary valves are found in the nature of their support by the underlying ventricles. The outflow tract of the right ventricle is exclusively muscular so that, throughout their circumference, the leaflets of the pulmonary valve are supported by infundibular musculature (Fig. 2.11). In this respect, however, it is also significant that the infundibulum is a free-standing structure and can be removed completely from the body of the right ventricle without damaging the outflow tract of the left ventricle. The leaflets of the aortic valve, in contrast, are attached only in part to the musculature of the left ventricle. Posteriorly, the aortic leaflets are in fibrous continuity with those of the mitral value (Fig. 2.8). This fibrous continuity does not alter the basic semilunar arrangement of the leaflets.

Major difficulties are encountered in describing the leaflets of the arterial valves in terms of anterior, posterior, right, and left coordinates when these structures are viewed relative to the overall position of the heart in the body. This is, again, the consequence of the oblique arrangement of both valves relative to the orthogonal axes of the body. It is much better, when naming the leaflets, to take note of two constant features. The first is that two leaflets (and sinuses) of the aortic valve face two leaflets of the pulmonary valve. These leaflets in both valves can be called the facing leaflets, while the third leaflet is then nonfacing. The second feature, virtually constant but showing very rare exceptions,[7] is that the coronary arteries arise from the two facing sinuses of the aortic valve. In normally constructed hearts, therefore, it is best to describe the right coronary, left coronary, and nonfacing (or noncoronary) sinuses (and leaflets) of the aortic valve (Fig. 2.13). When describing the pulmonary valve, it is best to consider oneself as standing in the nonfacing sinus and looking toward the aorta. The sinuses (and leaflets) are then well described as being to the right hand or left hand of the observer (Fig. 2.14). This latter convention works irrespective of the orientation of the arterial trunks one to the other, and so has equal utility in congenitally malformed hearts or in those in which the coronary arteries take anomalous origins.[8]

THE PATHOLOGY OF VALVULAR STENOSIS

Valves within the heart become stenotic as a consequence of either congenital or acquired disease. With the burgeoning use of interventional techniques, it is likely that, at some time or in some place, all varieties of valvular stenosis will be subjected to balloon dilatation. It is not possible in a chapter of this kind, however, to provide descriptions of all these variations. To attempt to do so would be to write a chapter on cardiac pathology, and is beyond our scope. Instead, therefore, we will concentrate upon those lesions that have been attacked most frequently to date, namely stenotic lesions of the mitral, aortic, and pulmonary valves. We will give only brief attention to the tricuspid valve, or to the topic of restenosis. The principles to be discussed, nonetheless, will be equally applicable in other, rarer, situations, such as dilatation of the left atrioventricular valve in atrioventricular septal defects or of the common valve found in the setting of a common arterial trunk, should these interventions ever be necessary.

Stenosis of the Mitral Valve

The mitral valve can be rendered stenotic by congenital malformations such as its overall miniaturization or absence of one commissure and papillary muscle as in the "parachute" arrangement.[9,10] These and other congenital lesions, rare in isolation in any case, are unlikely to be amenable to balloon dilatation, requiring sophisticated surgical techniques for even attempted repairs during infancy and childhood.[11] It is stenosis due to rheumatic disease that is most likely to bring the mitral valve to the attention of the interventional cardiologist, particularly in the setting of the third world. Rheumatic disease has a particular predilection for the mitral valve, afflicting it most frequently of all the valves, though often in combination with the aortic valve.

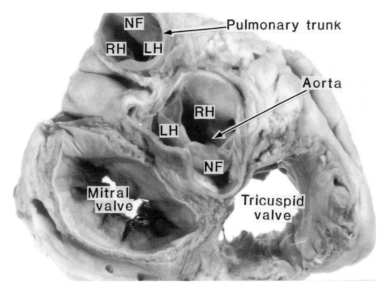

Figure 2.13 This view of the superior aspect of the dissected base of the heart shows how the sinuses of the pulmonary trunk face those of the aorta. Each sinus, therefore, can be designated as being to the right hand (*RH*) or left hand (*LH*) of the observer standing, figuratively speaking, within the nonfacing (*NF*) sinus (see Fig. 2.14).

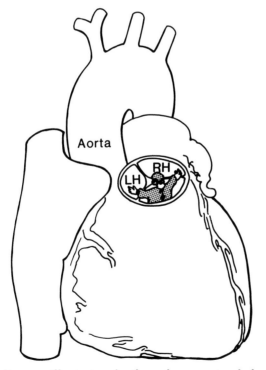

Figure 2.14 This diagram illustrates, for the pulmonary trunk, how the sinuses and valvular leaflets are designated as being to the right hand or left hand of the observer standing within the nonfacing sinus. The same convention is applicable to the aorta. (see Fig. 2.13).

The disease produces an inflammatory reaction affecting the connective tissues of both leaflets and cords, with fibrosis being the end result. Recurrent attacks may further damage the valvular apparatus and may cause further scarring of the affected structures. In due time, the valvular deformity may become further complicated by calcifications. The nature of the disease dictates that the degree of involvement of the valve will depend largely on the severity of the initial attack and the number of recurrences. Thus, the pathologic sequels may vary considerably. The leading phenomenon, however, is the fibrosis which renders the leaflets thickened and less mobile. The ends of the commissures may become glued together, although not necessarily to the same extent (Fig. 2.15). The effect, nonetheless, is to narrow the principal orifice of the mitral valve and to render it stenotic. In more advanced cases, the tendinous cords are involved, leading to fibrotic thickening and fusion with neighboring cords, thus causing narrowing and even total obliteration of the intercordal space (Fig. 2.16). Eventually, this process may lead to a funnel-shaped valvular stenosis, with the functional orifice being severely narrowed and displaced deeply into the ventricular cavity (Fig. 2.17).

Clearly, the effects of balloon dilatation will be determined largely by the state of deformity of the diseased mitral valve.[12,13] In case of fusion of the commissural ends, together with fibrosis of the leaflets, balloon dilatation may split the fused commissural ends, thereby improving the mobility of the leaflets.[14] This effect is, basically, comparable to that achieved by the surgeon performing commissurotomy. The rigidity of the leaflets, nevertheless, may be the limiting factor as far as immediate success is concerned. In the long term, it may be anticipated that the deformed valve will restenose at the sites of the split ends of the commissure.

The success of balloon dilatation may be hampered further by the presence of calcification. Calcification has a tendency to occupy the sites of the commissural ends, contributing to the stenosis and, at the same time, inhibiting appropriate opening after balloon dilatation. Once the cords are severely involved, leading to a funnel-

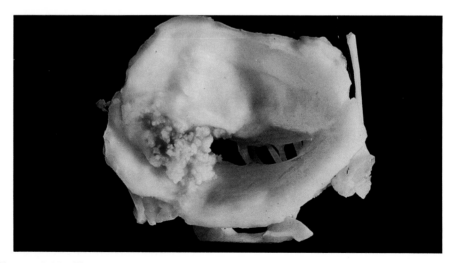

Figure 2.15 This resected mitral valve, from a patient with chronic rheumatic disease, has extensive commissural fusion but with sparing of the intercordal spaces.

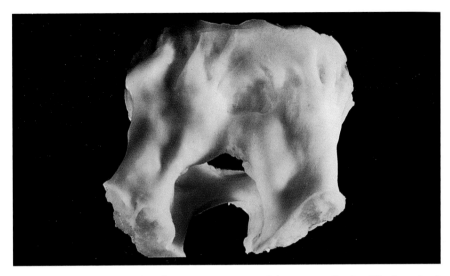

Figure 2.16 In this mitral valve, again removed from a patient with chronic rheumatic heart disease, there is commissural fusion and obliteration of the intercordal spaces.

shaped deformity, an inflated balloon within the displaced orifice may produce tears in the weakest sites of the surrounding walls. Under these circumstances, the tear may be either in the plane of the commissure or at other sites.[15] Such tears originate in the most apical part of the funnel-shaped valve, extending upward toward the atrio-ventricular junction (Fig. 2.18). A tear outside the commissural plane could cause

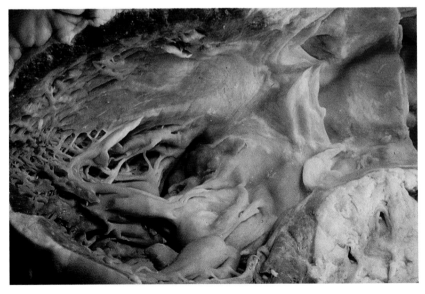

Figure 2.17 The mitral valve in this patient with chronic rheumatic heart disease shows typical funnel-shaped stenosis. The principal orifice is displaced apically and is hardly visible (compare with Fig. 2.8).

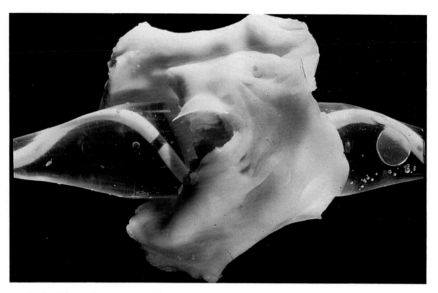

Figure 2.18 This photograph shows the mitral valve illustrated in Figure 2.16 after a balloon has been inflated within the valvular orifice subsequent to its surgical removal. The balloon produced a tear within the intercordal spaces instead of splitting the stenotic orifice at the sites of commissural fusion. Such a change is likely to produce severe valvular regurgitation should it occur during balloon dilatation in life.

serious and acute valvular insufficiency.[12] Adequate evaluation of the pathology of the rheumatic valve, with particular emphasis on the involvement of cords and the presence of a funnel-shaped deformity, is therefore essential in selecting the most appropriate patients for balloon dilatation. Cross-sectional echocardiography is a most helpful tool in this respect.

Stenosis of the Aortic Valve

Stenosis of the aortic valve can, like stenosis affecting the mitral valve, be of congenital or acquired origin. It is much more likely that aortic stenosis of congenital origin will be presented to the interventional cardiologist for balloon dilatation. Congenital stenosis, nonetheless, can take various forms. The most severe variant is critical stenosis presenting in the neonatal period. This is almost always of the so-called unicuspid and unicommissural pattern (Fig. 2.19). Careful examination of the sinusal structure of patients presenting in this fashion shows that the apparent formation of a valve with only one commissure is derived from abnormal development of a structure which, initially, possessed three commissures.[16] The persisting commissure is almost always the one separating the noncoronary and left coronary leaflets of the valve. This commissure then extends backward like a keyhole toward the area of fibrous continuity with the leaflets of the mitral valve. (Fig. 2.20). There is evidence of the other commissures in the form of persistence of the interleaflet triangles which separate the noncoronary and right coronary sinuses of the aorta from each other and from the left coronary sinus. There is no upward tenting of the line of attachment of the leaflets, however, so that, in contrast to the normal valve, the abnormal leaflets are attached in a fashion much more akin to that of the mythical annulus (Fig. 2.21). The

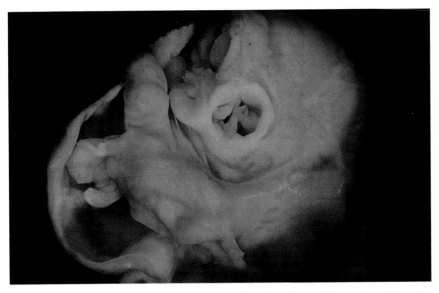

Figure 2.19 This shows a so-called "unicuspid and unicommissural" aortic valve as seen from above. The valve has one patent commissure, pointing backward toward the posterior extension of the left ventricular outflow tract (see Fig. 2.7), with rudimentary formation of the other two commissures.

leaflets themselves are also abnormal and thickened and, almost always, the aortic root itself is narrowed and hypoplastic. Careful measurements show that, in contrast to the normal valve, in which the free edge of each leaflet is longer than the circumferential arc of each sinus (Fig. 2.21, *upper*), the length of each leaflet in the apparently unicuspid valve is shorter than the arc of sinus between the putative commissures (Fig. 2.21, *lower*). The opening of the valve is itself restrictive and, in addition to the valvular problems, there are often fibroelastotic changes in the wall of the left ventricle (Fig. 2.20). Often these changes also involve the mitral valve.[17] It could well be the extent of these associated malformations that determines the eventual success of any attempt to relieve the valvular stenosis, be the attempt surgical or balloon dilatation.

The so-called unicuspid and unicommissural pattern can also be found as the cause of aortic stenosis presenting in later childhood, or even in adult life. The changes are less severe but still represent acquired change in a valve which, initially, was formed on the template of a trifoliate and trisinuate structure. The associated malformations are, self-evidently, much less extreme when the lesion manifests in later life, and the chances of successful dilatation are that much more increased.

Aortic stenosis of congenital origin presenting in later life is almost always due to change in a so-called bicuspid valve. Careful examination of the sinusal structure of aortic valves with two leaflets, as with the unicuspid variant, shows that, almost always, they too are formed on a trifoliate template.[18] Again, as with the unicuspid pattern, the rudimentary commissure usually has evidence beneath it of a vestigeal interleaflet triangle, and the commissure itself is often represented by an obvious raphe (Fig. 2.22). The conjoint leaflet can be formed by fusion of the two coronary leaflets or by

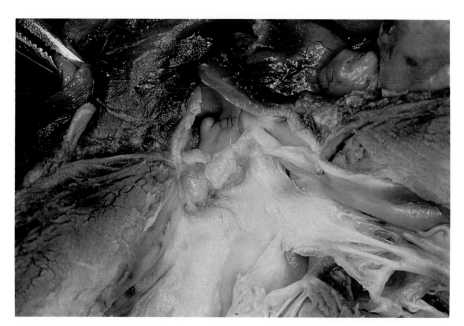

Figure 2.20 In this heart from an infant with critical aortic stenosis, the aortic outflow tract has been opened through an anterior incision and spread to show the attachment of the valvular leaflets. The arrangement is as depicted in Figure 2.19. There is one patent commissure which points toward the crux of the heart. The other commissures are reduced markedly in height, so that the leaflets are attached in more annular fashion than normal. Note also the ventricular fibroelastosis. (Reproduced by kind permission of Dr. Audrey Smith, Institute of Child Health, University of Liverpool.)

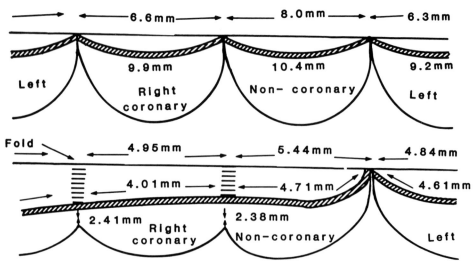

Figure 2.21 This diagram illustrates measurements taken from a series of normal hearts from infants (*upper*) and another series of hearts with critical aortic stenosis (*lower*). The measurements show the abnormal arrangement of all components of the valve, but particularly that the dimensions of the free edges of the leaflets are less than those of the sinuses which support them, in contrast to the arrangement in the normal. (Reproduced by kind permission of Drs. Roxane McKay and Audrey Smith, Institute of Child Health, University of Liverpool.)

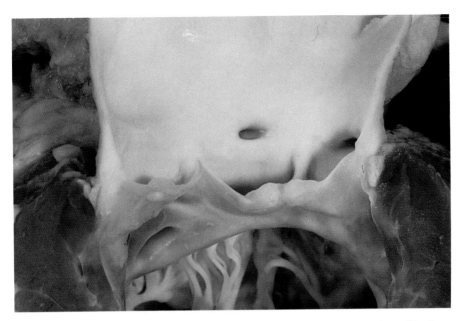

Figure 2.22 This picture shows an aortic valve with two leaflets, produced by fusion of one commissure during fetal growth. The rudimentary commissure is represented by the obvious raphe. This particular valve is not stenotic.

fusion of the noncoronary leaflet with either of the coronary leaflets. In a small minority of cases, even careful examination reveals presence of only two sinuses, and the leaflets themselves show no evidence that a rudimentary commissure or raphe has formed. These features are of minimal significance to relief of stenosis because the bicuspid valve, in itself, is not stenotic.[19] It is the superimposed acquired changes that bring the bicuspid valve to the attention of the cardiologist, either with stenosis, with prolapse, or as the seat of endocarditis.

Acquired stenosis of the aortic valve, therefore, takes one of two basic types. The most frequent variety, in the developed world, is valvular stenosis related to degenerative changes, which lead to fibrosis and secondary calcifications. Such degenerative changes may occur either in the congenitally bicuspid aortic valve (Fig. 2.23) or in an aortic valve with three leaflets (Fig. 2.24). The pathogenesis of the degenerative changes is due to "wear and tear." In the aortic valve with three leaflets, equality in proportional surface area of the three valve leaflets is the exception rather than the rule. Almost always, one or two of the leaflets are larger than the remaining leaflets, thus leading again to an inequal division of the diastolic pressure load over the leaflets.[20] The inequality in distribution of force enhances the natural phenomenon of disintegration of the connective tissue core of the leaflets, leading to fibrosis of the leaflets together with calcifications. Fusion of the ends of the commissures also occurs with time, but it is not the earliest and most dominant feature.

The second major cause for acquired stenosis is rheumatic disease (Fig. 2.25). The same mechanism that produces disease of the mitral valve also causes the deformity of the leaflets of the aortic valve. The process is thus accompanied by extensive fibrosis of the leaflets and fusion of the ends of the commissures. Commissural fusion may occur to such an extent that the valve, when observed from the aortic side, may appear

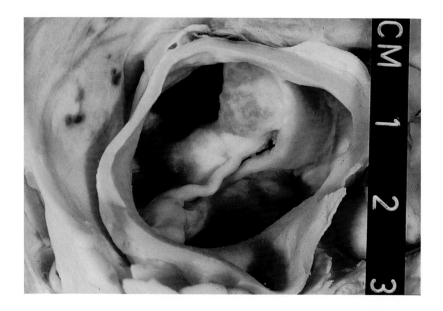

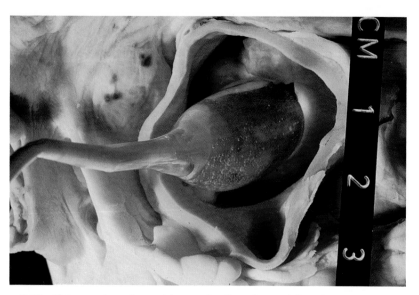

Figure 2.23 This aortic valve with two leaflets (*upper*) has become stenotic as a consequence of severe degeneration and calcification. Inflation of a balloon within the valve after its removal (*lower*) has opened the fused commissures.

to represent a congenitally bicuspid lesion. The fused ends of commissures, however, can almost always be properly identified and distinguished from the raphe observed in the conjoint leaflet of a truly congenitally bicuspid valve.

When contemplating balloon dilatation of a stenosed aortic valve, therefore, it is important to determine whether the underlying disorder is that of a degenerative process or of rheumatic disease.[21] In the latter instance, the incidence of fusion of the commissural ends is higher. It is this feature which, to a large extent, will determine

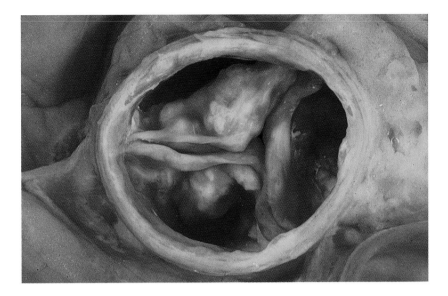

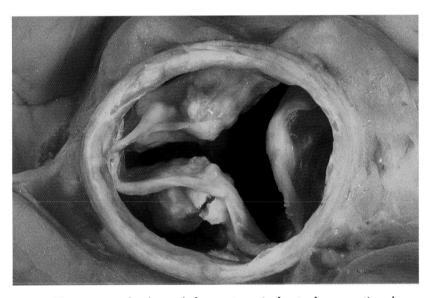

Figure 2.24 This aortic valve (*upper*) shows stenosis due to degenerative changes of aging. The leaflets are thickened by fibrosis and calcification, these being particularly prominent on the inner aspect. Inflation of a balloon within the valve after death (*lower*) has crushed many of the calcific deposits and opened the valvular orifice, although the leaflets remain immobile.

the immediate success of the balloon dilatation. In cases of degenerative valvular stenoses, the lack of fusion at the ends of the commissures often minimizes the effect of the balloon. It is the extent of dystrophic calcifications that usually becomes the ultimate limiting factor. Crushing the calcium deposits within the diseased leaflets should improve the mobility of the leaflets but, at the same time, may produce tears in the leaflets. Such tears can cause serious valvular insufficiency, as well as producing thrombotic or calcific embolic complications.

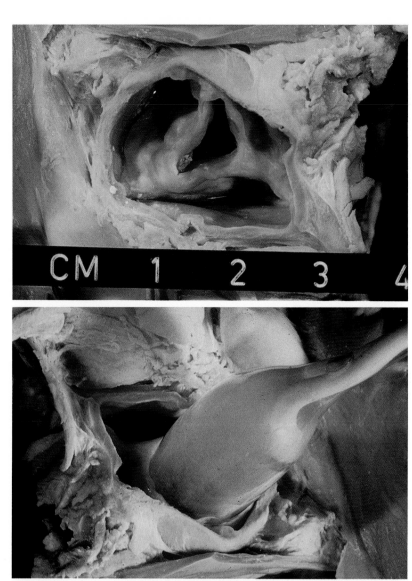
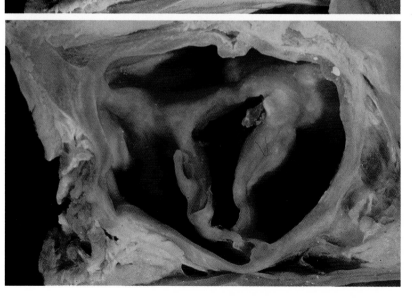

Stenosis of the Pulmonary Valve

Of all forms of valvular stenosis, it is in treatment of pulmonary valvular stenosis that balloon dilatation has established itself as the treatment of choice. Even in the pulmonary valve, however, some forms of stenosis are more amenable to dilatation than others. The form least amenable to dilatation is that produced by dysplastic leaflets. In this variant, seen most frequently as part of a syndrome such as Noonan's syndrome, it is the mere bulk of the dysplastic leaflets that obstructs the valvular orifice, commissural fusion being rare (Fig. 2.26). Relief of obstruction, therefore, can be achieved only by compressing the mucoid leaflets. More frequently, stenosis of the pulmonary valve is due to uniform fusion of the three commissures. This produces a stenotic orifice supported by a dome of conjoined leaflets (Fig. 2.27). The extent of stenosis depends initially on the degree of fusion of the commissures. The commissural fusion is then exacerbated by tethering of the fused ends of the commissures to the wall of the arterial trunk at the sinutubular junction. When extreme, this commissural tethering pinches the junction and can markedly narrow the orifices to the sinuses, producing so-called bottle-shaped sinuses.[22] From the anatomic observations, it seems that dilatation will be most successful before the tethering to the arterial wall has time to become severe. It is also well established that valvular stenosis can promote infundibular hypertrophy, so that the full benefits of dilatation may not become apparent until the infundibular musculature has a chance to regress. The morphologic findings also indicate that pulmonary atresia with an intact ventricular septum, when produced by an imperforate valvular membrane, is the endpoint of the spectrum of pulmonary valvular stenosis. Cases of critical pulmonary stenosis presenting in the neonatal period often show the same degree of dysplasia and thickening of the tricuspid valve as is seen in pulmonary atresia. These cases are, nonetheless, still amenable to balloon dilatation as, indeed, are cases of valvular pulmonary atresia if the valvular membrane is first perforated by laser.[23]

Stenosis of the Tricuspid Valve

Isolated tricuspid stenosis is a rare event. When it is seen, stenosis at the right atrioventricular junction is usually part and parcel of chronic rheumatic disease primarily affecting other valves, notably the aortic and mitral valves. When the tricuspid valve is involved in the rheumatic process, the changes are as described for the other valves (see above), with commissural fusion and obliteration of intercordal spaces being the leading features. When involved in this fashion, the valve is just as amenable to balloon dilatation as are the other valves, with the same problems and caveats as described above.

Congenital stenosis of the tricuspid valve is extremely rare except when the valve is distorted by Ebstein's malformation.[24] This can affect the normally located valve, or the morphologically tricuspid valve guarding the left atrioventricular junction when

Figure 2.25 In this aortic valve (*upper*), stenosis is the consequence of rheumatic disease, with eccentric fusion of the commissures producing an appearance that mimics the congenitally bicuspid arrangement (see Fig. 2.23). The *middle* panel shows a balloon that was inflated within the valve after death. The *lower* panel shows the extensive laceration of the thickened and fibrotic leaflets, with opening of two of the commissures.

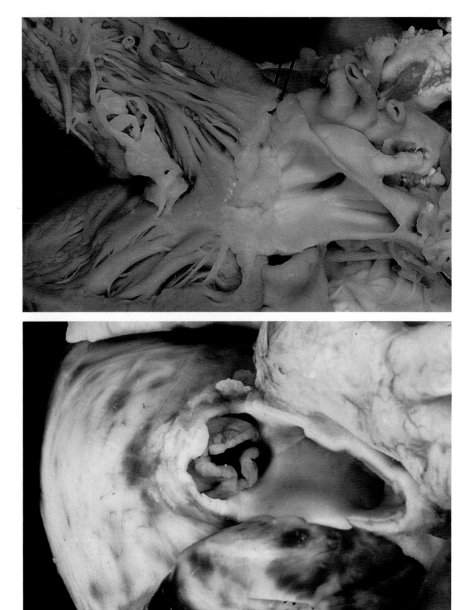

Figure 2.26 This heart (*upper*) is from an infant with Noonan's syndrome. The stenosis at the pulmonary valve is due to dysplastic changes within the leaflets rather than commissural fusion. The *lower* photograph shows another dysplastic valve that underwent balloon dilatation during life. The commissures are widely open, but the bulk of the leaflets leaves residual stenosis.

the atrioventricular connections are discordant ("corrected transposition"). In either event, the line of attachment of the leaflets, notably the mural and septal ones, is displaced from the atrioventricular junction toward the apex of the heart. The valvular leaflets often close at the junction of the inlet and apical trabecular components, and such a valvular orifice can be competent (Fig. 2.28). More usually, it is stenotic,

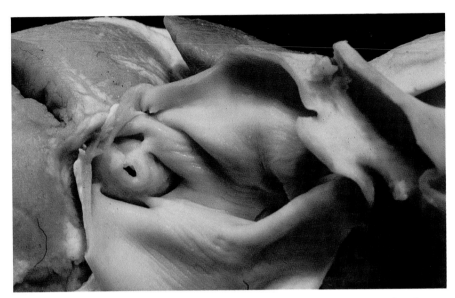

Figure 2.27 This opened pulmonary trunk from an infant with critical pulmonary stenosis reveals severe doming of the valve, with marked commissural fusion producing a pinhole meatus. Dilatation of such a valve is just as likely to tear or avulse the leaflets as to split the commissures.

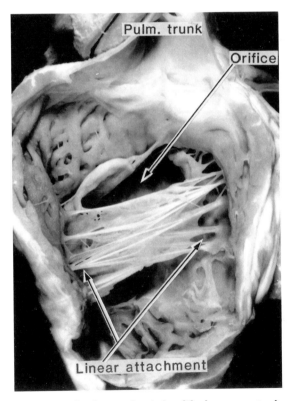

Figure 2.28 This photograph shows the infundibular aspect of a tricuspid valve severely deformed by Ebstein's malformation. There is linear attachment of the anterosuperior leaflet with a stenotic valvar orifice formed at the site of the initial anteroseptal commissure. On anatomic grounds, it would seem risky to attempt to dilate such a valve with a balloon.

regurgitant, or both. If stenotic, it is possible to envision the orifice being enlarged by balloon dilatation, but the anatomic arrangement would tend to suggest that such a maneuver would carry a high risk of inducing gross regurgitation.

Valvular Restenosis

The potential for restenosis after balloon dilatation will be related to the initial disease process responsible for the valvular deformity. Restenosis should not be anticipated to be a major problem for lesions of congenital origin, providing, of course, that the initial dilatation was adequate. Regurgitation due to tearing of the leaflets or disruption from their semilunar attachments is more likely to be a problem. Restenosis is likely to occur in patients with chronic rheumatic disease, and also with lesions produced by "wear and tear." There is no reason, however, why such valves that undergo restenosis should not be equally amenable to repeated balloon dilatation.

Acknowledgements: We are indebted to Dr. Siew Yen Ho, Mrs. Lucienne Kilpatrick, and Mr. Aldrin Sweeney for their help in the preparation of the illustrations. We are particularly grateful to Drs. Roxane McKay and Audrey Smith from the Institute of Child Health, University of Liverpool, for permission to quote early results from our ongoing study of the morphology of critical aortic stenosis presenting in infancy.

REFERENCES

1. Yacoub M: Anatomy of the mitral valve chordae and cusps. In: Kalmanson D, ed. *The Mitral Valve. A Pluridisciplinary Approach*. London: Edward Arnold, 1976, pp 15–20.
2. Lam JHC, Ranganathan N, Wigle ED, et al: Morphology of the human mitral valve, I: chordae tendineae: a new classification. *Circulation*. 41:449–458, 1970.
3. Silver MD, Lam JHC, Ranganathan N, et al: Morphology of the human tricuspid valve. *Circulation*. 43:333–348, 1971.
4. Anderson RH: Editorial note. The anatomy of arterial valvar stenosis. *Int J Cardiol*. 26:355–359, 1990.
5. Perloff JK, Roberts WC: The mitral apparatus. Functional anatomy of mitral regurgitation. *Circulation*. 46:227–239, 1972.
6. Becker AE, de Wit APM: Mitral valve apparatus. A spectrum of normality relevent to mitral valve prolapse. *Br Heart J*. 42:680–689, 1980.
7. Ishikawa T, Otsuka T, Suzuki T: Anomalous origin of the left main coronary artery from the noncoronary sinus of Valsalva. *Pediatr Cardiol*. 11:173–174, 1990.
8. Anderson RH: Editorial. Description of the origins and epicardial course of the coronary arteries in complete transposition. *Cardiol Young*. 1:11–12, 1991.
9. Becker AE: Valve pathology in the paediatric age group. In: Anderson RH, Macartney FJ, Shinebourne EA, et al, eds. *Paediatric Cardiology*, Vol 5. Edinburgh:Churchill Livingstone, 1983, pp 345–360.
10. Thiene G, Frescura C, Daliento L: The pathology of the congenitally malformed mitral valve. In: Marcelletti C, Anderson RH, Becker AE, et al, ed. *Paediatric Cardiology*,Vol 6. Edinburgh:Churchill Livingstone, 1986, pp 225–239.
11. Carpentier A, Branchini B, Cour JC, et al: Congenital malformations of the mitral valve in children. Pathology and surgical treatment. *J Thorac Cardiovasc Surg*. 72:854–866, 1976.
12. Kaplan JD, Isner JM, Karas RH, et al: In vitro analysis of mechanisms of balloon valvuloplasty of stenotic mitral valves. *Am J Cardiol*. 59:318–323, 1987.

13. McKay RG, Lock JE, Safian RD, et al: Balloon dilation of mitral stenosis in adult patients: postmortem and percutaneous mitral valvuloplasty studies. *J Am Coll Cardiol.* 9:723–731, 1987.

14. Thiene G, Turri M, Daliento L, et al: Morphological determinants of successful balloon valvoplasty in chronic rheumatic valvar disease. In: Crupi G, Parenzan L, Anderson RH, eds. *Perspectives in Pediatric Cardiology*, Vol 2, Pt 3 – Pediatric cardiac surgery. Mount Kisco, NY: Futura Publishing Company Ltd, 1990, pp 134–137.

15. Sadee AS, Becker AE: In vitro balloon dilatation of mitral valve stenosis: the importance of subvalvar involvement as a cause of mitral valve insufficiency. *Br Heart J.* 65:277–279, 1991.

16. Anderson RH, Devine WA, Ho SY, et al: The myth of the aortic annulus: the anatomy of the subaortic outflow tract. *Ann Thorac Surg.* 52:640–646, 1991.

17. Leung MP, McKay R, Smith A, et al: Critical aortic stenosis in early infancy. Anatomic and echocardiographic substrates of successful open valvotomy. *J Thorac Cardiovasc Surg.* 101:526–535, 1991.

18. Angelini A, Ho SY, Anderson RH, et al: The morphology of the normal aortic valve as compared with the aortic valve having two leaflets. *J Thorac Cardiovasc Surg.* 98:362–367, 1989.

19. Edwards JE: The congenital bicuspid aortic valve. *Circulation.* 23:485–488, 1961.

20. Vollebergh FEMG, Becker AE: Minor congenital variations of cusp size in tricuspid aortic valves. Possible link with isolated aortic stenosis. *Br Heart J.* 39:1006–1011, 1977.

21. Becker AE, Hoedemaker G: Balloon valvuloplasty in congenital and acquired heart disease: morphologic considerations. *Z Kardiol.* 76 (suppl 6):73–79, 1987.

22. Milo S, Fiegal A, Shem-Tov A, et al: Hour-glass deformity of the pulmonary valve: a third type of pulmonary valve stenosis. *Br Heart J.* 60:128–133, 1988.

23. Qureshi SA, Rosenthal E, Tynan M, et al: Transcatheter laser-assisted balloon pulmonary valve dilation in pulmonic valve atresia. *Am J Cardiol.* 67:428–430, 1991.

24. Leung MP, Baker EJ, Anderson RH, et al: Cineangiographic spectrum of Ebstein's malformation: its relevance to clinical presentation and outcome. *J Am Coll Cardiol.* 11:154–161, 1988.

CHAPTER 3

Pathophysiology of Valvular Stenosis

SING SAN YANG
VLADIR MARANHAO
HARRY GOLDBERG

MITRAL STENOSIS

The mitral valve, mitral annulus, chordae tendineae, and papillary muscles are considered to be a functional unit called the mitral complex[1] or mitral apparatus.[2] Structural alteration or functional disturbance in any of these components may cause significant hemodynamic derangement.

The mitral valve consists of two leaflets, anterior and posterior, which are attached to the annulus and encircle the orifice to form a funnel protruding into the left ventricular cavity. These two leaflets are connected by commissures. The numerous chordae tendineae arise from papillary muscles and attach to the mitral leaflets along their free edges or to the bodies of leaflets on the ventricular side. Blood flows through the mitral valve by way of a principal orifice and several secondary orifices.[3] The former has, as its anterior and posterior borders, the respective leaflets and lateral borders, each papillary muscle and the respective chordae. The secondary orifices consist of numerous spaces between the chordae tendineae. Thickening or calcification of the mitral leaflets and commissural fusion form the basis for the narrowing of the principal orifice (valvular stenosis), whereas chordal fusion accounts for the obliteration of the secondary orifices (subvalvular stenosis). In addition, extensive annular calcification has been implicated in significant narrowing of the mitral orifice at the annular level.[4-6]

If blood flow through the mitral orifice is obstructed, left atrial pressure rises sufficiently to propel the blood through the stenotic orifice, thereby producing a mitral valve gradient. The left atrial pressure pulse (Fig. 3.1) is characterized by a prominent *a* wave caused by vigorous atrial contraction and a slow *y* descent. Diastasis is absent because of the resistance to left atrial emptying and the continuous flow throughout left ventricular filling. In mild mitral stenosis, the mitral valve gradient is mainly or solely in early diastole and presystole, and the mean left atrial pressure is mildly increased. With increasing severity of mitral stenosis the mean left atrial pressure rises further, the height of *a* wave approaches that of the *v* wave, and the mitral valve gradient is present throughout diastole. The left atrial hypertension

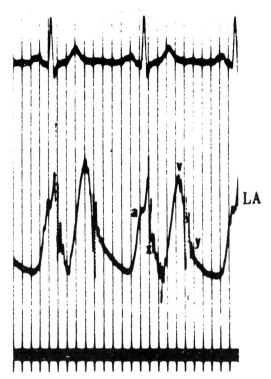

Figure 3.1 Left atrial pressure pulse in mitral stenosis, showing a prominent *a* wave, a slow *y* descent, and the absence of diastasis. *a—A* wave; *v—V* wave; *x—X* descent; *y—Y* descent.

results in distention of the left atrial chamber and passive congestion of the pulmonary veins and pulmonary capillaries. With a sufficient increase in pulmonary blood volume, lung compliance decreases and consequently the work of breathing is increased: *dyspnea*. An enlarged left atrium favors development of atrial fibrillation which, in turn, predisposes the left atrium to thrombus formation. Long-standing pulmonary venous congestion evokes pulmonary vascular changes, narrowing the arteriolar lumens and leading to pulmonary hypertension. The right ventricle hypertrophies, dilates, and may eventually fail.

Pulmonary Venous Hypertension

The symptom of dyspnea in mitral stenosis is caused by the pulmonary venous hypertension and pulmonary capillary engorgement caused by the elevated left atrial pressure and increased mitral valve gradient.

The mitral valve gradient rises with increasing severity of mitral stenosis at a given cardiac output. There are, however, many other factors that can affect the mitral valve gradient and thereby lead to dyspnea in mitral stenosis. According to Gorlin's formula, for a given mitral valve area the mitral valve gradient is proportional to the square of the mitral valve flow,[7] which is equal to the cardiac output divided by the diastolic filling period. Conditions that increase cardiac output, such as exercise, excitement, infection, fever, hyperthyroidism, or pregnancy, or conditions that shorten the diastolic filling period by increasing heart rate, such as tachycardia, exercise, infection, fever, or hyperthyroidism, raise the mitral valve flow, thereby significantly elevating the mitral valve gradient and left atrial pressure and leading to pulmonary capillary engorgement and dyspnea. (When the heart rate increases, the fraction of the cardiac cycle occupied by diastole is decreased, thereby cutting short the time available for atrial emptying.) Thus the onset of atrial tachyarrhythmia (eg, atrial tachycardia, atrial flutter, atrial fibrillation) may precipitate dyspnea and pulmonary edema in previously asymptomatic patients.[8] These patients respond dramatically to measures that slow down the ventricular rate, such as administration of digitalis or beta-blocking agents. Notable also is the development of pulmonary edema during the third trimester in pregnant women with noncritical mitral stenosis; the mitral valve flow increases significantly because of the higher cardiac output, heart rate, and blood volume.[9] The symptoms of pulmonary venous hypertension invariably subside postpartum.

The increase in left atrial pressure in mitral stenosis results not only from the impedance to left atrial emptying but also from the left atrial stiffness. Thus a noncompliant left atrium may be associated with a higher left atrial pressure and mitral valve gradient than a compliant left atrium. This phenomenon is exemplified by the case of tight mitral stenosis with a relatively small left atrium in which the marked increase in left atrial pressure and mitral valve gradient reflects not only the severity of mitral stenosis but also the stiffness of the small left atrium.

The normal mitral valve area in an adult is about 4 to 6 cm². In mild mitral stenosis with a mitral valve area of over 2.5 cm², exercise is usually well tolerated since there is no significant rise in left atrial pressure and therefore the mitral valve gradient. With a reduction of mitral valve area to 2 cm², patients who are asymptomatic at rest may experience dyspnea during strenuous exertion. When the mitral valve area falls below 1.5 cm², mild to moderate exertion causes dyspnea. Below the critical area of 1 cm², even mild exertion is not tolerated. At this level of obstruction, a mitral valve gradient of approximately 20 mmHg and a mean left atrial pressure of about 25 mmHg are required to maintain a normal cardiac output. It is estimated that a small (25%) increase in cardiac output and in heart rate such as occurs during normal activities or excitement may cause a modest (40%) increase in the mitral valve flow and consequently a doubling of the mitral valve gradient and a marked increase in pulmonary capillary pressure.[10] In moderate to severe mitral stenosis, exercise may double the cardiac output and hence quadruple the mitral valve gradient, elevating the pulmonary capillary pressure sufficiently to induce pulmonary edema.[11]

Pulmonary Hypertension

The pulmonary arterial pressure in mitral stenosis is not always directly related to the left atrial pressure because of the unpredictable behavior of the pulmonary vascular resistance.[12] A mild rise in left atrial pressure is usually associated with normal or slightly increased pulmonary vascular resistance and pulmonary arterial pressure. With a higher left atrial pressure, the pulmonary vascular resistance may be normal or increased, at times out of proportion to the level of left atrial pressure.

Three possible mechanisms cause pulmonary hypertension in patients with mitral stenosis:

1. an obligatory increase in the pulmonary arterial pressure in response to the

backward transmission of the elevated left atrial pressure *(passive pulmonary hypertension)*

2. Arteriolar constriction *(reactive pulmonary hypertension)*
3. Medial hypertrophy and intimal fibrosis of the small pulmonary arteries and arterioles *(obliterative pulmonary hypertension)*.

In passive pulmonary hypertension, which occurs in most patients with mitral stenosis, the increase in pulmonary arterial pressure is predictable, the pulmonary arterial − left atrial pressure gradient being about 10 mmHg.[9] In reactive pulmonary hypertension, pulmonary arterial pressure elevation is out of proportion to the increase in left atrial pressure. This condition is usually reversible after successful mitral valve surgery, with a return of normal left atrial pressure.[13,14] Reactive pulmonary hypertension seldom occurs in patients with mitral stenosis not severe enough to cause a left atrial hypertension of 20 to 25 mmHg or more (Fig. 3.2).[15] It is not well understood, however, why only one third of patients with tight mitral stenosis develop reactive pulmonary hypertension. In some patients, reactive pulmonary hypertension results from long-standing left atrial hypertension, but in others the onset may be early, without previous symptoms of severe pulmonary venous hypertension such as

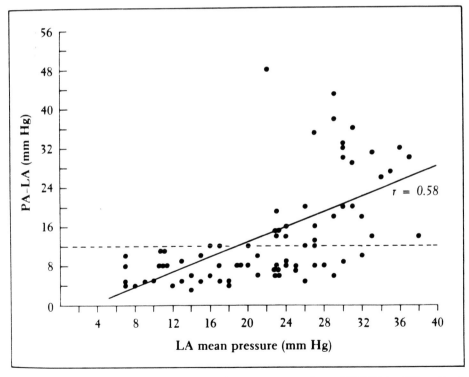

Figure 3.2 Pulmonary artery-left atrial pressure gradient (PA-LA) in 100 patients with mitral stenosis. Note that the gradient remains normal unless the mean left atrial (LA) pressure is 20 to 25 mmHg or more. On the other hand, it may be normal in some patients with considerable elevated left atrial pressure. (From: Dalen JE, Alpert JS: *Valvular Heart Disease*. 2nd ed. Boston: Little Brown, 1987, p. 57. With permission.)

orthopnea and paroxysmal nocturnal dyspnea. In Wood's series, the latter occurred in 78% of subjects with severe reactive pulmonary hypertension.[16]

Chronic pulmonary venous hypertension may lead to obliterative changes in the pulmonary vascular bed, namely, medial hypertrophy and intimal fibrosis of the small pulmonary arteries and the arterioles. These changes were always associated with a pulmonary vascular resistance exceeding 260 dynes·seconds·cm^{-5}·m^2, but there was no linear relationship between the severity of medial hypertrophy and the pulmonary vascular resistance.[17] As with reactive pulmonary hypertension, medial hypertrophy and intimal fibrosis are reversible after successful corrective mitral valve surgery.[18]

The increase in pulmonary vascular resistance and pulmonary arterial pressure protects the pulmonary capillary bed from excessive engorgement by opposing right ventricular emptying, hence decreasing right ventricular filling and venous return, (cardiac output). This protective effect is most beneficial during exercise when the increased venous return, not matched by an equal amount of flow into the left ventricle, would cause an inordinate increase in left atrial and pulmonary capillary pressures and produce pulmonary edema if some blood were not stored in the systemic veins and the right atrium. However, a high pulmonary vascular resistance achieves this goal by subjecting the right ventricle, a volume-adapted chamber, to a pressure overload, which leads to hypertrophy and eventual failure.

Left Ventricular Performance

Cardiac output is maintained in patients with mild mitral stenosis and rises appropriately with exercise. In moderately severe mitral stenosis, some reduction of cardiac output occurs, both at rest and with exercise, yet in some patients cardiac output may be well preserved, producing an inordinately large mitral valve gradient. In severe mitral stenosis with a high pulmonary vascular resistance, right ventricular failure, or both, cardiac output is often markedly reduced; exercise may not increase it and may even decrease it. The mitral valve gradient is then smaller than expected, and the presenting symptoms then are those of low cardiac output.

Reduction in cardiac output in mitral stenosis may be due to pulmonary arteriolar constriction, right ventricular failure secondary to pulmonary hypertension, left ventricular dysfunction, or any combination of these conditions. Of left ventricular dysfunction, several possible mechanisms have been postulated:

1. A reduction in preload resulting from impeded left ventricular filling, leading the left ventricle to operate at the lower end of the Frank-Starling curve,[19] with consequent low cardiac output and ejection fraction.

2. An increase in afterload resulting from reduced wall thickness.[20]

3. A rheumatic inflammatory process involving the myocardium with a resultant diffuse[21] or localized[22] hypokinesis.

4. Extension of the fibrotic process from the mitral valve into the adjacent posterobasal segment.[23]

5. Increased right ventricular volume and pressure causing the septum to bulge into the left ventricular cavity, further reducing left ventricular filling.

6. A reduction in coronary blood flow due to associated coronary artery disease or coronary embolism.

Atrial Fibrillation

Atrial tachyarrhythmia, especially atrial fibrillation, is an important complication of mitral stenosis because of its potential as a precipitator of pulmonary venous hypertension and its impact on the incidence of systemic embolism.

Atrial contribution to cardiac output is approximately 30%. Its deprivation with the onset of atrial fibrillation causes a reduction of 20% or more in cardiac output.[24] Atrial fibrillation also raises mean left atrial pressure because effective atrial contraction is absent[24] and a rapid ventricular rate is frequently associated.

Atrial fibrillation may be paroxysmal or chronic. The paroxysmal form may occur early when mitral stenosis is still relatively mild. It presents with episodes of marked elevation in pulmonary venous pressure — even up to pulmonary edema levels — and subsides upon administration of digitalis or a beta blocker. Chronic atrial fibrillation is usually associated with tight mitral stenosis, but it may occur in association with active myocarditis, coronary artery disease, mitral regurgitation, or left ventricular dysfunction.

The incidence of atrial fibrillation in mitral stenosis increases with age.[25] It also correlates with left atrial size.[26] In the series of Henry and associates,[26] of 117 patients with left atrial size smaller than 40 mm, there were only three with atrial fibrillation, but 80 of 148 patients with left atrial size larger than 40 mm had atrial fibrillation. In addition, atrial fibrillation contributes to further left atrial enlargement and development and perpetuation of the left and right atrial enlargement.[27]

Atrial fibrillation is a major risk factor for systemic embolism in patients with mitral stenosis. The majority of patients with mitral stenosis are in atrial fibrillation when they develop systemic embolism, 75% of which are cerebral.[16] There is, however, no consistent correlation between the severity of mitral stenosis and systemic embolism.

AORTIC STENOSIS

Valvular aortic stenosis is the most common form of left ventricular outflow obstruction, others being supravalvular aortic stenosis and subvalvular aortic stenosis. This lesion is frequently associated with aortic regurgitation and when coexisting with mitral valvular lesion it is invariably rheumatic in origin. Isolated valvular aortic stenosis occurs more frequently than other valvular lesions.[28] Valvular aortic stenosis may be either congenital or acquired (Fig. 3.3).[29] In congenital aortic stenosis, the aortic valve is either unicuspid, bicuspid, tricuspid, or a dome-shaped diaphragm. Acquired aortic stenosis may result from rheumatic fever (rheumatic aortic stenosis), fibrosis and calcification of the congenitally unicuspid or bicuspid aortic valve, degenerative wear and tear of the normal tricuspid aortic valve (degenerative calcific aortic stenosis, or, less frequently, from familial hypercholesterolemia,[30,31] systemic lupus erythematosus,[32] or rheumatoid heart disease.

The basic hemodynamic alteration in aortic stenosis is the systolic overloading of the left ventricle imposed by the obstruction to the left ventricular outflow. To maintain a normal cardiac output, the left ventricular systolic pressure rises sufficiently to propel the blood through the narrowed orifice, producing an aortic valve gradient, and the systolic ejection period is prolonged. Increased systolic pressure and a prolonged systolic ejection period combine to increase the tension time index[33] an

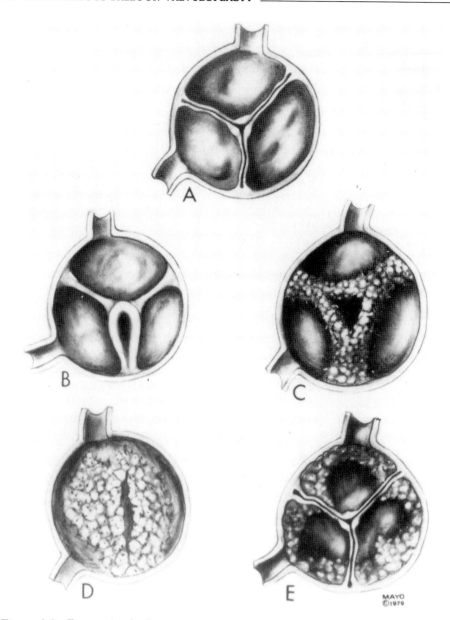

Figure 3.3 Types of valvular aortic stenosis. *A*, Normal aortic valve. *B*, Congenital aortic stenosis. *C*, Rheumatic aortic stenosis. *D*, Calcific bicuspid aortic stenosis, *E*, Calcific senile aortic stenosis. (From: Fuster V et al: Clinical approach and management of acquired valvular heart disease. *Cardiovasc Clin.* 10 (3): 126, 1980. With permission.)

index of myocardial O_2 consumption. In time, left ventricular hypertrophy develops as a compensatory mechanism and the left ventricular wall stress shifts back toward normal, the degree of improvement depending on the adequacy of wall thickening. A typical left ventricular pressure pulse in significant aortic stenosis shows a round peak in contrast to a normal flattened peak (Fig. 3.4). With severe aortic stenosis, end-diastolic pressure rises because of impaired left ventricular compliance secondary to

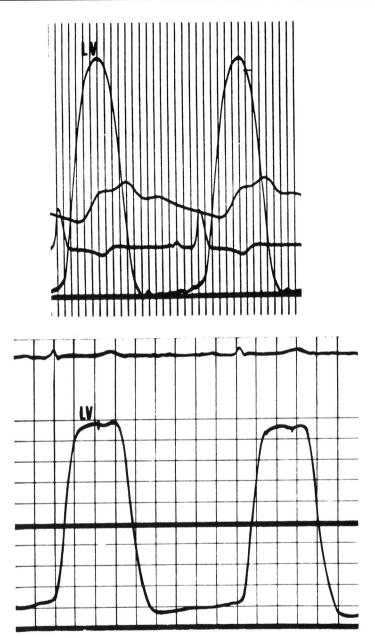

Figure 3.4 Left ventricular pressure pulse. *Top*, Aortic stenosis. *Bottom*, Normal. Note a flattened peak in normal and a round peak in aortic stenosis. *LV*—left ventricle.

left ventricular hypertrophy with or without left ventricular dilatation or failure.[34-36] The left atrial *a* wave becomes prominent owing to enhanced left atrial contraction and impaired left ventricular compliance. The aortic pressure has a slow systolic rise and a prolonged ejection time (Fig. 3.5), reflecting a slow and prolonged left ventricular ejection. The anacrotic notch is prominent and becomes lower with increasing severity of stenosis.

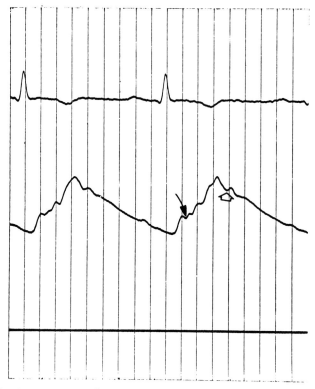

Figure 3.5 Aortic pressure pulse in aortic stenosis, showing a low anacrotic notch (*black arrow*), a slow systolic rise, and a prolonged ejection time. The *white arrow* denotes the dicrotic notch. The time-line interval is 0.1 sec.

Left Ventricular Systolic Overload

The normal aortic valve area in adults is 2.6 to 3.5 cm².[37] Narrowing of the aortic orifice imposes an obstruction to left ventricular ejection with a consequent increase in systolic left ventricular pressure and a prolongation of the systolic ejection period to maintain a normal cardiac output. In mild aortic stenosis in which the valve area is reduced by less than 50%, there may be no significant systolic pressure gradient across the obstruction nor any increase in left ventricular work. With a reduction in aortic valve area to about 1.0 cm² (approximately less than one-third normal size), the left ventricular systolic pressure increases to overcome the added impedance, and a sizable systolic gradient is produced across the obstruction. An aortic valve area of less than 0.75 cm² in average-sized adults (equivalent to 0.4 cm²/m², or approximately less than one-quarter normal size), a peak systolic gradient in excess of 50 mmHg in association with a normal cardiac output is considered to be critical.[38] The left ventricular systolic pressure may attain 300 mmHg or higher in severe aortic stenosis (aortic valve area < 0.75 cm²). The left ventricular hypertrophy that develops in response to systolic overload is usually concentric and rarely asymmetric, with asymmetry being an adaptive mechanism rather than the manifestation of coexisting cardiomyopathy.[39] The increase in left ventricular wall thickness tends to normalize the initially elevated left ventricular wall stress. In those with left ventricular failure and dilatation, and in the absence of adequate left ventricular wall thickening, the left ventricular wall stress may remain elevated.

When the left ventricle is severely hypertrophied in aortic stenosis, vigorous left atrial contraction is required for adequate diastolic filling.[40] A large left atrial *a* wave as well as an elevated left ventricular end-diastolic pressure is produced without an increase in mean left atrial pressure.[41] The *atrial kick* or *booster pump* function of the left atrium thus remarkably enhances the left ventricular diastolic filling, raising the left ventricular end-diastolic pressure sufficiently to render left ventricular contraction effective while maintaining normal mean left atrial pressure in the face of the raised atrial *a* wave. Development of atrial fibrillation or atrioventricular dissociation thus deprives these patients of an effective atrial kick, possibly leading to acute pulmonary edema.

The cardiac output remains normal at rest in most patients with severe aortic stenosis,[42] but it often shows a subnormal response to exercise. The aortic valve gradient may rise only slightly with exercise because the prolonged systolic ejection period caused by the increased heart rate tends to compensate for the increase in cardiac output. In later stages of the disease cardiac output and the aortic valve gradient fall, while left atrial, pulmonary capillary, right ventricular, and right atrial pressures rise.

Syncope in aortic stenosis is almost always exertional. It represents an event of reduced cerebral perfusion due to pronounced arterial hypotension resulting from peripheral vasodilatation in the face of inability to increase the cardiac output.[43] Activation of the baroreceptor in the wall of the left ventricle by sudden changes in left ventricular pressure has been implicated in the peripheral vasodilatation.[44,45]

Mitral regurgitation may develop in later stages of the disease as a result of left ventricular dilatation. Mitral regurgitation, when coexisting, tends to be intensified by the aortic stenosis as there is a large pressure difference between the left ventricle and the left atrium during systole.

Rarely, the markedly hypertrophied ventricular septum may encroach on the right ventricular cavity, producing right ventricular outflow tract obstruction, the so-called Bernheim syndrome.[46] The existence of such an entity has been disputed.[47]

Controversies remain concerning the nature of the contractile function of the chronically pressure-overloaded, hypertrophied left ventricle in patients with aortic stenosis. In isolated heart muscle and intact animal hearts, the severely and acutely pressure-overloaded, hypertrophied, and failing heart was shown to have decreased contractile function.[48-52] In experimental animals, the myocardial depression was directly related to the severity of systolic overload, the presence of congestive heart failure, and the duration of the overload.[48,51,53,54] Gunther and Grossman,[55] however, on the basis of their finding of an inverse correlation between wall stress and ejection fraction and velocity of fiber shortening (Fig. 3.6), suggested that poor left ventricular performance in patients with aortic stenosis may be related to increased wall stress due to inadequate wall thickening, resulting in afterload mismatch.[56] Fifer and associates,[57] studying the rate of stress development as a function of developed stress, noted nearly identical findings in patients with aortic stenosis (both compensated and overtly in failure with a depressed ejection fraction) and in control subjects, concluded that the contractile function of the left ventricle is not impaired in chronic pressure overload hypertrophy. Douglas and associates[58] and DePace and associates,[59] using echocardiographic measurements and left ventricular pressure data nonsimultaneously obtained at cardiac catheterization, derived an inverse relationship

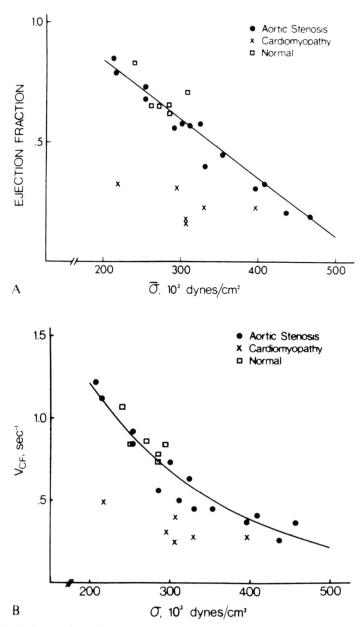

Figure 3.6 Relationships between wall stress and ejection phase indices (ejection fraction and mean velocity of circumferential fiber shortening) for three patient groups. Common to normal patients and to patients with aortic stenosis is an inverse relationship between wall stress and ejection phase indices. In contrast, patients with cardiomyopathy showed depressed values for ejection phase indices for any corresponding wall stress. $\bar{\sigma}$—mean wall stress. V_{CF}—mean circumferential fiber shortening velocity. (From: Gunther S, Grossman W: Determinants of ventricular function in pressure-overload hypertrophy in man. *Circulation.* 59:685, 1979. With permission of the American Heart Association, Inc.)

between wall stress and ejection phase indices. Others consider intrinsic depression of the contractility of the hypertrophied myocardium to be the cause of left ventricular systolic dysfunction.[60-62] Huber and associates[61] demonstrated in their series of 76 patients with pure or predominant aortic stenosis that both altered contractility and increased afterload are operative in depressing left ventricular ejection performance. In this view, whether or not hypertrophy is adequate or inadequate in maintaining normal systolic wall stress, advanced myocardial hypertrophy leads to depression of myocardial contractility.

Adverse Consequences of Compensatory Left Ventricular Hypertrophy

Left ventricular hypertrophy that develops as a compensation for pressure overload imposed by aortic stenosis has its costs, namely reduced diastolic compliance (increased wall stiffness) and increased myocardial O_2 consumption. Resistance to diastolic filling due to stiffness of the left ventricle (diastolic dysfunction) necessitates an enhanced left atrial contraction with consequent prominent left atrial *a* wave and an elevated left ventricular end-diastolic pressure (atrial kick). In some patients with severe aortic stenosis, mean left atrial pressure and therefore pulmonary venous pressure are elevated sufficiently to cause dyspnea and even pulmonary edema. Congestive heart failure in most patients with aortic stenosis results from impaired diastolic left ventricular compliance.[63] In these patients, abnormal diastolic relaxation is evident while the systolic function may be normal.[63-65] They may eventually develop systolic dysfunction, with a reduction in cardiac output and ejection fraction and other indices of systolic function.[66]

Increased myocardial O_2 consumption results from increased left ventricular work caused by increased left ventricular mass, elevated left ventricular systolic pressure, and a prolonged systolic ejection period. The coronary blood flow is hampered by a shortening of diastole, during which most of the myocardial perfusion takes place, and by an enhanced impedance to flow. Flow is impeded during systole because the contracting hypertrophied myocardium mechanically compresses the intramural vessels. During diastole flow is impeded because the coronary perfusion pressure — the difference between the aortic and left ventricular mean diastolic pressure — is reduced by an increase in left ventricular end-diastolic pressure. Together, increased myocardial O_2 consumption and reduced coronary blood flow predispose patients with aortic stenosis to imbalance between myocardial O_2 demand and supply, with resultant myocardial ischemia and angina pectoris[67-70] even in the absence of coronary artery disease.[71,72] The subendocardium is especially vulnerable for several reasons. It is subjected to severe compressive forces; intercapillary distances are great; vasodilator reserve is impaired; and the subendocardial: subepicardial flow ratio is reduced.

PULMONIC STENOSIS

Pulmonic stenosis may be classified into three types: valvular, supravalvular, and subvalvular, according to the level of obstruction. *Supravalvular pulmonic stenosis* is the obstruction of the pulmonary trunk or its branches. *Subvalvular* pulmonic stenosis may be of either the infundibular variety or due to a double-chambered right ventricle caused by anomalous muscle bundles. *Valvular pulmonic stenosis* is the most common form of right ventricular outflow obstruction and is mostly congenital,[73] occurring in approximately eight to ten percent of all congenital cardiac defects.[74-77] It is one of the more common obstructive cardiac malformations that allow survival to adulthood.[78-80] The congenitally stenotic pulmonic valve is usually tricuspid or less frequently bicuspid, with thickening and fusion of the cusps, giving rise to a dome-shaped appearance with a central or eccentric orifice. Rarely, it is dysplastic, with marked thickening and rigidity of cusps devoid of commissural fusion.[81-84] Acquired pulmonic stenosis is rare and includes rheumatic pulmonic stenosis, carcinoid pulmonic stenosis and external compression of the pulmonic valve — for example by an aneurysm of sinus of Valsalva or by tumors.[85] Poststenotic dilatation of the main and left pulmonary arteries is common.[86]

The principal hemodynamic derangement in pulmonic stenosis is systolic overloading of the right ventricle consequent to obstruction to right ventricular outflow. The right ventricular systolic pressure is increased and a pulmonic valvular gradient is thus produced. The right ventricular pressure pulse is characterized by a sharp upstroke to a late peak, followed by a rapid decline. With an intact ventricular septum and in the absence of right ventricular failure, the right ventricular systolic hypertension varies directly with the severity of the stenosis.[79] In severe pulmonic stenosis it may exceed that of the left ventricle, and the pulmonic valvular gradient may reach a level of 200 mmHg or more. To assess the degree of obstruction properly by the pulmonic valvular gradient, however, correlation with the pulmonary blood flow is necessary. A severe obstruction may be associated with a relatively small pulmonic valvular gradient because of low pulmonary blood flow related to right ventricular failure. Conversely, in a high output state, a relatively mild obstruction may present with a large pressure gradient. In the presence of normal cardiac output, the severity of pulmonic stenosis may be graded according to the right ventricular systolic pressure[87] or the ratio of the peak right ventricular pressure to peak systemic arterial pressure.[88] By the former system, pulmonic stenosis is graded mild with a right ventricular systolic pressure of less than 50mm Hg, moderate between 50 and 100 mmHg and severe above 100 mmHg.

In general, clinical manifestation of pulmonic stenosis depends on the degree of obstruction. Patients with mild pulmonic stenosis are asymptomatic and the condition may not progress in severity.[89] The cardiac output remains normal at rest in most patients with significant pulmonic stenosis and fails to increase normally with exercise. With moderate stenosis, patients may experience dyspnea and fatigue on exertion. In severe pulmonic stenosis, even moderate exercise is not tolerated. Strenuous exertion in these patients may at times precipitate syncope and even sudden death, especially in children. An inability to increase the cardiac output in response to augmented metabolic demand with exercise probably accounts for these symptoms.

Right ventricular hypertrophy develops as a compensatory mechanism for the increased right ventricular pressure work. When the capacity for compensatory hypertrophy is exhausted in severe pulmonic stenosis, the Frank-Starling mechanism is activated, with right ventricular dilatation and augmented contraction. When this mechanism is exhausted, pump failure results, exhibiting low cardiac output, elevated right ventricular end-diastolic pressure and mean right atrial pressure, and tricuspid regurgitation. The right atrial hypertension is transmitted backward to produce systemic venous congestion. The patient may then experience cyanosis either from a right-to-left shunt across the foramen ovale which is rendered open (central cyanosis) or from a high peripheral oxygen extraction due to low cardiac output (peripheral cyanosis). The systemic arterial saturation is decreased in central cyanosis and normal in peripheral cyanosis. Small right ventricular cavity size (severe right ventricular hypertrophy) with decreased compliance may also contribute to the central cyanosis.[90]

TRICUSPID STENOSIS

Tricuspid stenosis is a rare condition. It is almost always rheumatic in origin,[91] occurring in about 15 to 30% of all patients with rheumatic valvular disease at necropsy,[92,93] but is clinically recognizable only in about five percent.[94] Less common causes of right ventricular inflow obstruction include tricuspid atresia, carcinoid syndrome, right atrial tumors, systemic lupus erythematosus, endocardial fibroelastosis, vegetations, constrictive pericarditis, and extracardiac tumors. Rheumatic tricuspid stenosis seldom exists as an isolated lesion and is usually associated with mitral valve disease[95,96] and, less frequently, with aortic valve disease.

Structural changes of rheumatic tricuspid stenosis are similar to those of mitral stenosis, with commissural fusion, often accompanied by leaflet and chordal thickening. In severe tricuspid stenosis, there is a marked right atrial dilatation and passive congestion of the liver and spleen.

The normal tricuspid valve area is approximately $7 cm^2$ in adults.[97] Mild tricuspid stenosis with an orifice circumference (normally 11 to 13 cm) of 8 cm or more may not be detected clinically.[98] (Assuming a circular orifice, the area enclosed is approximately more than $5 cm^2$.) A tricuspid valve area of less than $1.5 cm^2$ is considered to represent significant tricuspid stenosis.

Obstruction to right ventricular inflow imposed by tricuspid stenosis causes an increase in right atrial diastolic pressure, producing a tricuspid valvular gradient. The right atrial pressure pulse in sinus rhythm is characterized by a prominent *a* wave which may even attain the level of the right ventricular systolic pressure. When atrial fibrillation develops, the *a* wave disappears and the *v* wave becomes prominent even in the absence of tricuspid regurgitation. The mean right atrial pressure then is greater than when sinus rhythm is present. The tricuspid valve gradient is usually small in tricuspid valve stenosis as compared to the mitral valve gradient in mitral stenosis, rarely exceeding 10 mmHg. A small mean diastolic gradient of 2 mmHg is sufficient to establish a diagnosis of tricuspid stenosis. This may not be easily detected if pullback pressure is recorded from the right ventricle to the right atrium and the nonsimultaneous right ventricular and right atrial pressures are compared. Either two catheters or a double-lumen catheter should be used to record both right ventricular and right atrial pressure pulses simultaneously from the same baseline, employing equisensitive gauges. A tricuspid valve gradient is augmented with an increase in tricuspid valve flow during inspiration (Fig. 3.7) or exercise. A mean tricuspid valve gradient in excess of 5 mmHg is usually associated with sufficient right atrial hypertension to cause systemic venous congestion (i.e., jugular venous congestion, ascites, edema).[99] The cardiac output, which is usually low at rest, does not rise during exercise. Even when mitral stenosis coexists, the left atrial, pulmonary arterial, and right ventricular pressures may remain normal or only mildly elevated.

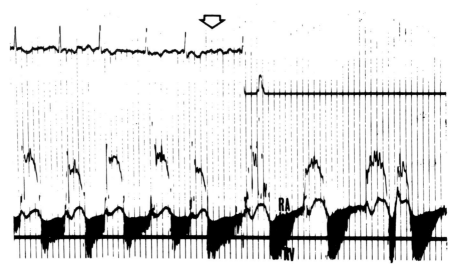

Figure 3.7 Inspiratory increase in tricuspid valvular gradient. *Arrow* indicates the beginning of inspiration. *RA*—right atrium. *RV*—right ventricle. (From: Yang SS et al: *From Cardiac Catheterization Data to Hemodynamic Parameters.* 3rd ed. Philadelphia: FA Davis Co, 1988, p 146. With permission.)

MULTIVALVULAR DISEASE

Involvement of more than one valve is common and is mostly of rheumatic origin. Different combinations of valvular stenosis and regurgitation of varied severities are possible and account for a wide range of clinical manifestations. Some of these regurgitant lesions are termed functional rather than organic because they are secondary to the hemodynamic effect of one or more proximal valve lesions. For example, mitral regurgitation may result from mitral annular dilatation in the later stage of aortic stenosis when the left ventricle dilates. Pulmonary hypertension secondary to aortic or mitral valve disease or both commonly leads to dilatation of the right ventricle with eventual tricuspid annular dilatation and consequent tricuspid regurgitation. Likewise, pulmonic regurgitation may occur when the pulmonic valve ring becomes dilated as a consequence of pulmonary hypertension.

Clinical and hemodynamic presentation of multivalvular lesions is determined by the relative severity of each individual lesion.[100] However, when two valvular lesions are almost equal in severity, the proximal lesion usually masks the distal lesion. Thus in combined aortic and mitral stenosis, for example, mitral stenosis protects the left ventricle from the pressure overload imposed by aortic stenosis, and the clinical manifestation is dominated by mitral stenosis.

In multivalvular lesions the selection of therapy, be it surgical or medical, must be made with utmost care, based on a full knowledge of each lesion. Failure to recognize all the involved valves may lead to a partial correction, leaving one or more significant lesions uncorrected—a hazardous, possibly life-threatening outcome. To establish a precise diagnosis in these patients, an extensive evaluation must be undertaken including noninvasive studies (especially two-dimensional and Doppler echocardiography) and right and left heart catheterization and angiocardiography.

Mitral Stenosis and Aortic Regurgitation

About two thirds of the patients with severe mitral stenosis have an early blowing diastolic murmur along the left sternal border, the vast majority of which represent mild aortic regurgitation.[101] In these patients the clinical manifestation is that of mitral stenosis. In only approximately 10% of patients with mitral stenosis, severe aortic regurgitation coexists,[102] recognizable usually by the wide pulse pressure, and by left ventricular dilatation and hyperkinesis. Severe aortic regurgitation is seldom combined with severe mitral stenosis, but when it occurs, aortic regurgitation can be unrecognized for lack of the typical aortic regurgitant murmur[103] and wide pulse pressure.[104] A dominant aortic regurgitation may obscure mitral stenosis. An opening snap and an accentuated S_1 provide clues to the diagnosis of mitral stenosis. On the other hand, an Austin-Flint murmur can be mistaken as the middiastolic murmur of mitral stenosis. Amyl nitrite will diminish the Austin-Flint murmur while it augments the mitral stenotic murmur. Two-dimensional and Doppler echocardiography are invaluable in identifying both lesions, and Doppler color flow imaging serves to semiquantitate aortic regurgitation. Ultimately, cardiac catheterization will disclose the mitral valve gradient, and contrast injection at the aortic root will demonstrate aortic regurgitation.

Aortic Stenosis and Mitral Regurgitation

The combination of aortic stenosis and mitral regurgitation is rather uncommon but hemodynamically devastating. Whereas mitral regurgitation is augmented by the increased left ventricular systolic pressure resulting from obstruction to left ventricular outflow, mitral regurgitation diminishes the left ventricular end-systolic volume, reducing the preload below the level necessary for adequate left ventricular performance. The result is a low forward output as well as severe left atrial and pulmonary venous hypertension.

The carotid pulse may not be typical of either lesion since the typical tardy upstroke of aortic stenosis is neutralized by the sharp upstroke of mitral regurgitation. The two systolic murmurs may be difficult to distinguish. Amyl nitrite tends to augment aortic stenotic murmur while diminishing the mitral regurgitation murmur. Two-dimensional echocardiography will demonstrate an enlarged left ventricle and left atrium while continuous Doppler echocardiography will yield an increased aortic valve flow velocity from which the aortic valve gradient can be derived. Doppler color flow imaging shows mitral regurgitation, which can be semiquantitated. Owing to decreased forward flow, the aortic valve gradient obtained by either Doppler or cardiac catheterization may be rather low, but the calculated aortic valve area should provide adequate estimate of the severity of aortic stenosis.

Mitral Stenosis and Aortic Stenosis

This combination is very common and is usually associated with some degree of regurgitation of either or both valves. In the series of 150 patients with combined aortic and mitral valvular disease reported by Zitnik et al[105], there were only 10 patients with pure aortic and mitral stenosis. The combination of severe aortic stenosis and mitral stenosis favors the clinical manifestation of mitral stenosis, those of aortic stenosis being masked.[105] The coexistence of severe mitral stenosis adds two mechanisms to reduce the cardiac output further in patients with severe aortic stenosis. First, the cardiac output may be low because of severe mitral stenosis. Second, the atrial *booster pump*, so important in left ventricular filling in aortic stenosis, is prevented from contributing by obstruction at the mitral valve level. A reduction in cardiac output leads to a lower left ventricular systolic pressure and a decreased aortic valve gradient, a lower incidence of angina, and delayed development of aortic calcification and left ventricular hypertrophy.[106] Clinical manifestations are dominated by those of mitral stenosis, namely, symptoms of pulmonary venous hypertension (dyspnea, orthopnea, hemoptysis, pulmonary edema), pulmonary arterial hypertension, atrial fibrillation, and systemic embolism. A typical S_4, sustained apical impulse, and slow carotid upstroke are absent, and ejection murmur may be of diminished intensity, whereas the middiastolic murmur of mitral stenosis as well as opening snap can be heard. Two-dimensional echocardiography yields evidences of aortic and mitral stenosis, and Doppler echocardiography provides flow velocity data from which pressure gradients across the respective valves can be derived. As with cardiac catheterization, the obtained aortic valve gradient is relatively low. However, the severity of aortic stenosis can be adequately estimated by the calculated aortic valve area.

Tricuspid Stenosis and Mitral Stenosis

Tricuspid stenosis is almost always of rheumatic origin and occurs in combination with other valvular lesions, mostly with mitral stenosis and less frequently with mitral regurgitation or aortic valvular disease. Mild tricuspid stenosis cannot be easily detected, especially when it coexists with one or more other valvular lesions. When both tricuspid stenosis and mitral stenosis are severe, mitral stenosis can be masked by tricuspid stenosis. The clinical presentations usually lack those of pulmonary venous hypertension, and are characterized by those of low cardiac output (fatigability and exercise intolerance) and peripheral venous hypertension (jugular venous distention, hepatosplenomegaly, ascites, edema). The mitral valve gradient may be rather low even if mitral stenosis is severe. Both flow data and pressure gradient are needed to calculate the mitral valve area by means of Gorlin's formula so that the severity of mitral stenosis can be adequately assessed. Two-dimensional echocardiography can be extremely helpful in establishing the diagnosis, and Doppler echocardiography can accurately estimate the transvalvular gradients across the respective valves. These data can be confirmed at cardiac catheterization.

Tricuspid Regurgitation in Combined Valvular Disease

Tricuspid regurgitation may be either organic, the result of intrinsic tricuspid valvular disease, or functional, secondary to pulmonary hypertension. Severe organic tricuspid regurgitation is mostly rheumatic in origin and is almost always associated with mitral or aortic valvular lesions. In these patients, clinical manifestations attributable to aortic and mitral valvular lesions can be masked by those of tricuspid regurgitation and the patients are less likely to experience symptoms of pulmonary venous hypertension.

ASSESSMENT OF VALVULAR STENOSIS

Proper management of patients with valvular stenosis requires that accurate assessment of valvular lesions be made, providing comprehensive information including

1. Diagnosis and etiology
2. Severity of the obstruction
3. Valve morphology (thickening/calcification and pliability of the involved cusps; annular calcification; commissural fusion; chordal involvement)
4. Coexistence and severity of regurgitation
5. Left and right ventricular size, hypertrophy, and wall motion
6. Complications such as endocarditis; thrombosis; functional tricuspid, mitral, or pulmonic regurgitation; pulmonary hypertension.
7. The presence of coronary artery disease.

Information thus obtained, combined with clinical symptoms and signs, is invaluable in deciding whether to follow up medically or to intervene surgically or nonsurgically using percutaneous balloon valvuloplasty in a given patient.

We have at our disposal several diagnostic techniques designed to acquire relevant morphologic and functional data: radiography, electrocardiography, echocardiography, ultrafast computed tomography, magnetic resonance imaging, and cardiac catheterization. Of these, cardiac catheterization is generally considered to be the *gold standard* against which all other techniques must be judged. Because of its invasive nature, however, it is not suitable for routine followup. Its role in evaluation prior to surgery or balloon valvuloplasty is being challenged, at least in some selected cases and possibly with increasing frequency, by echocardiography.

Estimation of the severity of valvular stenosis by cardiac catheterization is based on the measured transvalvular gradient (see previous subsections on each valve) and the calculated valve area (except in the case of pulmonic stenosis). The generally used pressure gradient criteria for the severity of valvular stenosis are applicable for patients with a normal cardiac output. Because of the flow dependency of the gradient, they are not valid in low output states. For example, a peak aortic valve gradient in excess of 50 mmHg is generally considered to indicate critical aortic stenosis,[38] but a small aortic valve gradient — in the range of 20 to 40 mmHg — does not necessarily rule out the possibility of severe aortic stenosis if the cardiac output is significantly reduced. The calculated aortic valve area using Gorlin's formula,[7] though it tends to underestimate the valve area in low output states,[107-109] can still help distinguish mild from severe obstruction. Exercise or administration of an inotropic agent temporarily increases the cardiac output and may improve the accuracy of area estimation by this method. Contrast ventriculography will demonstrate chamber dimensions and systolic ventricular contraction and allows for estimation of the ejection fraction as well as assessment of atrioventricular regurgitation (ie, mitral or tricuspid regurgitation), if present.

Echocardiography has witnessed a remarkable technological development, supplementing the standard imaging modality (M-mode and two-dimensional echocardiography) with Doppler echocardiography (continuous-wave and pulsed-wave), color-flow imaging, transesophageal echocardiography, and intravascular echocardiography. It is unchallenged in its ability to image the valves, especially the aortic, mitral, and tricuspid valves. It detects and assesses thickening/calcification and pliability of the leaflets and allows for measurement of orifice area, especially in the case of mitral stenosis. Chordal fusion can be detected and its severity evaluated. These findings, together with the degree of valve calcification and leaflet mobility, help screen those who are poor candidates for balloon mitral valvuloplasty.[110,111] Surgically, valve replacement is preferable to commissurotomy for these patients. Also important to surgeons is the sizing of the valve annulus, for use in estimating the size of the valve prosthesis to be implanted.

The valvular gradient can be obtained practically from any valve, using the valve flow velocity spectrum recorded with continuous-wave Doppler and applying the modified Bernoulli equation which relates flow velocity (in m/s) to pressure gradient (mmHg)[112]:

$$\text{pressure gradient} = 4 \times (\text{velocity})^2$$

This equation usually yields accurate results if the ultrasound beam aligns closely with the blood flow jet (ie, within 20°).

Orifice area for the aortic and mitral valves can be estimated by means of the valve flow velocity spectrum. For the mitral valve, the pressure half-time (time required for the pressure gradient to fall from peak to half its value) obtained from the velocity spectrum is used in the equation[113]:

$$\text{Area (cm}^2) = 220/\text{half-time(ms)}$$

The correlation between mitral valve area determined by the Doppler half-time method and that determined by cardiac catheterization[114-118] ranged from fair ($r = 0.51$) to excellent ($r = 0.95$) and the twice the standard error of regression equation estimate ranged between 0.30 to 0.80 cm^2. The correlation was poor immediately following balloon mitral valvuloplasty,[119,120] and this was attributed to altered left atrial pressure and compliance.[121] Other possible contributing factors include measurement errors in dealing with a small pressure gradient, underestimation of forward output related to the use of the Fick method of cardiac output determination, and iatrogenically induced left-to-right shunting at the atrial level.[117] The mitral valve calculation using the Gorlin formula immediately following balloon mitral valvuloplasty correlated best with Doppler pressure half-time when calculated with the atrial septostomy occluded.[122] The half-time method tends to overestimate mitral valve area if there is an increased left ventricular end-diastolic pressure due to aortic regurgitation and to conditions associated with impaired left ventricular compliance. The presence of mitral regurgitation does not invalidate this method.[113]

The use of a Doppler-derived aortic valve gradient in estimating the severity of aortic stenosis needs some consideration. Optimal positioning of the transducer and angling of the ultrasound beam is not always possible and may lead to underestimation of the pressure gradient. Not uncommonly, a relatively low pressure gradient is obtained even in the presence of severe aortic stenosis, because the cardiac output is low. Reliance on pressure gradient alone can therefore lead to misjudgment of the severity of aortic stenosis unless the mean aortic valve gradient is at least 50 mmHg. The use of the peak gradient is to be discouraged because it consistently overestimates the catheterization-derived mean and peak-to-peak gradients. The aortic valve area can be reliably estimated by the continuity equation method.[123-125] This involves measuring the left ventricular outflow tract diameter (D, in cm), recording the flow velocity spectrum from both the left ventricular outflow tract and the aortic valve, and calculating the aortic valve area as follows:

$$AVA = \pi\left(\frac{D}{2}\right)^2 \frac{V_{of}}{V_v}$$

where V_{of} and V_v are mean velocities from the left ventricular outflow tract by pulsed Doppler and aortic valve by continuous-wave Doppler, respectively. There is good ($r = 0.71$) to excellent ($r = 0.94$) correlation between Doppler estimates of aortic valve area and those determined by cardiac catheterization, but the twice the standard error of regression equation estimate ranged from 0.20 to 0.80 cm^2, suggesting a potential for significant error in some patients.[123-128] The method is valid even when there is an associated severe aortic regurgitation.[129]

Transesophageal echocardiography is strongly recommended prior to balloon mitral valvuloplasty to rule out a left atrial clot.[130,131] It can be used during balloon mitral valvuloplasty to guide and monitor the course of the catheter as a safeguard.[132-134]

Comparison of cardiac catheterization and Doppler echocardiography in the evaluation of severity of aortic and mitral stenoses has generally indicated good correlations between these techniques.[125,127,134-137] However, discrepancies exist in individual cases and opinions differ as to what extent Doppler echocardiography can substitute for cardiac catheterization in management decision making.[126,138-143] A prospective study of 189 consecutive patients was recently published. There were 110 patients with pure aortic stenosis or mixed aortic stenosis and aortic regurgitation, and 39 with pure mitral stenosis or mixed mitral stenosis and mitral regurgitation. Doppler echocardiography and cardiac catheterization were in agreement in 90% and 83%, respectively, of patients with mitral stenosis and aortic stenosis.[143]

REFERENCES

1. Silverman ME, Hurst JW: The mitral complex. Interaction of the anatomy, physiology, and pathology of the mitral annulus, mitral valve leaflets, chordae tendineae, and papillary muscles. *Am Heart J.* 76:399–418, 1968.

2. Perloff JK, Roberts WC: The mitral apparatus: functional anatomy of mitral regurgitation. *Circulation.* 46:227–239, 1972.

3. Bonnabeau RC Jr, Stevenson JE, Edwards JE: Obliteration of the principal orifice of the stenotic mitral valve: a rare form of "restenosis." *J Thorac Cardiovasc Surg.* 49:264–268, 1965.

4. Hammer WJ, Roberts WC, DeLeon AC Jr: "Mitral stenosis" secondary to combined "massive" mitral anular calcific deposits and small, hypertrophied left ventricles. Hemodynamic documentation in four patients. *Am J Med.* 64:371–376, 1978.

5. Hakki A-H, Iskandrian AS: Obstruction to left ventricular inflow secondary to combined mitral annular calcification and idiopathic hypertrophic subaortic stenosis. *Cathet Cardiovasc Diagn.* 6:191–196, 1980.

6. Osterberger LE, Goldstein S, Khaja F, et al: Functional mitral stenosis in patients with massive mitral annular calcification. *Circulation.* 64:472–476, 1981.

7. Gorlin R, Gorlin SG: Hydraulic formula for calculation of the area of the stenotic mitral valve, other cardiac valves, and central circulatory shunts. Part I. *Am Heart J.* 41:1–29, 1951.

8. Mitchell JH, Shapiro W: Atrial function and the hemodynamic consequences of atrial fibrillation in man. *Am J Cardiol.* 23:556–567, 1969.

9. Bader RA, Bader ME, Rose DJ, et al: Hemodynamics at rest and during exercise in normal pregnancy as studied by cardiac catheterization. *J Clin Invest.* 34:1524–1536, 1955.

10. Braunwald E, Turi ZG: Pathophysiology of mitral valve disease. In: Ionescu MI, Cohn LH, eds. *Mitral Valve Disease: Diagnosis and Treatment*, London:Butterworths, 1985, pp 4–5.

11. Nakhjavan FK, Katz MR, Maranhao V, et al: Analysis of influence of catecholamine and tachycardia during supine exercise in patients with mitral stenosis and sinus rhythm. *Br Heart J.* 31:753–761, 1969.

12. Donald KW: Pulmonary vascular resistance in mitral valvular disease. In: Adams WR, Veith I, eds. *Pulmonary Circulation.* New York:Grune & Stratton, 1959, p 286.

13. Aryanpur I, Paydar M, Shakibi JG, et al: Regression of pulmonary hypertension after mitral valve surgery in children. Operative management of rheumatic mitral valve disease. *Chest.* 71:354–360, 1977.

14. Dexter L, McDonald L, Rabinowitz M, et al: Medical aspects of patients undergoing surgery for mitral stenosis. *Circulation.* 9:758–770, 1954.

15. Dalen JE: Mitral stenosis. In: Dalen JE, Alpert JS, eds. *Valvular Heart Disease.* 2nd ed. Boston:Little Brown, 1987, p 57.

16. Wood P: An appreciation of mitral stenosis, Part I: clinical features. *Br Med J.* 1:1051–1063, 1954.

17. Jordan SC, Hicken P, Watson DA, et al: Pathology of the lungs in mitral stenosis in relation to respiratory function and pulmonary hemodynamics. *Br Heart J.* 28:101–107, 1966.

18. Heath D, Edwards JE: The pathology of hypertensive pulmonary vascular disease. A description of six grades of structural changes in the pulmonary arteries with special reference to congenital cardiac septal defects. *Circulation.* 18:533–547, 1958.

19. Braunwald E, Ross J Jr: Applicability of Starling's law of the heart to man. In: Evans JR, guest ed. Symposium: Structure and function of heart muscle. *Circ Res.* 15(suppl II):II-169–II-178, 1964.

20. Gash AK, Carabello BA, Cepin D, et al: Left ventricular ejection performance and systolic muscle function in patients with mitral stenosis. *Circulation.* 67:148–154, 1983.

21. Silverstein DM, Hansen DP, Ojiambo HP, et al: Left ventricular function in severe pure mitral stenosis as seen at the Kenyatta Hospital. *Am Heart J.* 99:727–733, 1980.

22. Dodge HT, Kennedy JW, Petersen JL: Quantitative angiographic methods in the evaluation of valvular heart disease. *Prog Cardiovasc Dis.* 16:1–23, 1973.

23. Heller SJ, Carleton RA: Abnormal left ventricular contraction in patients with mitral stenosis. *Circulation.* 42:1099–1110, 1970.

24. Thompson ME, Shaver JA, Leon DF: Effect of tachycardia on atrial transport in mitral stenosis. *Am Heart J.* 94:297–306, 1977.

25. Deverall PB, Olley PM, Smith DR, et al: Incidence of systemic embolism before and after mitral valvotomy. *Thorax.* 23:530–536, 1968.

26. Henry WL, Morganroth J, Pearlman AS, et al: Relation between echocardiographically determined left atrial size and atrial fibrillation. *Circulation.* 53:273–279, 1976.

27. Keren G, Etzion T, Sherez J, et al: Atrial fibrillation and atrial enlargement in patients with mitral stenosis. *Am Heart J.* 114:1146–1155, 1987.

28. Roberts WC: Valvular, subvalvular, and supravalvular aortic stenosis: Morphologic features. *Cardiovasc Clin.* 5(1):97–126, 1973.

29. Fuster V, Brandenburg RO, Giuliani ER, et al: Clinical approach and management of acquired valvular heart disease. *Cardiovasc Clin.* 10(3):125–159, 1980.

30. Narang NK, Andrew AMR, Chaudhury HR, et al: Aortic stenosis due to familial hypercholesterolemic xanthomatosis. A case report with brief review of literature. *Indian Heart J.* 30:189–192, 1978.

31. Deutscher S, Rockette HE, Krishnaswami V: Diabetes and hypercholesterolemia among patients with calcific aortic stenosis. *J. Chronic Dis.* 37:407–415, 1984.

32. Lerman BB, Thomas LC, Abrams GD, et al: Aortic stenosis associated with systemic lupus erythematosus. *Am J Med.* 72;707–710, 1982.

33. Sarnoff SJ, Braunwald E, Welch GH, et al: Hemodynamic determinants of oxygen consumption of the heart with special reference to the tension-time-index *Am J Physiol.* 192:148–156, 1958.

34. Oldershaw PJ, Dawkins KD, Ward DE, et al: Diastolic mechanisms of impaired exercise tolerance in aortic valve disease. *Br Heart J.* 49:568–573, 1983.

35. Hess OM, Ritter M, Schneider J, et al: Diastolic stiffness and myocardial structure in aortic valve disease before and after valve replacement. *Circulation.* 69:855–865, 1984.

36. Murakami T, Hess OM, Gage JE, et al: Diastolic filling dynamics in patients with aortic stenosis. *Circulation.* 73:1162–1174, 1986.

37. McMillan IKR: Aortic stenosis. A postmortem cinephotographic study of valve action. *Br Heart J.* 17:56–62, 1955.

38. Morrow AG, Roberts WC, Ross J Jr, et al: Obstruction to left ventricular outflow. Current concepts of management and operative treatment. *Ann Intern Med.* 69:1255–1286, 1968.

39. Hess OM, Schneider J, Turina M, et al: Asymmetric septal hypertrophy in patients with aortic stenosis: an adaptive mechanism or a coexistence of hypertrophic cardiomyopathy? *J Am Coll Cardiol.* 1:783–789, 1983.

40. Scott DK, Marpole DGF, Bristow JD, et al: The role of left atrial transport in aortic and mitral stenosis. *Circulation.* 41:1031–1041, 1970.

41. Braunwald E, Frahm CJ: Studies on Starling's law of the heart, IV: observations on the hemodynamic functions of the left atrium in man. *Circulation.* 24:633–642, 1961.

42. Grossman W, Baim DS: *Cardiac Catheterization, Angiography, and Intervention.* 4th ed. Philadelphia:Lea & Febiger, 1991, p 569.

43. Flamm MD, Braniff BA, Kimball R, et al: Mechanism of effort syncope in aortic stenosis. *Circulation.* 36(suppl II):II-109, 1967.

44. Johnson AM: Aortic stenosis, sudden death, and the left ventricular baroreceptors. *Br Heart J.* 33:1–5, 1971.

45. Mark AL: The Bezold-Jarisch reflex revisited: clinical implications of inhibitory reflexes originating in the heart. *J Am Coll Cardiol.* 1:90–102, 1983.

46. Russek HI, Zohman BL: The syndrome of Bernheim as a clinical entity. *Circulation.* 1:759–765, 1950.

47. White PD: *Heart Disease.* 4th ed. New York: Macmillan, 1951, p 649.

48. Spann JF Jr, Buccino RA, Sonnenblick EH, et al: Contractile state of cardiac muscle obtained from cats with experimentally produced ventricular hypertrophy and heart failure. *Circ Res.* 21:341–354, 1967.

49. Spann JF Jr, Covell JW, Eckberg DL, et al: Contractile performance of the hypertrophied and chronically failing cat ventricle. *Am J Physiol.* 223:1150–1157, 1792.

50. Cooper G IV, Satava RM Jr, Harrison CE, et al: Mechanism for the abnormal energetics of pressure-induced hypertrophy of cat myocardium. *Circ Res.* 33:213–223, 1973.

51. Coulson RL, Yazdanfar S, Rubio E, et al: Recuperative potential of cardiac muscle following relief of pressure overload hypertrophy and right ventricular failure in the cat. *Circ Res.* 40:41–49, 1977.

52. Newman WH, Webb JG: Adaptation of left ventricle to chronic pressure overload: response to inotropic drugs. *Am J Physiol.* 238:H134–H143, 1980.

53. Williams JF Jr, Potter RD: Normal contractile state of hypertrophied myocardium after pulmonary artery constriction in cat. *J Clin Invest.* 54:1266–1272, 1974.

54. Sasayama S, Ross J Jr, Franklin D, et al: Adaptations of the left ventricle to chronic pressure overload. *Circ Res.* 38:172–178, 1976.

55. Gunther S, Grossman W: Determinants of ventricular function in pressure overload hypertrophy in man. *Circulation.* 59:679–688, 1979.

56. Ross J Jr: Afterload mismatch and preload reserve: a conceptual framework for the analysis of ventricular function. *Prog Cardiovasc Dis.* 18:255–264, 1976.

57. Fifer MA, Gunther S, Grossman W, et al: Myocardial contractile function in aortic stenosis as determined from the rate of stress development during isovolumic phase. *Am J Cardiol.* 44:1318–1325, 1979.

58. Douglas PS, Reichek N, Hackney K, et al: Contribution of afterload, hypertrophy and geometry to left ventricular ejection fraction in aortic valve stenosis, pure aortic regurgitation and idiopathic dilated cardiomyopathy. *Am J Cardiol.* 59:1398–1404, 1987.

59. DePace NL, Ren J-F, Iskandrian AS, et al: Correlation of echocardiographic wall stress and left ventricular pressure and function in aortic stenosis. *Circulation.* 67:854–859, 1981.

60. Spann JF, Bove AA, Natarajan G, et al: Ventricular performance, pump function and compensatory mechanisms in patients with aortic stenosis. *Circulation.* 62:576–582, 1980.

61. Huber D, Grimm J, Koch R, et al: Determinants of ejection performance in aortic stenosis. *Circulation.* 64:126–134, 1981.

62. Wisenbaugh T, Booth D, DeMaria A, et al: Relationship of contractile state to ejection performance in patients with chronic aortic valve disease. *Circulation.* 73:47–53, 1986.

63. Dineen E, Brent BN: Aortic valve stenosis: comparison of patients with to those without chronic congestive heart failure. *Am J Cardiol.* 57:419–422, 1986.

64. Nishimura RA, Housmans PR, Hitle LK, et al: Assessment of diastolic function of the heart: background and current applications of Doppler echocardiography, I: physiologic and pathophysiologic features, II: clinical studies. *Mayo Clin Proc.* 64:71–81, 181–204, 1989.

65. Diver DJ, Royal HD, Aroesty JM, et al: Diastolic function in patients with aortic stenosis: influence of left ventricular load reduction. *J Am Coll Cardiol.* 12:642–648, 1988.

66. Schlant RC, Nutter DO: Heart failure in valvular heart disease. *Medicine.* 50:421–451, 1971.

67. Kennedy JW, Twiss RD, Blackmon JR, et al: Quantitative angiocardiography, III: relationships of left ventricular pressure, volume, and mass in aortic valve disease. *Circulation.* 38:838–845, 1968.

68. Buckberg G, Eber L, Herman M, et al: Ischemia in aortic stenosis: hemodynamic prediction. *Am J Cardiol.* 35:778–784, 1975.

69. Johnson LL, Sciacca RR, Ellis K, et al: Reduced left ventricular myocardial blood flow per unit mass in aortic stenosis. *Circulation.* 57:582–590, 1978.

70. Lombard JT, Selzer A: Valvular aortic stenosis: a clinical and hemodynamic profile of patients. *Ann Intern Med.* 106:292–298, 1987.

71. Bertrand ME, Lablanche JM, Tilmant PY, et al: Coronary sinus blood flow at rest and during isometric exercise in patients with aortic valve disease. Mechanism of angina pectoris in presence of normal coronary arteries. *Am J Cardiol.* 47:199–205, 1981.

72. Marcus ML, Doty DB, Hiratzka LF, et al: Decreased coronary reserve. A mechanism for angina pectoris in patients with aortic stenosis and normal coronary arteries. *N Engl J Med.* 307:1362–1366, 1982.

73. Kirshenbaum HD: Pulmonary valve disease. In: Dalen JE, Alpert JS, eds. *Valvular Heart Disease.* 2nd ed. Boston:Little Brown, 1987, p 403.

74. Watson H: *Paediatric Cardiology.* St. Louis:CV Mosby, 1968, pp 510–511.

75. Gasul BM, Arcilla RA, Lev M: *Heart Disease in Children.* Philadelphia:JB Lippincott, 1966, p 764.

76. Keith JD, Rowe RD, Vlad P: *Heart Disease in Infancy and Childhood.* 3rd ed. New York:Macmillan, 1978, p 761.

77. Abrahams DG, Wood P: Pulmonary stenosis with normal aortic root. *Br Heart J.* 13:519–548, 1951.

78. Hoffman JIE, Christianson R: Congenital heart disease in a cohort of 19,502 births with long-term follow-up. *Am J Cardiol.* 42:641–647, 1978.

79. Feldman T, Borow KM: Adults with pulmonic stenosis: management. *J Cardiovasc Med.* 9:711–719, 1984.

80. Kaplan S, Adolph RJ, Murphy DJ: Pulmonic valve stenosis. In: Roberts WC, ed. *Adult Congenital Heart Disease.* Philadelphia:FA Davis Co, 1987, pp 477–491.

81. Koretzky ED, Moller JH, Korns ME, et al: Congenital pulmonary stenosis resulting from dysplasia of valve. *Circulation.* 40:43–53, 1969.

82. Linde LM, Turner SW, Sparkes RS: Pulmonary valvular dysplasia. A cardiofacial syndrome. *Br Heart J.* 35:301–304, 1973.

83. Patterson DF, Haskins ME, Schnarr WR: Hereditary dysplasia of the pulmonary valve in beagle dogs. Pathologic and genetic studies. *Am J Cardiol.* 47:631–641, 1981.

84. Schneeweiss A, Blieden LC, Shem-Tov A, et al: Diagnostic angiocardiographic criteria in dysplastic stenotic pulmonic valve. *Am Heart J.* 106:761–762, 1983.

85. Seymour J, Emanuel R, Pattinson N: Acquired pulmonary stenosis. *Br Heart J.* 30:776–785, 1968.

86. Perloff JK: Congenital pulmonic stenosis. In: *The Clinical Recognition of Congenital Heart Disease.* 3rd ed. Philadelphia:WB Saunders Co, 1987, p 188.

87. Wood P: *Diseases of the Heart and Circulation.* 3rd ed. Philadelphia: JB Lippincott, 1968, p 501.

88. Gasul BM, Arcilla RA, Lev M: *Heart Disease in Children. Diagnosis and Treatment.* Philadelphia: JB Lippincott, 1966, p 765–766.

89. Levine OR, Blumenthal S: Pulmonic stenosis. *Circulation.* 32(suppl III):III-33–III-41, 1965.

90. Williams JCP, Barratt-Boyes BG, Lowe JB: Underdeveloped right ventricle and pulmonary stenosis. *Am J Cardiol.* 11:458–468, 1963.

91. Edwards JE: The spectrum and clinical significance of tricuspid regurgitation. *Practical Cardiol* 6(2):86–95, 1980.

92. Chopra P, Tandon HD: Pathology of chronic rheumatic heart disease with particular reference to tricuspid valve involvement. *Acta Cardiol.* 32:423–434, 1977.

93. Edwards WD, Peterson K, Edwards JE: Active valvulitis associated with chronic rheumatic valvular disease and active myocarditis. *Circulation.* 57:181–185, 1978.

94. Kitchin A, Turner R: Diagnosis and treatment of tricuspid stenosis. *Br Heart J.* 26:354–379, 1964.

95. Wooley CF, Fontana ME, Kilman JW, et al: Tricuspid stenosis. Atrial systolic murmur, tricuspid opening snap, and right atrial pressure pulse. *Am J Med.* 78:375–384, 1985.

96. Ockene IS: Tricuspid valve disease. In: Dalen JE, Alpert JS, eds. *Valvular Heart Disease.* 2nd ed. Boston:Little Brown, 1987, p 389.

97. Rackley CE, Wallace RB, Edwards JE, et al: Tricuspid valve disease. In: Hurst JW. *The Heart.* 7th ed. New York:McGraw-Hill, 1990, p 856.

98. White PD: *Heart Disease.* 4th ed. New York:Macmillan, 1951, pp 694–695.

99. Braunwald E: Valvular heart disease. In: *Heart Disease. A Textbook of Cardiovascular Medicine.* 3rd ed. Philadelphia:WB Saunders Co, 1988, p 1069.

100. Paraskos JA: Combined valvular disease. In: Dalen JE, Alpert JS, eds. *Valvular Heart Disease.* 2nd ed. Boston:Little Brown, 1987, p 439.

101. Brest AN, Udhoji V, Likoff W: A re-evaluation of the Graham-Steell murmur. *N Engl J Med.* 263:1229–1231, 1960.

102. Segal J, Harvey WP, Hufnagel CA: Clinical study of one hundred cases of severe aortic insufficiency. *Am J Med.* 21:200–210, 1956.

103. Segal BL, Likoff W, Kaspar AJ: "Silent" rheumatic aortic regurgitation. *Am J Cardiol.* 14:628–632, 1964.

104. Cohn LH, Mason DT, Ross J Jr, et al: Preoperative assessment of aortic regurgitation in patients with mitral valve disease. *Am J Cardiol.* 19:177–182, 1967.

105. Zitnik RS, Piemme TE, Messer RJ, et al: The masking of aortic stenosis by mitral stenosis. *Am Heart J.* 69:22–30, 1965.

106. Schattenberg TT, Titus JL, Parkin TW: Clinical findings in acquired aortic valve stenosis. Effect of disease of other valves. *Am Heart J.* 73:322–325, 1967.

107. Ubago JL, Figueroa A, Colman T, et al: Hemodynamic factors that affect calculated orifice areas in the mitral Hancock xenograft valve. *Circulation.* 61:388–394, 1980.

108. Gaspar J, Cohn LH, Collins JJ, et al: Overestimation of aortic stenosis with Gorlin equation in low flow states (abstr.). *J Am Coll Cardiol.* 1:639, 1983.

109. Cannon SR, Richard KL, Crawford M: Hydraulic estimation of stenotic orifice area: a correction of the Gorlin formula. *Circulation.* 71:1170–1178, 1985.

110. Reid CL, Chandraratna PAN, Kawanishi DT, et al: Influence of mitral valve morphology on double-balloon catheter balloon valvuloplasty in patients with mitral stenosis: analysis of factors predicting immediate and 3-month results. *Circulation.* 80:515–524, 1989.

111. Abascal VM, Wilkins GT, Choong CY, et al: Mitral regurgitation after percutaneous balloon mitral valvuloplasty in adults: evaluation by pulsed Doppler echocardiography. *J Am Coll Cardiol.* 11:257–263, 1988.

112. Holen J, Aaslid R, Landmark K, et al: Determination of pressure gradient in mitral stenosis with a non-invasive ultrasound Doppler technique. *Acta Med Scand.* 199:455–460, 1976.

113. Hatle L, Angelson B, Tromsdal A: Noninvasive assessment of atrioventricular pressure half-time by Doppler ultrasound. *Circulation.* 60:1096–1104, 1979.

114. Stamm RB, Martin RP: Quantification of pressure gradients across stenotic valves by Doppler ultrasound. *J Am Coll Cardiol.* 2:707–718, 1983.

115. Smith MD, Handshoe R, Handshoe S, et al: Comparative accuracy of two-dimensional echocardiography and Doppler pressure half-time methods in assessing severity of mitral stenosis in patients with and without prior commissurotomy. *Circulation.* 73:100–107, 1986.

116. Nakatani S, Masuyama T, Kodama K, et al: Value and limitations of Doppler echocardiography in the quantification of stenotic mitral valve area: comparison of the pressure half-time and the continuity equation methods. *Circulation.* 77:78–85, 1988.

117. Come PC, Riley MF, Diver DJ, et al: Noninvasive assessment of mitral stenosis before and after percutaneous balloon mitral valvuloplasty. *Am J Cardiol.* 61:817–825, 1988.

118. Gonzalez MA, Child JS, Krivokapich J: Comparison of two-dimensional and Doppler echocardiography and intracardiac hemodynamics for quantification of mitral stenosis. *Am J Cardiol.* 60:327–332, 1987.

119. Wilkins G, Thomas J, Abascal V, et al: Failure of the Doppler pressure halftime to accurately demonstrate change in mitral valve area following percutaneous miral valvotomy (abstr.). *J Am Coll Cardiol.* 9:218A, 1987.

120. Reid C, McKay C, Chandraratna P, et al: Mechanism of increase in mitral valve area by double-balloon catheter balloon valvuloplasty in adults with mitral stenosis: echocardiographic–Doppler correlation (abstr.). *J Am Coll Cardiol.* 9:217A, 1987.

121. Thomas JD, Wilkins GT, Abascal V, et al: The transmitral pressure half-time is significantly affected by left atrial pressure and compliance: observations in 21 patients undergoing percutaneous balloon mitral valvotomy (abstr.). *J Am Coll Cardiol.* 9:218A, 1987.

122. Manga P, Brandis S, Singh S: Effect of occlusion of atrial septostomy on calculations of mitral valve area post balloon mitral valvuloplasty (abstr.). *J Am Coll Cardiol.* 17:339A, 1991.

123. Skjaerpe T, Hegrenaes L, Hatle L: Noninvasive estimation of valve area in patients with aortic stenosis by Doppler ultrasound and two-dimensional echocardiography. *Circulation.* 72:810–818, 1985.

124. Zoghbi WA, Farmer KL, Soto JG, et al: Accurate noninvasive quantification of stenotic aortic valve area by Doppler echocardiography. *Circulation.* 73:452–459, 1986.

125. Oh JK, Taliercio CP, Holmes DR Jr, et al: Prediction of the severity of aortic stenosis by Doppler aortic valve area determination: prospective Doppler–catheterization correlation in 100 patients. *J Am Coll Cardiol.* 11:1227–1234, 1988.

126. Otto CM, Pearlman AS, Comess KA, et al: Determination of the stenotic aortic valve area in adults using Doppler echocardiography. *J Am Coll Cardiol.* 7:509–517, 1986.

127. Teirstein P, Yeager M, Yock PG, et al: Doppler echocardiographic measurement of aortic valve area in aortic stenosis: a noninvasive application of the Gorlin formula. *J Am Coll Cardiol.* 8:1059–1065, 1986.

128. Nishimura RA, Holmes DR Jr, Reeder GS, et al: Doppler evaluation of results of percutaneous aortic balloon valvuloplasty in calcific aortic stenosis. *Circulation.* 78:791–799, 1988.

129. Grayburn PA, Smith MD, Harrison MR, et al: Pivotal role of aortic valve area calculation by the continuity equation for Doppler assessment of aortic stenosis in patients with combined aortic stenosis and regurgitation. *Am J Cardiol.* 61:376–381, 1988.

130. Griffen DL, Sheikh KH, Harrison JK, et al: Clinical value of pre-procedure transesophageal and transthoracic echocardiography in candidates for balloon mitral valvuloplasty. *Circulation.* 82(suppl III):III-500, 1990.

131. Manning WJ, Reis GJ: Use of transesophageal echocardiography to detect left atrial thrombi prior to percutaneous mitral valvuloplasty: a prospective study. *Circulation.* 82(suppl III):III-546, 1990.

132. Chirillo F, Ramondo A, Dan M, et al: Transesophageal echocardiography during percutaneous balloon mitral valvuloplasty. *Circulation.* 82(suppl III):III-46, 1990.

133. Kyo S, Hung J-S, Omoto R, et al: Intraoperative monitoring of catheter balloon percutaneous mitral valvuloplasty by biplane transesophageal echocardiography. *Circulation.* 82:(Suppl III):III-80, 1990.

134. Milner MR, Goldstein SA, Lindsay J, et al: Transesophageal echocardiographic guidance for percutaneous balloon mitral valvuloplasty. *Circulation.* 82(suppl III):III-81, 1990.

135. Yeager M, Yock PG, Popp RL: Comparison of Doppler-derived pressure gradient to that derived at cardiac catheterization in adults with aortic valve stenosis: implications for management. *Am J Cardiol.* 57:644–648, 1986.

136. Smith MD, Dawson PL, Elion JL, et al: Correlation of continuous wave Doppler velocities with cardiac catheterization gradients: an experimental model of aortic stenosis. *J Am Coll Cardiol.* 6:1306–1314, 1985.

137. Harrison MR, Gurley JC, Smith MD, et al: A practical application of Doppler echocardiography for the assessment of severity of aortic stenosis. *Am Heart J.* 115:622–628, 1986.

138. Jaffe WM, Roche AHG, Coverdale HA, et al: Clinical evaluation versus Doppler echocardiography in the quantitative assessment of valvular heart disease. *Circulation.* 78:267–275, 1988.

139. Miller FA Jr: Aortic stenosis: most cases no longer require invasive hemodynamic study. *J Am Coll Cardiol.* 13:551–553, 1989.

140. Currie PJ, Seward JB, Reeder GS, et al: Continuous wave Doppler echocardiographic assessment of severity of calcific aortic stenosis: a simultaneous Doppler–catheter correlative study in 100 adult patients. *Circulation.* 71:1162–1169, 1985.

141. Otto CM, Pearlman AS: Doppler echocardiography in adults with symptomatic aortic stenosis. Diagnostic utility and cost-effectiveness. *Arch Intern Med.* 148:2553–2560, 1988.

142. Otto CM, Pearlman AS, Gardner CL: Hemodynamic progression of aortic stenosis in adults assessed by Doppler echocardiography. *J Am Coll Cardiol.* 13:545–550, 1989.

143. Slater J, Gindea AJ, Freedberg RS, et al: Comparison of cardiac catheterization and Doppler echocardiography in the decision to operate in aortic and mitral valve disease. *J Am Coll Cardiol.* 17:1026–1036, 1991.

CHAPTER **4**

Clinical Evaluation

JOSEPH K. PERLOFF
LAWRENCE A. YEATMAN

An important objective of the clinical cardiovascular evaluation is to resolve whether a given patient is likely to qualify for percutaneous balloon valvuloplasty. It is this initial judgment that determines whether or not to proceed with more refined investigations, and which of these investigations are most relevant. This chapter focuses on acquired and congenital stenosis of native cardiac valves (mitral, tricuspid, aortic, and pulmonic) and on bioprosthetic valves (aortic, mitral, tricuspid, pulmonic, and valved conduits). In each category, the history, physical signs, scalar electrocardiogram, and radiograph (chest roentgenograms, fluoroscopy, angiocardiograms) are assessed for the light that might be shed on whether or not percutaneous balloon valvuloplasty is an appropriate option.

NATIVE CARDIAC VALVES

Mitral Stenosis

In his classic treatise on *rheumatic heart disease*, published in 1924,[1] Carey Coombs described mitral stenosis as follows:

> The normal mitral orifice is a flexible opening with a caliber which admits the whole of two fingers; but in mitral stenosis it is a narrow, hard-lipped chink barely large enough for the passage of a lead pencil. . . . Instead of a channel varying in caliber with the varying calls imposed upon it by the several phases of the cardiac cycle, there is a rigid aperture which is sometimes a mere slit between the stiffened curtains.

Coombs drew attention to dyspnea (especially paroxysmal dyspnea or cardiac asthma), systemic emboli originating in "clot from the appendix of the left auricle," cough as the lungs become congested, and hemoptysis "which is so common a feature of established mitral stenosis."[1] Paul Wood, in his seminal monograph, "An Appreciation of Mitral Stenosis," elaborated on the symptoms so related, giving them physiological meanings from which diagnostic inferences could be drawn.[2] Because progression of the disease and the associated symptoms are often insidious, patients may initially be unaware of subtle but tangible limitations to which they have become accustomed. How far can a patient walk on the level ground in pleasant weather? Against cold wind? On a warm humid day? Uphill? Is there a history of recurrent dry nocturnal cough? What matters is that the patient is in fact symptomatic, albeit New York Heart Association Class II. Because the morbidity and mortality of balloon mitral valvuloplasty is less than that of open valvotomy (and much less than mitral replacement), there is an inclination to relax the stringency of symptomatic requirements for interventional catheterization. This is especially so in females of childbearing age. Rheumatic mitral stenosis poses a formidable risk during pregnancy, and previously asymptomatic or mildly symptomatic women with rheumatic mitral stenosis may first experience pulmonary edema during the course of gestation, sometimes in the late first trimester.[3] That risk is materially diminished by anticipatory balloon dilatation of the stenotic mitral valve, and interventional catheterization can be a very successful alternative to mitral valve surgery during pregnancy, even if operation takes the form of emergency closed valvotomy.[4]

The pink frothy sputum of pulmonary edema is only one form of hemoptysis in mitral stenosis.[2] Blood streaked sputum may accompany winter bronchitis; intermittent episodes of copious hemoptysis unaccompanied by chest pain originate in varicosed bronchial veins caused by the high pulmonary venous pressure of mitral stenosis; hemoptysis associated with pleuritic pain is a feature of pulmonary embolism with infarction in pulmonary hypertensive mitral stenosis with right ventricular failure and peripheral edema.[2]

One of the most feared complications of percutaneous balloon mitral valvuloplasty is stroke caused by dislodgement and embolization of a left atrial thrombus. Accordingly, in a patient with a history of a systemic embolus, especially a recent embolus, not necessarily cerebral, one must be cautious in recommending balloon valvuloplasty. Any patient with mitral stenosis and atrial fibrillation — even in the absence of the history of systemic embolization — should be given anticoagulant therapy for an appropriate period in anticipation of balloon valvuloplasty, and that patient *must* have a transesophageal echocardiogram to exclude the presence of a left atrial thrombus[5] (see also Chapter 11).

The history should include meticulous queries regarding infective endocarditis. A recent or relatively recent history contraindicates percutaneous balloon mitral valvuloplasty.

In 1806, Jean-Nicholas Corvisart described the murmur of mitral stenosis: "Among the several specific signs which permit recognition of this affection is a peculiar murmur . . . , difficult to describe, which shows that the blood is passing through an orifice which is not large enough in proportion to the quantity of blood to which it must give passage."[6] Auscultation, properly applied and rigorously analyzed, is one of the most important bases for judging whether a given patient with rheumatic mitral stenosis is properly selected for balloon dilatation. The information from cardiac auscultation is important on three counts: first to provide evidence of a critical reduction in orifice size of the mitral valve; second as an index of mitral leaflet mobility, especially mobility of the anterior leaflet; and third, for detection of significant coexisting mitral regurgitation.[7] But let us put auscultation in the context of the cardiovascular physical examination as a whole. In pure mitral stenosis, the arterial pulse is normal or small, and the rhythm is sinus or atrial fibrillation. In sinus rhythm, a large jugular venous A wave together with a palpable right ventricular impulse and a palpable second heart sound at the left base (pulmonary closure) are features of pulmonary hypertension.[7] The left ventricular impulse, however elusive, must be meticulously sought in the left lateral decubitus position because it is at that site that the bell of the stethoscope should be applied to elicit the auscultatory signs of mitral stenosis which might otherwise be subtle if not absent.[7] Parenthetically, but importantly, a prominent left ventricular impulse warns of significant coexisting mitral regurgitation and cautions against balloon valvuloplasty. The intensity of the first heart sound, especially the first major audible component, depends largely on the position of the bellies of the mitral leaflets, particularly the anterior leaflet, at the time the left ventricle begins to contract, and upon the mobility (pliability) of the anterior leaflet.[7] Accordingly, a loud first heart sound in mitral stenosis implies that the anterior mitral leaflet is mobile and maximally recessed into the left ventricle at the onset of ventricular systole (high left atrial pressure) (Fig. 4.1). A loud, early opening snap reinforces this conclusion, indicating that a mobile anterior leaflet is abruptly recessed into the left ventricular cavity in early diastole by the high left atrial pressure.[7] A presystolic murmur is an important auscultatory sign of mitral stenosis but not necessarily of its severity (Fig. 4.1). More important is the duration of the mid-diastolic murmur of mitral stenosis in atrial fibrillation. A mid-diastolic murmur that begins with a prominent opening snap and continues up to a loud first heart sound even after long diastolic cycle lengths predicts a significant end-diastolic

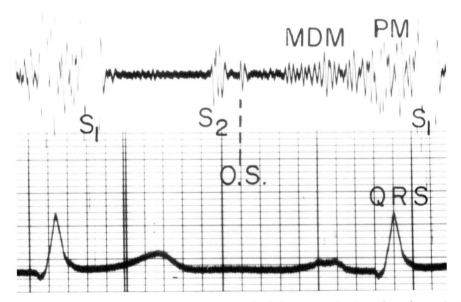

Figure 4.1 Phonocardiogram recorded over the left ventricular impulse of a patient with pure rheumatic mitral stenosis and mobile mitral leaflets. The first heart sound (S₁) is loud. There is no systolic murmur. The second heart sound (S₂) is followed by a prominent opening snap (O.S.) The S₂-O.S. interval is short (60 ms). A mid-diastolic murmur (MDM) is followed by a presystolic murmur (PM) that rises in crescendo to the next loud first heart sound. The loud first heart sound and opening snap indicate that the anterior mitral leaflet is mobile. The short S₂-O.S. interval indicates that a high left atrial pressure causes early opening movement of the anterior mitral leaflet into the left ventricular cavity.

gradient, reflecting the basic hemodynamic fault of severe mitral stenosis.[7] Conversely, a mid-diastolic murmur introduced by a third heart sound and ending before the first heart sound implies that the degree of stenosis is not significant, especially if the murmur of mitral regurgitation coexists.

The physical examination should also focus on the configuration of the bony thorax. Because percutaneous balloon mitral valvuloplasty is performed by means of transseptal left-heart catheterization, significant musculoskeletal abnormalities, especially kyphoscoliosis, make the procedure more risky if not technically untenable.

The electrocardiogram in sinus rhythm shows the broad bifid P waves of delayed depolarization of an enlarged left atrium (see Chapter 5). A tall peaked initial component of the P wave together with electrocardiographic evidence of right ventricular hypertrophy are features of pulmonary hypertensive mitral stenosis but bear no relationship to the mobility of the mitral valve or whether it is amenable to balloon dilatation. In atrial fibrillation, the suspicion of pulmonary hypertension rests only on QRS evidence of right ventricular hypertrophy, which may take the form of no more than a vertical frontal plane electrical axis.

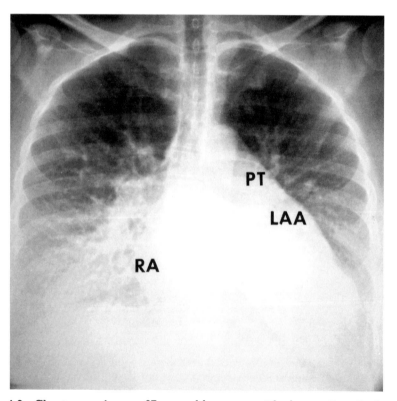

Figure 4.2 Chest x-ray from a 37-year-old woman with rheumatic mitral stenosis and pulmonary edema (typical radiographic picture) during the 33rd week of pregnancy. The patient underwent balloon dilatation of her mitral valve under transesophageal echocardiographic monitoring. The pulmonary trunk (*PT*) is moderately convex, and the right atrium (*RA*) is enlarged. There is a prominent left atrial appendage (*LAA*).

Cardiac fluoroscopy, apart from that required during cardiac catheterization, has fallen out of use but was once a valuable means of identifying mitral valve calcium and, when performed with a barium esophogram, of identifying left atrial enlargement. All else being equal, absence of fluoroscopic evidence of mitral valve calcium is a favorable sign for balloon valvuloplasty, whereas dense calcification warns against success.

Chest roentgenograms for the evaluation of rheumatic mitral valve disease at one time included four views — posteroanterior, lateral, and both obliques — with a barium esophogram. Posteroanterior and lateral roentgenograms remain routine and should be read meticulously (Figs. 4.2 and 4.3). Kerley "B" lines together with an ill-defined right hilus and venous redistribution to the apices are radiologic signs of the high left atrial (and pulmonary venous) pressure of severe mitral stenosis. A convex pulmonary trunk and an enlarged right atrium (posteroanterior view) together with an enlarged right ventricle (lateral view) are radiologic signs of pulmonary hypertension (Fig. 4.3). Enlargement of the left atrial appendage is a feature of *rheumatic* mitral valve disease and is best identified in the posteroanterior view. The size of the left atrium in rheumatic mitral stenosis is generally moderate rather than marked (see Fig. 4.2) and is best assessed in the lateral projection as a convex density beneath the left bronchus (Fig. 4.3). The foregoing radiologic signs identify obstruction of the mitral orifice but shed little or no light on whether the obstruction is amenable to balloon dilatation. Obvious calcification of the mitral valve, best seen in the lateral projection, makes the prospect of successful balloon dilatation vanishingly small, although the absence of radiologic calcium does not ensure that the stenotic valve is mobile.

Left ventriculography was previously used to evaluate the mobility and thickness of the mitral leaflets and the extent of subvalvular shortening. Angiocardiography is now

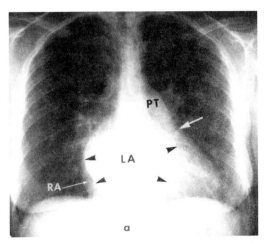
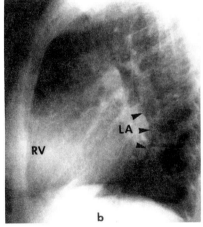

Figure 4.3 Chest roentgenograms from a 32-year-old woman with pure rheumatic mitral stenosis and pulmonary hypertension. *a*, The posteroanterior view shows the double density of the enlarged left atrium (*LA*), the straight left border caused by the left atrial appendage (*white arrow*), and a convex pulmonary trunk (*PT*). The *small white arrow* identifies an enlarged right atrium (*RA*). *b*, The lateral projection shows the enlarged left atrium (*LA*) beneath the left bronchus. No mitral valve calcium is seen radiologically. An enlarged right ventricle (*RV*) encroaches on the retrosternal space.

seldom employed to assess the degree of mitral stenosis or the mobility of the stenotic valve, having given way to transthoracic and transesophageal echocardiography.

Anatomic types of *congenital mitral stenosis* in the presence of a functionally adequate left ventricle include, in approximate order of frequency: (1) "typical" congenital mitral stenosis characterized by short chordae tendineae, fibrous reduction in or obliteration of interchordal spaces, and a variable decrease in interpapillary muscle distance, (2) parachute mitral valve, (3) anomalous mitral arcade, (4) supravalvular stenosing ring, (5) accessory mitral valve tissue, and (6) anomalous left ventricular muscle bundles or large obstructing papillary muscles.[8] Most of these anatomic variations are unsuitable for balloon dilatation and will not be elaborated on further (see Chapter 8).

Tricuspid Stenosis

Rheumatic tricuspid stenosis almost always occurs in the setting of coexisting mitral stenosis.[9] The first feature that might arouse suspicion is the history in a patient with known mitral stenosis but with a relative paucity of acute paroxysmal symptoms such as pulmonary edema, paroxysmal nocturnal dyspnea, and the "pulmonary apoplexy" type of hemoptysis.[9] Attenuation of the paroxysmal symptoms of mitral stenosis is believed to be due to curtailment of abrupt increases in pulmonary blood flow by the proximal obstruction at the tricuspid orifice. The physical signs, however, provide the highest index of suspicion of tricuspid stenosis. The typical tricuspid stenotic jugular venous pulse in sinus rhythm consists of an A wave of unusual magnitude, occasionally reaching the angle of the jaw, a relatively small V wave, and a gentle, usually imperceptible Y descent (Fig. 4.4).[7,9] This jugular venous configuration is virtually diagnostic of triscuspid stenosis in a patient with rheumatic mitral stenosis, provided the physical signs of pulmonary hypertension are absent. In atrial fibrillation, the jugular venous pulse exhibits a tall V wave with an inappropriately slow Y descent (Fig. 4.5). Auscultatory evidence of coexisting mitral stenosis is almost always present, an important point because it is difficult if not impossible to assign an opening snap to the stenotic tricuspid valve unless there is immobilizing mitral valve calcification, a feature not identifiable at the bedside. The most useful auscultatory sign of tricuspid stenosis is the murmur itself.[9] In sinus rhythm, the tricuspid stenotic murmur is presystolic, occurring in the absence of a perceptible mid-diastolic murmur because the tricuspid gradient is usually negligible until the powerful right atrium contracts (Fig. 4.6). The presystolic murmur of tricuspid stenosis can be distinguished from that of mitral stenosis on two counts (Fig. 4.6): (1) the tricuspid murmur is crescendo–decrescendo in shape and fades toward the first heart sound and (2) most important, the tricuspid stenotic murmur selectively increases during inspiration because the presystolic gradient increases in response to an increase in right atrial contractile force in the face of an inspiratory decline in right ventricular end-diastolic pressure.[7,9] In atrial fibrillation, the presystolic murmur is replaced by a mid-diastolic murmur that need not reach the first heart sound but that selectively increases during inspiration. These elegant physical signs serve to identify the presence and degree of tricuspid stenosis, but do they shed light on amenability of the stenotic valve to balloon dilatation? The stenotic tricuspid valve is seldom calcified, so selection for balloon valvuloplasty must rest on other criteria. A tall V wave with brisk Y descent and a lower left (or right) sternal edge systolic murmur that increases with inspiration indicate significant tricuspid regurgitation, and warn against success.

The typical electrocardiogram of rheumatic tricuspid stenosis in sinus rhythm shows an impressive right atrial P wave with little or no electrocardiographic evidence of right ventricular hypertrophy, implying that the right atrium contracts against a resistance at the tricuspid orifice, not in a thick-walled pulmonary hypertensive right ventricle (see Chapter 5). The chest x-ray shows radiologic signs of mitral stenosis,

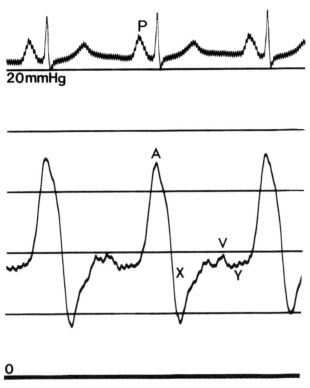

Figure 4.4 Right atrial pressure pulse that was reflected in the jugular venous pulse of a patient with rheumatic tricuspid stenosis in sinus rhythm. There is a large A wave, a conspicuous X descent, and a V wave with a blunted Y descent. Note the peaked P wave in the accompanying electrocardiogram.

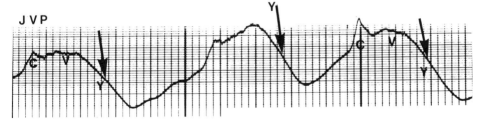

Figure 4.5 Jugular venous pulse (*JVP*) from a patient with rheumatic tricuspid stenosis in atrial fibrillation. A tall V wave crest is followed by an attenuated Y descent (*arrows*) owing to obstruction at the stenotic tricuspid orifice. The C wave is the impact of the carotid pulse.

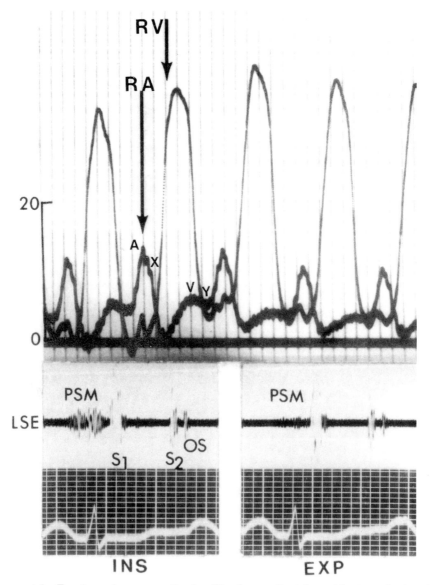

Figure 4.6 Tracings from a patient with rheumatic tricuspid stenosis in sinus rhythm. The upper tracing is a simultaneous right ventricular (*RV*) and right atrial (*RA*) pressure pulse during inspiration (*INS*) and expiration (*EXP*). The right atrial pressure pulse exhibits a tall A wave, a brisk X descent, and a V wave followed by a gentle Y descent. During inspiration, the gradient increases owing to a simultaneous fall in right ventricular diastolic pressure together with an increase in the A wave. The phonocardiogram at the lower left sternal edge (*LSE*) records a crescendo-decrescendo presystolic murmur (*PSM*) that selectively increases during inspiration as the gradient increases, and decreases if not vanishes altogether during expiration as the gradient declines. The loud first heart sound (S_1) and opening snap (*OS*) are caused by coexisting rheumatic mitral stenosis.

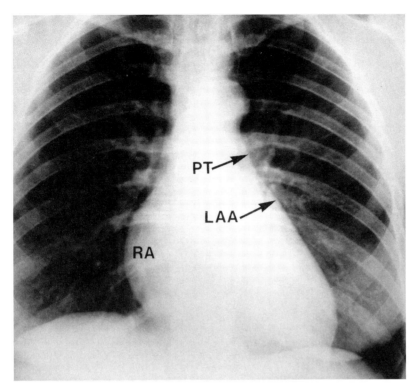

Figure 4.7 Posteroanterior chest x-ray from a 33-year-old woman with rheumatic tricuspid stenosis and mitral stenosis. The right atrium (*RA*) is distinctly enlarged but the pulmonary trunk (*PT*) is inconspicuous, indicating that the right atrial enlargement is not due to pulmonary hypertension. *LAA*—left atrial appendage.

but there is a distinctive increase in *right* atrial size in the absence of radiologic signs of pulmonary hypertension (relatively inconspicuous pulmonary trunk) (Fig. 4.7).[9]

Aortic Valve Stenosis

Stenosis of the aortic valve can be congenital or acquired, noncalcific or calcific. Response to balloon aortic valvuloplasty differs appreciably according to the morphologic characteristics of the valve.

A *bicuspid aortic valve* is the most common congenital abnormality to which that structure is subject (Fig. 4.8).[8, 10] The bicuspid aortic valve, which was first sketched by Leonardo da Vinci,[11] occurs in an estimated 2% of the population[8, 10] and is often functionally normal at birth. Bicuspid aortic stenosis in adults typically is caused by calcification of an initially functionally normal congenital bicuspid aortic valve. (Fig. 4.8). This form of calcific aortic stenosis accounts for approximately one half of cases of surgically important pure aortic stenosis in adults.[12] The patients are typically male with an estimated sex ratio of approximately 4:1.[10] If the valve is functionally normal at birth, there is little in the early history that calls attention to the lesion unless it announces itself because of susceptibility to infective endocarditis. A history

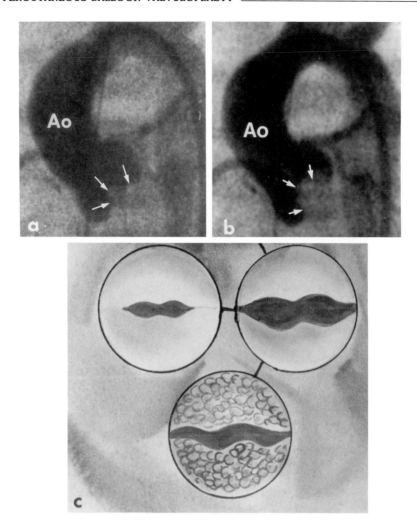

Figure 4.8 Lateral thoracic aortogram (*a*) and (*b*) in a patient with typical mobile, dome congenital bicuspid aortic stenosis. *Arrows* point to abrupt cephalad opening of the mobile valve reflected in the aortic ejection sound. There is poststenotic dilatation of the aortic root (*Ao*). (*c*) Illustration of three bicuspid aortic valves. The *upper left* shows bicuspid aortic stenosis due to failure of commissural separation. *Upper right* shows a functionally normal bicuspid aortic valve without commissural fusion, the best result that can be achieved with balloon valvuloplasty. The *lower* illustration represents calcific aortic stenosis of a previously functionally normal bicuspid aortic valve without commissural fusion. The calcified valve does not generate an ejection sound.

of the gradual development of a conspicuous murmur awaits significant thickening and calcification of the bicuspid valve, a condition which, as a rule, progresses insidiously over decades. Effort dyspnea, chest oppression, lightheadedness or effort-induced syncope reflect severity, although sudden death is not a feature of calcific bicuspid aortic stenosis in relatively young adults with normal coronary arteries. The

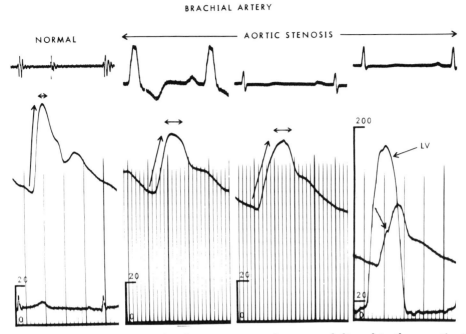

Figure 4.9 Brachial arterial pulses in a normal young adult and in three patients with aortic valve stenosis. The aortic stenotic pulse exhibits a relatively small pulse pressure, a slow rate of rise, a sustained peak and a gentle fall. In the fourth panel, there is an anacrotic notch (*arrow*) midway up the ascending limb of the arterial pulse. *LV*—left ventricle.

arterial pulse tends to reflect the degree of obstruction, with a slow rise and sustained peak indicating severe stenosis (Fig. 4.9).[7] A sustained left ventricular impulse accompanied by presystolic distention (augmented contraction of the left atrium) reinforces the impression of severity.[7] A systolic thrill, maximal at the right base, is seldom present unless the degree of obstruction is at least moderate to marked, depending upon body build. A fourth heart sound is the auscultatory counterpart of presystolic distention of the left ventricle, and has the same physiologic significance (Fig. 4. 10).[13] Both the duration and frequency composition of the systolic murmur are important. All else being equal, the longer the murmur, the more severe the obstruction (Fig. 4.10). Importantly, the frequency composition of the murmur tends to be the same (relatively impure) at the right base and at the apex in contrast to Gallavardin dissociation (described below) for calcified trileaflet aortic valves in older adults.[7,14] These physical signs identify aortic stenosis but not its etiologic type. However, if auscultation detects a convincing aortic ejection sound (Fig. 4.10), typically heard best at the site of the left ventricular impulse, a bicuspid aortic valve is a legitimate diagnostic conclusion.[7,8,15] The presence of the ejection sound not only focuses attention on *bicuspid* aortic stenosis but indicates mobility of the valve, a sign that sets the stage for but does not guarantee the success of balloon dilatation. Paradoxical splitting of the second heart sound is a feature of severity of obstruction and of leaflet mobility (Fig. 4.11).[7,15]

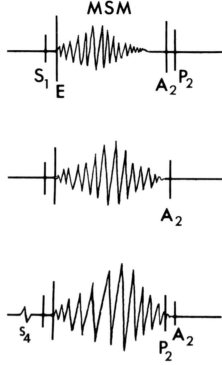

Figure 4.10 Illustrations of auscultatory signs (from top to bottom) of mild, moderate, and severe congenital aortic valve stenosis. Mild: an ejection sound (*E*) introduces a short midsystolic murmur (*MSM*) that peaks in early systole. The second sound splits normally, and the aortic component (*A₂*) is prominent. Moderate: the ejection sound introduces a longer midsystolic murmur with a later systolic peak. The second sound (*A₂*) is single. Severe: a fourth heart sound (*S₄*) precedes the first heart sound which is followed by an ejection sound that introduces a long midsystolic murmur with a late systolic peak. The second heart sound is paradoxically split (*A₂* follows *P₂*). As severity increases, the murmur remains symmetric (diamond-shaped), despite an increased length.

The electrocardiogram in young adults with bicuspid aortic stenosis often but not invariably mirrors the degree of obstruction to left ventricular outflow (see Chapter 5). If the P wave shows a left atrial abnormality, especially in a relatively young adult, it is reasonable to conclude that the degree of aortic stenosis is sufficient to call upon the left atrium to contract with greater force in response to the increase in left ventricular mass. The electrocardiographic diagnosis of left ventricular hypertrophy is most secure in the presence of both voltage and repolarization criteria, the latter of which may in part reflect a disparity between left ventricular mass and coronary flow, rather than coexisting coronary artery disease as might be expected in older subjects with calcific aortic stenosis of any etiology.

If the chest roentgenograms show a greater degree of convexity of the ascending aorta (poststenotic dilatation) than is appropriate for age, bicuspid aortic stenosis can be suspected (Fig. 4.12).[8] The left ventricular silhouette should be examined in the posteroanterior projection for increased convexity and for displacement to the left and below the ipsilateral hemidiaphragm. In the lateral projection, the position of the left

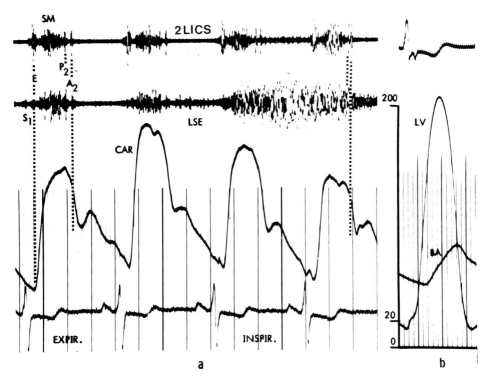

Figure 4.11 Tracings from a 62-year-old man with severe congenital bicuspid aortic valve stenosis and relatively little calcium deposition. The mobility of the bicuspid stenotic valve is reflected in the phonocardiograms as an aortic ejection sound (E) and persistent audibility of the aortic component (A_2) of the second heart sound which is paradoxically split (P_2 before A_2). *CAR*—carotid pulse. *EXPIR*—expiration. *INSPIR*—inspiration. *SM*—systolic murmur. *2LICS*—second left intercostal space. *LSE*—lower left sternal edge. The panel on the *right* shows the left ventricular (LV) and brachial arterial (BA) pressure pulses, recording the gradient and the typical configuration of the aortic stenotic pressure pulse.

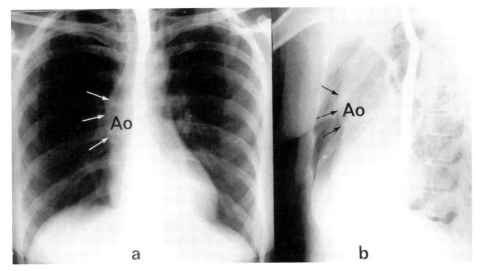

Figure 4.12 *a*, Posteroanterior and *b*, lateral chest x-rays from a 36-year-old man with typical aortic valve stenosis and a gradient of 55 mmHlg. There is conspicuous poststenotic dilatation of the aortic root (*Ao*) (*arrows*).

ventricular silhouette in its posterior projection should be compared with the inferior vena caval shadow, which is normally behind the junction of the left ventricle and diaphragm. The lateral projection is most suitable for identifying calcium in the aortic valve and for determining left atrial size beneath the left bronchus. In addition to detection of valvular calcium per se, the pattern of calcium deposition is sometimes revealing. A bicuspid aortic valve is occasionally recognized by one of several patterns, ranging from the bulbous or clublike configuration of the calcified raphe to calcification of both leaflets manifested by a circle or semicircle with the bulbous raphe pointing toward its center (Fig. 4.13).[8] Fluoroscopy, seldom employed except during cardiac catheterization, refines the radiologic detection of the aortic valve calcium. Angiocardiography is useful on two counts, first to exclude coexisting coronary artery disease in older males with fibrocalcific obstruction of a bicuspid aortic valve, and second to shed light on the morphology of the valve and the degree of mobility (aortic root angiography).

In children and adolescents with noncalcified mobile bicuspid stenotic valves, balloon dilatation increases orifice size by splitting the two fused commissures.[16] If successful, the result is analogous to if not identical with the result of direct surgical repair without valve replacement. Balloon valvuloplasty has also been used successfully in selected patients with recurrent aortic stenosis after surgical valvotomy in childhood. By contrast, the adult with bicuspid aortic stenosis experiences limited success in response to balloon dilatation because there is little or no commissural

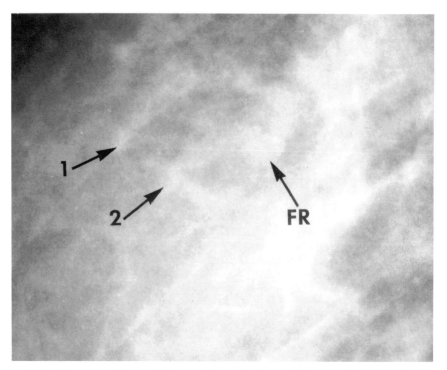

Figure 4.13 Closeup of lateral chest radiograph from a 77-year-old man with calcific bicuspid aortic stenosis. *Arrows* marked (*1*) and (*2*) point to calcium in the two aortic leaflets, and the *third arrow* points to calcium in the false raphe (*FR*).

fusion; obstruction is due chiefly, if not exclusively, to fibrocalcific thickening of the leaflets.[16]

A second variety of congenital aortic valve stenosis is designated *unicuspid unicommissural* because the free edge of a single (unicuspid) leaflet orginates from a single commissural attachment at the aortic wall, proceeds across the aortic orifice without making additional contact with the wall, bends on itself, and returns to reinsert at the same point from which it originated, thus forming one commissure (unicommissural).[8,17] The typical unicommissural valve is intrinsically stenotic at birth, but if the free edge is sufficiently redundant and the single commissure is not fused, obstruction is initially mild or absent (functionally normal) but then develops in young adulthood when valve mobility is reduced by fibrosis and calcification.[17] Except as a matter of probability (or improbability), it is difficult if not impossible to distinguish fibrocalcific obstruction of a previously functionally normal unicommissural unicuspid aortic valve in adults from fibrocalcific obstruction of an initially functionally normal bicuspid aortic valve (see above).

It is important to distinguish *discrete subaortic stenosis* from bicuspid aortic stenosis in young adults. The localized crescent-shaped membrane located immediately below the aortic valve responds poorly if at all, and the long, narrow fibromuscular channel is not amenable to balloon dilatation. The chief feature that is likely to set the stage for distinguishing discrete subaortic stenosis from bicuspid aortic stenosis is auscultation.[8] An aortic ejection sound is *not* a feature of discrete subaortic stenosis, and the murmur of aortic regurgitation is much more likely to be present in discrete subvalvular obstruction because of the relatively high incidence of coexisting abnormalities of the aortic valve. Intrinsically stenotic bicuspid aortic valves in infants and children are seldom associated with regurgitation, but during the development of fibrocalcific obstruction of a previously functionally normal bicuspid aortic valve, stenosis and regurgitation not uncommonly coexist.

Calcific aortic stenosis in adults above age 60 years constitutes the second major category of surgically important aortic stenosis in adulthood.[12,14] In the hydraulically ideal trileaflet aortic valve (leaflet equality), total diastolic force is equally distributed among the three equal leaflets. When there is leaflet *inequality*, total diastolic force is *unequally* distributed. The fibrocalcific aging process is believed to proceed more rapidly in a leaflet or leaflets that bear the greatest hemodynamic stress.[18] Accordingly, congenital leaflet inequality appears to play a role in enhancing the process of "normal" aging and in converting normal trileaflet aortic valves into calcific aortic stenosis. Patients with this form of "acquired" obstruction to left ventricular outflow are generally above age 60 years, with an equal sex distribution rather than male dominance.[14] There is no history of murmur in early and midadult life. Once obstruction develops, symptoms may be similar if not identical to those described above in younger adults with calcified bicuspid aortic stenosis. In the older patient with acquired calcification of a previously normal trileaflet aortic valve, however, chest oppression is more likely to be associated with coronary artery disease, and syncope is much more likely to herald sudden death because of the ischemia related to coexisting coronary arterial obstruction. The systemic blood pressure and arterial pulse are often misleading in older subjects with calcific aortic stenosis.[14] The pulse pressure is not necessarily small, the rate of rise is not necessarily slow, and the crest of the pulse is not necessarily prolonged (Fig. 4.14). This is so because the decrease in compliance (reduced distensibility characteristics) of the ascending aorta and brachiocephalic arteries serves to amplify the systolic blood pressure and increase the

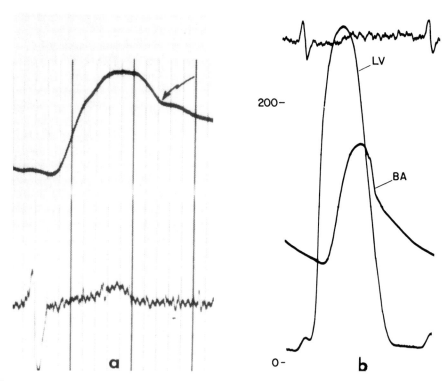

Figure 4.14   *a*, Indirect carotid arterial pulse tracing showing the typical slow rate of rise, broad crest and slurred dicrotic notch (*arrow*) of severe aortic valve stenosis in a young adult. *b*, Simultaneous left ventricular (*LV*) and brachial arterial (*BA*) pressure pulses from an 81-year-old man with severe calcific aortic stenosis. The brachial arterial systolic pressure is 172 mmHg with an increase in pulse pressure, a relatively normal rate of rise, and a nonsustained crest.

rate of rise of the arterial pulse (Fig. 4.15).[7,14] An increased anteroposterior chest dimension in older adults may seriously compromise precordial palpation and auscultation. Accordingly, a systolic thrill may be present only in the suprasternal notch and above the clavicles, and the left ventricular impulse may be relatively inconspicuous if not absent altogether even in the left lateral decubitus position. In patients with a significant increase in anteroposterior chest dimension the systolic murmur is often disarmingly soft and short at the right base, and is heard conspicuously only in the suprasternal notch or above the clavicles. Nevertheless, auscultation can be virtually diagnostic of fibrocalcific thickening of a previously normal trileaflet aortic valve in older subjects, whether the valve is sclerotic or stenotic. In 1925, Louis Gallavardin described the dissociation between a noisy, impure systolic murmur at the right base and a pure musical murmur at the apex (Fig. 4.16).[19] The right basal component of the murmur originates within the aortic root because of turbulence caused by the high velocity jet. The pure, musical component of the murmur is heard over the left ventricular impulse and is ascribed to periodic high frequency vibrations of fibrocalcific leaflets without commissural fusion.[7,14] The musical component of the apical midsystolic murmur is sometimes dramatically loud.

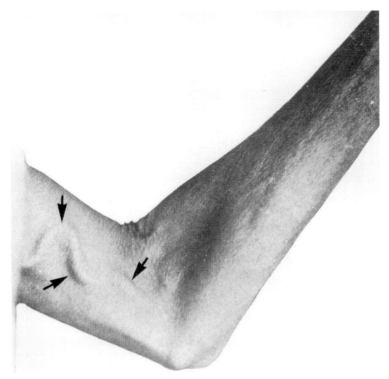

Figure 4.15 Increased pulse pressure in a thickened, serpentine brachial artery of Monckeberg's sclerosis visible beneath the skin of the antecubital fossa (*arrows*). From Cabot RC: *Physical Diagnosis*. New York: William Wood and Co, 1915 (Courtesy of Dr. Sherman M. Mellinkoff, UCLA Medical Center).

Intensity of the murmur, especially at the apex, is not necessarily a reflection of severity; duration is more likely to be an index of severity unless mitral regurgitation coexists. Gallavardin dissociation is diagnostically distinctive of fibrocalcific thickening of a previously normal trileaflet aortic valve, seldom occurring with bicuspid calcific aortic stenosis. An aortic ejection sound is consistently absent, and the aortic component of the second sound is soft or inaudible. A fourth heart sound is common (Fig. 16B) but may relate to the patient's age rather than to the severity of aortic stenosis.[13]

The electrocardiogram is not necessarily an accurate reflection of the degree of obstruction (see Chapter 5). A left atrial P wave abnormality is common in older patients without aortic stenosis, indicating delayed depolarization of a normal-sized left atrium. The amplitude of the R wave may be reduced by an increase in anteroposterior chest dimensions, and repolarization abnormalities may reflect coronary artery disease rather than left ventricular hypertrophy.

Although the clinical signs, including the electrocardiogram, may not shed adequate light on the severity of calcific trileaflet aortic stenosis, a simple but useful diagnostic intervention is fluoroscopy conducted during cardiac catheterization. Mild or absent fluoroscopic calcification is presumptive evidence of a "sclerotic" but nonstenotic trileaflet aortic valve, whereas the presence of dense calcification signifies

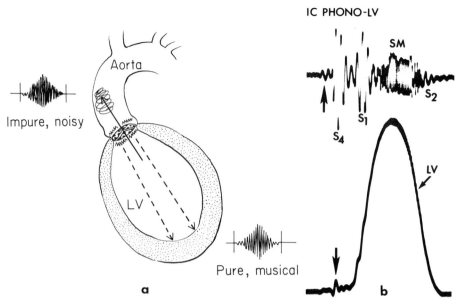

Figure 4.16 *a*, Schematic illustration of "Gallavardin dissociation" of the murmurs associated with a fibrocalcific nonfused trileaflet aortic valve in older adults. The impure, noise midsystolic murmur at the right base originates within the aortic root because of turbulence caused by the high velocity jet. The pure, musical midsystolic murmur at the apex results from periodic high frequency vibrations originating in the fibrocalcific but mobile nonfused leaflets and radiates selectively into the left ventricular cavity (*LV*). *b*, Intracardiac left ventricular (*LV*) phonocardiogram with simultaneous pressure pulse from an elderly patient with calcific aortic stenosis of a previously normal trileaflet aortic valve. The phonocardiogram shows a remarkably prominent fourth heart sound (S_4) preceded by low frequency vibrations (inaudible) of left atrial contraction per se. The systolic murmur is the typical musical Gallavardin murmur transmitted into the left ventricular cavity from periodic vibrations of the nonfused fibrocalcific aortic leaflets. The *arrow* on the left ventricular pressure pulse identifies presystolic distention palpable at the bedside.

appreciable obstruction, with few exceptions. The chest roentgenograms may disclose a conspicuous ascending aorta due to age rather than due to poststenotic dilatation. An increase in left ventricular size may be influenced by coronary artery disease, and an increase in left atrial size by coexisting mitral regurgitation. It goes without saying that clearly identifiable calcification of the aortic valve in the lateral projection carries the implications mentioned in regard to fluoroscopy. The relative contributions of aortic stenosis and coronary artery disease are sometimes difficult if not impossible to establish without comprehensive assessment including two-dimensional Doppler echocardiography, thallium imaging, and cardiac catheterization with coronary angiography.[20]

The clinical distinction between adults with calcific *bicuspid* aortic stenosis and those with calcific *trileaflet* aortic stenosis is important because the response to balloon dilatation differs between the two.[21,22] Balloon valvuloplasty may reduce the gradient in calcific trileaflet aortic stenosis, increase the orifice size, and relieve symptoms, at least in the short term, by producing fractures or fissures within the calcified leaflets, resulting in hinge points that apparently allow increased leaflet mobility. The morphologic differences between the calcified trileaflet aortic valve and the calcified bicuspid aortic valve are believed to account for the poorer response to balloon valvuloplasty of the latter, which is less likely to develop mobile hinge points.[16,23,24]

Now let us turn to *rheumatic aortic stenosis*. Carey Coombs wrote, "Rheumatic invasion of these aortic valves, then, spoils their function. . . . That it may sometimes so stiffen them that they are likely to become a hindrance to the systolic discharge of the ventricular contents is clear enough from anatomical evidence."[1] Rheumatic fever may lead to aortic stenosis without calcification by causing fusion of the commissures. The direct effects of rheumatic fever on the aortic valve may be mild, but the stage is then set for subsequent calcification with progressive obstruction, combining commissural fusion with fibrocalcific thickening of the leaflets. There is a relatively uniform consensus that anatomically isolated aortic valve disease is seldom if ever rheumatic.[10] Accordingly, initial clinical suspicion of rheumatic aortic stenosis depends on a history of rheumatic fever or its equivalents (not uncommonly unavailable in patients with rheumatic heart disease), or on identification of coexisting rheumatic mitral valve disease. The physical signs are seldom those of aortic stenosis alone, and the thickened but noncalcified stenotic rheumatic aortic valve does not generate an aortic ejection sound. Balloon dilatation may force separation of the fused commissures, but less readily than in pliant, thin, fused bicuspid leaflets.[22] Balloon valvuloplasty is less likely to succeed if the obstruction is caused chiefly by fibrocalcific thickening rather than by fusion of rheumatic aortic leaflets. Balloon dilatation is even less likely to be efficacious if a rheumatic stenotic aortic valve is calcified. This is true whether the calcium is deposited on a valve with commissural fusion or whether late degenerative calcification is the major cause of obstruction. The electrocardiogram, chest x-rays, and angiographic features focus chiefly on evidence of coexisting rheumatic mitral valve disease, stenosis, incompetence, or a combination thereof.

Aortic valve replacement is the time-tested treatment for calcific aortic stenosis. Balloon valvuloplasty is not a competing therapeutic modality but a palliative procedure whose benefits are limited in degree and in duration.[22] Selection of adults with calcific aortic stenosis for balloon valvuloplasty is based chiefly if not entirely on clinical considerations.[25] Balloon dilatation can resolve a *therapeutic* dilemma in elderly patients who face an urgent need for major noncardiac surgery such as abdominal aortic aneurysm or gastrointestinal bleeding.[26] Balloon valvuloplasty sometimes contributes to the resolution of a *diagnostic* dilemma in elderly patients with severe calcific aortic stenosis and marked left ventricular failure or cardiogenic shock.[27] An increase in aortic valve area following balloon valvuloplasty may allow sufficient left ventricular recovery to clarify the relative contributions of obstruction to left ventricular outflow versus left ventricular dysfunction, and to determine whether aortic valve replacement might be useful. In a patient who refuses aortic valve replacement, temporary relief of symptoms following balloon valvuloplasty followed by recurrence of symptoms, together with lack of long-term benefit of nonsurgical treatment, may help the patient decide on aortic valve replacement.[22] Patients with rheumatic mitral and aortic valve disease not uncommonly develop hemodynamically significant obstructive lesions of those valves during different time courses.[22] Balloon aortic valvuloplasty might delay the need for reoperation in a patient with previous mitral valve repair. Balloon aortic valvuloplasty is a legitimate consideration under certain clinical circumstances that make aortic valve replacement undesirable: advanced chronologic and physiological age, or refusal of aortic valve replacement by a frail symptomatic patient age 75 years or older. In the face of an unresolved issue of limited life expectancy from other causes (malignancy, recent cerebrovascular accident), balloon aortic valvuloplasty as palliation may provide the time necessary for determining whether or not aortic valve replacement is feasible.[22] Emergency balloon dilatation has been employed in an attempt to reverse acute hemodynamic decompensation that develops during cardiac catheterization for aortic stenosis.

Congenital Pulmonary Valve Stenosis

Isolated congenital stenosis of the pulmonary valve is typically represented by a conical or dome-shaped structure with a narrow outlet at its apex.[8,28] Three rudimentary raphes extend from the central opening to the wall of the pulmonary artery. Balloon dilatation is the treatment of choice for dome-shaped mobile stenotic pulmonary valves (Fig. 4.17).[16,29-32] The history usually begins in infancy if not at birth, because the anatomic and physiological conditions necessary for the generation of the murmur are usually present at birth. The soft murmurs of mild obstruction may be overlooked or considered innocent for many years. With the exception of pinpoint pulmonary valve stenosis in neonates, survival into adolescence and adulthood is the rule, even though signs of the anomaly date from birth or early infancy.[8] Importantly, the normal pulmonary valve orifice increases linearly with age and body surface area, so patients with typical dome pulmonary valve stenosis experience an increase in orifice size with age and growth.[8] This pattern is sometimes modified by the development of secondary hypertrophic (infundibular) obstruction (Fig. 4.17); nor should it be forgotten that with advancing age, fibrous thickening and even calcification are occasionally responsible for reducing valve mobility and increasing the degree of

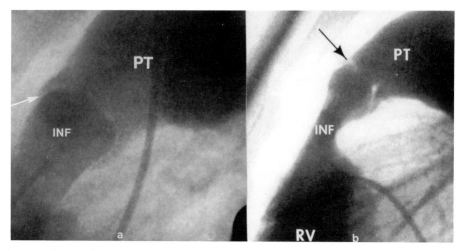

Figure 4.17 Right ventriculograms (*RV*) in two patients with pulmonary valve stenosis. *a*, The mobile, stenotic pulmonary valve domes (*arrow*) but the infundibulum (*INF*) does not narrow in systole. There is conspicuous poststenotic dilatation of the pulmonary trunk (*PT*). *b*, In addition to the mobile stenotic pulmonary valve (*arrow*), there is conspicuous systolic narrowing of the infundibulum (*INF*). The pulmonary trunk (*PT*) is dilated.

obstruction.[8] An appreciable number of patients with moderate to severe pulmonary valve stenosis remain virtually asymptomatic into early adulthood.[8] Dyspnea and fatigue are the most common symptoms. Patients sometimes experience giddiness, lightheadedness, or syncope, especially with effort. Syncope followed by death is exceptional but not unknown.

The jugular venous pulse is a useful index of the degree of obstruction based upon the amplitude of the A wave (Figs. 4.18*a* and 4.19*b*).[7,8] Exercise and excitement augment the A wave, whereas bedrest has the opposite effect. A giant A wave that "leaps to the eye, towering above and dwarfing the other waves of the venous pulse,"[28] is even more impressive when compared with the normal or small arterial pulse that accompanies severe pulmonary valve stenosis. Powerful right atrial contraction is delivered into the inferior vena cava and transmitted to the liver as a presystolic liver pulse. Precordial palpation detects a right ventricular impulse and, if there is an increased force of right atrial contraction, presystolic distention of the right ventricle (Fig. 4.18*b*). The thrill accompanying typical pulmonary valve stenosis is maximal in the second or occasionally third left interspace with radiation upward and toward the left because the intrapulmonary jet is directed toward the left pulmonary artery.[7] When severe pulmonary valve stenosis is accompanied by significant secondary

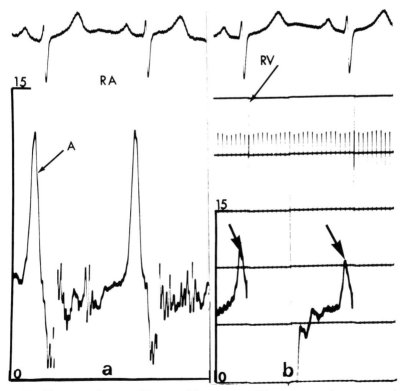

Figure 4.18 Tracings from a 47-year-old woman with severe pulmonary valve stenosis. *a*, Right atrial (*RA*) pressure pulse that was reflected in the jugular venous pulse, displaying a large A wave. *b*, Right ventricular (*RV*) pressure pulse showing prominent presystolic distention (*arrow*) detected by palpation at the lower left sternal edge and the subxyphoid region.

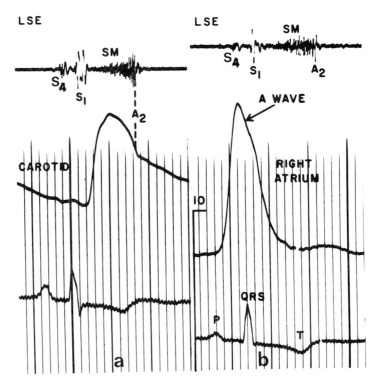

Figure 4.19 Tracings from a patient with severe pulmonary valve stenosis. The phonocardiogram was recorded from the lower left sternal edge (*LSE*). *a*, The tracing shows a prominent fourth heart sound S_4. S_1—first heart sound, *SM*—systolic murmur, A_2—aortic component of the second heart sound. *b*, Simultaneous tracing from the right atrium records a large A wave that was reflected in the jugular venous pulse and coincided with presystolic distention of the right ventricle and the fourth heart sound (S_4).

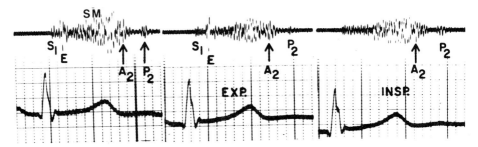

Figure 4.20 Phonocardiogram from a 21-year-old woman with pulmonary valve stenosis and a transvalvular gradient of 80 mmHg. The first heart sound (S_1) is followed by a prominent ejection sound (*E*) that virtually disappears during casual inspiration (*INSP*). The systolic murmur (*SM*) peaks late and envelops the aortic component of the second heart sound (A_2). The pulmonic component (P_2) is delayed and soft. The phonocardiogram was recorded from the second left interspace. *EXP*—expiration.

infundibular hypertrophy, the thrill tends to be maximal in the third or even fourth left interspace.[7,8] The nonauscultatory physical signs together with the length and configuration of the pulmonic stenotic murmur are accurate reflections of the degree of obstruction,[8] but it is the presence of a clearly audible pulmonic ejection sound that predicts the success of balloon dilatation (Figs. 4.20 and 4.21). The ejection sound is recognized by its high-pitched, sharp, clicking quality, by its maximal intensity in the second left interspace, and by its distinctive, selective decrease during inspiration and increase during expiration.[7,28] The ejection sound is a characteristic feature of congenital mobile dome-shaped pulmonary valve stenosis, serving an important function in identifying this form of obstruction and in suggesting that the valve is mobile and potentially amenable to balloon dilatation. The magnitude of stenosis is the major determinant of the duration of right ventricular ejection, which in turn determines the length of the systolic murmur (Figs. 4.20 and 4.21). If the length of the pulmonic

PULMONIC STENOSIS

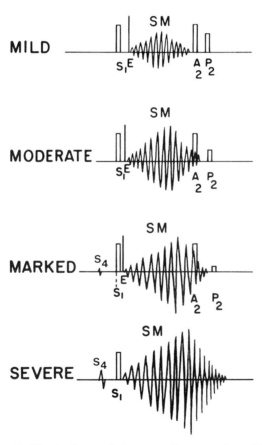

Figure 4.21 Schematic illustrations of phonocardiograms in mild to severe pulmonary valve stenosis. S_1—first heart sound, E—ejection sound, SM—systolic murmur, A_2—aortic component of the second heart sound, P_2—pulmonic component of the second heart sound, S_4—fourth heart sound.

stenotic murmur is related to the aortic component of the second heart sound, the relative durations of right and left ventricular ejection can be compared.[8] In selecting patients for potential balloon valvuloplasty, the location of maximal intensity of the systolic murmur is important because a relatively low location is likely to be associated with secondary subvalvular hypertrophy. Balloon dilatation of the mobile valve can still proceed, but a postdilatation gradient caused by infundibular hypertrophy may persist and respond to propranolol before gradually decreasing if not vanishing altogether.[16,33] The large jugular venous A wave with presystolic distention of the right ventricle is a feature of significant obstruction to right ventricular outflow, and a fourth heart sound reinforces this conclusion (see Fig. 4.19). The intensity of the pulmonic component of the second heart sound ranges from normal to inaudible as severity ranges from mild to severe (Figs. 4.20 and 4.21). Nevertheless, so long as there is a clearly audible ejection sound (abrupt cephalad doming of the stenotic valve), balloon dilatation is feasible. The soft or inaudible pulmonic component of the second sound is not a reflection of leaflet immobility but instead of low closing pressure.

The electrocardiogram is, as a rule, a relatively accurate reflection of the degree of obstruction to right ventricular outflow (see Chapter 5). In mild pulmonary valve stenosis, the only abnormality may be persistence of upright T waves in right precordial leads. As the degree of obstruction increases, the P wave becomes peaked (right atrial abnormality), the electrical axis in the frontal plane becomes vertical if not rightward, and voltage and repolarization criteria for right ventricular hypertrophy become progressively evident.[8] The severity of pulmonary stenosis correlates fairly well with the R/S ratio in leads V_1 and V_6, and with the height of the R wave in V_1. In mild pulmonary valve stenosis, an initial rS may be followed by a terminal r' wave, producing an rSr' pattern that is difficult to distinguish from normal. In severe pulmonary stenosis, the R wave in lead V_1 is tall and monophasic, followed by ST segment depressions and asymmetric T wave inversions in the right precordial leads.

The most distinctive features of the chest roentgenograms are poststenotic dilatation of the pulmonary trunk, disproportionate dilatation of the left branch, and an increase in right atrial and right ventricular sizes (Fig. 4.22).[8] Poststenotic dilatation is an important and often striking feature of typical dome-shaped pulmonary valve stenosis. This radiologic sign encourages the belief that the valve is in fact the dome type and potentially amenable to balloon dilatation, depending upon mobility and the severity of obstruction. Right ventriculography, especially in the lateral projection, identifies the mobile stenotic valve doming upward in systole with a central jet through the stenotic orifice (Figs. 4.17 and 4.22b). The cine–right ventriculogram may also disclose secondary hypertrophic subpulmonic stenosis with dynamic systolic narrowing of the outflow tract (Figs. 4.17 and 4.22b). It is important to diagnose hypertrophic subpulmonic stenosis before proceeding with balloon dilatation. Fluoroscopy and cineradiography serve to identify the occasional older adult with calcific pulmonic stenosis. The calcium is sometimes seen on the plain films as well. Repeat balloon valvuloplasty has proved efficacious in selected patients with pulmonary valve restenosis.[31]

A much less common variety of pulmonary stenosis is caused by a *dysplastic valve* represented by marked thickening of three distinct leaflets (disorganized myxomatous tissue) without commissural fusion.[8] It is necessary to recognize when a dysplastic pulmonic valve is causing the obstruction to right ventricular outflow because that type of valve is much less responsive to balloon dilatation.[16,29] Suspicion of a

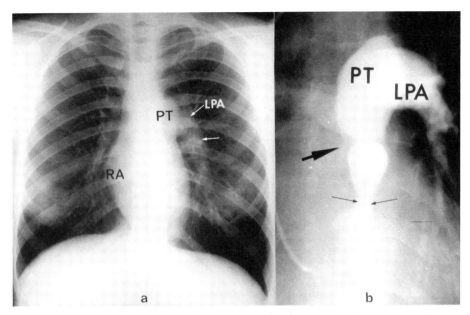

Figure 4.22 *a,* X-ray from a patient with typical pulmonary valve stenosis. There is conspicuous poststenotic dilatation of the pulmonary trunk (*PT*) with disproportionate dilatation of the left pulmonary artery (*LPA*). *RA*—right atrium. *b,* Right ventriculogram from another patient with typical pulmonary valve stenosis showing poststenotic dilatation of the pulmonary trunk (*PT*) with disproportionate dilatation of the proximal left branch (*LPA*). The large black *arrow* points to the stenotic pulmonary valve. Smaller *arrows* identify systolic narrowing of the infundibulum.

dysplastic pulmonic valve is heightened if the physical appearance suggests the Noonan syndrome characterized by short stature, delayed sexual development, web neck, low posterior hairline, low-set ears, micrognathia, hypertelorism, inguinal hernia, undescended testes, and dystrophic nails.[8] Because the dysplastic valve is immobile, auscultation discloses no pulmonic ejection sound and an inaudible pulmonic component of the second sound even when the degree of obstruction is not severe.

Bicuspid stenotic pulmonary valves seldom occur in isolation. In Fallot's tetralogy, the pulmonic valve is frequently bicuspid and responsible for additional obstruction to right ventricular outflow, but balloon dilatation is, for all practical purposes, not efficacious in this setting, so the topic will not be discussed further.

BIOPROSTHETIC VALVES

There are three categories of prostheses: valves, patches, and conduits.[34,35] The term "bioprosthesis" refers to a device that consists either entirely of natural materials or of combinations of synthetic and biologic materials. Exogenous bioprosthetic materials are secured from human cadavers (homografts) or animal sources (xenografts). The following remarks focus on bioprosthetic valves.

Homografts

Homografts are obtained fresh and placed in antibiotic solutions for relatively immediate use, or they are cryopreserved and stored in liquid nitrogen for later use.[34,36,37] Homograft cardiac bioprostheses presently in use consist of aortic and pulmonary valves excised in continuity with their annulus and great artery. Hemodynamic characteristics of homograft valves are optimal because their "natural" attachments permit insertion without reduction of orifice size or annular area. Calcification of the contiguous wall of aortic or pulmonary homografts is relatively frequent but has no apparent ill effect.[34,36,37] Homograft valve function is usually excellent for 15 to 20 years after installation, after which a 10 to 20% incidence of homograft failure begins, with continued failure (fibrocalcific thickening) beyond 20 years.[36] The chief index of suspicion of fibrocalcific thickening of a homograft valve that might be amenable to balloon dilatation is an increase in the duration of the associated systolic murmur. The length of the murmur is what arouses suspicion of progressive obstruction that may be amenable to balloon dilatation. It is therefore important to characterize the systolic murmur clearly just after the valve is inserted. Because normally functioning homograft valves do not generate sounds as they open (analogous to normal outflow valves), it is the closing sound (or its absence) that relates to mobility or immobility.

Xenografts

Exogenous bioprosthetic materials from animal sources — xenografts — are prepared and preserved by fixing the tissue with glutaraldehyde or other chemical fixatives, by exposing the tissues to high pressures, or by a combination of these two processes.[34] The most important xenograft cardiac bioprostheses are the porcine aortic and bovine

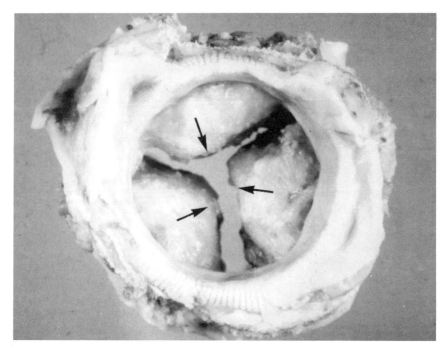

Figure 4.23 Fibrocalcific degeneration of an Ionescu-Shiley pericardial bioprosthetic aortic valve removed from a 19-year-old male 4 years after insertion. The specimen is seen from its ventricular aspect. All three leaflets (*arrows*) are calcified.

pericardial valves that are composite biologic and synthetic devices hand sewn to a synthetic, cloth-covered stent.[38] These xenografts have the advantages of wide ranges of size, ready availability, and sewing rings that are part of the stenting device. A shortcoming is that the stent and sewing ring reduce the effective valve orifice in comparison to that of the native annulus, so that pressure gradients in excess of 15 to 20 mmHg across xenograft valves in the aortic position are relatively frequent, especially in small patients. Long-term function of xenografts is not as good as that of homograft valves and is significantly related to the patient's age at the time of placement (Fig. 4.23). When a xenograft valve is inserted in patients aged 35 years or older, the failure rate 10 years after implantation falls to between 10 and 20%. Xenografts possess even greater durability in patients over 65 years of age. These features should be taken into account in assessing the probability of xenograft obstruction that might be responsive to balloon dilatation.[39,40]

In addition to the general characteristics of prosthetic valves already outlined, there are important differences in how prosthetic valves perform in different locations.[34] Bioprostheses are preferred for replacement of right-sided valves (Fig. 4.24). Xenograft bioprosthetic valves are usually preferred for replacement of the tricuspid valve (or systemic atrioventricular valve). Homograft valves may be preferred for replacement of the pulmonary valve, but there is limited experience using homograft

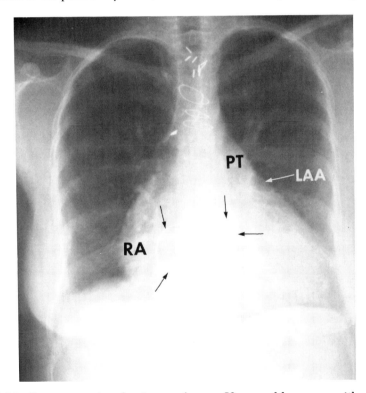

Figure 4.24 Posteroanterior chest x-ray from a 56-year-old woman with rheumatic mitral stenosis and tricuspid stenosis. The mitral valve had been replaced with a 33-mm Bjork-Shiley valve, and the tricuspid valve had been replaced with a 35-mm porcine valve. The mitral prothesis continued to function as designed, but the tricuspid prosthesis developed degenerative obstruction. The right atrium (*RA*) is conspicuously enlarged. The left cardiac border is straight because of the left atrial appendage (*LAA*). *PT*—pulmonary trunk.

valves sewn to a stent for tricuspid valve replacement. A homograft valve in the systemic arterial circulation offers the advantages of increased durability in comparison to that of a xenograft valve and less risk of thromboembolism in comparison to that of a mechanical valve. In the aortic location, homograft valves are being inserted frequently, according to availability. However, the use of homograft valves in the mitral position is limited, and poses formidable technical problems.

Extracardiac Conduits

A conduit or "tube graft" can be valved or nonvalved.[34] Nonvalved conduits are used for connections between the right ventricle and the pulmonary artery when a low to normal postoperative pulmonary arterial pressure is anticipated. Such conduits are not dealt with here. Synthetic conduits containing mechanical or bioprosthetic valves have been used extensively and with considerable success, although complication rates are relatively high.[41] Pseudointimal thickening related to the use of cloth conduits is apparently increased considerably by the presence of a valve within the conduit.[34] Pseudointimal proliferation near the prosthetic valve is believed to be due to turbulence and may result in obstruction of the conduit per se or obstruction or dysfunction of the valve within the conduit. The distinction is important, because conduit obstruction may be amenable to balloon dilatation, but valvular obstruction is not.[41,42] A progressive increase in the length of a systolic murmur can be caused by obstruction of the conduit, by obstruction of the valve within it, or both. Homograft valve conduits represent a significant step forward because natural arterial walls are not subject to pseudointimal thickening, because progressive internal obstruction of the homograft conduit is uncommon, and because the homograft valve leaflets are not prone to the same degree of degeneration as are the glutaraldehyde-preserved leaflets of the xenograft valve. Homograft valve conduits are expected to last longer than 15 to 20 years before valve dysfunction occurs, and it is hoped that balloon dilatation of an obstructed homograft valve in right-sided conduits will permit further longevity of the prosthesis. An increase in the length of a murmur within the conduit can be assigned to the valve rather than the conduit alone. However, external compression may alter the function of the prosthesis because the homograft valve does not have a rigid annulus. Compression can either distort the prosthesis and render the valve incompetent or compress the conduit itself. A long systolic murmur may therefore be a reflection of conduit compression that is not amenable to balloon dilatation.[41]

Progressive obstruction of a bioprosthesis in the tricuspid location in sinus rhythm is suspected by an increase in the A wave in the jugular venous pulse and by a lower left sternal edge presystolic murmur that selectively augments during inspiration. With the advent of atrial fibrillation, the A wave disappears, the V wave crest increases, the Y descent remains gentle, and the lower left sternal edge murmur that augments with inspiration is confined to middiastole. Obstruction of a bioprosthesis is likely to come to light sooner in the mitral location than in the tricuspid location because of the symptoms induced by pulmonary venous congestion.[39,40] Middiastolic or presystolic murmurs across the obstructed systemic atrioventricular valve prosthesis are, as a rule, less readily identified than are the diastolic murmurs of equivalent degrees of obstruction in patients with native mitral valve stenosis. The absence of an opening sound of the prosthesis has no bearing on the auscultatory assessment of the presence or degree of obstruction or of valve mobility.

For further discussion of balloon dilatation of conduits and conduit valves the reader is referred to Chapter 18.

REFERENCES

1. Coombs CF: *Rheumatic Heart Disease*. Bristol: John Wright & Sons Ltd, 1924.

2. Wood P: An appreciation of mitral stenosis, Part I: clinical features. *Br Med J*. 1:1051–1063, 1954.

3. Perloff JK: Pregnancy and cardiovascular disease. In: Braunwald E, ed. *Heart Disease*. 3rd ed. Philadelphia: WB Saunders Co, 1988, pp 1848–1869.

4. Mangione JA, de M Zuliani MF, Del Castillo JM, et al: Percutaneous double balloon mitral valvuloplasty in pregnant women. *Am J Cardiol*. 64:99–102, 1989.

5. Kronzon I, Tunick PA, Glassman E, et al: Transesophageal echocardiography to detect atrial clots in candidates for percutaneous transseptal mitral balloon valvuloplasty. *J Am Coll Cardiol*. 16:1320–1322, 1990.

6. Corvisart JN: Essai sur les maladies et les lésions organiques de coeur et des gros vaisseaux. Paris: 1806, p. 236. (ref 297 In McKusick VA: *Cardiovascular Sound in Health and Disease*. Baltimore: Williams & Wilkins Co, 1958).

7. Perloff JK: *Physical Examination of the Heart and Circulation*. 2nd ed. Philadelphia: WB Saunders Co, 1990.

8. Perloff JK: *Clinical Recognition of Congenital Heart Disease*. Philadelphia: WB Saunders Co, 1987.

9. Perloff JK, Harvey WP: Clinical recognition of tricuspid stenosis. *Circulation*. 22:346–364, 1960.

10. Roberts WC: The congenitally bicuspid aortic valve. A study of 85 autopsy cases. *Am J Cardiol*. 26:72–83, 1970.

11. Da Vinci L: *Leonardo on the Human Body*. New York: Dover Publications, 1983.

12. Subramanian R, Olson LJ, Edwards WD: Surgical pathology of pure aortic stenosis: a study of 374 cases. *Mayo Clin Proc*. 59:683–690, 1984.

13. Caulfield WH, de Leon AC Jr, Perloff JK, et al: The clinical significance of the fourth heart sound in aortic stenosis. *Am J Cardiol*. 28:179–182, 1971.

14. Roberts WC, Perloff JK, Costantino T: Severe valvular aortic stenosis in patients over 65 years of age. A clinicopathologic study. *Am J Cardiol*. 27:497–506, 1971.

15. Perloff JK: Clinical recognition of aortic stenosis. The physical signs and differential diagnosis of the various forms of obstruction to left ventricular outflow. *Progr Cardiovasc Dis*. 10:323–352, 1968.

16. Jarmakani JM, Isabel-Jones JB: Cardiac catheterization as a therapeutic intervention. In: Perloff JK, Child JS, eds. *Congenital Heart Disease in Adults*. Philadelphia: WB Saunders Co, 1991, pp 224–238.

17. Falcone MW, Roberts WC, Morrow AG, et al: Congenital aortic stenosis resulting from a unicommissural valve. Clinical and anatomic features in twenty-one adult patients. *Circulation*. 44:272–280, 1971.

18. Vollebergh FEMG, Becker AE: Minor congenital variations of cusp size in tricuspid aortic valves. Possible link with isolated aortic stenosis. *Br Heart J*. 39:1006–1011, 1977.

19. Gallavardin L, Ravault P: Le souffle de rétrécissement aortique pent changer de timbre et devenir musical dans sa propagation apexienne. *Lyon Med*. 135:523–529, 1925.

20. Perloff JK: Assessment of structural abnormalities and blood flow. In: Hurst JW, ed. *The Heart*. 7th ed. New York: McGraw-Hill, 1990, pp. 301–319.

21. Lababidi Z: Aortic balloon valvuloplasty. *Am Heart J*. 106:751–752, 1983.

22. Kulick DL, Kawanishi DT, Reid CL, et al: Catheter balloon valvuloplasty in adults, Part I: Aortic stenosis. *Curr Probl Cardiol*. 15:353–395, 1990.

23. Holland K, Santinga J, Lee L, et al: Angiographic determination of valve type predicts

hemodynamic response to percutaneous balloon aortic valvuloplasty. *Circulation*. 76 (suppl IV):IV-189, 1987.

24. Isner JM: Aortic valvuloplasty: are balloon-dilated valves all they are "cracked" up to be? *Mayo Clin Proc*. 63:830–834, 1988.

25. Meliones JN, Beekman RH, Rocchini AP, et al: Balloon valvuloplasty for recurrent aortic stenosis after surgical valvotomy in childhood: immediate and follow-up studies. *J Am Coll Cardiol*. 13:1106–1110, 1989.

26. Levine MJ, Berman AD, Safian RD, et al: Palliation of valvular aortic stenosis by balloon valvuloplasty as preoperative preparation for noncardiac surgery. *Am J Cardiol*. 62:1309–1310, 1988.

27. Desnoyers MR, Salem DN, Rosenfield K, et al: Treatment of cardiogenic shock by emergency aortic balloon valvuloplasty. *Ann Intern Med*. 108:833–835, 1988.

28. Abrahams DG, Wood P: Pulmonary stenosis with normal aortic root. *Br Heart J*. 13:519–548, 1951.

29. Marantz PM, Huhta JC, Mullins CE, et al: Results of balloon valvuloplasty in typical and dysplastic pulmonary valve stenosis: Doppler echocardiographic follow-up. *J Am Coll Cardiol*. 12:476–479, 1988.

30. Sherman W, Hershman R, Alexopoulos D, et al: Pulmonic balloon valvuloplasty in adults. *Am Heart J*. 119:186–190, 1990.

31. Ali Khan MA, Al-Yousef S, Moore JW, et al: Results of repeat percutaneous balloon valvuloplasty for pulmonary valvar restenosis. *Am Heart J*. 120:878–881, 1990.

32. Rao PS: Balloon pulmonary valvuloplasty: a review. *Clin Cardiol*. 12:55–74, 1989.

33. Thapar MK, Rao PS: Significance of infundibular obstruction following balloon valvuloplasty for valvar pulmonic stenosis. *Am Heart J*. 118:99–103, 1989.

34. Haas G, Laks H, Perloff JK: The selection, use, and long-term effects of prosthetic materials. In: Perloff JK, Child JS: *Congenital Heart Disease in Adults*. Philadelphia: WB Saunders Co, 1991, pp 213–223.

35. Drinkwater DC, Laks H, Perloff JK: Surgical considerations: operation and reoperation. In: Perloff JK, Child JS. *Congenital Heart Disease in Adults*. Philadelphia: WB Saunders Co, 1991, pp 193–212.

36. Shabbo FP, Wain WH, Ross DN: Right ventricular outflow reconstruction with aortic homograft conduit: analysis of the long-term results. *Thorac Cardiovasc Surg*. 28:21–25, 1980.

37. Kay PH, Ross DN: Fifteen years' experience with the aortic homograft: the conduit of choice for right ventricular outflow tract reconstruction. *Ann Thorac Surg*. 40:360–364, 1985.

38. Magilligan DJ Jr, Lewis JW Jr, Stein P, et al: The porcine bioprosthetic heart valve: experience at 15 years. *Ann Thorac Surg*. 48:324–330, 1989.

39. Feit F, Stecy PJ, Nachamie MS: Percutaneous balloon valvuloplasty for stenosis of a porcine bioprosthesis in the tricuspid valve position. *Am J Cardiol*. 58:363–364, 1986.

40. Calvo OL, Sobrino N, Gamallo C, et al: Balloon percutaneous valvuloplasty for stenotic bioprosthetic valves in the mitral position. *Am J Cardiol*. 60:736–737, 1987.

41. Agarwal KC, Edwards WD, Feldt RH, et al: Clinicopathological correlates of obstructed right-sided porcine-valved extracardiac conduits. *J Thorac Cardiovasc Surg*. 81:591–601, 1981.

42. Lloyd TR, Marvin WJ Jr, Mahoney LT, et al: Balloon dilation valvuloplasty of bioprosthetic valves in extracardiac conduits. *Am Heart J*. 114:268–274, 1987.

CHAPTER **5**

Electrocardiographic Evaluation

E. WILLIAM HANCOCK

GENERAL ASPECTS

The electrocardiogram (ECG) plays a limited direct role in balloon valvuloplasty for valvular stenosis, but it remains a basic clinical tool in the evaluation of the patient. The clinical assessment of patients with valvular stenosis rests primarily on the history, the physical examination, and the echocardiogram, with cardiac catheterization and angiography as a confirmatory step. The ECG has played a major part in the past in assessing the severity of valvular stenosis and is still useful as a step in the clinical evaluation. The information from the ECG is independent of the other methods of study, and it can often be helpful in deciding whether the more elaborate and expensive procedures such as echocardiography and cardiac catheterization need to be carried out.

Valvular Disease and Cardiac Enlargement

Valvular stenosis causes enlargement (hypertrophy and dilatation) of the cardiac chambers that are proximal to the obstructed valve. The effect is greatest in the chamber that is immediately proximal to the diseased valve, ie, the left ventricle in aortic stenosis, the left atrium in mitral stenosis, the right ventricle in pulmonary valve stenosis, and the right atrium in tricuspid stenosis. However, any of the upstream chambers are likely to become enlarged in advanced disease. Thus, in aortic stenosis there is often left atrial enlargement, and sometimes enlargement of the right-sided chambers. Right ventricular and right atrial enlargement often develop in patients with mitral stenosis, and enlargement of the right atrium as well as the right ventricle is often seen in patients with pulmonary valve stenosis.

The enlargement of the cardiac chambers in valvular stenosis is principally the result of increased pressure work. The pressure work leads to myocardial hypertrophy. The hypertrophy may take the form of increased wall thickness, with the cavity retaining its normal diameter; this condition is seen primarily in the ventricles and is usually termed *concentric hypertrophy*. Often, however, there is some dilatation of the chamber as well, and in some cases the dilatation may be considerable. Since the introduction of echocardiography, which permits useful measurements in vivo of the thickness of the right and left ventricular walls, there has been a tendency to define chamber hypertrophy only in terms of increased thickness of the wall. Cardiac chambers that are dilated but have a normal wall thickness are sometimes spoken of as being dilated but not hypertrophied. However, such a chamber is truly hypertrophied as well as dilated, a condition that is usually termed *eccentric hypertrophy*. A cardiac chamber that is dilated but not hypertrophied would have a less than normal wall thickness. This occurs in the right and left atrium in advanced stages of valvular stenosis, probably because the muscle has undergone degeneration and fibrous replacement. In early stages of mitral and tricuspid stenosis the atria are hypertrophied and not necessarily greatly dilated. This condition is less easily recognized by echocardiography than by electrocardiography, because the former is not well suited to the accurate measurement of variations in thickness of the atrial walls.

The ECG and Cardiac Enlargement

Factors Influencing the QRS Voltage

The major hallmark in the electrocardiogram of chamber enlargement is increased voltage, ie, increase in the voltage of the QRS complex when the ventricles are enlarged and increase in the voltage of the P wave when the atria are enlarged.[1] Although a positive relation between the ECG voltage and the mass of the myocardium may be expected intuitively to occur, the factors that affect the voltage are not well understood. Factors other than the mass of the myocardium clearly affect the voltage significantly. The ECG voltage diminishes with age, not only between childhood and adult life but also over the succeeding decades of later adult life. Men have a higher voltage than women, and thin people have a higher voltage than stout people. Young black men have a higher voltage than young white men. Additional factors may affect the proximity of the chest electrodes to the heart and thereby affect the ECG voltage, among them pulmonary emphysema, pericardial effusion, and previous mastectomy.

Cardiac Dilatation vs Increased Wall Thickness

When enlargement of a cardiac chamber does cause an increase in the ECG voltage, it is not clear whether the increased voltage is most clearly related to the total mass of the myocardium of that chamber, to the thickness of its wall, or to the dimensions of its cavity. Studies correlating the several dimensions of the left ventricle with the ECG have given somewhat conflicting results on this issue. Antman and associates concluded that both dilatation and increased wall thickness had an effect on the voltage, but that dilatation was more important.[2] Devereux and associates concluded, however, that the total mass of the myocardium and the thickness of the wall were the important determinants, with dilatation playing a considerably smaller role.[3] Both of these studies included patients with a wide variety of conditions underlying the left ventricular enlargement. Murphy and associates found that different etiologies of left ventricular enlargement gave different values for the sensitivity of several ECG criteria for enlargement.[4] The QRS voltage was more closely related to the degree of hypertrophy in patients with aortic stenosis or hypertension than it was in patients with coronary artery disease or idiopathic cardiomyopathy. Thus, it is unclear whether the ECG reflects the thickness of the wall, the dimension of the cavity, or the total mass of the myocardium. The terms enlargement and hypertrophy, when used with reference to ECG patterns, are virtually interchangeable.

Conduction Delay Resulting From Enlargement

Increased voltage is not the only effect of enlargement of the cardiac chambers on the ECG. Conduction delay is another important feature. Conduction delay can reflect simply the increased mass of muscle, which requires a longer time to be activated even though the activation process may spread over the heart with a normal velocity. More important is an increase in fibrous tissue that often accompanies hypertrophy, with the likelihood that the presence of fibrous tissue can delay the velocity of the spread of electrical activation.

Abnormalities of the ST Segments and T Waves

Another aspect of the ECG in patients with enlargement of the cardiac chambers is the abnormality of the ST segment and the T wave. The T wave axis moves toward a position that is farther from the axis of the QRS complex than normal. This can be described in terms of a widening of the QRS-T angle. The most typical abnormality is inversion of the T wave in those leads that have predominant R waves that reflect the activation of the enlarged chamber. There is also a downsloping depression of the ST segment, with an upward convex pattern. The abnormality is often loosely referred to as "strain," following Barnes' description of its occurrence primarily in patients with uncontrolled hypertension.[5]

Many authors have considered ischemia to be the cause of the secondary ST-T abnormality, postulating that the hypertrophied ventricle was unable to increase its coronary blood supply to the extent necessary to supply the increased muscle mass adequately. Other theories, however, suggest the possible source of the ST-T abnormality in a prolonged duration of the action potential of the outer layers of the ventricular wall, such that the sequence of repolarization of the various layers of myocardium is significantly altered.[6,7] The prolonged duration of the action potential could result from the increased pressure within the ventricular wall. This issue remains controversial.

Left Ventricular Enlargement

The changes in the ECG that reflect left ventricular enlargement include increased voltage of the QRS complex, a mild degree of delay in activation of the left ventricle, a tendency to left axis deviation, abnormality of the ST segments and T waves, and evidence of left atrial abnormality. Increased QRS voltage is the most specific of these abnormalities for hypertrophy. The other features can be caused by a wide variety of other myocardial abnormalities. The several types of abnormality may be considered separately or may be combined into a point scoring system.

QRS Voltage in Adults

The measurement of QRS voltage for the assessment of left ventricular hypertrophy is a complex matter. No single measurement has proved to be optimal. Indeed, a large number of measurements have been proposed (Table 5.1). At least five or six of these are in common use. In general, QRS voltage criteria have relatively low sensitivity for the detection of left ventricular enlargement, as judged either by measurement of the weight of the chamber at autopsy or by echocardiographic estimation of the left

Table 5.1 SELECTED QRS VOLTAGE CRITERIA FOR LEFT VENTRICULAR HYPERTROPHY IN ADULTS

Measurement	Threshold
R wave amplitude, lead 1	13 mm
R wave lead 1 + S wave lead 3	25 mm
(R-S) lead 1 + (S-R) lead 3	17 mm
S wave lead aVR	14 mm
R wave lead aVL	7 mm
R wave lead aVF	19 mm
S wave lead V1	24 mm
S wave lead V3	25 mm
R wave lead V5	26 mm
R wave lead V6	20 mm
S wave V1 + R wave V5 or V6	35 mm
S wave V3 + R wave aVL	
Men	28 mm
Women	20 mm

ventricular wall thickness and cavity diameter. Furthermore, the criteria must be made age-specific to be useful. Further refinements would also adjust for gender, ethnicity, body weight, chest wall thickness, and lung volume.

The Sokolow and Lyon index, in which the S wave amplitude in lead V_1 is added to the larger of the R wave amplitudes in V_5 or V_6, is the single most useful criterion.[8] The upper normal limit is 35 mm (3.5 mV) in people over the age of 35 years. Some authors use a modified Sokolow and Lyon index in which the deeper S wave in V_1 or V_2 is added to the R wave in V_5 or V_6; however, the upper normal limit for this index would be approximately 45 mm in people over the age of 35 years, and this index would not improve the sensitivity or the specificity.

The amplitude of the R wave in lead aVL is a single measurement that has considerable value. Sokolow and Lyon suggested an upper normal limit of 11 mm (1.1 mV), but the sensitivity would be only about 10% at this threshold. At a threshold of 7 mm (0.7 mV) the sensitivity improves to 23%, with a specificity of 96%. One qualification in the use of this measurement is that if the QRS axis is abnormally leftward, an amplitude of about 13 mm (1.3 mV) should be required to diagnose left ventricular hypertrophy.

The sum of the amplitudes of the R wave in lead 1 and the S wave in lead 3, with an upper normal limit of 25 mm (2.5 mV), is another simple index of considerable value. A more complex index proposed by Sir Thomas Lewis $(R_1 - S_1) + (S_3 - R_3)$ provides better discrimination, with a sensitivity of about 18%.[9] The upper normal limit for this index is 17 mm (1.7 mV). Criteria that use the voltage in the limb leads are particularly useful in elderly patients.

A more recently proposed voltage index combines the R wave amplitude in lead aVL and the S wave amplitude in lead V_3 (10). The upper normal limit is 28 mm in men and 20 mm in women. This is the only commonly used criterion that takes advantage of the known differences in QRS voltage between adult men and women.

Another voltage measurement that may be useful is the total amplitude of the QRS complexes in all 12 leads.[11,12]

QRS Voltage in Children

The QRS voltage in infants and children differs greatly from that in adults. Criteria for left ventricular hypertrophy must be based on the range of normal voltage for specific age groups. Simplified ranges are given in Tables 5.2 and 5.3. Between ages 16 and 35 years it is rather unreliable to use the QRS voltage alone as an indication of left ventricular hypertrophy, because the normal range is wide enough to encompass most of the range of high voltages that are encountered in left ventricular hypertrophy.

Conduction delay in the enlarged ventricle may be manifested as a slight prolongation of the total duration of the QRS complex. This is rarely of much value in the diagnosis of left ventricular hypertrophy; slight changes are nonspecific, and a marked prolongation is usually considered to represent bundle branch block or some other form of primary intraventricular conduction defect. The most convenient measurement of prolonged ventricular activation due to ventricular enlargement is the interval from the beginning of the QRS complex to the peak of the R wave in V_5 or V_6. The upper normal limit for this measurement, termed the *intrinsicoid deflection* or *ventricular activation time*, is approximately 0.04 s. The use of this measurement is derived from studies using leads directly on the surface of the heart, where the arrival of the wave of excitation at the site of the electrode is marked by the end of the upward

Table 5.2 MAXIMUM NORMAL VALUES FOR THE AMPLITUDE OF R WAVES IN SELECTED ECG LEADS IN CHILDREN AND YOUNG ADULTS

Age	ECG Lead								
	1	2	3	aVL	aVF	V_1	V_2	V_5	V_6
0–1 mo	8	14	16	7	14	25	30	30	21
1–6 mo	13	24	20	8	20	20	30	30	20
6–12 mo	16	27	20	10	16	20	28	30	20
1–3 yr	16	23	20	10	20	18	25	36	24
3–8 yr	15	22	20	10	19	18	26	36	24
8–12 yr	15	24	24	10	20	16	22	36	24
12–16 yr	13	24	24	12	21	16	19	33	22
16–34 yr	13	25	22	9	24	14	21	33	21

Table 5.3 MAXIMUM NORMAL VALUES FOR AMPLITUDE OF S WAVES IN SELECTED ECG LEADS IN CHILDREN AND YOUNG ADULTS

Age	ECG Lead				
	1	V_1	V_2	V_5	V_6
0–1 mo	10	20	35	30	12
1–6 mo	9	18	30	26	6
6–12 mo	9	16	30	20	4
1–3 yr	8	27	34	16	4
3–8 yr	8	30	38	14	4
8–12 yr	8	26	38	17	4
12–16 yr	8	24	48	16	5
16–34 yr	6	23	36	14	13

deflection and the beginning of the downward deflection, the intrinsic deflection. Prolongation of the ventricular activation time is mainly useful when the measurement is combined with at least one QRS voltage abnormality, since an isolated prolongation of ventricular activation time is probably more likely to indicate disease of the conduction system alone.

Left Axis Deviation

A tendency to left axis deviation is often listed as a criterion of left ventricular enlargement, although it is doubtful whether enlargement in itself truly deviates the axis very far leftward. The normal QRS axis of 0 to 90° reflects the large predominance of the mass of the left ventricle over the mass of the right ventricle in the normal heart. When the left ventricle becomes hypertrophied, the predominance of the mass of the left ventricle is hardly different from the normal ratio. Left anterior fascicular block, on the other hand, causes abnormal left axis deviation by delaying the activation of the lateral and superior region of the left ventricle. In adults with the common forms of heart disease, there is a close relation between left ventricular enlargement and left anterior fascicular block, to the extent that abnormal left axis deviation is a useful marker for left ventricular enlargement.

In children the predominance of the left ventricle over the right ventricle is less than in adults, and the range of the normal QRS axis is smaller than in adults. Thus, left axis deviation is more often a useful indication of left ventricular enlargement in children than it is in adults.

Abnormalities of the ST Segments and T Waves

The most characteristic abnormality of the ST segments and T waves is the pattern of downsloping depression of the ST segment and deep inversion of the T wave that is often termed the strain pattern (Fig. 5.1). In fact, a wide variety of repolarization abnormalities occur in left ventricular hypertrophy, but many of these patterns are relatively nonspecific. Many patients show only repolarization abnormalities with normal QRS voltage. Since myocardial ischemia, intraventricular conduction delay, and digitalis can cause similar repolarization abnormalities, it is often appropriate to interpret such changes as consistent with hypertrophy, digitalis, ischemia, or (if there is any prolongation of the QRS duration or the ventricular activation time) intraventricular conduction delay.

In young adults with left ventricular hypertrophy, the QRS axis is often in the range of 60 to 90°, rather than the range of 30° to −30° that is more usual in older patients. In the presence of a rightward axis, the abnormalities of the ST segments and the T waves are often more prominent in the inferior limb leads than in the lateral limb leads or in the precordial leads (Fig. 5.2). These young patients are also more likely to show prominent Q waves in the lateral leads, reflecting septal hypertrophy, whereas older patients more often show diminished or absent Q waves in the lateral leads, reflecting myocardial fibrosis.

Scoring Systems for Left Ventricular Hypertrophy

Because many individual measurements have some value in indicating left ventricular hypertrophy but are applicable in relatively few patients, it is useful to combine several criteria into point scoring systems or other complex formulae. Few clinicians or electrocardiographers find such formulas useful enough to warrant their routine

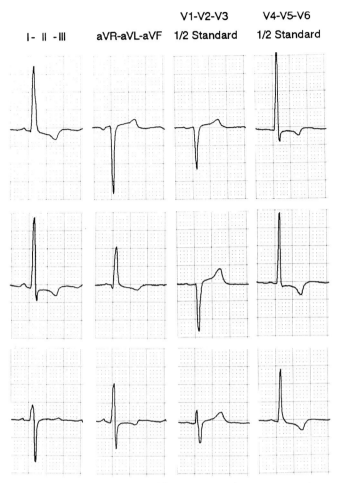

Figure 5.1 12-lead ECG in a 45-year-old woman with severe aortic stenosis. All of the standard QRS voltage criteria are exceeded. In addition, the abnormalities of the ST segments and T waves are characteristic. The axis lies in the leftward portion of the normal range. The pattern is characteristic of relatively severe left ventricular hypertrophy as it is seen in adults in the older age groups with systolic (pressure) overloading of the left ventricle.

clinical use, but they can easily be incorporated into computer programs. With the ever widening use of computer-assisted ECG interpretation, the formulas have achieved greater use in recent years.

The most widely used point scoring system is that of Romhilt and Estes (Table 5.4).[13] This system includes the QRS voltage in either the limb leads or the precordial leads, along with considerable emphasis on ST-T abnormalities and P wave abnormalities. It has a sensitivity of approximately 60%, with a very high specificity. The Romhilt and Estes system has been widely used in clinical research. MacFarlane and Lawrie have modified it by specifying different ranges of QRS voltage for men and women in four different age groups.[14]

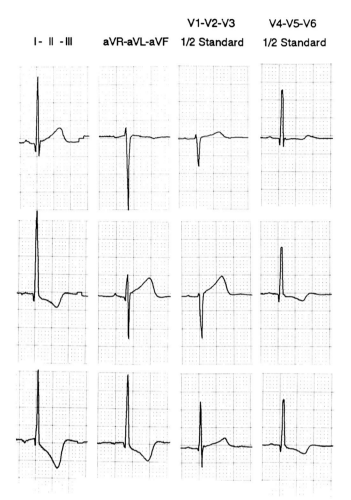

Figure 5.2 12-lead ECG in a 36-year-old man with severe aortic stenosis. The QRS axis is approximately 70° in the frontal plane. The secondary abnormalities of the ST segments and T waves are most prominent in the inferior limb leads.

Casale and associates developed regression equations based on the QRS voltage in leads aVL and V_3, the T wave in lead V_1, the QRS duration, and the P wave in lead V_1.[10] Different formulas for men and women and for patients in sinus rhythm and atrial fibrillation are provided.

Systolic and Diastolic Overload Patterns

Systolic (pressure) overwork of the left ventricle has been considered to cause a different ECG pattern of hypertrophy than diastolic (volume) overwork. The principal difference is that depression of the ST segment and inversion of the T wave occur predominantly in pressure overwork, whereas in volume overwork the T waves remain upright and are even taller than usual. Another difference is that there are unusually deep, but narrow, Q waves in those leads that have tall R waves in patients with volume overwork. In contrast, patients with left ventricular hypertrophy due to

Table 5.4 THE ROMHILT-ESTES SCORING SYSTEM

Criterion	Threshold	Points
QRS Voltage		
R or S wave in any limb lead	20 mm or more	3
or		
S in V_1 or S in V_2	30 mm or more	
or		
R in V_5 or R in V_6	30 mm or more	
ST-T Abnormalities		
Typical of LVH, without digitalis	Present	3
or		
Typical of LVH, with digitalis	Present	1
P Wave Abnormality		
P terminal force in lead V_1	1×1 mm	3
QRS Axis		
Left axis deviation	$-30°$ or more	2
QRS Duration		
Total QRS duration	0.090 s or more	1
Ventricular activation time V_5 or V_6	0.050 s or more	1

A total of 5 points indicates a high probability of left ventricular hypertrophy

pressure overwork often have less conspicuous septal Q waves, even in instances where the QRS duration and the ventricular activation time are normal.

The electrocardiographic differences between pressure and volume overwork are best seen in children and young adults with congenital heart disease, particularly when conditions with left-to-right shunts such as simple ventricular septal defect or patent ductus arteriosus are compared with congenital aortic valve stenosis. Differences between aortic stenosis and aortic regurgitation are also seen. Older adult patients do not show consistently different ECG patterns in aortic stenosis and aortic regurgitation.

Left Ventricular Hypertrophy and Intraventricular Conduction Delay

LEFT BUNDLE BRANCH BLOCK. The diagnosis of left ventricular hypertrophy in the presence of complete left bundle branch block has traditionally been considered difficult or impossible. The problem has been muddled by the fact that nearly all patients with left bundle branch block have left ventricular hypertrophy at autopsy, even though some living patients are seen who appear to have normal structure and function of the left ventricle despite the presence of left bundle branch block. Studies in recent years with echocardiography indicate that some of the same QRS voltage criteria that are useful in identifying left ventricular hypertrophy in the presence of normal ventricular activation are equally useful in the presence of left bundle branch block.[15-17] The point scoring systems should not be used, however, since the abnormalities of the ST segments and the T waves can be secondary to the intraventricular conduction delay.

LESSER DEGREES OF INTRAVENTRICULAR CONDUCTION DELAY.   Many ECGs show patterns that combine certain of the features of left ventricular hypertrophy and left bundle branch block (Fig. 5.3). They have in common an increased QRS voltage, some widening of the QRS complex, absent Q waves in leads V_5 and V_6, and typical secondary ST-T abnormalities. The QRS complex is 0.12 to 0.14 s in duration, which is wide enough to represent complete left bundle branch block, but there is little or no notching or slurring of the QRS complex. Such patterns are usually seen in patients who have organic heart disease of a type that would be expected to cause left ventricular enlargement. Since the presence of left ventricular hypertrophy can be inferred with high accuracy in such cases, it is reasonable to interpret ECGs of this type as left ventricular hypertrophy with associated intraventricular conduction delay, even though they meet the usual stated criteria for left bundle branch block. When

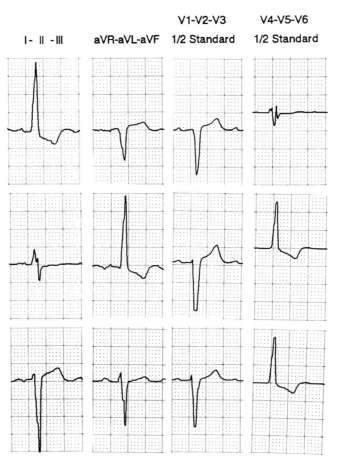

Figure 5.3 12-lead ECG in a 65-year-old woman with severe aortic stenosis. The characteristic increased QRS voltage and secondary abnormalities of the ST segments and T waves are evident. In addition, the QRS complex is widened to approximately 0.12 sec and the ventricular activation time is prolonged to approximately 0.06 sec in leads V_5 and V_6. Such patterns are best designated as left ventricular hypertrophy with secondary repolarization abnormality and associated intraventricular conduction delay.

there is also abnormal left axis deviation it is appropriate to add this to the description, rather than diagnose left anterior fascicular block, since the intraventricular conduction delay is not limited to the left anterior fascicle.

Right Ventricular Hypertrophy

Like left ventricular hypertrophy, the ECG diagnosis of right ventricular hypertrophy rests on several types of abnormality, including increased QRS voltage, axis deviation, delayed ventricular activation, secondary ST-T abnormalities, and P wave abnormalities. In general the electrocardiographic diagnosis of right ventricular hypertrophy is even less sensitive than that for left ventricular hypertrophy because of the relatively small contribution of the right ventricle to the genesis of the QRS complex. The right ventricle has less than 20% of the total ventricular myocardial mass; it probably requires at least a twofold increase in right ventricular mass to alter the right and left ventricular balance appreciably. Overt ECG patterns of right ventricular hypertrophy are seen consistently in congenital conditions in which the pressure work of the right ventricle is equal to or greater than that of the left ventricle, and has been so since birth. In these conditions the right ventricular dominance that was present in fetal and neonatal life has not regressed. On the other hand, in many conditions that are acquired during adult life the pressure work of the right ventricle remains less than that of the left ventricle, and the ECG patterns of right ventricular hypertrophy are less overt.

QRS Voltage

The most direct result in the ECG of right ventricular hypertrophy is an increase in the amplitude of those QRS forces that reflect activation of the right ventricle.[18] This activation proceeds in a direction that is anterior, downward, and rightward, but the anterior direction predominates. Lead V_1 is the lead that is closest to the right ventricle and also the lead that most directly reflects the anteriorly directed forces of right ventricular activation. Thus, lead V_1 is the lead that is most likely to show evidence of right ventricular hypertrophy, in the form of an abnormally tall R wave.

Additional QRS voltage criteria that are useful in the diagnosis of right ventricular hypertrophy in adults are given in Table 5.5. An amplitude of more than 5 to 7 mm

Table 5.5 SELECTED QRS VOLTAGE CRITERIA FOR RIGHT VENTRICULAR HYPERTROPHY IN ADULTS

Criterion	Threshold
R wave V_1	>7 mm
S wave V_1	<2 mm
R:S ratio V_1	>1.0
S wave V_5, V_6	>7 mm
R wave V_5, V_6	<5 mm
R:S ratio V_5, V_6	<1.0
R wave V_1 + S wave V_5, V_6	>10.5 mm
Ventricular activation time, lead V_1	>0.04s
Right axis deviation	>110°

Table 5.6 DIFFERENTIAL DIAGNOSIS OF PROMINENT R WAVE IN LEAD V$_1$

Condition	QRS Duration	Timing of Peak R Wave	T Wave in V$_1$
Right ventricular hypertrophy	Up to 0.12	Early	Often inverted
Right bundle branch block	More than 0.12	Late	Inverted
Posterior infarction	Normal	Early	Upright
Early transition	Normal	Early	Usually upright
Wolff-Parkinson-White syndrome	More than 0.1	Variable	Variable

(5.0 to 7.0 mV) in lead V$_1$ can usually be taken as evidence of right ventricular hypertrophy. However, the ratio of R wave to S wave amplitude in lead V$_1$ is a more useful index. The R:S ratio should be less than 1.0 in adults. The differential diagnosis of an R:S ratio greater than 1.0 includes right bundle branch block, posterior infarction, and a normal or positional early precordial transition. Several additional features in the ECG, as well as clinical features, are usually sufficient to resolve this differential diagnosis (see Table 5.6).

QRS Voltage in Children

Tables 5.2 and 5.3 summarized the range of normal amplitude of the R and S waves in selected leads that are useful in assessing right ventricular hypertrophy. Table 5.7 gives the range of normal R:S ratio in lead V$_1$ in children. The R wave can exceed the S wave amplitude in normal children up to approximately 8 years of age.

In the most typical instances, the peak R wave in lead V$_1$ in patients with right ventricular hypertrophy is early in the QRS complex, unlike the situation in right bundle branch block where it is late in the QRS complex. Right ventricular hypertrophy may, however, present an RSR' pattern, where the R' is the peak R wave. Right ventricular hypertrophy that causes this pattern is usually relatively mild and/or is due to a condition that is primarily one of dilatation of the right ventricle, as in atrial septal defect. The RSR' pattern also tends to reflect hypertrophy that mainly involves the infundibular (outflow) area of the right ventricle. The infundibular area is among the last regions of the heart to be activated, so that increased QRS forces from this area are represented as late R waves, often as an R' in lead V$_1$. Incomplete right bundle branch block is often invoked to explain ECG patterns with RSR' in lead V$_1$ that are in fact due to right ventricular hypertrophy.

QRS Axis	Terminal Slur of QRS	Clinical Setting
Rightward	None or slight	Pulmonary vascular disease, mitral stenosis, or pulmonary stenosis
Variable	Prominent	Variable
Often leftward	None	Angina or myocardial infarction
Normal	None	Usually normal
Variable	Variable	Normal or paroxysmal tachycardia

Table 5.7 RANGE OF NORMAL R:S RATIO IN LEAD V$_1$ IN CHILDREN AND YOUNG ADULTS

Age	R:S ratio, Lead V$_1$
0–1 mo	0.3–19
1–6 mo	0.3–12
6–12 mo	0.3–6.0
1–3 yr	0.3–2.0
3–8 yr	0.1–2.0
8–12 yr	0.1–1.0
12–16 yr	0.1–1.0
16–34 yr	0.1–1.0

The QR Pattern in V$_1$

Another feature of right ventricular hypertrophy is the pattern of a small Q wave followed by a tall R wave in lead V$_1$. The Q wave reflects hypertrophy of the right ventricular portion of the ventricular septum. The septum is activated in both the right-to-left and left-to-right directions, from Purkinje branches of both the right and left proximal bundle branches, but the left-to-right normally predominates. Thus, the initial deflection in lead V$_1$ is normally upright. Loss of the normal initial R wave in lead V$_1$ caused by septal infarction or to left bundle branch block is usually easily differentiated from right ventricular hypertrophy. Another reason for a Q wave in lead V$_1$ is dilatation of the right atrium, related to a condition such as severe tricuspid regurgitation, such that the V_1 position lies over the right atrium rather than the right ventricle. In this situation the entire V_1 complex is usually negative.

Right Axis Deviation

Deviation of the QRS axis rightward is an important sign of right ventricular hypertrophy, more so than is leftward deviation as a sign of left ventricular hypertrophy. This reflects the fact that right ventricular hypertrophy alters the balance of right and left ventricular mass in a qualitative way, whereas left ventricular hypertrophy causes only a quantitative change in the balance, perpetuating the normal left ventricular dominance. The right axis deviation that results from right ventricular hypertrophy is often mild, falling just outside the normal range or near the upper limit of the normal range. However, it is exceptional to see left axis deviation in the presence of right ventricular hypertrophy.

Prominent S Waves in Left Precordial Leads

A third feature of the QRS complex in right ventricular hypertrophy is the persistence of prominent S waves across the precordial leads through V_6. An S wave that is 7 mm or more in amplitude is a useful indication of right ventricular hypertrophy. The prominent S waves reflect increased representation of forces that activate the right ventricle late in the QRS complex.

Abnormalities of the ST Segments and T waves

Abnormalities of the ST segments and T waves, much like the "strain" pattern in left ventricular hypertrophy, also occur in right ventricular hypertrophy, most prominently in the right precordial leads. In contrast with left ventricular hypertrophy, it is relatively unusual to see right ventricular hypertrophy manifested solely by ST-T abnormalities in chronic cardiopulmonary syndromes. The ST-T abnormalities in right ventricular hypertrophy are probably less likely to result from myocardial ischemia than those of left ventricular hypertrophy; their occurrence in situations of markedly increased pressure overwork of the right ventricle favors the theory of altered action potential duration and sequence of repolarization as the mechanism for such changes.

Right Atrial Abnormality

Evidence of right atrial abnormality occurs frequently in patients with right ventricular hypertrophy. This occurs primarily in conditions with pressure overwork of the right ventricle, and it reflects the reduced diastolic compliance of the right ventricle, the elevated right ventricular end-diastolic pressure, and the consequent pressure overwork of the right atrium.

Scoring Systems for Right Ventricular Hypertrophy

Although the multiplicity of criteria for right ventricular hypertrophy would suggest value for a point scoring system, such a system has not been developed to a stage of general usefulness.

Right Ventricular Hypertrophy and Intraventricular Conduction Delay

In complete right bundle branch block the voltage of the R' wave in lead V_1 can be very high in patients without right ventricular hypertrophy. This reflects the fact that the period of 0.09 to 0.12 s of the QRS complex in complete right bundle branch block represents activation of the right ventricle that is unopposed by any simultaneous forces activating the left ventricle. Therefore, it is unreliable to use voltage criteria to diagnose right ventricular hypertrophy in the presence of complete right bundle branch block. However, some ECGs in patients with severe right ventricular hypertrophy also meet the conventional criteria for complete right bundle branch block. It is best to refer to these patterns as having right ventricular hypertrophy with secondary repolarization abnormality and associated intraventricular conduction delay.

Left Atrial Abnormality

Hemodynamic overload of the left atrium causes changes in the P waves that reflect atrial myocardial hypertrophy, dilatation, or conduction delay. In the electrocardiographic sense, enlargement of the atrium may connote hypertrophy, dilatation, or a combination; in fact, conduction delay within the atrium may be more important than either as a cause of the abnormalities of the P wave. Hence, the noncommittal term atrial abnormality may be preferable to the terms hypertrophy, dilatation, enlargement, or overload, which are virtually synonymous when used in an electrocardiographic context.[19]

Left atrial abnormality is characterized by a delay in activation of the left atrium and an increase in amplitude of the forces that represent left atrial activation. The three cardinal features of the abnormal P wave result directly from this.

1. The total P wave duration is prolonged, because the left atrial activation always finishes later than right atrial activation and constitutes the terminal portion of the P wave.
2. The P wave becomes twin-peaked, because the peaks of the right and left atrial activation are farther separated in time than they are normally.
3. The terminal portion of the P wave is increased in amplitude and is directed more leftward and posteriorly than normal.

Duration of the P Wave
The duration of the P wave should be measured in lead 2, because this lead is most nearly parallel to the mean direction of atrial activation and is least likely to be isoelectric at either the beginning or the end of the P wave. A P wave duration of 0.12 s or greater is a useful indicator of left atrial abnormality.

Since the P wave and P-R interval both vary with age and heart rate, it is useful to consider the ratio of the P wave duration to the P-R segment, the Macruz index.[20] A value for the Macruz index of 1.6 or greater is a good indicator of left atrial abnormality.

Notching of the P Wave
Separation of the peaks that represent right and left atrial activation results in a twin-peaked effect, or notching of the P wave. This sign is especially significant when the two peaks are separated by 0.04 s or more. In a typical case the second peak is higher than the first. Notched P waves are less useful in diagnosis than the other measurements because the phenomenon is somewhat subjective and is dependent on high

I - II - III   V1 - V2 - V6

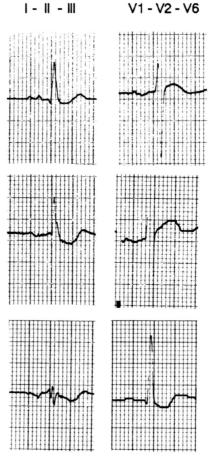

Figure 5.4 Leads I, II, III, and V_1, V_2, V_6 in a patient with mitral stenosis. The P waves are wide and notched and have a leftward axis, but the voltage of the P wave is not conspicuously increased. Such a pattern is more one of intraatrial conduction delay than of left atrial pressure overload as such.

fidelity ECG recording technique. Prominent widening and notching of the P wave, without conspicuous increase in the voltage, probably connotes intraatrial conduction delay more than pressure overload as such (Fig. 5.4).

Abnormality of the P Terminal Force
The most useful of all the criteria for identification of left atrial abnormality is the P terminal force in lead V_1, or the area of the terminal negative portion of the P wave in that lead[21] (Fig. 5.5). A terminal negative component that is 1 mm in duration (0.04 s) and 1 mm in amplitude (0.1 mV) correlates well with the presence of left atrial overload, especially in valvular heart disease such as mitral stenosis. The amplitude is easily measured, but the duration is more difficult, because many P waves slope gradually upward back to the baseline. It may be necessary to extrapolate the first portion of the upslope as a straight line to estimate the duration. A common error is to suppose that any P wave that is purely or predominantly negative in lead V_1 repre-

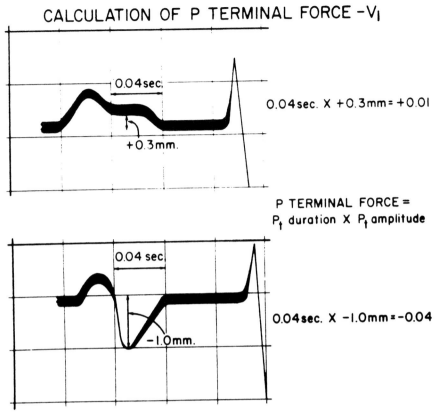

CALCULATION OF P TERMINAL FORCE $-V_1$

$0.04\,\text{sec.} \times +0.3\,\text{mm} = +0.01$

P TERMINAL FORCE =
P$_t$ duration X P$_t$ amplitude

$0.04\,\text{sec.} \times -1.0\,\text{mm} = -0.04$

Figure 5.5 Calculation of the P terminal force in lead V_1. The amplitude and duration of the P wave are measured separately for the initial and terminal components. The P terminal force is the amplitude multiplied by the duration for each component. In the upper example the P terminal force is positive, while in the lower example it is negative. (From: Morris JJ Jr et al: P-wave analysis in valvular heart disease. *Circulation*. 29: 242–252, 1964. With permission.)

sents left atrial abnormality; the abnormal P terminal force must be a full 1 mm both in amplitude and duration to achieve the optimal sensitivity and specificity for the diagnosis of left atrial abnormality.

Technical Problems in P Wave Analysis
Refinement of the ECG criteria for left atrial abnormality has been difficult because of two problems. The standard ECG recording techniques give P waves that are usually barely 1 mm in amplitude and 2 mm in duration. The calibration factors were chosen to display the QRS complex and the T waves optimally, sacrificing a high fidelity display of the P wave. Amplified recordings may be used but are not readily available in the clinical setting. In addition, high amplitude recordings of the P wave are plagued by an unfavorable signal-to-noise ratio. Furthermore, the filters employed by modern ECG recorders may further degrade the fidelity of the P wave in the interest of eliminating artifacts.

The second difficulty is that of the reference standard used to evaluate ECG criteria. Echocardiographic measurements of the diameter of the atrial cavity have been most often used in recent years as a reference standard. However, the echocardiographic diameter is only one aspect of the atrial abnormality, and not necessarily the most important aspect.[22] Variables such as the diastolic compliance of the left ventricle, the left ventricular end-diastolic pressure, and the left atrial mean pressure would probably be more closely related to the ECG changes, but these are more dynamic quantities and change in response to such variables as cardiac output, heart rate, and intravascular volume status.

Right Atrial Abnormality

Right atrial abnormality (enlargement, hypertrophy, overload) prolongs the duration and increases the amplitude of the right atrial portion of the P wave. Since the right atrial activation always begins first, and ends before the end of the left atrial activation, prolongation of the right atrial component does not prolong the total duration of the P wave. Also, instead of separating the two peaks and causing notching of the P wave, delay of the right atrial activation causes the two peaks to be more simultaneous than usual. The simultaneous peaks of right and left atrial activation cause a summation of the P wave voltage, resulting in a tall but narrow P wave. The tall narrow P wave often takes on the appearance of a sharp peak that is recognizable as the hallmark of right atrial abnormality. A P wave amplitude of 2.5 mm or greater in leads 2, 3, or aVF is a useful indicator of right atrial abnormality.

Since the process of activation of the right atrium is directed anteriorly as well as downward, the increased amplitude of the P wave in lead V_1 is upright. The peaked upright P wave is often more prominent in lead V_2 than in V_1.

Right atrial abnormality is more marked in conditions such as pulmonary valve stenosis or primary pulmonary hypertension, in which there is no septal defect communicating with the left side of the heart, than it is in conditions such as the tetralogy of Fallot or Eisenmenger's syndrome, in which such defects are present. This difference occurs even though similar levels of right ventricular systolic pressure, often equal to the systemic pressure level, are present. The difference is that the septal defect provides a limit on the increased afterload that the right ventricle is subject to — in exercise, for example.

P Pulmonale

The P wave that reflects right atrial overload, occurring in conditions such as pulmonary hypertension, pulmonary valve stenosis, or tricuspid stenosis, can be differentiated from the P wave that occurs in various forms of diffuse chronic lung disease, often referred to as P pulmonale. The essential characteristic of P pulmonale is the rightward axis of the P wave, sufficiently rightward for the P wave to be inverted in lead aVL. The rightward axis of the P wave reflects a low diaphragm and a vertical position of the heart because of an overinflated lung. The right atrium is not dilated in most instances of P pulmonale.[23]

Pseudo Left Atrial Abnormality

In some patients, including those with either right atrial overload or with P pulmonale, the P wave may be wholly or predominantly inverted in V_1, thereby suggesting left atrial abnormality. This condition, termed pseudo-P-mitrale, can be recognized by the absence of prolongation of the P wave and the appearance in the limb leads of the characteristic right atrial abnormality.

THE ECG IN AORTIC STENOSIS

The ECG is abnormal in nearly all adult patients with aortic stenosis that is severe enough to require balloon valvuloplasty or surgery. [24,25] The most commonly used Sokolow-Lyon criterion ($S_{V_1} + R_{V_5 \text{ or } V_6}$) is met in 80 to 90% of such cases, and all but a few patients have abnormalities of the ST segments and T waves as well. The ECG has been found to play an important role in a noninvasive point scoring system for evaluating the severity of aortic stenosis.[26] Those patients with aortic stenosis who do have a normal or near-normal ECG usually have a degree of stenosis that is in the moderate rather than the most severe category. In elderly patients who have no symptoms but are identified by routine screening for a systolic murmur, followed up by Doppler echocardiographic estimation of the pressure gradient, the ECG shows definite evidence of left ventricular hypertrophy less frequently[27]. Thus a normal ECG does not rule out significant aortic stenosis, but is certainly an unusual finding.

Echocardiography in optimal circumstances is undoubtedly superior to the ECG in detecting left ventricular hypertrophy. However, because of the difficulty in obtaining satisfactory echocardiographic studies in many patients, particularly elderly patients, the ECG is equally valuable as a clinical tool in day-to-day practice.[28] The thickness of the left ventricular wall can be normal in severe aortic stenosis, even in technically optimal echocardiographic studies; this is most likely to occur when there is some dilatation of the left ventricle.[29]

QRS Voltage as an Indication of the Pressure Gradient
Classification of those adult patients who have significant aortic stenosis into moderate and severe groups on the basis of the ECG is not reliable, however, even though a positive correlation does exist between the pressure gradient and aortic valve area and both the QRS voltage and abnormalities of the ST segments and T waves. Siegel and Roberts noted that the sum of QRS amplitudes in all 12 leads (in mm) approximated the peak systolic pressure in the left ventricle (in mmHg).[11] Thus, subtracting the systolic pressure measured in the arm from the total QRS amplitude in 12 leads gave an approximation of the peak-to-peak aortic systolic pressure gradient. The relationship is useful, but the scatter of values is too wide to allow use of this formula as a reliable indicator of the gradient in individual patients.

Aortic Stenosis in Children
In children with congenital aortic valve stenosis, the ECG is somewhat more likely to be normal than it is in adults with calcific aortic stenosis. A multiinstitutional study on the natural history of congenital heart disease provided considerable information on this issue.[30] The study included 441 patients ranging from 2 to 21 years of age. The stenosis was considered severe in 22 per cent, moderate in 25 per cent, mild in 33 per cent, and trivial in 20 per cent. The most helpful ECG correlation was with the T wave in lead V_6, which was abnormal in about 50 per cent of the severe group and 25 per cent of the moderate group, but was abnormal in less than 5 per cent of those with peak-to-peak systolic gradient smaller than 50 mm Hg. The moderate or severe cases with normal T waves usually showed increased amplitude of the R wave in lead V_6 and a Q wave in V_6 that was absent or less than the usual amplitude.

From the data in the natural history study, Wagner and associates[30] suggested a formula for estimating the pressure gradient from the ECG and the loudness of the systolic murmur:

$$\begin{array}{cccc} \text{LV} - \text{AO gradient} = 13 \times \text{grade of murmur} + & \text{R}_{V_6} & - 6 \times \text{Q}_{V_6} & - 9 \\ \text{(mmHg)} & \text{(scale of 0 to 6)} & \text{(mm)} & \text{(mm)} \end{array}$$

Values of less than 30 were always associated with pressure gradients measured at cardiac catheterization that were in the nonsurgical range, and only 4% of patients with scores less than 45 had measured gradients of 80 mmHg or more.

Overall, about 15% of children with aortic stenosis that is severe enough to require surgery or balloon valvuloplasty have normal or near-normal ECGs. However, increased voltage with normal T waves is consistent with either mild or severe aortic stenosis in children. Young men aged 15 to 30 years are particularly likely to have a nondiagnostic ECG in the presence of aortic stenosis, because their normal range of QRS voltage is very wide and overlaps much of the range of values that occurs in left ventricular hypertrophy. The ECG is more reliable in younger children and in infants.

Treadmill exercise tests often show depression of the ST segments in children with aortic stenosis who have normal ST segments and T waves in the resting ECG, similar to the findings in adults with coronary artery disease. Kveselis and associates considered this finding to be one of the three basic indications for intervention in valvular aortic stenosis, along with the presence of symptoms and of a documented systolic pressure gradient of substantial size.[31]

Coronary Artery Disease and Myocardial Infarction

Associated coronary artery disease is often present in patients over the age of 40 with calcific aortic stenosis, and its detection is difficult, short of coronary arteriography. Myocardial infarction patterns in the resting ECG should be a useful indicator of the presence of coronary artery disease, since aortic stenosis alone rarely causes myocardial infarction, even though it does commonly cause angina pectoris. However, left ventricular hypertrophy alone causes a decrease or loss of the initial R wave in leads V_1 and V_2. Thus, "poor R wave progression" in leads V_1 to V_3, and even QS complexes in leads V_1 and V_2, have virtually no diagnostic specificity for the diagnosis of anteroseptal infarction in patients with aortic stenosis. However, pathologic Q waves in leads V_4 to V_6, and in the inferior limb leads, have much the same correlation with myocardial infarction that they have in the absence of left ventricular hypertrophy. Pathologic Q waves in these leads are associated with occlusive coronary arterial lesions in more than 90% of instances.[32]

Regression of Left Ventricular Hypertrophy

The mass of the left ventricle decreases significantly after successful aortic valve replacement for aortic stenosis. This regression typically amounts to 25 to 35%, and the resulting value for mass is typically near the upper limit of normal.[33] Regression of the ECG evidence of left ventricular hypertrophy also occurs, particularly in children, who lose the abnormalities of the ST segments and T waves in up to 80% of instances, and revert to a normal ECG in about one third of cases.[34] Adults show less complete regression of the ECG patterns of left ventricular hypertrophy than this, probably because of the greater degree of myocardial fibrosis and remodeling of the fibrous skeleton of the left ventricle that occurs in adults.

THE ECG IN PULMONARY VALVE STENOSIS

Pulmonary valve stenosis with an intact ventricular septum, especially in children, is probably the most straightforward example of a close correlation between the range of ECG evidences that reflect a hemodynamic disorder and the anatomic and physiological severity of the disorder itself.[35-37] Pulmonary valve stenosis leads to concentric hypertrophy of the right ventricle, with dilatation playing little or no role in most cases. Associated myocardial fibrosis is also minimal in most instances, at least in children. With an intact ventricular septum, the right ventricular peak systolic pressure can exceed the systemic arterial pressure, and thus can be increased over a nearly tenfold range of elevated values. The ECG changes may even have value beyond their correlation with the right ventricular peak systolic pressure or the pulmonary valve systolic pressure gradient, because the ECG measurements correlate somewhat better with measures such as the stroke work of the right ventricle, the total pulmonary valve resistance, and the calculated pulmonary valve area than with the simple pressure measurements alone.[38] ECGs typical of moderate and very severe degrees of pulmonary stenosis are shown in Figures 5.6 and 5.7.

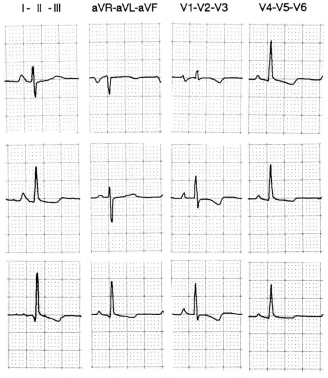

Figure 5.6 12-lead ECG in a 26-year-old woman with a right ventricular peak systolic pressure of 95 mmHg. There is borderline evidence of right atrial abnormality, borderline right axis deviation, and a low amplitude but predominant R wave in V_1, as well as a marked abnormality of the ST segments and T waves in both the limb leads and the precordial leads.

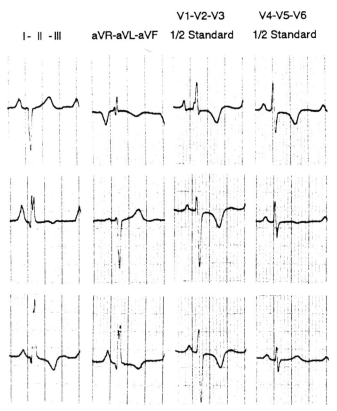

Figure 5.7 12-lead ECG in a 21-year-old man with very severe pulmonary stenosis. A marked right atrial abnormality is present, as well as severe right axis deviation (130°), a virtually pure R wave of 15-mm amplitude in lead V_1, and marked abnormalities of the ST segment and T waves in the right and mid precordial leads.

Although any of the usual ECG criteria for right ventricular hypertrophy apply in patients with pulmonary valve stenosis, most of the useful correlation is obtained with a few simple measurements. These include the amplitude of the R wave in lead V_1, the presence of a Q wave in V_1, the axis of the QRS complex in the limb leads, the presence of inversion of the T wave in lead aVF, and the amplitude of the S waves in leads 1 and V_6 (Table 5.8). Findings that virtually assure the presence of a severe lesion include an R wave taller than 20 mm in lead V_1, a QR pattern in V_1, an S wave greater than 15 mm in lead 1, and an inverted T wave in lead aVF.

The QRS axis is also useful in a negative sense, because an axis in the normal or leftward range essentially rules out a severe degree of isolated pulmonary valve stenosis.

Patients with mild right axis deviation and moderate prominence of R in V_1, S in V_6, and S in lead 1, with normal T waves, can have variable degrees of severity of pulmonary valve stenosis. Ellison and associates proposed a formula for predicting the pulmonary valvular systolic pressure gradient from several ECG measurements, as follows[39]:

Table 5.8 ECG FEATURES IN PULMONARY VALVE STENOSIS, BY GRADE OF SEVERITY

ECG Item	Pulmonary Systolic Pressure Gradient, mmHg			
	<25	25–49	50–79	>79
QRS Axis				
270–89	47	55	10	1
90–119	21	61	28	20
120–269	5	33	62	79
QR in V_1	0	0	0	12
R Wave in V_1				
<10	62	101	44	23
10–19	10	45	39	54
>19	1	3	17	77
S Wave in V_6				
<3	31	48	10	17
3–8	40	94	77	80
>8	2	7	13	57
S Wave in 1				
<10	71	136	64	52
10–14	2	13	34	52
>15	0	0	2	49
Inverted T Wave in aVF	1	0	0	26

$$\text{Gradient} = R_{V_1} + S_{V_6} + 60\,\frac{S_1}{R_1 + S_1} + T_{aVF} + T_{V_1} + 10$$

$$T_{aVF} = \quad \begin{aligned} &0 \text{ if flat or upright} \\ &50 \text{ if inverted} \end{aligned}$$

$$T_{V_1} = \quad \begin{aligned} &0 \text{ if flat or upright} \\ &-10 \text{ if inverted and } R_{V_1} < 10 \text{ mm} \\ &+15 \text{ if inverted and } R_{V_1} > 10 \text{ mm} \end{aligned}$$

The degree of correlation between the measured gradient and the values predicted by this formula was low enough to indicate that the formula should not be used by itself as a predictor, but the principles involved are useful.

Special note of the T wave in lead V_1 should be made. When the R wave in lead V_1 is taller than 10 mm, an inverted T wave gives additional evidence of severe pulmonary stenosis. However, when the R wave in V_1 is smaller than 10 mm, an inverted T wave in V_1 is not an additional sign of severity, but is a sign that suggests mild disease, being the normal polarity of the T wave in children.

Regression of the ECG evidence of right ventricular hypertrophy after both surgical treatment and balloon valvuloplasty has been well documented.[40] The regression is not seen fully until approximately 6 months have elapsed. This corresponds to the time during which the secondary pressure gradient due to functional obstruction of the right ventricle by hypertrophied infundibular muscle regresses.

THE ECG IN MITRAL STENOSIS

The characteristic changes in the ECG in patients with mitral stenosis are the abnormalities of the P wave that reflect left atrial pressure overload and the evidence of right ventricular hypertrophy that reflects pulmonary hypertension. The most characteristic pattern includes both of these elements (Fig. 5.8).

The P waves are abnormal in most patients with mitral stenosis that is severe enough to warrant surgery or balloon valvuloplasty.[41,42] The occurrence of entirely normal P waves in a patient with mitral stenosis and significant symptoms should

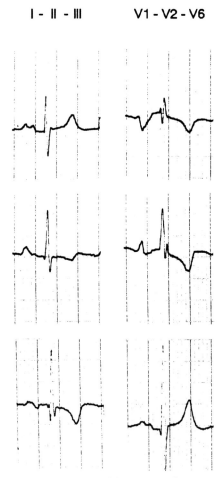

I - II - III   V1 - V2 - V6

Figure 5.8   12-lead ECG in a 50-year-old man with severe mitral stenosis. The P wave is broad and notched in the limb leads and has a markedly abnormal negative P terminal force in lead V_1. The QRS axis is rightward, at 90°, and the R:S ratio in lead V_1 is slightly over 1.0. The prominence of the initial component of the P wave in lead 2 and the prominent upright P initial force in lead V_2 suggest right atrial abnormality as well, probably secondary to pulmonary hypertension and right ventricular hypertrophy.

suggest a complicating feature, such as dyspnea due to primary lung disease or a psychological problem that leads to exaggeration of the symptoms.

Among patients with significant degrees of mitral stenosis, however, the relation between various measurements of the P waves and the severity of the stenosis is not very close.[22] Also, the presence of atrial fibrillation is not closely related to the grade of severity of the mitral stenosis, but is more closely related to the patient's age and to the duration of the disease. Patients with pure or predominant mitral regurgitation are as likely to have abnormal P waves, or atrial fibrillation, as patients with pure or predominant mitral stenosis.

Regression of the abnormalities of the P wave after successful surgical mitral valvotomy has been well documented, and it serves as a simple indicator of hemodynamic success.[43,44] Similar regression has been reported following percutaneous balloon mitral valvuloplasty (Fig. 5.9).[45]

In contrast with the P wave, evidence of right ventricular hypertrophy is useful in assessing the severity of mitral stenosis, since pulmonary hypertension occurs primarily in those with relatively severe stenosis.[46-48] A simple determination of the axis of the QRS complex in the limb leads is particularly useful, since the great majority of patients with pure or predominant mitral stenosis of significant degree have an axis that is to the right of 60°. An axis to the left of 60° usually indicates mild stenosis, predominant mitral regurgitation, or an additional factor such as hypertension or aortic valvular disease.

Overt patterns of right ventricular hypertrophy, such as those with an axis to the right of 120°, an R wave exceeding 5 mm in V_1, or an R wave clearly taller than the S wave in V_1, is usually a reliable indicator of pulmonary hypertension in patients with mitral stenosis, with a mean pressure in the pulmonary artery exceeding 30 mmHg at rest and a total pulmonary vascular resistance exceeding 800 dynes·seconds·cm^{-5}. Right axis deviation in the range of 100° to 120°, an R wave slightly greater than the S wave in V_1, an S wave greater than the R wave in V_5, or an R wave greater than the Q wave in aVR are also good indicators of pulmonary hypertension.

Many patients with mitral stenosis have a QRS axis of approximately 90° and approximately equal R and S waves in V_1. In these cases the stenosis is usually at least moderate, but falls within a broader range of severities. In addition, patients with mixed mitral stenosis and regurgitation, or even predominant mitral regurgitation, may have patterns of this type and may have significant pulmonary hypertension.

The presence of clear evidence of left ventricular hypertrophy in the ECG is not consistent with pure mitral stenosis of significant degrees. It suggests the presence of additional factors such as significant mitral regurgitation, hypertension, or aortic valve disease.

THE ECG IN TRICUSPID STENOSIS

Tricuspid stenosis is usually a rheumatic valvular lesion that occurs in patients with mitral stenosis, who often have aortic valvular disease as well.[49-51] The ECG thus reflects a balance of the effects of double or triple valvular lesions. Women are even more subject to tricuspid stenosis, relative to men, than they are to mitral stenosis. A surprising proportion, usually more than 50%, are in sinus rhythm when they present with symptoms of tricuspid stenosis.

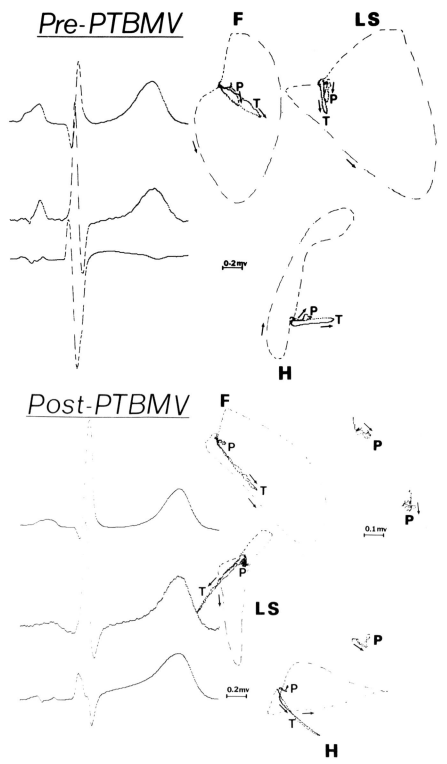

Figure 5.9 Vectorcardiograms before (top) and after (bottom) percutaneous trans-septal balloon mitral valvuloplasty (PTBMV). Note size of P-loop after PTBMV was so reduced in amplitude that it had to be enlarged to twice its size for better visualization. *F*—frontal plane, *LS*—left sagittal plane, *H*—horizontal plane. (From: Chen C et al: Percutaneous transseptal balloon mitral valvuloplasty: the Chinese experience in 30 patients. *Am Heart J.* 115: 937–947, 1988. With permission.)

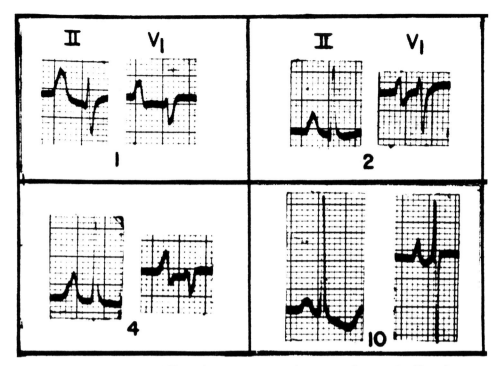

Figure 5.10 Leads 11 and V$_1$ in four patients with tricuspid stenosis. The characteristic features are the tall peaked P waves in lead II and the increased upright P initial force in lead V$_1$, without evidence of right ventricular hypertrophy. P waves taller than the QRS complex in the same lead are also characteristic. (Modified from: Perloff JK, Harvey WP: Clinical recognition of tricuspid stenosis. Circulation. 22: 346–364, 1960. With permission.)

The hallmark in the ECG of tricuspid stenosis is the P wave that reflects right atrial pressure overload.[52,53] The P wave is taller than 3 mm in lead 2 and shows an increased positive initial force in leads V$_1$ and V$_2$ (Fig. 5.10). Such a P wave is not specific for tricuspid stenosis, since it may also reflect pulmonary hypertension and right ventricular hypertrophy secondary to mitral stenosis. However, a particular feature of the P wave in patients with tricuspid stenosis is a prominent picture of right atrial pressure overload without evidence of right ventricular hypertrophy. In the most characteristic instances, the P wave is larger than the QRS complex in certain leads.

Q waves in V$_1$ often occur on the basis of right atrial dilatation, because the heart is rotated toward the left and the V$_1$ electrode position lies over the right atrium rather than over the right ventricle. This is often seen in tricuspid regurgitation but is much less common in the rarer cases of pure or predominant tricuspid stenosis.

The carcinoid heart syndrome can cause tricuspid valve stenosis, and some cases have been treated with balloon valvuloplasty.[54-56] The P waves are not particularly prominent in these patients, perhaps because the right atrial pressure overload has not been sustained over many years, or perhaps because the carcinoid tissue is heavily deposited on the right atrium as well as the tricuspid valve and prevents atrial muscular hypertrophy from developing.

REFERENCES

1. Surawicz B: Electrocardiographic diagnosis of chamber enlargement. *J Am Coll Cardiol.* 8:711–724, 1986.

2. Antman EM, Green LH, Grossman W: Physiologic determinants of the electrocardiographic diagnosis of left ventricular hypertrophy. *Circulation.* 60:386–396, 1979.

3. Devereux RB, Phillips MC, Casale PN, et al: Geometric determinants of electrocardiographic left ventricular hypertrophy. *Circulation.* 67:907–911, 1983.

4. Murphy ML, Thenabadu PN, de Soyza N, et al: Sensitivity of electrocardiographic criteria for left ventricular hypertrophy according to type of cardiac disease. *Am J Cardiol.* 55:545–549, 1985.

5. Barnes AR, Whitten MB: Study of T-wave negativity in predominant ventricular strain. *Am Heart J.* 5:14–67, 1929.

6. Cowan JC, Hilton CJ, Griffiths CJ, et al: Sequence of epicardial repolarisation and configuration of the T wave. *Br Heart J.* 60:424–433, 1988.

7. Franz MR, Bargheer K, Rafflenbeul W, et al: Monophasic action potential mapping in human subjects with normal electrocardiograms: direct evidence for the genesis of the T wave. *Circulation.* 75:379–386, 1987.

8. Sokolow M, Lyon TP: The ventricular complex in left ventricular hypertrophy as obtained by unipolar precordial and limb leads. *Am Heart J.* 37:161–186, 1949.

9. Lewis T: Observations upon ventricular hypertrophy, with especial reference to preponderance of one or other chamber. *Heart.* 5:367–402, 1914.

10. Casale PN, Devereux RB, Alonso DR, et al: Improved sex-specific criteria of left ventricular hypertrophy for clinical and computer interpretation of electrocardiograms: validation with autopsy findings. *Circulation.* 75:565–572, 1987.

11. Siegel RJ, Roberts WC: Electrocardiographic observations in severe aortic valve stenosis: correlative necropsy study to clinical, hemodynamic, and ECG variables demonstrating relation of 12-lead QRS amplitude to peak systolic transaortic pressure gradient. *Am Heart J.* 103:210–221, 1982.

12. Odom H II, David JL, Dinh H, et al: QRS voltage measurements in autopsied men free of cardiopulmonary disease: a basis for evaluating total QRS voltage as an index of left ventricular hypertrophy. *Am J Cardiol.* 58:801–804, 1986.

13. Romhilt DW, Estes EH Jr: A point-score system for the ECG diagnosis of left ventricular hypertrophy. *Am Heart J.* 75:752–758, 1968.

14. MacFarlane PW, Lawrie TDV: *Comprehensive Electrocardiology. Theory and Practice in Health and Disease.* New York: Pergamon Press, 1989.

15. Kafka H, Burggraf GW, Milliken JA: Electrocardiographic diagnosis of left ventricular hypertrophy in the presence of left bundle branch block: an echocardiographic study. *Am J Cardiol.* 55:103–106, 1985.

16. Klein RC, Vera Z, DeMaria AN, et al: Electrocardiographic diagnosis of left ventricular hypertrophy in the presence of left bundle branch block. *Am Heart J.* 108:502–506, 1984.

17. Cokkinos DV, Demopoulos JN, Heimonas ET, et al: Electrocardiographic criteria of left ventricular hypertrophy in left bundle-branch block. *Br Heart J.* 40:320–324, 1978.

18. Flowers NC, Horan LG: Subtle signs of right ventricular enlargement and their relative importance. In: Schlant RC, Hurst JW, eds. *Advances in Electrocardiography.* New York: Grune & Stratton, 1972, pp. 297–308.

19. Genovesi-Ebert A, Marabotti C, Palombo C, et al: Electrocardiographic signs of atrial overload in hypertensive patients: indexes of abnormality of atrial morphology or function? *Am Heart J.* 121:1113–1118, 1991.

20. Macruz R, Perloff JK, Case RB: A method for the electrocardiograhic recognition of atrial enlargement. *Circulation.* 17:882–889, 1958.

21. Morris JJ Jr, Estes EH Jr, Whalen RE, et al: P-wave analysis in valvular heart disease. *Circulation.* 29:242–252, 1964.

22. Saunders JL, Calatayud JB, Schulz KJ, et al: Evaluation of ECG criteria for P-wave abnormalities. *Am Heart J.* 74:757–765, 1967.

23. Reeves WC, Hallahan W, Schwiter EJ, et al: Two-dimensional echocardiographic assessment of electrocardiographic criteria for right atrial enlargement. *Circulation.* 64:387–391, 1981.

24. Hancock EW, Fleming PR: Aortic stenosis. *Q J Med.* 29:209–234, 1960.

25. Nylander E, Ekman I, Marklund T, et al: Severe aortic stenosis in elderly patients. *Br Heart J.* 55:480–487, 1986.

26. Nitta M, Nakamura T, Hultgren HN, et al: Noninvasive evaluation of the severity of aortic stenosis in adults. *Chest.* 91:682–687, 1987.

27. Aronow WS, Kronzon I: Prevalence and severity of valvular aortic stenosis determined by Doppler echocardiography and its association with echocardiographic and electrocardiographic left ventricular hypertrophy and physical signs of aortic stenosis in elderly patients. *Am J Cardiol.* 67:776–777, 1991.

28. Dancy M: Comparison of electrocardiographic and echocardiographic measures of left ventricular hypertropy in the assessment of aortic stenosis. *Br Heart J.* 55:155–161, 1986.

29. Bergeron GA, Schiller NB: Implications of normal left ventricular wall thickness in critical aortic stenosis. *Chest.* 90:380–382, 1986.

30. Wagner HR, Weidman WH, Ellison RC, et al: Indirect assessment of severity in aortic stenosis. In: Nadas AS, Ellison RC, Weidman WH, eds. Pulmonary stenosis, aortic stenosis, ventricular septal defect: clinical course and indirect assessment. Report from the Joint Study on the Natural History of Congenital Heart Defects. *Circulation.* 56(suppl I):I-20–I-23, 1977.

31. Kveselis DA, Rocchini AP, Rosenthal A, et al: Hemodynamic determinants of exercise-induced ST-segment depression in children with valvar aortic stenosis. *Am J Cardiol.* 55:1133–1139, 1985.

32. Hancock EW: Aortic stenosis, angina pectoris, and coronary artery disease. *Am Heart J.* 93:382–393, 1977.

33. Kurnik PB, Innerfield M, Wachspress JD, et al: Left ventricular mass regression after aortic valve replacement measured by ultrafast computed tomography. *Am Heart J.* 120:919–927, 1990.

34. Tveter KJ, Foker JE, Moller JH, et al: Long-term evaluation of aortic valvotomy for congenital aortic stenosis. *Ann Surg.* 206:496–503, 1987.

35. Rocchini AP, Emmanouilides GC: Pulmonary stenosis. In: Adams FH, Emmanouilides GC, Riemenschneider TA, eds. *Moss' Heart Disease in Infants, Children, and Adolescents.* 4th ed. Baltimore: Williams & Wilkins, 1989, pp 308–338.

36. Witham AC, Rainey RL, Edmonds JH Jr: Prediction of right ventricular pressure in pulmonic stenosis from sponge vectorcardiogram and electrocardiogram. *Am Heart J.* 75:187–199, 1968.

37. Cayler GG, Ongley P, Nadas AS: Relation of systolic pressure in the right ventricle to the electrocardiogram. *N Engl J Med.* 258:979–982, 1958.

38. Bassingthwaighte JB, Parkin TW, DuShane JW, et al: The electrocardiographic and hemodynamic findings in pulmonary stenosis with intact ventricular septum. *Circulation.* 28:893–905, 1963.

39. Ellison RC, Freedom RM, Keane JF, et al: Indirect assessment of severity in pulmo-

nary stenosis. In: Nadas AS, Ellison RC, Weidman WH, eds. Pulmonary stenosis, aortic stenosis, ventricular septal defect: clinical course and indirect assessment. Report from the Joint Study on the Natural History of Congenital Heart Defects. *Circulation.* 56(suppl I):I-14–I-20, 1977.

40. Rao PS: Balloon pulmonary valvuloplasty: a review. *Clin Cardiol.* 12:55–74, 1989.

41. Fraser HRL, Turner R: Electrocardiography in mitral valvular disease. *Br Heart J.* 17:459–483, 1955.

42. Thomas P, DeJong D: The P wave in the electrocardiogram in the diagnosis of heart disease. *Br Heart J.* 16:241–254, 1954.

43. Mounsey P: The atrial electrocardiogram as a guide to prognosis after mitral valvotomy. *Br Heart J.* 22:617–628, 1960.

44. Calatayud JB, Saunders JL, Schulz KJ, et al: P wave changes after open heart mitral commissurotomy for isolated mitral stenosis. *Angiology.* 19:238–246, 1968.

45. Chen C, Lo Z, Huang Z, et al: Percutaneous transseptal balloon mitral valvuloplasty: the Chinese experience in 30 patients. *Am Heart J.* 115:937–947, 1988.

46. Butler PM, Leggett SI, Howe CM, et al: Identification of electrocardiographic criteria for diagnosis of right ventricular hypertrophy due to mitral stenosis. *Am J Cardiol.* 57:639–643, 1986.

47. Semler HJ, Pruitt RD: An electrocardiographic estimation of the pulmonary vascular obstruction in 80 patients with mitral stenosis. *Am Heart J.* 59:541–547, 1960.

48. Pruitt RD, Robinson JG: The electrocardiographic findings in patients undergoing surgical exploration of the mitral valve. *Am Heart J.* 52:880–886, 1956.

49. Kitchin A, Turner R: Diagnosis and treatment of tricuspid stenosis. *Br Heart J.* 26:354–379, 1964.

50. Ribeiro PA, Al Zaibag M, Sawyer W: A prospective study comparing the haemodynamic with the cross-sectional echocardiographic diagnosis of tricuspid stenosis. *Eur Heart J.* 10:120–126, 1989.

51. Yousof AM, Shafei MZ, Endrys G, et al: Tricuspid stenosis and regurgitation in rheumatic heart disease: a prospective cardiac catheterization study in 525 patients. *Am Heart J.* 110:60–64, 1985.

52. Killip T III, Lukas DS: Tricuspid stenosis. Clinical features in 12 cases. *Am J Med.* 24:836–852, 1958.

53. Perloff JK, Harvey WP: Clinical recognition of tricuspid stenosis. *Circulation.* 22:346–364, 1960.

54. Thorson AH: Studies on carcinoid disease. *Acta Med Scand.* 334(suppl):1–132, 1958.

55. Roberts WC, Sjoerdsma A: The cardiac disease associated with the carcinoid syndrome (carcinoid heart disease). *Am J Med.* 36:5–34, 1964.

56. Mullins PA, Hall JA, Shapiro LM: Balloon dilatation of tricuspid stenosis caused by carcinoid heart disease. *Br Heart J.* 63:249–250, 1990.

CHAPTER 6

Echocardiographic Evaluation

CHUNGUANG CHEN
VIVIAN M. ABASCAL

Introduced in the past few years, percutaneous balloon valvuloplasty has been used to relieve severe stenosis of mitral, aortic, pulmonary, and tricuspid valves and, in many instances, as an alternative to cardiac surgery.[1-3] This procedure requires precise evaluation of valve morphology and function for pre-procedure decision making and post-procedure evaluation of patients. Although cardiac catheterization offers information about hemodynamic status, valve function, or both, it has only a limited value in assessing valve morphology.[4,5] Moreover, catheterization is costly and carries a small but definite risk of morbidity and mortality.[6] It is therefore less than ideal for repeat assessment in followup of patients who have undergone percutaneous balloon valvuloplasty. Two-dimensional echocardiography is a noninvasive tool for evaluating morphologic characteristics of the valvular and subvalvular apparatus[7,8] and valve annular size.[9] Doppler echocardiography provides functional information on transvalvular flow velocity, which can be used to derive pressure gradients across the valves, and to calculate regurgitant flow.[10] Mitral valve area can be either obtained from two-dimensional echocardiography[11] or derived from Doppler pressure half-time studies,[10] whereas the aortic valve area can be calculated by means of the continuity principle by a combination of Doppler and two-dimensional echocardiographic data.[12] Thus, echocardiography is currently the most widely used technique for assessing results of percutaneous balloon valvuloplasty. Many studies have now been done to evaluate (1) the accuracy of echocardiographic methods in assessing pressure gradient and valve area before and after percutaneous balloon valvuloplasty; (2) the relationship between echocardiographic valvular morphology and results of percutaneous balloon valvuloplasty. Following is a detailed discussion of advantages and limitations of echocardiography, its recent developments in evaluating results of percutaneous balloon valvuloplasty, and its clinical utility in patient selection for the valvuloplasty procedure.

MITRAL STENOSIS

In patients with mitral stenosis, symptoms of dyspnea and fatigue give some indication of the severity of the stenosis, but these symptoms are often difficult to quantify and do not always reflect genuine reductions in mitral valve area. Moreover, associated multiple valvular lesions may change the characteristics of the auscultatory findings on physical examination. Thus, in clinical decision making, a sophisticated noninvasive imaging technique with or without cardiac catheterization is often required. Echocardiography enhances evaluation of patients with mitral stenosis considerably and is very helpful in selecting therapeutic options for patient management. For patients being considered for percutaneous balloon mitral valvuloplasty, echocardiography can be helpful in defining the severity of the stenosis; the morphologic characteristics of the valve apparatus; and other causes of obstruction at the mitral level such as left atrial myxoma, significant associated lesions such as severe mitral regurgitation or aortic disease, and, more important, left atrial thrombus.

Assessment of Severity

Two-Dimensional Echocardiography

Although the value of M-mode echocardiography in the detection of mitral stenosis has been well established, this technique is unable to estimate mitral valve area.[13-17] Two-dimensional echocardiography, conversely, has been shown to provide measurements of true anatomic mitral valve area.[18-21] Doming of the mitral leaflets can be typically observed in apical four-chamber, two-chamber, and parasternal long-axis views. The mobile middle portion of a doming mitral valve forms an angle in diastole with a concavity toward the left atrial side and restricted separation at the tip of the valve. Therefore, to avoid the possibility of overestimating the size of the orifice, the transducer should be so positioned that the perpendicular plane of the mitral orifice at the tip of the mitral valve is obtained in the parasternal short-axis view. The mitral valve area should be measured at the smallest orifice of the valve in the parasternal short-axis view by scanning from the left atrium to the left ventricle and recording the lowest level of the mitral valve tip with the entire circumference of the mitral orifice (Fig. 6.1). To avoid an error in planimetry,[18-23] attention should be paid to adjusting optimal gain settings. High gain settings may underestimate the valve area because of the "blooming" effect from the thickened leaflets. Conversely, low gain settings may lead to image dropout and consequently to falsely large estimates of the orifice size. The measurement should be taken in early diastole when the mitral valve is maximally open. To limit the error in planimetry, the lowest imaging depth (12–16 cm) that just includes the mitral valve should be used to obtain the measurement. At least three measurements in sinus rhythm and five measurements in atrial fibrillation should be obtained to minimize the error resulting from beat-to-beat variation. Many studies have demonstrated that when an adequate quality of echo images could be obtained, planimetry of mitral valve area correlated well with the mitral valve area calculated from catheterization data using the Gorlin formula[18-22] or direct surgical examination.[24] The correlation coefficients ranged from 0.83 to 0.95 and the standard error of regression equation estimate of the catheterization-derived mitral valve area (SEE, 0.21–0.25 cm^2) was usually acceptable (Fig. 6.2). The correlation between catheterization data and two-dimensional echocardiographic measurement remains good in patients after percutaneous balloon mitral valvuloplasty.[25] However, when the mitral valve is extensively distorted or severely calcified, or both, accurate two-dimensional echocardiographic measurement of mitral valve area may not be possible, especially after surgical commissurotomy.[22] Thus, two-dimensional echocardiographic measurement of the mitral valve area is technically demanding, requires

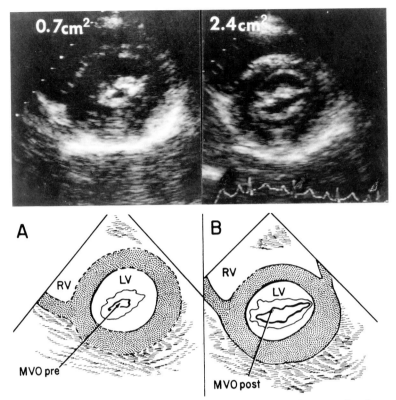

Figure 6.1 Mitral valve area measured by planimetry of the mitral valve orifice in early diastole from a parasternal short-axis view before (*left*) and after (*right*) balloon valvuloplasty. Panel *A* shows the small orifice (0.7 cm²) before valvuloplasty (*MVO pre*). Panel *B* shows the orifice significantly larger (2.4 cm²) after the procedure (*MVO post*), with cleavage along the commissures. (From: Wilkins GT et al: Percutaneous balloon dilatation of the mitral valve: an analysis of echocardiographic variables related to outcome and the mechanism of dilatation. *Br Heart J.* 60:299–308, 1988. With permission.)

experience and expertise, and may not be feasible in some patients. It has been reported that, because of technically inadequate studies, two-dimensional echocardiographic measurement of mitral valve area was not possible in 8 to 15% of patients.[18-23]

Doppler Echocardiography
Continuous-wave Doppler echocardiography can record transmitral diastolic flow velocity profile (Fig. 6.3). The Doppler recording can be obtained from the apical approach with the use of either an imaging or a nonimaging transducer. The transducer should be adjusted by visual and auditory monitoring to record the maximal velocity across the mitral valve. The smallest angle between the stream direction of mitral blood flow and the Doppler ultrasound beam should be used to record the mitral velocity profile. The color Doppler flow mapping technique is very useful in aligning the ultrasound beam to the direction of transmitral flow, although one should keep in mind that the stenotic flow jet is three-dimensional. The transmitral flow

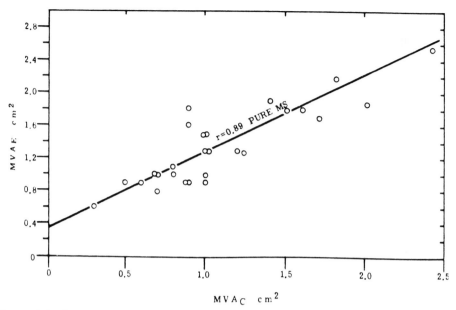

Figure 6.2 Relationship between mitral valve area calculated by the Gorlin formula at the time of cardiac catheterization (MVA_C) and mitral valve area measured by echocardiographic planimetry (MVA_E) (From Wann LS et al: Determination of mitral valve area by cross-sectional echocardiography. *Ann Intern Med.* 88:337–341, 1978. With permission.)

velocities can then be converted into pressure gradients using the simplified Bernoulli equation:

$$\Delta P = 4V^2$$

where ΔP is the pressure gradient in mmHg and V is the transmitral velocity in m/s[26,27] Both maximal and mean pressure gradients correlated well with those obtained from the simultaneous measurements at catheterization.[10,28] The correlation coefficient was 0.97,[10] and the standard error of estimate of the true pressure gradient ranged from 2 to 4 mmHg by Doppler measurement.[10,28] Although the mean diastolic transmitral pressure gradient in some degree reflects severity of mitral stenosis, the pressure gradient (ΔP) depends not only on the mitral valve area (MVA) but also on cardiac output and heart rate, as stated in Gorlin's formula[29]:

$$\text{MVA} = 38.5 \times \frac{\text{mitral diastolic flow}}{\sqrt{\Delta P}}$$

Therefore, the mitral valve area must also be measured.

The diastolic transmitral velocity profile obtained by Doppler echocardiography can be used to derive pressure half-time (Fig. 6.4) and thereby mitral valve area. The pressure half-time — time required for the left atrioventricular pressure gradient to fall to half of its maximal early diastolic value — was originally developed with catheterization data by Libanoff and Rodbard[30] and then applied by Hatle and colleagues to the emerging field of Doppler echocardiography,[31] where it has rapidly gained acceptance as an accurate estimate of mitral valve area in both native and prosthetic valves. The time required for the pressure gradient to fall to its half value $T_{\frac{1}{2}}$ is inversely

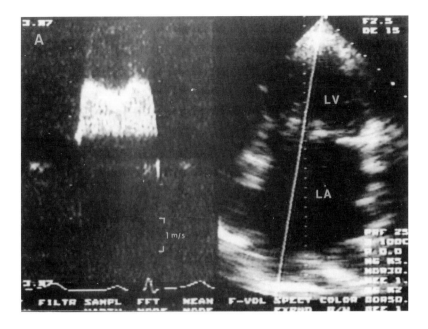

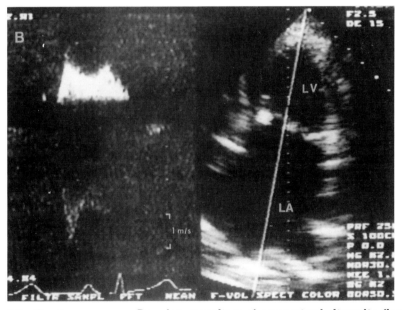

Figure 6.3 Continuous-wave Doppler recording of transmitral diastolic flow velocity profile from the apex using an imaging transducer in a patient with mitral stenosis before and after balloon valvuloplasty. Panel *A* shows a maximal velocity of 2 m/s before the procedure. Panel *B* shows a drop in maximal velocity to 1.3 m/s after balloon dilatation of the valve. Transmitral flow velocity can be converted into pressure gradients using the simplified Bernoulli equation: $\Delta P = 4 V^2$. ΔP — Pressure gradient in mmHg. *V*—velocity in m/s. *LA*—left atrium. *LV*—left ventricle.

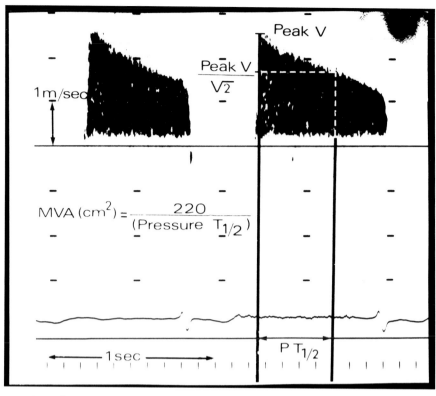

Figure 6.4 Continuous-wave Doppler velocity profile from a patient with mitral stenosis. The pressure half-time is the time required for the pressure to fall to its half value (PT$_{\frac{1}{2}}$) and can be measured as the time during which the peak velocity (*Peak V*) decays to Peak V/$\sqrt{2}$. Mitral valve area (*MVA*) can be calculated from PT$_{\frac{1}{2}}$) using *MVA* = 220/PT$_{\frac{1}{2}}$ where 220 is an empirical constant.

related to the mitral valve area (MVA) and is expressed in an empirical formula developed by Hatle and associates:

$$MVA = \frac{220}{PT_{\frac{1}{2}}}$$

The empirical constant 220 proposed by Hatle's group was originally derived by relating Doppler-derived pressure half-time and mitral valve area derived from catheterization data in 20 patients with mitral stenosis.[10] Using the empirical constant 220, a number of studies have demonstrated that mitral valve area can be accurately estimated by Doppler pressure half-time when catheterization-derived data is used as the gold standard. The correlation coefficient between Doppler-derived mitral valve areas and those derived from cardiac catheterization ranged from 0.81 to 0.90 with a standard error of estimate of 0.18 to 0.21 cm^2 in patients with mitral stenosis.[22,28,32] It has been suggested that the pressure half-time method is more accurate than two-dimensional planimetry in patients with distorted and calcified valve leaflets after surgical commissurotomy.[22] Another potential advantage of the Doppler pressure half-time method over two-dimensional echocardiography is apparent in patients with atrial fibrillation, in whom maximal early diastolic opening may be difficult to discern by two-dimensional echocardiography if the patient has very irregular rhythms.[21,22,31]

It was previously believed that pressure half-time is independent of cardiac output, heart rate, left atrial pressure, and mitral regurgitation, but studies have now demonstrated that the relationship between mitral valve area[10] and pressure half-time is more complex.[32-39] Using computer simulation and an in vitro fluid dynamic model, Thomas and associates described this more complicated relationship of the pressure half-time $(T_{\frac{1}{2}})$[33,34] and the mitral value area (MVA), as stated in the formula:

$$T_{\frac{1}{2}} = \frac{11.6 \; C_n \; \sqrt{\Delta Po}}{MVA}$$

Here $T_{\frac{1}{2}}$ was predicted to vary inversely with MVA but also to vary directly with net left atrial and ventricular compliance (C_n) and the square root of the initial peak transmitral pressure gradient (ΔPo). In many clinical situations, a balance may be obtained by a predictable change in initial peak pressure gradient and net left atrial and ventricular compliance in opposite directions. Thus, a reliable estimate of the mitral valve area is achieved by the simplified relationship between the pressure half-time and the mitral valve area proposed by Hatle and associates.[10] However, in the case of percutaneous balloon mitral valvuloplasty, Thomas and associates[33] demonstrated that with valvuloplasty the initial peak transmitral pressure gradient was significantly reduced—by 36% on average, the left atrial compliance was doubled, and conversely, the left ventricular compliance tended to decrease so that the net compliance rose by 42%. In their study, although the increase in the product of C_n and $\sqrt{\Delta Po}$ by 9% was on average not statistically significant, the wide variability in individual patients led to the poor predictive accuracy of the mitral valve area as measured by pressure half-time immediately after valvuloplasty. The poor correlation $(r = 0.36-0.71; SEE = 0.35-0.49 \; cm^2)$ between mitral valve area and pressure half-time immediately after mitral valvuloplasty was also observed by others[32,36,40,41] (Fig. 6.5). This poor relationship appears also to be related to changes in volume load immediately after the valvuloplasty procedure.[39] Thus, pressure half-time is an unreliable measure of the mitral valve area shortly after balloon mitral valvuloplasty.

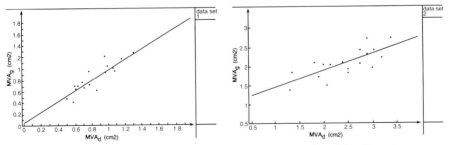

Figure 6.5 Correlation between mitral valve area calculated by Doppler pressure half-time (MVA_d) and that obtained by Gorlin formula (MVA_g) at the time of catheterization, before (*left*) and after balloon valvuloplasty (*right*). (From: Chen C et al: Reliability of the Doppler pressure half-time method for assessing effects of percutaneous mitral balloon valvuloplasty. *J Am Coll Cardiol.* 13:1309–1313, 1989. With permission.)

Timing of the measurement is key to its accuracy, as demonstrated in a study using simultaneous recordings of hemodynamic and Doppler data. If Doppler pressure half-time was measured 24 to 48 hours after balloon mitral valvuloplasty, a fairly good correlation (r = 0.84; SEE = 0.20 cm²) was observed between mitral valve areas derived from Doppler pressure half-time and those from catheterization data.[32] A similarly good correlation was also obtained 3 to 6 months after balloon mitral valvuloplasty.[24,25] Therefore, these results suggest that one should not use the pressure half-time method to estimate mitral valve area within 24 hours after percutaneous balloon mitral valvuloplasty, but may use it 24 to 48 hours after the procedure to obtain clinically accurate measurement of the mitral valve area.

Using the continuity principle, mitral valve area (MVA) can be calculated:

$$MVA = \frac{SV}{V}$$

where SV is stroke volume and can be obtained by Doppler and two-dimensional echocardiography. The transmitral velocity integral, V, can be obtained from continuous-wave Doppler. This method has been shown to be independent of the peak transmitral gradient and net left atrioventricular compliance and thus superior to the pressure half-time method.[42] However, reproducibility of this method may be strongly dependent on the echocardiographer's experience. Furthermore, this method is more time-consuming than the pressure half-time method. For clinical practice, therefore, mitral valve area determined by the continuity principle may be used only in situations in which the pressure half-time method is not reliable.

Color Doppler Flow Mapping

Although the color Doppler flow mapping technique is useful for quantifying valvular regurgitation, this technique is not often used to derive qualitative data in valvular stenosis. In mitral stenosis, a narrow diastolic jet (Fig. 6.6) with an aliasing velocity color profile (mosaic pattern) can be observed through the stenotic mitral orifice, indicating a reduced mitral orifice and increased transmitral flow velocity. It has been suggested that diastolic jet widths through the mitral orifice in two orthogonal apical planes can be used to estimate mitral valve area, assuming that the mitral orifice has an elliptical shape. In a preliminary study, Monterroso and associates[43] demonstrated that using color jet widths obtained from two-chamber and four-chamber views, the mitral valve area can be estimated with good correlation to that derived from catheterization (r = 0.85; SEE = 0.20 cm²). This alternative method may be useful in the situation in which two-dimensional echocardiographic planimetry of mitral valve area is not possible — for example, suboptimal echo quality in parasternal views, and when the Doppler pressure half-time method is inaccurate — for example in severe aortic regurgitation or immediately after valvuloplasty. However, whether changes in the color Doppler algorithm and gain settings will affect the accuracy of the measurement is yet to be determined.

A novel concept of flow acceleration proximal to a narrow orifice has been used to quantify mitral stenosis.[44] The mitral valve area calculated by means of this concept correlated well with catheterization-derived mitral valve area (r = 0.87). However, whether the morphology of the mitral valve and its inlet will influence the accuracy of the calculation is still unknown.

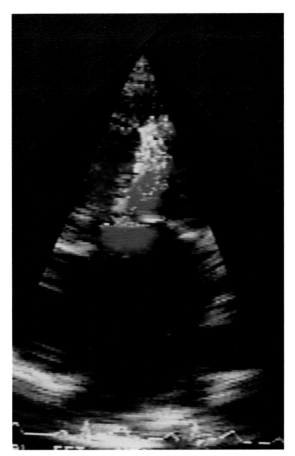

Figure 6.6 Color flow mapping from the apical four-chamber view in a patient with mitral stenosis showing aliasing (*blue pattern*) color profile indicating increased transmitral flow velocity as the blood approaches the stenotic orifice.

Echocardiographic Morphology as Related to Outcome After Balloon Valvuloplasty

Percutaneous balloon mitral valvuloplasty has achieved excellent results in the majority of patients with severe mitral stenosis.[45-63] Different balloon dilating techniques and balloon dilating diameters have influenced the results of this procedure.[54,58] The double-balloon and Inoue-balloon techniques have shown a greater increase in mitral valve area than the single-balloon technique in which the single balloon is 25 mm or less in diameter.[58,61,62] Even when double-balloon or Inoue-balloon techniques are used, an insufficient increase in valve area is reported in a certain subgroup of patients.[42,46,48,56-63] This finding may be related to pathologic changes of the valvular and subvalvular structures and to the mechanism of balloon valvuloplasty.

Percutaneous balloon mitral valvuloplasty, like closed surgical commissurotomy, increases mitral valve area by splitting fused commissures.[64-67] Before balloon mitral valvuloplasty was introduced, the classic indication for surgical commissurotomy was

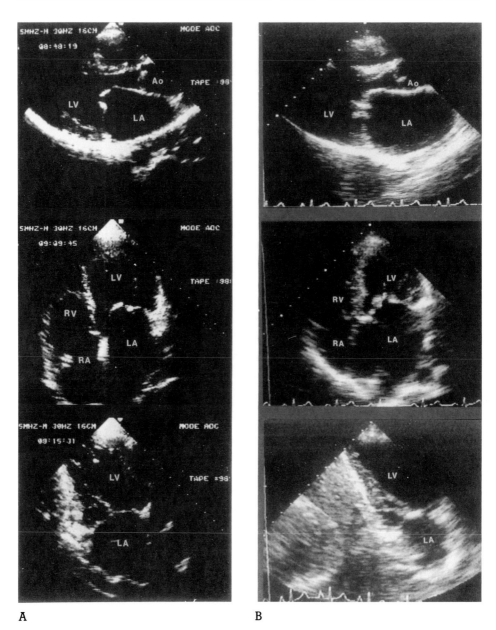

A   B

Figure 6.7 *A,* Echocardiographic parasternal long-axis view (*upper panel*), apical (four-chamber (*middle panel*) and slightly modified two-chamber view (*lower panel*) on a patient with a highly mobile, minimally thickened and calcified mitral valve. There is minimal subvalvular disease. The total echocardiographic score is 4. *LA*— left atrium. *LV*—left ventricle. *RA*—right atrium. *RV*—right ventricle. *B,* Same echocardiographic views as in *A* showing mitral valve morphology in a patient with moderate valve thickening and calcification. There is moderate involvement of the subvalvular apparatus. The total echocardiographic score is 7. *LA*—left atrium. *LV*— left ventricle. *RA*—right atrium. *RV*—right ventricle.

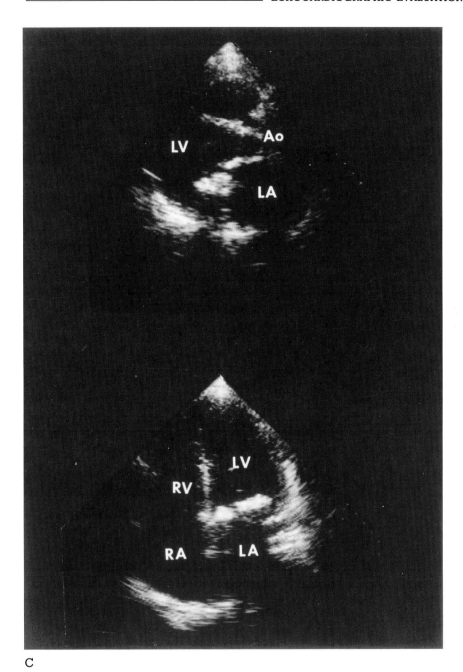

C

Figure 6.7 (Continued) *C*, Echocardiographic parasternal long-axis view and apical four-chamber view on a patient with marked thickening and calcification of the mitral leaflets. The echocardiographic score is 14. *LA*—left atrium. *LV*—left ventricle. *RA*—right atrium. *RV*—right ventricle. *Ao*—aorta.

**Table 6.1 GRADING OF MITRAL VALVE CHARACTERISTICS FROM
THE ECHOCARDIOGRAPHIC EXAMINATION**

Grade	Mobility	Subvalvar thickening
1	Highly mobile valve with only leaflet tips restricted	Minimal thickening just below the mitral leaflets
2	Leaflet mid and base portions have normal mobility	Thickening of chordal structures extending up to one third of the chordal length
3	Valve continues to move forward in diastole, mainly from the base	Thickening extending to the distal third of the chords
4	No or minimal forward movement of the leaflets in diastole	Extensive thickening and shortening of all chordal structures extending down to the papillary muscles

The echocardiographic score was obtained by analyzing mitral leaflet mobility, valvular and subvalvular thickening and valvular calcification which were graded from 1 to 4 on the basis of the above criteria. The total echocardiographic score (0 to 16) was obtained by adding the individual scores.

Source: From Wilkins GT, et al: Percutaneous balloon dilatation of the mitral valve: an analysis of echocardiographic variables related to outcome and the mechanism of dilatation. *Br Heart J.* 60:299–308, 1988. With permission.

pure mitral stenosis without severe calcification as identified by x-ray fluoroscopy.[68] It is generally agreed that the results of closed surgical mitral commissurotomy are less favorable in patients with mitral valve calcification; however, most (94%) patients with valve calcification do have a satisfactory increase in mitral valve orifice size by closed surgical commissurotomy.[69] However, mitral value replacement is required more frequently in patients with calcified valves (33%) than in those with noncalcified valves (15%), indicating less favorable long-term results.[70]

Two-dimensional echocardiography is a reliable tool for assessing mitral valvulor and subvalvular morphologic changes[71-73] and can provide information about valve thickness, mobility, calcification, and changes in the subvalvular apparatus. A number of studies have been performed to identify the morphologic characteristics of the subgroup of patients in whom balloon valvuloplasty may not be beneficial. Several echocardiographic systems for assessing mitral valve morphology have been suggested. The most widely accepted is the echo score system proposed by Abascal and Wilkins and associates.[74,75] By this system valve thickening, valve calcification, valve immobility, and subvalvular thickening are each graded from 1+ to 4+ (mild, moderate, moderately severe, and severe), yielding a maximum total echocardiographic score of 16 (Fig. 6.7; Table 6.1). The more severe the valvular pathologic changes the higher the echocardiographic score a patient will have. Considering fusion of subvalvular structure as an important part of subvalvular rheumatic involvement, Chen and associates[60] modified the subvalvular grading method so that thickening extending only from the tip of mitral leaflets to one third of the chordal length was graded as I. Thickening of the subvalvular structure extending more than one third and more than two thirds of the chordal length were grades II and III, respectively. Grade IV was considered only if both the following features were

Thickening	Calcification
Leaflets near normal in thickness (4–5 mm)	A single area of increased echo brightness
Mid-leaflets normal, considerable thickening of margins (5–8 mm)	Scattered areas of brightness confined to leaflet margins
Thickening extending through the entire leaflet (5–8 mm)	Brightness extending into the mid-portion of the leaflets
Considerable thickening of all leaflet tissue (>8–10 mm)	Extensive brightness throughout much of the leaflet tissue

present: (1) extensive thickening observed in all subvalvular structures involving chords and papillary muscles, and (2) no apparent separation of chords connecting anteromedial and posterolateral papillary muscles observed in multiple views (Fig. 6.8).

For all assessments, some technical points for imaging valve and subvalvular structures should be emphasized. It is important to examine mitral valvular and subvalvular structures extensively in multiple standard and tilted parasternal long-axis views and apical two- or four-chamber-views.[72,75] Efforts should be made to image subvalvular structures in their maximal length, usually in a view midway in orientation between the parasternal and apical planes.[60]

There have been controversial reports regarding whether valvular and subvalvular structural features affect the increase in mitral valve area by balloon mitral valvuloplasty.[25,60,61,63,76] Examination of pathologic specimens has revealed that balloon dilatation usually enlarges the mitral valve orifice by splitting the commissures.[64-67] By performing in vitro studies using mitral valves excised intact at the time of mitral valve replacement, Kaplan and associates[65] showed that the presence of extensive calcific deposits did not preclude adequate opening of a stenotic mitral orifice. Surprisingly, Ribeiro and associates,[66] in similar studies, found that commissural splitting occurred preferentially in calcified mitral commissures (81%) as opposed to noncalcified commissures (56%). The severity of the calcification in these valves was not assessed, however. Most clinical studies have found calcification of the commissures, rigid valve leaflets, and subvalvular diseases to be associated with a smaller mitral valve area following balloon valvuloplasty.[25,60,61,63]

Studies have also been performed to determine what degree of severity of valvular and subvalvular disease as assessed by two-dimensional echocardiography precludes a satisfactory immediate result of balloon mitral valvuloplasty. In a large series of 130 patients, Abascal and associates[59] reported that 84% (61/73) of patients with an echocardiographic score of 8 or less had a good outcome as defined by a final valve area of 1.5 cm^2 or more and an increase in valve area of 25% or more by valvuloplasty. In contrast, 58% (33/57) of patients with an echocardiographic score of 8 or more had a

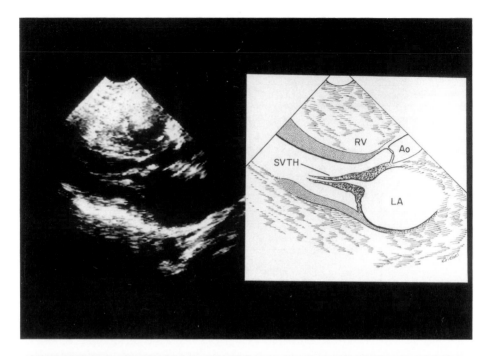

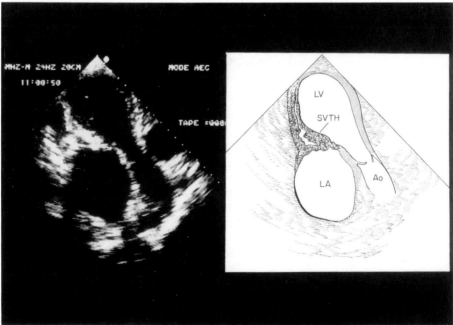

Figure 6.8 Top, Echocardiographic parasternal long-axis view in a patient with moderate thickening of the mitral valve leaflets and involvement of the subvalvular apparatus extending into the papillary muscles. Bottom, Echocardiographic apical long-axis view in a patient with severe subvalvular disease. There is extensive thickening and calcification of all subvalvular structures. *LA*—left atrium. *LV*—left ventricle. *SVTH*—subvalvular thickening. *Ao*—aorta. RV—right ventricle.

suboptimal result as defined by final valve area less than 1.5 cm^2 or an increase in valve area less than 25% (p < 0.001). The sensitivity of an echocardiographic score of 8 or less for predicting a good outcome was 72% and the specificity was 73%. Although the total echocardiographic score and the severity of valvular thickening correlated best with an absolute increase in mitral valve area after balloon valvuloplasty, there was substantial scatter in the data (Fig. 6.9). Similar results were reported by Chen and associates.[60] It is not surprising that the reliability of echocardiographic morphologic features for predicting results of percutaneous balloon valvuloplasty is not optimal, because results of a valvuloplasty also relate to a number of other factors: dilating balloon diameter and its relation to mitral annular size, learning curve of those performing the balloon valvuloplasty procedure, and differences in balloon dilating techniques.[45-63] Furthermore, difficulty in grading the severity of subvalvular disease by echocardiography may attenuate the reliability of echocardiographic scoring of subvalvular disease for predicting the balloon valvuloplasty results.[60,72]

Balloon valvuloplasty is not effective in treating severe subvalvular disease when it is the dominant cause of mitral stenosis because it does not split the chordal fusion present in such disease. Reid and associates[63] observed that the presence of subvalvular disease tended to be associated with a smaller increase in the valve area but did not preclude satisfactory results of mitral valvuloplasty using the double-balloon technique. However, these investigators did not grade the severity of valvular or subvalvular disease. Both thickening and fusion of subvalvular structures are the

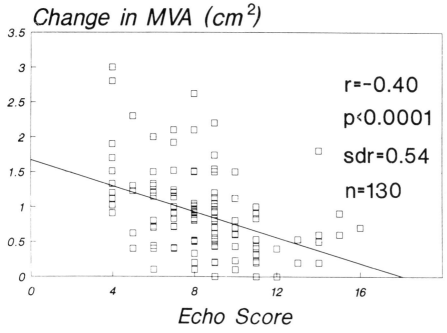

Figure 6.9 Relationship between the total echocardiographic score and the increase in mitral valve area after balloon mitral valvuloplasty. Although the correlation is significant (r = −0.40, p < 0.0001), there is substantial scatter in the data. (From: Abascal VM et al: Prediction of successful outcome in 130 patients undergoing percutaneous balloon mitral valvotomy. *Circulation*. 82:448–456, 1990. With permission of the American Heart Association, Inc.)

important features of subvalvular disease and are the dominant cause of mitral stenosis in 5 to 10% of patients[77,78] (see Fig. 6.8). Accordingly, Chen and associates[60] modified their system for echo grading of subvalvular disease by defining severe subvalvular disease as having both extensive thickening and nondetectable diastolic separation of tethered chords. Using this modified grading system for assessing severity of subvalvular disease, it has been demonstrated that severity of subvalvular disease is correlated negatively with mitral valve area following balloon valvuloplasty (multiple r = −0.65; p < 0.0002).[60] Three of four patients with severe mitral subvalvular disease of grade IV had only a small increase in mitral valve area following balloon valvuloplasty (≤ 1.5 cM^2) and the remaining patient had a mitral valve area of 1.6 cm^2 after valvuloplasty. However, most patients with moderate severity of subvalvular disease of grade III or less had a satisfactory result following balloon valvuloplasty. Thus, subvalvular disease less than grade IV does not preclude a satisfactory increase in mitral valve area.

In the study of Chen and associates[60] the total echocardiographic score had a weaker correlation with mitral valve area after balloon valvuloplasty than did sub-valvular disease. Multiple regression analysis showed that the total echocardiographic score is not an independent factor predicting suboptimal results of balloon mitral valvuloplasty. In young patients with rheumatic mitral stenosis, severe subvalvular disease is not always associated with severe thickening or calcification of the valve. In our own experience, one 18-year-old patient with severe subvalvular disease of grade IV had grade II thickening without calcification and grade I immobility of the valve (a total echocardiographic score of 7). This patient had a valve area of only 1.3 cm^2 with mitral regurgitation of grade II after valvuloplasty despite use of the double-balloon technique with an effective balloon diameter of 2.7 (1.8 + 1.5) cm.* Therefore, severe subvalvular disease limits the benefits of this procedure in two ways: (1) by inadequate enlargement of the mitral valve area by valvuloplasty and (2) by frequently leading to increased mitral regurgitation (to be discussed later in the section on mitral regurgitation after balloon valvuloplasty).

Differences in study populations may affect the relationship between the echocardiographic scoring system and mitral valve area after balloon valvuloplasty. In the study reported by Chen and associates,[60] the patients were younger (mean age = 36 ± 10 yrs) and may have had more severe rheumatic involvement of the valve and subvalvular structure and less calcification of the valve. Thus, the subvalvular disease becomes the most important factor related to the results of balloon valvuloplasty. In contrast, in the study reported by Abascal and associates[59] the patients were older (mean age = 55 ± 17 yrs) and may have had more severe mitral valve calcification, which in turn causes more thickening and immobility of the mitral valve and thus shows a greater total echocardiographic score. Consequently, total echo score and valve thickening are more important predictors than subvalvular disease in the Abascal study. Obviously, heavy calcification of mitral valve would prevent the commissure from being split like balloon aortic valvuloplasty in the calcified aortic valve, while mild calcification should have no significant influence on the splitting of commissural fusion by balloon valvuloplasty. Therefore, it is conceivable that either severe exten-

---

* The effective balloon diameter of a combination of two dilatation balloons was calculated according to the formula proposed by Yeager (Yeager SB: Balloon selection for double balloon valvotomy. *J Am Coll Cardiol.* 9:467–468, 1987).

sive calcification of the valve or severe subvalvular disease could lead to insufficient increase in mitral valve area by balloon valvuloplasty.

Assessment of Mitral Regurgitation

Doppler echocardiography is a very sensitive method for detecting mitral regurgitation, which is defined by a high velocity systolic flow in the left atrium with a sensitivity of 95% and a specificity of 90%.[79-85] Severity of mitral regurgitation can also be estimated by pulsed-wave[80] or color Doppler methods[86-88] or by combination of pulsed-wave Doppler and two-dimensional and M-mode echocardiography.[83,89]

Pulsed-wave Doppler
The Doppler examination should be performed in multiple parasternal and apical views, and the sample volume of pulsed-wave Doppler should carefully and progressively move from the mitral valve to the top of the left atrium to assess the extent of the regurgitant jet. Clinically useful semiquantitation of mitral regurgitation can be achieved by this approach using the extension of the jet. Mitral regurgitation can be graded from 1+ to 4+ by pulsed-wave Doppler mapping.[80] Mitral regurgitation grade 1+ represents abnormal systolic flow that extends to the proximal quarter of the left atrium, grade 2+ represents systolic flow detected halfway up the left atrium, grade 3+ represents systolic flow extending to the proximal three quarters of the left atrium, and grade 4+ represents regurgitant flow extending beyond three quarters of the atrium (Fig. 6.10). Pulsed Doppler–graded severity of mitral regurgitation has been shown to correlate well with angiographic assessment.[80] Although moderately severe or severe mitral regurgitation is not usually missed by pulsed Doppler technique, very eccentrically directed (wall) mitral regurgitant jets may not be reliably quantified by pulsed-wave Doppler mapping because three-dimensional distribution of the regurgitant jet is altered by the jet's hitting or emerging along the left atrial wall.[90-92]

Doppler, M-mode, and Two-dimensional Modalities Combined
By the continuity principle, in patients without aortic valve disease, the mitral regurgitant fraction can be derived by subtracting the total diastolic mitral flow from the aortic systolic flow and then dividing this difference by the diastolic mitral flow. A combination of M-mode, two-dimensional, and Doppler echocardiographic data is used in the calculation. However, this method is time-consuming, and a regurgitant fraction can be measured in up to 17% of normal patients without mitral regurgitation because the measurement error of aortic or mitral flow is 5 to 10%[83,89,93,94] Thus, this method is not used routinely.

Color Doppler Flow Mapping
With the color Doppler flow mapping technique, regurgitant jets (Fig. 6.11) can be visualized in real-time, and jet area and length easily measured.[86-88] Jet morphology (free vs. wall jet) can also be assessed (Fig. 6.11). It should be noted that to image the mitral regurgitant jet fully, echocardiographic recording should be taken in multiple views including an apical four-chamber view with and without the aorta, an apical two-chamber view with and without the aorta, and parasternal long-axis and short-axis views at the mitral valve and the aorta levels. Effort should be made to image the maximal jet size by adjusting transducer position to obtain an echocardiographic view

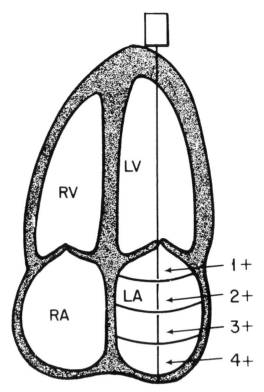

Figure 6.10 Diagram showing grading of the severity of mitral regurgitation according to the extent of the regurgitant jet within the left atrium. *Grade 1+*—Abnormal systolic flow that extends to the proximal quarter of the left atrium. *Grade 2+*—Regurgitant flow detected halfway up to the left atrium. *Grade 3+*—Systolic flow extending to the proximal three-quarters of the left atrium. *Grade 4+*—Regurgitant flow extending beyond three-quarters of the left atrium. *LA*—left atrium. *LV*—left ventricle. *RA*—right atrium, *RV*—right ventricle. (From: Abascal VM et al: Mitral regurgitation after percutaneous balloon mitral valvuloplasty in adults: evaluation by pulsed Doppler echocardiography. *J Am Coll Cardiol.* 11:257-2:-63, 1988. With permission.)

parallel to the jet direction and by using nonstandard tilted views in some cases. Maximal regurgitant jet area or ratio of the regurgitant jet area to the left atrial area correlated fairly well with the degree of mitral insufficiency assessed by left ventriculogram.[87,88] This correlation is best when three orthogonal planes are used to assess the regurgitant jet area.[87] A ratio of jet area to left atrial area of less than 20% represents mild mitral regurgitation, 20 to 40% indicates moderate regurgitation, more than 40% represents moderately severe mitral regurgitation, and more than 60% represents severe mitral regurgitation.

More recent studies have shown far less consistency, however. Spain[95] performed color Doppler flow mapping in 47 patients undergoing cardiac catheterization with left ventriculography and found that when the maximal jet area was measured as the largest clearly definable flow disturbance in the parasternal and apical views, a maximal jet area of more than 8 cm^2 from any of these views predicts severe mitral

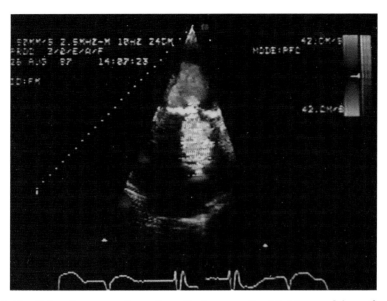

Figure 6.11 Color flow mapping of a mitral regurgitant jet imaged from the apical four-chamber view.

regurgitation with only moderate sensitivity (82%) and specificity (94%). This jet area correlated poorly with catheterization-derived regurgitant volume and fraction. The relationship between regurgitant volume and jet area is far more complex than originally recognized. For example, in vitro studies have demonstrated that the color Doppler jet area depends not only on the flow rate but also on driving pressure, regurgitant orifice size, instrument gain settings, chamber constraint, and wall impingement.[90-92,96-103] In patients with mitral regurgitation, in a dog model of mitral regurgitation, and in an in vitro flow model, Chen and associates demonstrated that when the mitral regurgitant jet was eccentrically spreading along the lateral, anterior, or septal left atrial wall (wall jet), these wall jets imaged on a two-dimensional plane usually appeared smaller than a centrally located free jet.[92] In patients with an eccentrically directed wall jet, very poor correlation was found between wall jet area and mitral regurgitant fraction.[90] Thus, when interpreting mitral regurgitation after balloon valvuloplasty, jet morphology (wall or free jets) should be considered in grading the severity of mitral regurgitation. Since size of free jet correlated fairly well with mitral regurgitant fraction or volume, color Doppler can be reliably used to semiquantitatively estimate the severity of mitral regurgitation in patients with free mitral regurgitant jets. An accurate method for estimating severity of mitral regurgitation in patients with wall jets is yet to be determined.

Valvular Morphology as Related to Mitral Regurgitation After Balloon Valvuloplasty

Mitral regurgitation is a recognized complication after closed surgical commissurotomy, documented angiographically in 8 to 20% of a large series of patients.[69-70] Those with calcified mitral valve as assessed by the surgeon during commissurotomy had a higher incidence of an increase in mitral regurgitation than those without calcification.[70] Angiographic documentation of an increase in mitral regurgitation occurred in 25 to 48% of patients after balloon valvuloplasty.[45-63,74] Mitral regurgitation is usually mild (less than grade 2+). Severe mitral regurgitation was rare, occurring in 0 to 5% of patients.[60-63] Since associated mitral regurgitation increases mortality and morbidity after surgical commissurotomy,[104] to predict which patient will develop mitral regurgitation, especially severe regurgitation, after balloon valvuloplasty is of great clinical importance.

Using an echocardiographic scoring system in patients with mitral stenosis who had undergone balloon valvuloplasty, Chen and associates[60] demonstrated a significant correlation between the total echocardiographic score of mitral valvular and subvalvular features and an increase in mitral regurgitation after valvuloplasty, although there was substantial scatter in the data. The multiple regression analysis showed that severity of subvalvular disease is one of the important independent factors correlating with the increase in mitral regurgitation by balloon valvuloplasty. Most (6/11) patients with severe subvalvular disease of grade III or more had an increase in mitral regurgitation after valvuloplasty, whereas only 6 of 27 patients with subvalvular disease of grade II or less showed an increase in mitral regurgitation (p < 0.05). Two patients with an increase in mitral regurgitation by two grades had severe subvalvular disease of grade IV as assessed by echocardiography.

The mechanism for an increase in mitral regurgitation after balloon valvuloplasty is not completely understood. The underlying rheumatic deformation of mitral leaflets and subvalvular fusion together with mitral commissural splitting may interact to cause incomplete closure of mitral leaflets during systole. As in surgical commissurotomy, it appears that the rupture of chordae tendineae and valve tear or detachment caused by balloon valvuloplasty are responsible for severe mitral regurgitation.

Selection of Balloon Size

Most studies indicate that an adequate size of dilating balloons is the prerequisite for achieving an optimal increase in the valve area, although oversized balloons may produce a higher incidence of mitral regurgitation after percutaneous balloon valvuloplasty.[58-62] Some authors use body surface area as a reference to select balloon size.[62] Using mitral ring size as a reference to select the balloon may prevent overdilating the mitral ring and causing severe mitral regurgitation.[60] Two-dimensional echocardiography can accurately measure the diameters of the mitral annulus.[105,106] The major axis diameter of the elliptical mitral annulus can be measured from the apical four-chamber view and the minor axis diameter from the parasternal long-axis view. It has been shown that the diameter of mitral annulus[106] measured from the apical four-chamber view is a useful parameter for selecting balloon size.[60] In a series of 38 consecutive patients undergoing mitral balloon valvuloplasty by the double-balloon technique, Chen and associates[60] observed that the mitral valve area $(0.9 \pm 0.3 \text{ cm}^2)$ was not adequately increased when the sum of two balloon diameters was 10% less than the mitral annulus size. The mitral valve area was not enlarged further by using a ratio of the sum of the diameters from two balloons and mitral annular diameter of more than 1.1, but the incidence of new or worsened mitral regurgitation after valvuloplasty did increase sharply (Fig. 6.12). This suggests that when the double-balloon technique is used, balloon size should be between 90% and 110% of the mitral annular size in the apical four-chamber view.

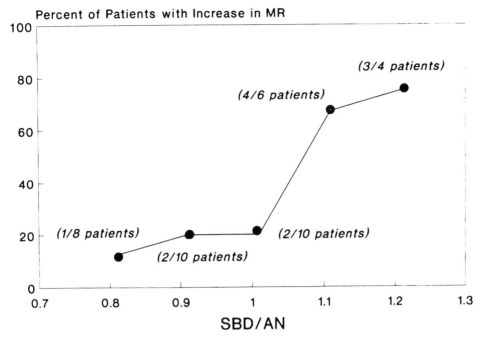

Figure 6.12 Relationship between the percentage of patients with an increase in mitral regurgitation (*MR*) produced by balloon valvuloplasty and the ratio of the sum of diameters from two dilating balloons used and mitral annulus diameter (*SBD/AN*). (From: Chen C et al: Value of two-dimensional echocardiography in selecting patients and balloon sizes for percutaneous balloon mitral valvuloplasty. *J Am Coll Cardiol.* 14:1651–1658, 1989. With permission.)

Patient Followup

Being noninvasive, convenient, and easily available, echocardiography is an ideal tool for repeat assessment of mitral valve area and severity of mitral regurgitation after balloon mitral valvuloplasty. Abascal and associates[59] followed 20 patients for 6 months after balloon mitral valvuloplasty and observed that 4 of 20 (20%) patients experienced restenosis as defined by a reduction of the mitral valve area of $>25\%$ (compared to the valve area immediately after valvuloplasty) and an area of <1.5 cm^2 at followup. The echocardiographic score in patients who exhibited restenosis was 11 ± 2, significantly higher than the score in those without restenosis (7 ± 2; p $<$ 0.002). All 4 patients with restenosis had an echocardiographic score of more than 8. Palacios and associates[62] further demonstrated that only 2 of 45 (4.4%) patients with echocardiographic scores < 8 had restenosis as defined by the criteria of Abascal and associates, whereas 7 of 10 (70%) patients with echocardiographic scores > 8 experienced restenosis at an average of 13 months' followup. The patients with high echocardiographic score also had severe symptoms of New York Heart Association function class III to IV (42% of patients in NYHA classes III and IV) at followup. Nobuyoshi and associates[61] found a similar relationship between echocardiographic and morphologic features and results of balloon mitral valvuloplasty in 97 patients at short-term (9 ± 4 months) followup after valvuloplasty. However, echocardiographic mitral valve and subvalvular features in their study were graded differently from the system proposed by Abascal and Wilkins.[25,75] In patients with pliable and semipliable mitral valves, both immediate and followup results including symptomatic improvement, mitral valve area, and incidence of mitral regurgitation were significantly better than those in patients with rigid valves.[61] In a preliminary report at 2 to 4 years' clinical followup (mean 20 ± 1) in 320 patients after balloon valvuloplasty, Palacios and associates[107] demonstrated that a greater number (80%) of patients with echocardiographic scores < 8 were free from total clinical events (death, mitral valve replacement, and NYHA class III or IV) than those (40%) with echocardiographic scores more than 8. The survival at the followup period was 99% in patients with echocardiographic scores < 8 and 75% in patients with echocardiographic scores > 8. There are still no data available to assess long-term effects of percutaneous balloon mitral valvuloplasty.

Using Doppler echocardiography in followup assessment of patients after balloon mitral valvuloplasty, Abascal and associates[25] showed that mitral regurgitation remained unchanged in 35% of patients and decreased at least by one grade in 55% of patients; 10% patients showed an increase in mitral regurgitation at 6 months followup. However, there are no long-term followup data regarding the natural history of mitral regurgitation after balloon valvuloplasty, especially in moderate mitral regurgitation.

Identification of Left Atrial Thrombus

Given the potentially devastating consequences of cardiogenic emboli, the identification of a left atrial thrombus (Fig. 6.13) is of major clinical relevance; during balloon mitral valvuloplasty, catheter manipulation in the left atrium may dislodge the left atrial thrombus and release systemic emboli. Thromboembolic complication has been reported to occur in 0 to 4.8% of patients undergoing balloon mitral valvuloplasty despite careful transthoracic echocardiographic exclusion of left atrial thrombus.[45-62,108-112] The embolism is believed to be caused by dislodging of the atrial thrombus, calcium, or excessive material of the rheumatic changes of the mitral valve. It was demonstrated that a thrombus in the left atrial appendage is often missed by transthoracic echocardiography[113,114] and that transesophageal echocardiography is a unique technique for its detection (Fig. 6.14). Kronzon and associates[113] performed both a transthoracic and a transesophageal echocardiogram in 19 consecutive candidates for percutaneous balloon mitral valvuloplasty and observed that in 5 of 19 (26%) patients transesophageal echocardiography revealed a thrombus in the left atrial appendage. In 3 of the 5, the thrombus extended to the atrial cavity, and transthoracic echocardiography revealed evidence of suspected thrombosis in only 1 patient. In a study by Chen and associates (unpublished data), transesophageal echocardiography was performed in 20 consecutive candidates without transthoracic echocardiographic evidence of a thrombus in the left atrium, and only 1 patient was found to have a left atrial thrombus. Therefore, the frequency of detection of a thrombus in the left atrium including appendage by transesophageal echocardiography in patients without any transthoracic echocardiographic evidence is yet to be defined in a large series of consecutive candidates for balloon valvuloplasty.[115] The appropriateness of transesophageal echocardiography for every candidate being considered for balloon mitral valvuloplasty is still uncertain.

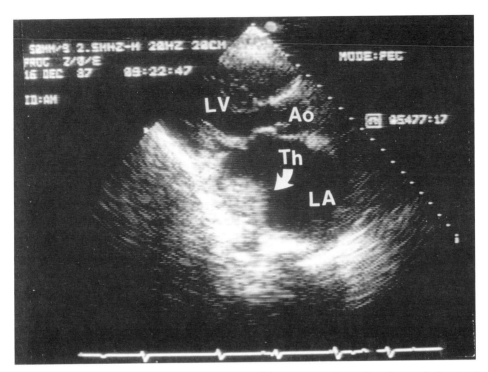

Figure 6.13 Echocardiographic parasternal long-axis view showing a left atrial thrombus in a patient with mitral stenosis. *LA*—left atrium. *LV*—left ventricle. *Ao*—aorta, *Th*—thrombus.

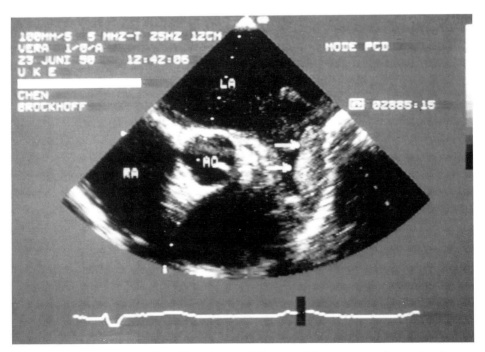

Figure 6.14 Left atrial thrombus (*arrows*) detected by transesophageal echocardiography. *Ao*—aorta. *LA*—left atrium. *RA*—right atrium.

Evaluation of Postvalvuloplasty Atrial Septal Defect

Most operators use the transseptal approach to introduce balloon catheters through the stenotic mitral valve during balloon mitral valvuloplasty. It was demonstrated in a canine study that persistence of a small (<5 mm) atrial septal defect was found after a transseptal puncture with a 7-mm catheter.[46] An iatrogenic atrial septal defect after balloon mitral valvuloplasty was reported to occur in 10 to 25% of patients.[45-63] Although the interatrial shunt was often small (Qs/Qp <1:1.5), acute creation of interatrial communication could be particularly damaging in patients with longstanding pulmonary hypertension secondary to mitral stenosis because the added volume overload in the right ventricle could theoretically lead to worsening hemodynamic consequences. Furthermore, an interatrial shunt may lead to inaccuracy in calculation of the mitral valve area by means of the thermodilution technique of measuring cardiac output.

Examining the immediate and long-term effects of small shunts and the possibility of spontaneous closure of the defect is therefore important. An oxygen stepup of > 7% by saturation or > 2% by content in the right atrium at cardiac catheterization has been conventionally used to define an interatrial shunt. This technique is insensitive for small shunts, however. It is also costly for followup of patients, and it carries some risk of the common complications of an invasive technique. Two-dimensional and M-mode echocardiography can detect the consequences of a left-to-right shunt (right ventricular dilatation and paradoxical motion of the interventricular septum) in moderate and large atrial septal defect.[116-118] A moderate-sized (>1.0 cm) defect of the interatrial septum may be directly identified by two-dimensional echocardiography. However, a small atrial septal defect (<5 mm) after balloon mitral valvuloplasty may not be recognized by two-dimensional technique. Doppler techniques permit noninvasive evaluation of intracardiac blood flow velocity and direction and have a widely established record of accuracy in the detection and quantification of atrial septal defects.[119-124] Come and associates[125] reported that an interatrial shunt was detected in 12 of 37 (32%) of patients after balloon mitral valvuloplasty by contrast or pulsed-wave Doppler echocardiography or both and in 9 of 37 (24%) of patients by oximetry. Echocardiographic and oximetric diagnoses of the presence or absence of an atrial septal defect were concurrent in 30 patients. One patient with a shunt of Qp/Qs = 1.2 was not identified by echocardiography. Five patients with echocardiographic findings of a left-to-right shunt had no diagnostic oxygen stepup in the right heart. Thus, pulsed-wave, color Doppler, and contrast echocardiography appear to be more sensitive for detecting small degrees of interatrial shunting.

Transesophageal color Doppler flow mapping technique has considerably enhanced detection of small interatrial left-to-right shunts (Fig. 6.15). The advantages of transesophageal over transthoracic echocardiography in the detection of left-to-right shunt flow are (1) the absence of anatomic obstacles between the ultrasound transducer and the interatrial septum, (2) nearly parallel alignment of the ultrasound beam with the shunting flow through the defect, and (3) better resolution characteristics with higher frequency (5 MHz) transducers.[124] Using transesophageal color Doppler technique, Yoshida and associates [124] detected an atrial left-to-right shunting flow in 13 of 15 (87%) patients, in 73% of patients, and in 47% of patients, respectively, at intervals of 1 day, 1 week, and 1 month after balloon mitral valvuloplasty. Only 2 of 15 patients with transesophageal echocardiographically–detected shunt could be identified by transthoracic echocardiography at 1 day, and the

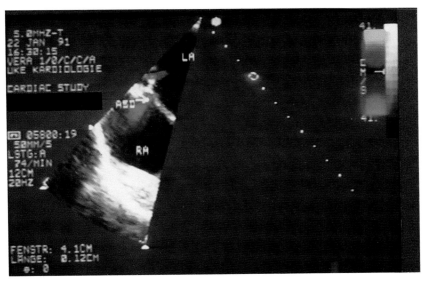

Figure 6.15 Color flow mapping of left-to-right shunt flow through the defect in atrial septum (ASD) in a patient immediately after percutaneous balloon mitral valvuloplasty imaged by transesophageal echocardiography. *LA*—left atrium. *RA*—right atrium.

shunt disappeared at 1 week after the procedure. However, the correlation between transesophageal color Doppler technique and other more sensitive techniques (such as the indicator dilution curve technique) used to detect shunts has not been tested. Long-term effects of a small shunting flow in patients after valvuloplasty are not totally clear. Using color Doppler echocardiography, Reid and associates[126] observed that a left-to-right shunt at the atrial level persisted in 42%, 33%, and 31% of patients at 1, 2, and 3 years of followup, respectively. Persistence of the shunt did not appear to correlate with symptomatic functional classes.

Transesophageal Echocardiography

As discussed earlier in this chapter, transesophageal echocardiography is more sensitive than transthoracic echocardiography in detecting left atrial thrombus before balloon valvuloplasty and in identifying atrial septal defects after valvuloplasty. Several studies have been conducted to examine (1) the possible advantages of the transesophageal over the transthoracic approach in assessing valvular structure of the mitral valve and (2) the utility of transesophageal echocardiography in monitoring balloon mitral valvuloplasty.

More detailed and accurate assessment of the mitral valve and subvalvular structures may help in selecting patients for successful balloon valvuloplasty and in averting major complications such as severe mitral regurgitation. Transesophageal echocardiography may provide additional information on morphologic characteristics of the mitral valve and the subvalvular structures if an adequate quality of transthoracic echocardiogram is not available (Fig. 6.16). Griffen and associates[127] compared echocardiographic scores of mitral valve morphology in 15 consecutive patients. They

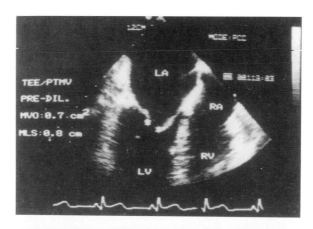

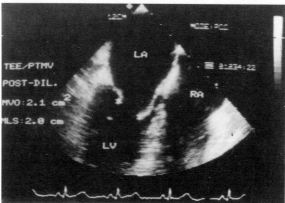

Figure 6.16 Four-chamber transesophageal echocardiograms obtained before (*upper*) and after (*lower*) percutaneous balloon mitral valvuloplasty. The maximal leaflet separation (*MLS*) was 0.8 cm before and 2.0 cm after valvuloplasty. The mitral valve orifice (*MVO*), as examined by Doppler echocardiography, was 0.7 cm² before and 2.1 cm² after valvuloplasty. *LA*—left atrium. *LV*—left ventricle. *RA*—right atrium. *RV*—right ventricle. (From: Erbel et al: *Transesophageal Echocardiography. A New Window To The Heart.* New York: Springer-Verlag, 1988. With permission.)

found that echocardiographic scores graded by monoplane transesophageal echocardiography (6.1 ± 1.3) were consistently lower than those (7.1 ± 2.1) graded using the transthoracic approach. Echocardiographic scores graded by transesophageal echocardiography correlated slightly better (r = 0.66) with the absolute change in mitral valve area after balloon valvuloplasty than scores graded by the transthoracic approach (r = 0.50). However, the patient group in this study was too small to permit any definite conclusions to be drawn. It is well known that monoplane transesophageal echocardiography is limited in imaging the posteromedial papillary muscle and the proximal portion of its related chordae tendineae and the posteromedial commissure of the mitral valve.[128,129] Thus, localized change of the mitral valve such as calcification and subvalvular disease might be missed if only the single-plane transesophageal transducer is used.[129] Nevertheless, in patients in whom the quality of precordial echocardiography has been inadequate, the transesophageal technique is certainly an alternative complimentary approach for assessment of mitral morphology.

Using biplane transesophageal echocardiography, more detailed assessment of mitral valve and subvalvular structure may be achieved. Wang and associates [129] used a biplane transesophageal, two-dimensional approach in sectioning seven cadavers and their hearts to produce nine transverse and six longitudinal transesophageal equivalent planes. They also performed transesophageal echocardiograms in 427 subjects, using either a uniplane or biplane transducer, and found the transverse plane of the left heart to be very useful for the study of transmitral flow dynamics, mitral valve movement, and the detection of mitral stenosis and mitral regurgitation. Since the commissures of the mitral valve are not linear, transthoracic imaging may be limited by the restricted windows. Thus, the transesophageal biplane approach appears to have advantages in detailed noninvasive assessment of mitral commissures and valve morphology. For balloon mitral valvuloplasty, it is very important to assess the subvalvular structure. The advantage of biplane transesophageal echocardiography in imaging subvalvular apparatus is, however, still unclear.

In a few centers, transesophageal echocardiography has also been used to monitor the percutaneous valvuloplasty procedure.[130,131] The interatrial septum, particularly that of the oval fossa, can be visualized by transesophageal echocardiography. When the tip of the transseptal needle reaches the atrial septum and some pressure is applied, the atrial septum changes its shape to a triangular configuration. In a study of 15 patients undergoing balloon mitral valvuloplasty while under general anesthesia, Visser and associates [131] showed that in 2 cases this monitoring was necessary to guide appropriate positioning of the transseptal puncturing device. Usually, experienced operators have no difficulty with the transseptal puncture under x-ray fluoroscopy. However, significant dilatation of the right atrium may make the transseptal puncture complicated and, in these cases, transesophageal monitoring may be helpful. Another potential use of transesophageal echocardiography may be to guide the positioning of the balloon catheter through the mitral valve to avoid unsuccessful inflation of the balloon catheters and perforation of the left ventricle. It has also been suggested that transesophageal monitoring shortens the x-ray exposure time during balloon valvuloplasty.[131] Transesophageal echocardiography provides an on-table (catheterization table) assessment of commissural separation and such complications as pericardial effusion by cardiac perforation, severe mitral regurgitation or rupture of chordae tendineae, and atrial septal defect; it is a valuable tool in clinical decision making. Obviously, transesophageal echocardiography is an adjunct to fluoroscopy and hemodynamic monitoring, providing important additional information during balloon valvuloplasty. Although there was one report of transesophageal monitoring in an awake patient,[130] transesophageal monitoring with the currently available probe (10–12 mm in diameter) can be performed only in patients under general anesthesia. Therefore, the advantages of this echocardiographic support should be weighed against the risk of general anesthesia.

Patient Selection and Echocardiography

What are the clinical implications of echocardiographic studies for patient selection in balloon mitral valvuloplasty? Patients with extensive calcification of the valve and extensive subvalvular disease are not expected to have sufficient increase in mitral valve area after balloon valvuloplasty, and severe mitral regurgitation caused by valvuloplasty is more likely to occur. There is also a high restenosis rate with poor clinical and hemodynamic improvement at intermediate-term followup in these patients. Clearly, balloon mitral valvuloplasty should not be considered for these patients if surgical valve replacement can be performed. To prevent catastrophic effects of arterial embolism, patients with atrial thrombi should not be considered as candidates for balloon valvuloplasty. Transthoracic echocardiography is therefore required for all candidates for balloon mitral valvuloplasty to exclude patients with atrial thrombi. Transesophageal echocardiography should be used if thrombi are suspected on the bases of the transthoracic echocardiogram. It is not clear whether all candidates for balloon mitral valvuloplasty should undergo transesophageal procedure to rule out thrombi in the left atrial appendage. (See also Chapter 11.)

AORTIC STENOSIS

After the initial description of balloon aortic valvuloplasty in children and young adults with congenital aortic stenosis in 1984,[132] Cribier and associates[133] in 1986 reported the extended use of this technique to treat elderly patients with symptomatic aortic stenosis. Aortic valve replacement is associated with considerable perioperative mortality ranging from 3%[134] to 18%[135] and with an even higher rate (24%) in patients who are more than 80 years of age.[136] The 1-year survival rate of untreated patients with symptomatic severe aortic stenosis is as low as 57% in contrast to 93% in age- and sex-matched controls.[137] Therefore, percutaneous balloon aortic valvuloplasty was initially performed with much enthusiasm and has been evaluated extensively for the palliation of elderly patients wih severe aortic stenosis.[138-145] Two-dimensional and Doppler echocardiography have been widely used to evaluate patients before, immediately after, and in long-term follow-up of balloon aortic valvuloplasty.

Assessment of Severity

Patients with systolic ejection murmurs are often referred for echocardiography to determine the causes of the murmurs, such as aortic valvular stenosis, subvalvular or supravalvular obstruction, or aortic sclerosis without significant stenosis seen especially in elderly and hypertensive patients.

M-mode and Two-dimensional Assessment

M-mode echocardiography can record two of three aortic valve leaflets, and two-dimensional echocardiography provides assessment of all three leaflets in parasternal short-axis views. If the valve is thickened, distinction can be made between aortic sclerosis and aortic stenosis. In aortic sclerosis without stenosis, the aortic valve leaflets are thickened but open adequately during systole. In contrast, in calcified aortic stenosis, aortic valve leaflets are frequently extensively thickened and have a restricted opening. In congenital aortic valve stenosis, the valve leaflets are usually thin, but typical doming can be observed during systole in the parasternal long-axis view of the left ventricular outflow tract and proximal ascending aorta. In the short-axis view of the aortic valve, the bicuspid aortic valve can be identified. Both of the thickened leaflets of the aortic valve and a reduced aortic opening with systolic doming can be observed in rheumatic aortic stenosis with or without calcification. Rheumatic aortic stenosis is almost always associated with mitral valve disease.

Although amplitude of the valve separation can be used for a rough estimate of the severity of stenosis, the amplitude of the opening (aortic excursion) measured in the parasternal long-axis view correlated only fairly well with the aortic valve area derived from catheterization data (r = 0.63; SEE = 0.22 cm^2).[146] Obviously, the aortic amplitude depends also on cardiac output and can be difficult to measure when the valve is extensively calcified and the leaflets of the valve are asymmetrically affected. In congenital aortic valve stenosis, measurement of leaflet separation should be taken at the tip of the aortic leaflets to avoid false measurement of the larger opening at the proximal part of the dome. The planimetry of the aortic valve opening at short axis is often difficult to obtain,[147] and in calcific aortic stenosis, it is almost impossible because of shadowing from the calcific material. Significant left ventricular hypertrophy usually indicates severe aortic stenosis[148] when other causes such as hypertension are ruled out. However, at advanced stages of the disease, the left ventricle becomes dilated. Thus, for reliable and accurate quantification of aortic stenosis, two-dimensional echocardiography is often inadequate.

Doppler Echocardiography

Doppler recording of transaortic velocity (Fig. 6.17) is very useful for quantification of aortic stenosis and provides calculations of the aortic valve area and the pressure gradient across the aortic valve. As in mitral stenosis, the simplified Bernoulli equation is used to convert aortic flow velocity into a pressure gradient.[10,27] The following are some important technical and terminological aspects to be considered for accurate interpretation of the Doppler-derived transaortic gradient.

1. *Limitations of the simplified Bernoulli equation:* The simplified Bernoulli equation ($\Delta P = 4V^2$) assumes that viscous friction and flow acceleration components of the complete Bernoulli equation are negligible[10]:

$$P_1 - P_2 = \underbrace{\frac{1}{2}\rho(v_2^2 - v_1^2)}_{\substack{\text{convective} \\ \text{acceleration}}} + \underbrace{\rho\int_1^2 \frac{d\vec{v}}{dt}d\vec{s}}_{\substack{\text{flow} \\ \text{acceleration}}} + \underbrace{R(\vec{v})}_{\substack{\text{viscous} \\ \text{friction}}}$$

where suffix 1 denotes the position of the fluid element in front of the valve, and suffix 2 in the valve jet; P is the pressure, $\vec{v}$ is the velocity vector of the fluid element along its path, and $d\vec{s}$ is the path element; ρ is mass density or density of blood. The Bernoulli equation states that the energy from the pressure drop across a stenosis is used to overcome the losses of energy from the viscous friction, flow acceleration, and convective acceleration of the flow. Viscous friction is small in large vessels with laminar flow, and the flow acceleration term is negligible when flow velocity is unchanging. Since aortic velocity is usually more than 4 m/s in significant aortic stenosis, the square of the velocity proximal to the aortic valve (V_1) (left ventricular outflow tract), which is usually less than 1.0 m/s, is more than 15 times smaller than the square of the transaortic velocity (V_2). Thus, velocity in the left ventricular outflow tract (V_1) is negligible. However, in cases of increased cardiac output and subaortic flow velocity such as in aortic stenosis associated with significant aortic regurgitation and in very mild aortic stenosis (transaortic velocity <2 m/s), V_1

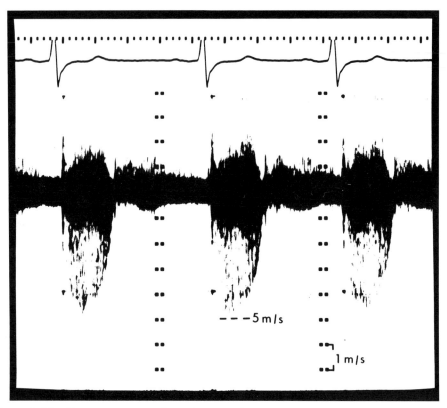

Figure 6.17   Continuous-wave Doppler recording of transaortic systolic flow velocity profile using a nonimaging transducer from the apex in a patient with calcific aortic stenosis. The peak velocity is 5 m/s; the estimated transaortic peak gradient is 100 mmHg using the modified Bernoulli equation.

can no longer be ignored and the simplified Bernoulli equation may overestimate the transaortic pressure gradient.

2. *Sampling angle of the ultrasound beam and experience of technicians:* The ultrasound beam should be aligned parallel to aortic flow direction (the center axis of the stenotic jet) because Doppler-measured velocity varies inversely with cosine of the angle between the Doppler beam and the direction of the blood flow

$$V = f_d \cdot c/2f_t \cdot \cos \Theta$$

where f_d = frequency shift, c = speed of sound in blood, f_t = transducer frequency, and Θ = the intercept angle between the ultrasound beam and the direction of blood flow. An angle of more than 20° between the ultrasound beam and the flow direction will cause significant underestimation of the pressure gradient.[10] To minimize the underestimation, effort should be made to obtain parallel alignment of the ultrasound beam to the aortic flow direction and to obtain the velocity profile by positioning the transducer at all three commonly used imaging approaches: at the apex, at the right upper sternal border, and at the suprasternal notch if possible. The maximal transaortic velocity from any of these three approaches is then used to calculate the gradient.

The average value of the maximal velocity should be determined from at least three beats. If an adequate Doppler velocity profile of the aortic flow cannot be obtained from the former three approaches, an adequate Doppler signal of the stenotic jet can sometimes be recorded at the left parasternal border. Since the noninmaging continuous-wave Doppler transducer is used in most clinical situations, the echocardiographer has to rely on acoustic signal monitoring to identify the peak transaortic velocity. An inexperienced echocardiographic technician may therefore not be able to record maximal velocity. With development of the combined transducer for pulsed-wave, continuous-wave, and color Doppler flow imaging and the transducer with a steerable continuous-wave Doppler beam under color Doppler guiding, the alignment of ultrasound beam to the center axis of the stenotic jet can be improved and the angle between the stenotic jet and the ultrasound beam can be corrected.

3. *Peak-to-peak gradient and instantaneous maximal gradient:* In aortic stenosis, a temporal inequality between peak left ventricular pressure and peak aortic pressure exists and the peak aortic pressure usually occurs later than the peak left ventricular pressure. Thus, the difference between the peak aortic pressure and peak left ventricular pressure (peak-to-peak pressure gradient), which is conventionally reported by a catheterization laboratory, should not be expected to be the same as the maximal instantaneous difference between aortic pressure and left ventricular pressure (maximal instantaneous pressure gradient).[149] Continuous-wave Doppler echocardiography records instantaneous velocity across the aortic valve and thereby the instantaneous pressure gradient across the aortic valve during systole. Maximal instantaneous pressure gradient and mean systolic pressure gradient (integration of entire systolic instantaneous pressure gradients divided by systolic time) can then be obtained using the recorded continuous-wave Doppler aortic velocity profile. Therefore, the catheterization-derived peak-to-peak pressure gradient is lower than the Doppler-derived maximal instantaneous pressure gradient, but the catheterization-derived mean gradient should be the same as the Doppler-derived mean gradient (Fig. 6.18).

Estimation of Aortic Valve Area

By combining echocardiographic and Doppler techniques, the aortic valve area can be estimated with the continuity equation.[150-154] Aortic valve area is not dependent on left ventricular performance or concomitant aortic regurgitation. Calculation of the aortic valve area is therefore particularly useful in patients with low cardiac output and severely depressed left ventricular function or with concomitant significant aortic regurgitation. The most widely accepted method for Doppler echocardiographic calculation of aortic valve area (Fig. 6.19) is by the continuity principle. The method uses the equality of the flow through the left ventricular outflow tract (LVOT), which is the product of LVOT area (A_{LVOT}) and the LVOT velocity integral (V_{LVOT}), and the transaortic flow, which is the product of aortic valve area (A_{AV}) and the transaortic velocity integral (V_{AV}):

$$A_{LVOT} \times V_{LVOT} = A_{AV} \times V_{AV}$$

This can be rearranged as:

$$A_{AV} = \frac{A_{LVOT} \times V_{LVOT}}{V_{AV}}$$

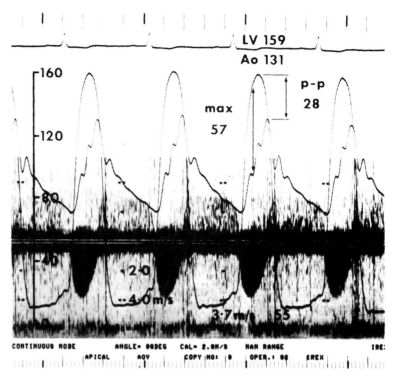

Figure 6.18 Simultaneous recording of left ventricular and aortic pressures and Doppler continuous-wave velocity profile in a patient with moderate aortic stenosis. Peak pressure gradients obtained by Doppler technique were similar to maximum catheter gradient (max). Peak-to-peak gradient (p–p) is measured from the cardiac catheterization data. (From: Currie PJ et al: Continuous-wave Doppler echocardiographic assessment of severity of calcific aortic stenosis: a simultaneous Doppler–catheter correlative study in 100 adult patients. *Circulation.* 71:1162–1169, 1985. With permission of the American Heart Association, Inc.)

The peak velocities across the LVOT and the aortic valve can be substituted for the velocity integrals. The LVOT area is calculated from the LVOT diameter assuming a circular shape of the LVOT. The LVOT diameter is measured immediately below the aortic valve.[12] The trailing-edge-to-leading-edge diameter is usually used to calculate the cross-sectional area. Special attention should be paid to obtaining LVOT velocity. The apical four-chamber view with aortic valve (5-chamber view) is most often used to record the LVOT blood flow velocity. Doppler sample volume should begin at the LVOT distal to the aortic valve and move toward the valve. As the sampling position is moved toward the aortic valve, the recorded velocity increases until approximately 1 to 2 cm proximal to the valve. The velocity is stable at this point, and the velocity for the LVOT should be measured there. Further adjustment of the sampling position toward the aortic valve will lead to recording of a sudden increase in velocity, and aliasing of the Doppler recorded blood velocity is usually observed.

Several studies have demonstrated excellent correlation between Doppler-derived data and catheterization-derived data for both the maximal instantaneous trans-

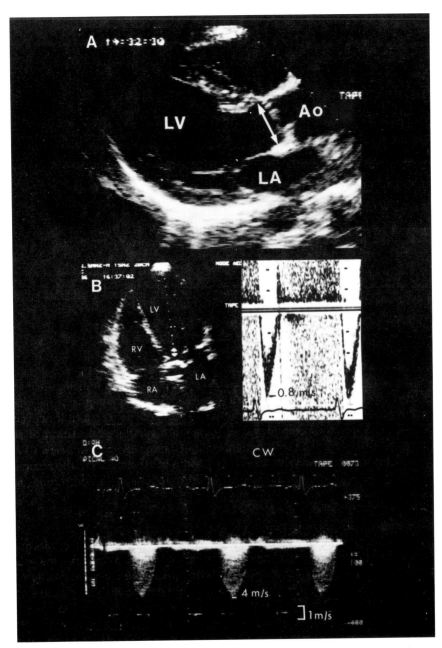

Figure 6.19 Calculation of aortic valve area using the continuity equation from two-dimensional and Doppler techniques in a patient with aortic stenosis. *Panel A,* Two-dimensional echocardiogram showing measurement of left ventricular outflow tract diameter. Left ventricular outflow tract area is then calculated assuming a circular shape. *Panel B,* Pulsed-wave Doppler flow velocity recorded at the left ventricular outflow tract from apical five-chamber view (See text.) *Panel C,* Continuous-wave Doppler of transaortic velocity recorded from the apex. The peak velocity is 4 m/s. *LA*—left atrium. *LV*—left ventricle. *Ao*—aorta, *RV*—right ventricle. *RA*—right atrium.

aortic gradient and the mean gradient (r = 0.92 and SEE = 15 mmHg for the maximal gradient; r = 0.93 and SEE = 10 mmHg for the mean gradient) (Fig. 6.20).[149,155-158] Similarly, the Doppler-derived aortic valve area correlated well with the catheterization-derived valve area (r = 0.80–0.89, SEE ±0.12–0.21cm²)[12] (Fig. 6.21). However, only a fair correlation (r = 0.61) was found between Doppler-derived aortic valve area and catheterization-derived area (Fig. 6.22) by Nishimura and associates.[159] It should be noted that in their study the echocardiographic measurements after balloon aortic valvuloplasty were performed 1 day after the procedure, whereas the hemodynamic measurements were taken immediately after the valvuloplasty procedure. It has been documented that the pressure gradient and aortic valve area change significantly within 24 hours after balloon valvuloplasty.[160-162] Therefore, this moderate correlation may be due to non-simultaneous measurements of catheterization and Doppler parameters. Unfortunately, there have been no published reports of simultaneous measurements of catheterization and Doppler parameters after balloon aortic valvuloplasty.

Color Doppler Flow Mapping

Although a narrow stenotic color Doppler jet can usually be recorded in aortic stenosis if the valve is not extensively calcified, color Doppler flow mapping is not routinely used for quantification of aortic stenosis. In a preliminary study,[163] aortic valve area was calculated by color Doppler jet width, assuming a circular stenotic orifice, and was found to correlate fairly well with aortic valve area. However, in an extensively calcified valve, the shadowing of the calcification often makes it difficult to view the color jet through the stenosis because color Doppler equipment usually has a tissue priority algorithm. The gain settings of color Doppler equipment may have a further influence on the accuracy of the measurement of the jet width. Importantly, limited axial resolution of color Doppler mapping may affect calculation of aortic valve area by the jet width. A measurement error of 2 mm will usually cause a 30–40% error in calculation of aortic valve area in a jet width of 10 mm. Thus, the accuracy of color Doppler jet width in quantification of aortic stenosis in clinical settings needs further investigation.

Transesophageal Echocardiography

Transthoracic Doppler echocardiography usually provides quantitative information about pressure gradients across the aortic valve and aortic valve area for grading severity of aortic stenosis. In about 5 to 10% of patients, an adequate quality of the Doppler velocity profile across aortic valve may not be obtainable by means of the transthoracic approach.[164,165] Transesophageal two-dimensional echocardiography has been used to measure the aortic valve area directly in its short-axis view.[164,165] Reportedly there is a good correlation between aortic valve orifice determined using transesophageal and the catheterization-derived aortic valve orifice area using Gorlin's formula (r = 0.92).[164] However, this planimetric method is not possible in about 17% of patients who have a severely calcified valve.

Transesophageal echocardiography with continuous-wave Doppler records the aortic velocity profile and thus is used to calculate the pressure gradients and aortic valve area. A preliminary report showed that there was a constant underestimation of pressure gradient by transesophageal measurement and only a fair correlation between maximal gradient measurements by catheterization and transesophageal Doppler (r = 0.64) was observed.[166] This may be due to difficulty in alignment of the

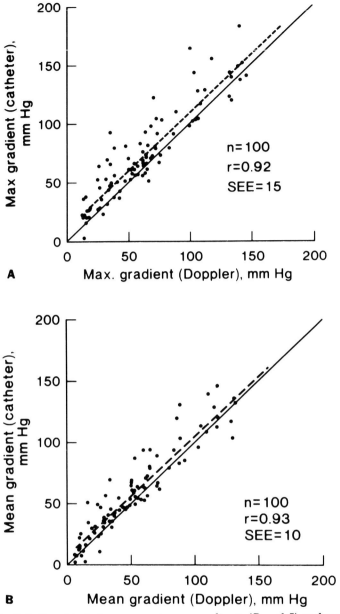

Figure 6.20 Relationship between maximum gradients (*Panel A*) and mean gradient (*Panel B*) measured at cardiac catheterization and those estimated by continuous-wave Doppler in 100 patients with aortic stenosis. (From: Currie PJ et al: Continuous-wave Doppler echocardiographic assessment of severity of calcific aortic stenosis: a simultaneous Doppler–catheter correlative study in 100 patients. *Circulation.* 71:1162–1169, 1985. With permission of the American Heart Association, Inc.)

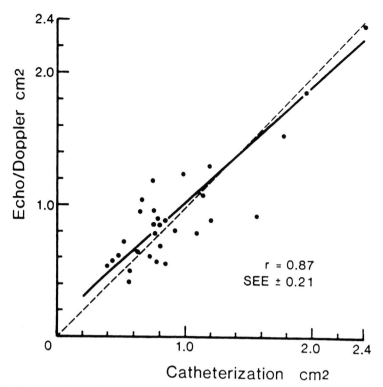

Figure 6.21 Correlation between echo/Doppler-derived valve areas and those calculated at the time of cardiac catheterization. (From Skjaerpe T et al: Noninvasive estimation of valve area in patients with aortic stenosis by Doppler ultrasound and two dimensional echocardiography. *Circulation.* 72:810–818, 1985. With permission of the American Heart Association, Inc.)

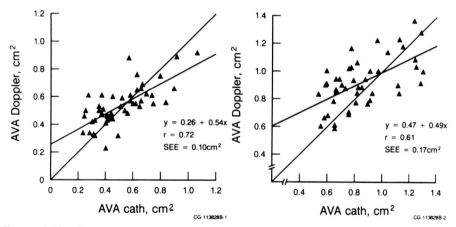

Figure 6.22 Correlation between Doppler-derived aortic valve area (*AVA Doppler*) and catheterization valve area (*AVA cath*) before (*left*) and after (*right*) balloon aortic valvuloplasty. (From: Nishimura RA et al: Doppler evaluation of results of percutaneous aortic balloon valvuloplasty in calcific aortic stenosis. *Circulation.* 78:791–799, 1988. With permission of the American Heart Association, Inc.)

ultrasound beam to the flow direction through the aortic valve. Further investigation is needed to reach a fair conclusion.

Assessment of Aortic Regurgitation

Two-dimensional and M-mode Echocardiography

In M-mode echocardiography a fine (high frequency) mitral valve flutter is a characteristic echocardiographic sign of aortic regurgitation if the jet is directed to the anterior mitral valve leaflet. Flutter on the left ventricular side of the endocardium of interventricular septum can be observed if a regurgitant jet is directed to the ventricular septum.[167-169] However, this M-mode echocardiographic sign has no value in quantifying the severity of the regurgitation. The premature diastolic closure of the mitral valve indicates acute severe aortic regurgitation[170,171] and may be useful in identifying severe acute aortic regurgitation after balloon aortic valvuloplasty. Two-dimensional echocardiography is useful in detecting aortic valve tear, prolapse, or other complications of balloon aortic valvuloplasty.

Doppler Echocardiography

Pulsed-wave and color Doppler echocardiography are very sensitive methods of detecting aortic insufficiency.[172-174] Minimal aortic regurgitation, which is detected by Doppler, may not be seen by angiography. The pulsed-wave Doppler sample is usually taken at apical four- or two-chamber views and begins immediately below the aortic valve. Care should be taken to distinguish mitral inflow and aortic regurgitant flow in patients with mitral stenosis and mitral prostheses with mitral inflow directed toward the left ventricular outflow tract. Continuous-wave Doppler is very helpful in this case. The velocity of an aortic regurgitant jet (Fig. 6.23) usually exceeds 2 to

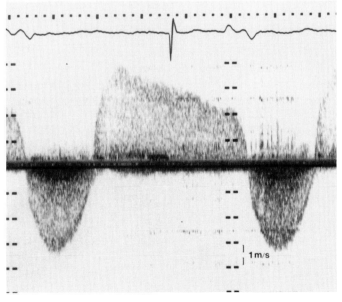

1 m/s

Figure 6.23 Continuous-wave Doppler velocity profile of a patient with both aortic stenosis and regurgitation. The peak velocity of the aortic regurgitant jet is 3.8 m/s.

3 m/s with a holodiastolic pattern including an isovolumic diastolic phase. The mitral inflow is usually less than 2 to 3 m/s with characteristic E and A waves in sinus rhythm. Color Doppler flow mapping is useful in directly visualizing regurgitant jet extent and morphology (broad or narrow, central or eccentric). Color regurgitant jets beginning from the very early diastole before mitral valve opening represent aortic regurgitant flow. Although the severity of aortic regurgitation can be graded semi-quantitatively by regurgitant jet extent from pulsed-wave Doppler and color Doppler echocardiography,[174,175] there is substantial scatter in the data when correlating Doppler-graded severity of aortic regurgitation and angiography-graded severity. Several grading systems have been proposed to assess severity of aortic regurgitation[174,175] Measurement of the regurgitant jet area derived from color Doppler in the short-axis view immediately below the aortic valve in the left ventricular outflow tract appears most promising.[176]

Color or pulsed-wave Doppler is more sensitive for detecting aortic regurgitation before or after balloon valvuloplasty and the severity of aortic regurgitation graded by color or pulsed-wave Doppler usually appears more severe than that graded by angiography.[146] By combining pulsed Doppler and two-dimensional data, the aortic regurgitant fraction can be calculated and used to estimate the severity of aortic regurgitation.[177-180] Calculation of the aortic regurgitant fraction from aortic flow (aortic velocity integral times aortic area derived from aortic annular diameter) and pulmonary flow (pulmonary velocity integral times pulmonary valve area derived from pulmonary annular diameter) is, however, not applicable in patients undergoing balloon aortic valvuloplasty because aortic annular area is no longer equivalent to aortic valve area in patients with calcific aortic stenosis.

The continuous-wave Doppler aortic regurgitant velocity profile represents changes in the pressure gradient between the ascending aorta and the left ventricle during entire diastole. In mild aortic regurgitation, the pressure gradient does not change dramatically: the slope of the diastolic regurgitant velocity decreases slowly and the time for the pressure gradient to fall to half its value (pressure-half time, (Fig. 6.24A) is long. In contrast, in severe aortic regurgitation, left ventricular diastolic pressure increases rapidly owing to large regurgitation flow into the left ventricle. Consequently, left ventricular pressure may be equal to the pressure in the ascending aorta at end-diastole so that the pressure gradient falls quickly and pressure half-time is shortened. The pressure half-time derived from the Doppler regurgitant velocity profile correlates well with semiquantitatively graded aortic regurgitation by angiography (I–IV).[181,182] There is considerable overlap of data between grade II and grade III aortic regurgitation, but severe aortic regurgitation usually has a pressure half-time of less than 270 ms (Fig. 6.24B). Limitations of this method are:

1. It is not uncommon that a complete, clearly delineated velocity profile cannot be obtained even in patients with severe aortic regurgitation.
2. The pressure half-time depends not only on regurgitant flow volume but also on the compliance of the left ventricle and the resistance of the systemic circulation. Since a complete aortic regurgitant velocity profile cannot usually be obtained in mild aortic regurgitation and in aortic stenosis with more than mild aortic regurgitation, these patients are not usually considered for balloon valvuloplasty.

There are no published data about the changes of aortic regurgitation assessed by the pressure half-time method after balloon valvuloplasty; however, the pressure half-

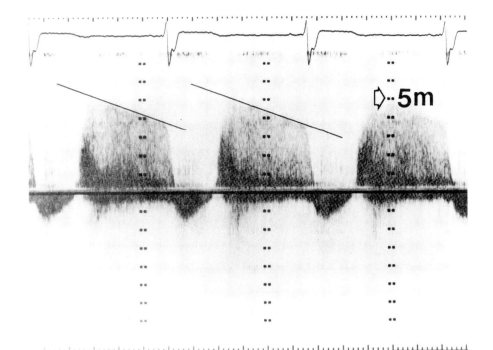

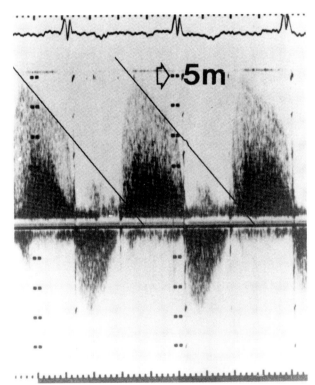

Figure 6.24 Continuous-wave Doppler velocity profile in two patients with aortic regurgitation with similar peak velocities (5 m/s). The deceleration rate (indicated by *line*), is markedly slower in *Panel A* (the pressure half-time is 520 ms indicating mild aortic regurgitation. In *Panel B,* the deceleration rate is rapid with a pressure half-time of 200 ms, indicating severe aortic regurgitation. (From St John Sutton M et al: Acquired aortic and pulmonary valve disease. In: St. John Sutton M, Oldershaw P. *Pediatric Echocardiography and Doppler.* Boston:Blackwell Scientific, 1989, p 256. Reprinted with permission of Blackwell Scientific Publications, Inc.)

time may be useful in assessing severity of aortic regurgitation if the regurgitation is more than mild after balloon valvuloplasty.

The ratio of forward flow to reverse flow in the aorta during diastole has also been used to estimate severity of aortic regurgitation and correlates fairly well with severity of aortic regurgitation.[183-187] This ratio correlated well with the aortic regurgitant fraction.[187]

Echocardiographic Morphology as Related to Outcome After Balloon Valvuloplasty

In calcific aortic stenosis, high echo reflection and shadowing of the calcification are usually observed. There have been no reports comparing degree of calcification of the valve and results of the balloon aortic valvuloplasty. Different morphologic characteristics represent the cause of the aortic stenosis: heavy calcification of aortic leaflets in severe degenerative aortic stenosis; pliable leaflets with commissural fusion in congenital aortic stenosis in young adults or children; and commissural fusion with thickened valve leaflets in rheumatic aortic stenosis.

Fairly good results have been reported in children and young adults with congenital aortic stenosis with pliable leaflets. Lababidi and associates reported that peak-to-peak aortic pressure gradient was decreased from 113 ± 48 to 32 ± 15 mmHg by balloon aortic valvuloplasty in 23 patients aged from 2 to 17 years with congenital aortic stenosis. These good results persisted at followup of 3 to 9 months.[132]

There have been few reports about results of balloon valvuloplasty in rheumatic aortic stenosis. Rheumatic aortic stenosis is usually associated with mitral valve disease (such as mitral stenosis). Thus, double-valve balloon valvuloplasty is performed in these patients. We have performed balloon valvuloplasty in 3 patients with both rheumatic aortic stenosis and mitral stenosis. The Doppler-derived aortic valve area increased from 0.6 ± 0.1 cm^2 to 1.5 ± 0.2 cm^2, and the instantaneous maximal pressure gradient decreased from 90 ± 8 mmHg to 20 ± 9 mmHg after balloon valvuloplasty. At 6 months to 1 year followup, no significant changes in valve area and pressure gradient were observed in 2 patients. One patient showed a decrease of aortic valve area from 1.4 to 1.1 cm^2 with a maximal gradient of 40 mmHg at 1 year followup.

Immediate and long-term results of balloon aortic valvuloplasty have been extensively investigated in calcific degenerative aortic stenosis.[133,137-146,159,160] Cribier and associates[138] reported on immediate results in 92 patients with severe calcific aortic stenosis and a mean age of 75 years. The calculated aortic valve area using Gorlin's formula increased from 0.49 ± 0.17 cm^2 to 0.93 ± 0.36 cm^2. Similar results have been reported by several authors[139,143,159] and the Mansfield Balloon Aortic Valvuloplasty Registry.[145] In this registry, which encompass 27 clinical centers and 492 patients, aortic valve area increased from 0.50 ± 0.18 cm^2 to 0.82 ± 0.30 cm^2 immediately after valvuloplasty and mean gradient decreased from 60 ± 23 mmHg to 30 ± 13 mmHg.[145] There was a great individual variation in increase in valve area after balloon aortic valvuloplasty from the published studies. Few factors have been demonstrated to possibly relate to the results of balloon aortic valvuloplasty, including balloon inflation time, double-balloon versus single-balloon technique, and exchange times of dilating balloons. Whether morphology of the valve can predict individual variation of the results in balloon aortic valvuloplasty has not been systematically assessed since transthoracic echocardiography very often cannot provide subtle morphologic differences in moderately to severely calcified aortic valves owing to the shadowing of calcification. Transesophageal echocardiography with biplane or multiplane probes may provide better morphological assessment of the aortic valve and may predict favorable results in a certain subgroup of patients and need further clinical investigations.

Recently, intracardiac ultrasound imaging has been used to better differentiate the morphologic characteristics of calcific aortic leaflets. This new imaging technique may identify underlying diseases of calcific aortic stenosis such as calcification that has developed from underlying bicuspid leaflets of the aortic valve. This may be helpful in distinguishing patients who may have good results of balloon valvuloplasty from those who may have poor results.[188] Although initial clinical improvement has been reported immediately after percutaneous balloon aortic valvuloplasty, longer-term followup has been less satisfactory. Safian and associates[139] as well as Nishimura and associates,[159] using Doppler echocardiography, reported restenosis in 50 to 60% of patients by 6 months. Mortality has also been reported to be high. Recent series that included severely ill elderly patients have reported a mortality of 4.9% at 24 hours reaching 7% within 7 days after the procedure.[145] More significantly, mortality has been as high as 28% at 6 months and 55% at 1 year in one series.[189] Although a small number of patients have persistent clinical improvement, because of the high rate of mortality and complications the use of balloon aortic valvuloplasty has been reserved for the palliation of symptoms in patients who are not surgical candidates because of other medical conditions. (See also Chapter 14)

PULMONARY VALVE STENOSIS

Relief of pulmonary valve stenosis by balloon dilatation during cardiac catheterization was first described in 1982 by Kan and associates.[190] Subsequently, the results of this procedure have been reported in several series of neonate and adult patients with a wide range of ages (1 day–76 years).[191-198] The usual mechanism of pulmonary valve stenosis is commissural fusion. In general, the immediate and intermediate results of balloon pulmonary valvuloplasty are comparable to those of surgical valvotomy.[191-198] However, a different mechanism of pulmonary valve stenosis, a dysplastic pulmonary valve, is reported to have a less favorable influence on the outcome of balloon pulmonary valvuloplasty.[199] Two-dimensional echocardiography is very useful in assessing pulmonary valve morphology[199,200] and thereby the mechanism of the stenosis. Doppler echocardiography can accurately measure the pressure gradient across the pulmonary valve or right ventricular outflow tract.[201-203]

Assessment of Severity

M-mode and Two-dimensional Echocardiography
Although M-mode recording of pulmonary valve motion shows a large "a" wave in patients with moderate to severe pulmonary stenosis, this M-mode echocardiographic sign is neither specific nor sensitive for the presence or severity of valvular stenosis.[204] In parasternal views, two-dimensional echocardiography can record two pulmonary leaflets (occasionally three leaflets in its short axis in children), the right ventricular outflow tract, and the pulmonary artery trunk and its bifurcation into right and left pulmonary arteries. Right ventricular outflow obstruction or supravalvular stenosis,

which may not be relievable by balloon valvuloplasty, can be easily recognized by two-dimensional echocardiography and differentiated from valvular stenosis. The annular size of pulmonary valve can be measured in the parastenal long-axis view of the pulmonary trunk (short-axis view of the aorta). Measurement of pulmonary annulus may be useful for selection of balloon size and detection of a dysplastic pulmonary valve. Normal pulmonary leaflets are thin, open widely, and lie parallel (often not visible) to the pulmonary artery wall during systole. Pulmonary valvular stenosis is almost always congenital in origin, though in rare instances it may be caused by rheumatic or carcinoid heart disease.

In most cases of congenital pulmonary valvular stenosis, the valve is tri-leaflet with fusion occurring along the commissures, narrowing the orifice at the tip of the valve (Fig. 6.25). Typically, two-dimensional echocardiography shows restricted opening of the leaflet tip and doming of the valve leaflets during systole. The valve leaflets are usually slightly thickened and appear redundant.[200] Congenital pulmonary valvular stenosis by commissural fusion is almost always associated with poststenotic dilatation of the main and even the secondary branches of the pulmonary artery.[199] Less frequently, congenital pulmonary valvular stenosis may be caused by a dysplastic valve. The dysplastic valve is usually not fused along the commissures but consists of considerably thickened and fibrotic valve leaflets often associated with a hypoplastic valve annulus. No systolic doming of the valve leaflets can be observed, and poststenotic dilatation is usually absent.[199] Although two-dimensional echocardiography provides important anatomic information, the severity of pulmonary stenosis can be assessed only indirectly on the basis of right ventricular hypertrophy, dilatation of the right ventricle, and abnormal position and motion of the interventricular septum.

Doppler Echocardiography

Reliable quantitation of pulmonary valvular stenosis can be provided by Doppler echocardiography. The pressure gradient can be obtained from the Doppler velocity profile,[201-203] and the pulmonary valve area can be calculated by using a combination of Doppler and two-dimensional echocardiographic data.[150] The Doppler velocity profile from the stenotic jet is recorded from the parasternal or subcostal view with the pulmonary valve and artery imaged in its long axis as the right ventricular outflow tract wrapping around the left ventricular outflow tract. Color Doppler echocardiography is very helpful in identifying the location of obstruction, in guiding alignment of the Doppler sampling beam parallel to the stenotic jet, or in correcting the angle. Pulsed-wave Doppler echocardiography is used when the stenosis is mild. Moderate or severe pulmonary stenosis usually causes aliasing of the velocity signal, however, so either continuous-wave or high pulse repetition Doppler must be used. The maximal and mean velocity is then converted into a maximal and mean pressure gradient by the simplified Bernoulli equation.[201,202] The Doppler-derived pressure gradient across the pulmonary valve has been shown to correlate well with the catheterization-derived gradient (r = 0.95), although Doppler echocardiography underestimates the gradient when the stenosis is severe.[201-203] To avoid influences of cardiac output and heart rate on pressure gradient measurement, the pulmonary valve area can be calculated by means of the continuity equation proposed by Kosturakis and associates[150]:

$$PVA = SV/(0.88 \times V_2 \times VET)$$

where PVA is the pulmonary valve area in cm^2; SV is the stroke volume in mL derived from the product of aortic flow integral and aortic valve area; V_2 is the maximal

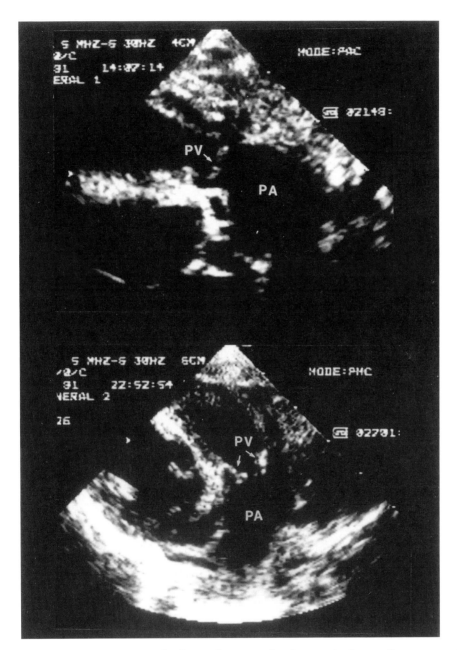

Figure 6.25 Two-dimensional echocardiogram of right ventricular outflow tract and pulmonary valve in a patient with congenital pulmonary valvular stenosis before (*top panel*) and after (*lower panel*) balloon dilatation of the valve. PV—pulmonary valve. PA—pulmonary artery.

velocity in cm/s distal to stenosis; VET is the ventricular ejection time in seconds; and 0.88 is a constant for correction of the difference of blood flow across the pulmonary and aortic valves. Valve areas derived by the Doppler method correlated well with those calculated by the Gorlin formula from catheterization data (r = 0.90; SEE = 0.08 cm²).[150] Therefore, Doppler echocardiography is very useful for assessing pressure gradient and pulmonary valve area before balloon valvuloplasty, immediately after valvuloplasty, and especially at followup. A further decrease in the pressure gradient across the right ventricular outflow tract has been reported at followup owing to regression of hypertrophy in the right ventricular outflow tract after percutaneous balloon pulmonary valvuloplasty.[205,206]

Echocardiographic Morphology as Related to Outcome After Balloon Valvuloplasty

As discussed earlier, pulmonary stenosis may be caused by commissural fusion of the leaflets, which reduces the orifice at the tip of the valve,[207] or by dysplasia of the valve leaflets (see Fig. 6.25), which obstructs flow, with or without a commissural component and often with a hypoplastic valve annulus.[199, 208-211] In a multicenter study conducted by the Valvuloplasty and Angioplasty of Congenital Anomalies Registry,[198] in 737 patients with typical valve stenosis with commissural fusion, the peak-to-peak pressure gradient between the right ventricle and the pulmonary artery was 71 ± 32 mmHg before valvuloplasty and reduced to 27 ± 20 mmHg after valvuloplasty. In contrast, in 46 patients with dysplastic pulmonary valve with or without Noonan's syndrome, reduction in the pressure gradient was from 74 ± 30 or 79 ± 35 mmHg before valvuloplasty to 42 ± 30 or 49 ± 20 mmHg after valvuloplasty. The reduction was significantly less than that in patients in whom the stenosis was caused by commissural fusion ($p < 0.05$). The results at followup are also less favorable for patients with dysplastic valve than for those with commissural fusion. Musewe and associates[199] reported on seven patients with dysplastic pulmonary valves who underwent balloon pulmonary valvuloplasty. The echocardiographic features in these patients were pronounced thickening of leaflets, leaflet immobility in diastole and systole, no dilatation of the sinuses of Valsalva in diastole, and supraannular narrowing.[199] Only one of these patients had a significant decrease in pressure gradient immediately after balloon valvuloplasty (from 96 to 60 mmHg) and at 6-month followup (23 mmHg). Echocardiographically, in addition to pronounced thickening of the valve indicating valvular dysplasia, this patient had commissural fusion of the valve as evidenced by doming of the valve and widening of one of the pulmonary sinuses of Valsalva in diastole.[199] Therefore, if dysplasia of the pulmonary valve is identified echocardiographically, balloon valvuloplasty is unlikely to improve hemodynamic function; but it should be attempted if commissural fusion is also present.

TRICUSPID VALVE STENOSIS

Tricuspid stenosis is not commonly seen. It is most often caused by rheumatic disease, which is always associated with mitral stenosis.[212] Carcinoid disease is a rare cause of tricuspid stenosis and is often associated with tricuspid regurgitation.[212] Successful balloon valvuloplasty for relief of rheumatic tricuspid stenosis has been reported.[213] Two-dimensional echocardiography can identify typical signs of tricuspid stenosis: valve thickening, restricted separation of the leaflet tip at diastole, and doming of the valve with dilatation of the right atrium[214-216] (Fig. 6.26). Color Doppler echocardiography reveals a narrow jet with a mosaic color pattern (increased velocity) through the tricuspid valve and is useful for aligning the continuous-wave Doppler beam or pulsed-wave Doppler sample to the stenotic jet for recording the velocity

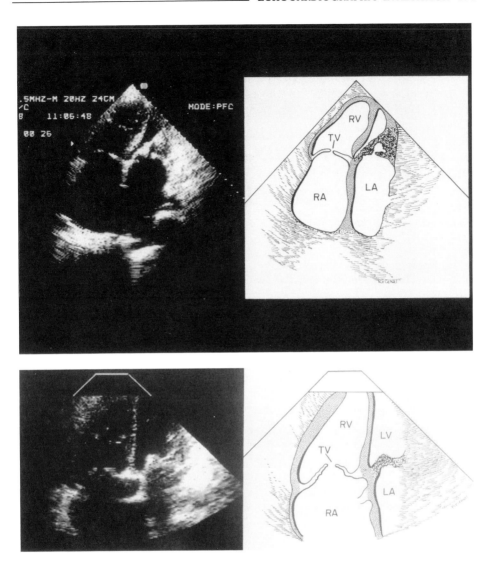

Figure 6.26 Two-dimensional echocardiogram of apical four-chamber view in a patient with rheumatic tricuspid stenosis before (*upper*) and after (*lower*) balloon dilatation of the stenotic valve. The patient also has mitral-stenosis. *TV*—tricuspid valve. *LA*—left atrium. *LV*—left ventricle. *RV*—right ventricle. *RA*—right atrium.

profile of the stenosis. The velocity profile recorded from pulsed-wave or continuous-wave Doppler is converted into a pressure gradient using the simplified Bernoulli equation; theoretically, the velocity profile can be used to calculate valve area by means of pressure half-time.[217,218] However, care should be taken to record the well-delineated velocity profile with the ultrasound beam aligned at the center of the stenotic jet and parallel to the jet direction. Because velocity or pressure gradient across the tricuspid valve is usually low, the measurement error is thus comparatively large. Color Doppler or pulsed-wave flow mapping is also very useful for detecting tricuspid regurgitation and grading its severity,[219] since concomitant severe tricuspid regurgitation is a contraindication for balloon tricuspid valvuloplasty.

CONCLUSIONS

The echocardiographic and Doppler examinations, as convenient, noninvasive diagnostic methods, are an integral part of the percutaneous balloon valvuloplasty procedure. Echocardiography not only offers a reliable means of diagnosing valvular stenosis, but it may be used both to select patients appropriate for balloon valvuloplasty and to exclude those for whom the procedure may be contraindicated. In many cases unique and critical information — for example subvalvular involvement in mitral stenosis — cannot be obtained from any other diagnostic modalities including cardiac catheterization. Subvalvular involvement in mitral stenosis not only predicts poor procedure results but also predisposes to induction or worsening of mitral regurgitation.[60,220] Color Doppler echocardiography, of course, is very useful in identifying patients with significant mitral regurgitation, either before or after balloon mitral valvuloplasty. It is also more sensitive than oximetry in the detection of iatrogenic atrial septal defects following percutaneous transseptal balloon mitral valvuloplasty.[221]

Echocardiographic and Doppler studies are essential for making appropriate clinical decisions regarding adults with symptomatic aortic stenosis. These methods have been well validated against invasive standards for determination of transaortic valvular gradients and valve areas when employed by experienced cardiologists. Cardiac catheterization provides no additional information beyond that provided by Doppler examination except in the case of patients with suspected or known coronary artery disease, for whom coronary arteriography is indicated.[222,223] Furthermore, the continuity equation for calculating aortic and mitral areas measures the physiological, or effective, orifice area. In contrast, areas calculated by the Gorlin formula give the anatomic area of the valve. Physiological area is a more important variable to consider clinically, because it is directly related to pressure and flow and therefore better reflects the patient's clinical hemodynamic status than does the anatomic area.[224]

For pulmonary or tricuspid stenosis, echocardiography/Doppler examination is highly accurate in making a diagnosis, determining the severity, assessing the valvular morphology, evaluating any coexisting subvalvular or multivalvular lesions, and measuring ventricular function. Prevalvuloplasty echocardiographic/Doppler data provide useful prognostic information on the anticipated long-term result after balloon valvuloplasty. Postvalvuloplasty, long-term followup of progression or regression of stenosis, ventricular function, and the severity of coexisting valvular regurgitation can also be accomplished with this noninvasive technique.

Overall, echocardiography and Doppler examinations are essential in the evaluation of patients with valvular heart disease in connection with percutaneous balloon valvuloplasty. They should allow for a more conservative application of cardiac catheterization in these patients.

Acknowledgment: The authors wish to thank Dr. Arthur E. Weyman, Director, Echocardiographic Laboratory, Massachusetts General Hospital, for contributing many of the illustrations used in this chapter.

REFERENCES

1. Block PC: Percutaneous balloon valvuloplasty. In: Hurst JW ed. *The Heart*. 7th ed. New York: McGraw-Hill, 1990, pp 2162–2176.

2. McKay RG, Grossman W: Balloon valvuloplasty. In: Grossman W, Baim DS, eds. *Cardiac Catheterization, Angiography and Intervention*. 4th ed. Philadelphia: Lea & Febiger, 1991, pp 511–533.

3. Roskamm H, Reindell H: *Herzkrankheiten. Pathophysiologie Diagnostik Therapie*. 3rd ed. Berlin: Springer-Verlag, 1989, pp 1180–1272.

4. Grossman W: *Profiles in Valvular Heart Disease*. In: Grossman W, Baim DS, eds. *Cardiac Catheterization, Angiography and Intervention*. 4th ed. Philadelphia: Lea & Febiger, 1991, pp 557–581.

5. Miller SW: *Cardiac Angiography*. 1st ed. Boston: Little Brown, 1984, pp 21–50.

6. Wyman RM, Safian RD, Portway V, et al: Current complications of diagnostic and therapeutic cardiac catheterization. *J Am Coll Cardiol*. 12:1400–1406, 1988.

7. Weyman AE. *Cross-sectional Echocardiography*. Philadelphia: Lea & Febiger, 1982, pp 150–165.

8. Tajik AJ, Seward JB, Hagler DJ, et al: Two-dimensional real-time ultrasonic imaging of the heart and great vessels. Technique, image orientation, structure identification, and validation. *Mayo Clin Proc*. 53:271–303, 1978.

9. Reid CL, Kawanishi DT, Chandraratna PA, et al: Doppler/two dimensional echocardiographic assessment of catheter balloon valvuloplasty for mitral stenosis: changes and correlations with cardiac catheterization. In: Bodner E. *Surgery for Heart Valve Disease*, London: ICR Publishers, 1990, pp 136–144.

10. Hatle L, Angelsen B: *Doppler Ultrasound in Cardiology: Physical Principles and Clinical Applications*. 2nd ed. Philadelphia: Lea & Febiger, 1985, pp 97–176.

11. Henry WL, Griffith JM, Michaelis LL, et al: Measurement of mitral orifice area in patients with mitral valve disease by real-time, two-dimensional echocardiography. *Circulation*. 51:827–831, 1975.

12. Skjaerpe T, Hegrenaes L, Hatle L: Noninvasive estimation of valve area in patients with aortic stenosis by Doppler ultrasound and two-dimensional echocardiography. *Circulation*. 72:810–818, 1985.

13. Effert S: Pre- and postoperative evaluation of mitral stenosis by ultrasound. *Am J Cardiol*. 19:59–65, 1967.

14. Zaky A, Nasser WK, Feigenbaum H: A study of mitral valve action recorded by reflected ultrasound and its application in the diagnosis of mitral stenosis. *Circulation*. 37:789–799, 1968.

15. Duchak JM Jr, Chang S, Feigenbaum H: The posterior mitral valve echo and the echocardiographic diagnosis of mitral stenosis. *Am J Cardiol*. 29:628–632, 1972.

16. Cope GD, Kisslo JA, Johnson ML, et al: A reassessment of the echocardiogram in mitral stenosis. *Circulation*. 52:664–670, 1975.

17. Hall R, Austin A, Hunter S: M-mode echogram as a means of distinguishing between mild and severe mitral stenosis. *Br Heart J*. 46:486–491, 1981.

18. Wann LS, Weyman AE, Dillon JC, et al: Determination of mitral valve area by cross-sectional echocardiography. *Am J Cardiol*. 39:278, 1977.

19. Wann LS, Weyman AE, Feigenbaum H, et al: Determination of mitral valve area by cross-sectional echocardiography. *Ann Intern Med*. 88:337–341, 1978.

20. Nichol PM, Gilbert BW, Kisslo JA: Two-dimensional echocardiographic assessment of mitral stenosis. *Circulation*. 55:120–128, 1977.

21. Martin RP, Rakowski H, Kleiman JH, et al: Reliability and reproducibility of two dimensional echocardiographic measurement of the stenotic mitral valve orifice area. *Am J Cardiol*. 43:560–568, 1979.

22. Smith MD, Handshoe R, Handshoe S, et al: Comparative accuracy of two-dimensional

echocardiography and Doppler pressure half-time methods in assessing severity of mitral stenosis in patients with and without prior commissurotomy. *Circulation.* 73:100–107, 1986.

23. Nanda NC, Gramiak R, Shah PM, et al: Mitral commissurotomy versus replacement: preoperative evaluation by echocardiography. *Circulation.* 51:263–267, 1975.

24. Reid C, McKay C, Chandraratna P, et al: Mechanism of increase in mitral valve area by double-balloon catheter balloon valvuloplasty in adults with mitral stenosis: echocardiographic–Doppler correlation. *J Am Coll Cardiol.* 9:217A, 1987.

25. Abascal VM, Wilkins GT, Choong CY, et al: Echocardiographic evaluation of mitral valve structure and function in patients followed for at least 6 months after percutaneous balloon mitral valvuloplasty. *J Am Coll Cardiol.* 12:606–615, 1988.

26. Hatle L, Brubakk A, Tromsdal A, et al: Noninvasive assessment of pressure drop in mitral stenosis by Doppler ultrasound. *Br Heart J.* 40:131–140, 1978.

27. Hatle L, Angelson BA, Tromsdal A: Non-invasive assessment of aortic stenosis by Doppler ultrasound. *Br Heart J.* 43:284–292, 1980.

28. Stamm RB, Martin RP: Quantification of pressure gradients across stenotic valves by Doppler ultrasound. *J Am Coll Cardiol.* 2:707–718, 1983.

29. Gorlin R, Gorlin SG: Hydraulic formula for calculation of the area of the stenotic mitral valve, other cardiac valves, and central circulatory shunts. Part I. *Am Heart J.* 41:1–29, 1951.

30. Libanoff AJ, Rodbard S: Atrioventricular pressure half-time: measurement of mitral valve orifice area. *Circulation.* 38:144–150, 1968.

31. Hatle L, Angelsen B, Tromsdal A: Noninvasive assessment of atrioventricular pressure half-time by Doppler ultrasound. *Circulation.* 60:1096–1104, 1979.

32. Chen C, Wang Y, Guo B, et al: Reliability of the Doppler pressure half-time method for assessing effects of percutaneous mitral balloon valvuloplasty. *J Am Coll Cardiol.* 13:1309–1313, 1989.

33. Thomas JD, Wilkins GT, Choong CYP, et al: Inaccuracy of mitral pressure half-time immediately after percutaneous mitral valvotomy. Dependence on transmitral gradient and left atrial and ventricular compliance. *Circulation.* 78:980–993, 1988.

34. Thomas JD, Weyman AE: Doppler mitral pressure half-time: a clinical tool in search of theoretical justification. *J Am Coll Cardiol.* 10:923–929, 1987.

35. Thomas JD, Choong CY, Weyman AE: Prolonged left ventricular relaxation lowers transmitral blood velocity: predictions of a fluid dynamics model with in vivo verification. *Circulation.* 76(suppl IV):IV-124, 1987.

36. Nakatani S, Masuyama T, Kodama K, et al: Value and limitations of Doppler echocardiography in the quantification of stenotic mitral valve area: comparison of the pressure half-time and the continuity equation methods. *Circulation.* 77:78–85, 1988.

37. Karp K, Teien D, Bjerle P, et al: Reassessment of valve area determinations in mitral stenosis by the pressure half-time method: impact of left ventricular stiffness and peak diastolic pressure difference. *J Am Coll Cardiol.* 13:594–599, 1989.

38. Flachskampf FA, Weyman AE, Gillam L, et al: Aortic regurgitation shortens Doppler pressure half-time in mitral stenosis: clinical evidence, in vitro simulation and theoretic analysis. *J Am Coll Cardiol.* 16:396–404, 1990.

39. Wisenbaugh T, Berk M, Essop R, et al: Effect of mitral regurgitation and volume loading on pressure half-time before and after balloon valvotomy in mitral stenosis. *Am J Cardiol.* 67:162–168, 1991.

40. Rahimtoola SH: Perspective on valvular heart disease: an update. *J Am Coll Cardiol.* 14:1–23, 1989.

41. Wilkins G, Thomas J, Abascal V, et al: Failure of the Doppler pressure halftime to accurately demonstrate change in mitral valve area following percutaneous mitral valvotomy. *J Am Coll Cardiol.* 9:218A, 1987.

42. Braverman AC, Lee TH, Lee RT: Mitral valve area determination during minor changes in hemodynamic state: superiority of the continuity equation. *J Am Coll Cardiol*. 17:155A, 1991.

43. Monterroso VH, Chen C, Rodriguez L, et al: Estimation of mitral valve area by color Doppler flow mapping. *Circulation*. 80(suppl II): II-167, 1989.

44. Rodriguez L, Monterroso V, Mueller L, et al: Validation of a new method for valve area calculation using the proximal isovelocity surface area in patients with mitral stenosis. *J Am Coll Cardiol*. 15:109A, 1990.

45. Lock JE, Khalilullah M, Shrivastava S, et al: Percutaneous catheter commissurotomy in rheumatic mitral stenosis. *N Engl J Med*. 313:1515–1518, 1985.

46. Inoue K, Owaki T, Nakamura T, et al: Clinical application of transvenous mitral commissurotomy by a new balloon catheter. *J Thorac Cardiovasc Surg*. 87:394–402, 1984.

47. Al Zaibag M, Ribeiro P, Al Kasab S, et al: Percutaneous double-balloon mitral valvotomy for rheumatic mitral-valve stenosis. *Lancet*. 1:757–761, 1986.

48. McKay RG, Lock JE, Keane JF, et al: Percutaneous mitral valvuloplasty in an adult patient with calcific rheumatic mitral stenosis. *J Am Coll Cardiol*. 7:1410–1415, 1986.

49. Palacios I, Block PC, Brandi S, et al: Percutaneous balloon valvotomy for patients with severe mitral stenosis. *Circulation*. 75:778–784, 1987.

50. Chen C, Chen J, Huang Z, et al: Percutaneous transseptal balloon mitral valvuloplasty: The Chinese experience in 21 patients. *J Am Coll Cardiol*. 9:83A, 1987.

51. McKay CR, Kawanishi DT, Rahimtoola SH: Catheter balloon valvuloplasty of the mitral valve in adults using a double-balloon technique. Early hemodynamic results. *JAMA*. 257:1753–1761, 1987.

52. McKay RG, Lock JE, Safian RD, et al: Balloon dilation of mitral stenosis in adult patients: postmortem and percutaneous mitral valvuloplasty studies. *J Am Coll Cardiol*. 9:723–731, 1987.

53. Mullins CE, Nihill MR, Vick GW III, et al: Double balloon technique for dilation of valvular or vessel stenosis in congenital and acquired heart disease. *J Am Coll Cardiol*. 10:107–114, 1987.

54. Chen C, Wang Y, Qing D, et al: Percutaneous mitral balloon dilatation by a new sequential single- and double-balloon technique. *Am Heart J*. 116:1161–1167, 1988.

55. Palacios IF, Block P: Percutaneous mitral balloon valvotomy (PMV): update of immediate results and follow-up. *Circulation*. 78(suppl II):II-489, 1988.

56. Rahimtoola SH: Catheter balloon valvuloplasty of aortic and mitral stenosis in adults: 1987. *Circulation*. 75:895–901, 1987.

57. Chen C, Wang Y, Lin Y, et al: Double-balloon technique for dilatation of rheumatic mitral stenosis. *Z Kardiol*. 77(suppl I):I-86, 1988.

58. Chen C, Wang Y, Duan Q, et al: Comparative results of percutaneous mitral balloon dilatation by various techniques *Circulation*. 78(suppl II):II-530, 1988.

59. Abascal VM, Wilkins GT, O'Shea JP, et al: Prediction of successful outcome in 130 patients undergoing percutaneous balloon mitral valvotomy. *Circulation*. 82:448–456, 1990.

60. Chen C, Wang X, Wang Y, et al: Value of two-dimensional echocardiography in selecting patients and balloon sizes for percutaneous balloon mitral valvuloplasty. *J Am Coll Cardiol*. 14:1651–1658, 1989.

61. Nobuyoshi M, Hamasaki N, Kimura T, et al: Indications, complications, and short-term clinical outcome of percutaneous transvenous mitral commissurotomy. *Circulation*. 80:782–792, 1989.

62. Palacios IF, Block PC, Wilkins GT, et al: Follow-up of patients undergoing percutaneous mitral balloon valvotomy. Analysis of factors determining restenosis. *Circulation*. 79:573–579, 1989.

63. Reid CL, Chandraratna AN, Kawanishi DT, et al: Influence of mitral valve morphology on double-balloon catheter balloon valvuloplasty in patients with mitral stenosis. Analysis of factors predicting immediate and 3-month results. *Circulation.* 80:515–524, 1989.

64. Reid CL, McKay CR, Chandraratna PAN, et al: Mechanisms of increase in mitral valve area and influence of anatomic features in double-balloon, catheter balloon valvuloplasty in adults with rheumatic mitral stenosis: a Doppler and two-dimensional echocardiographic study. *Circulation.* 76:628–636, 1987.

65. Kaplan JD, Isner JM, Karas RH, et al: In vitro analysis of mechanisms of balloon valvuloplasty of stenotic mitral valves. *Am J Cardiol.* 59:318–323, 1987.

66. Ribeiro PA, Zaibag MA, Rajendran V, et al: Mechanism of mitral valve area increase by in vitro single and double balloon mitral valvotomy. *Am J Cardiol.* 62:264–269, 1988.

67. Block PC, Palacios IF, Jacobs ML, et al: Mechanism of percutaneous mitral valvotomy. *Am J Cardiol.* 59:178–179, 1987.

68. Rusted IE, Sheifley CH, Edwards JE, et al: Guides to the commissures in operations upon the mitral valve. *Proc Mayo Clin.* 26:297–305, 1951.

69. John S, Bashi VV, Jairaj PS, et al: Closed mitral valvotomy: early results and long-term follow-up of 3724 consecutive patients. *Circulation.* 68:891–896, 1983.

70. Rutledge R, McIntosh CL, Morrow AG, et al: Mitral valve replacement after closed mitral commissurotomy. *Circulation.* 66(suppl I):I-162–I-166, 1982.

71. Rijsterborgh H, Roelandt J: Doppler assessment of aortic stenosis: Bernoulli revisited. *Ultrasound Med Biol.* 13:241–248, 1987.

72. Sahn DJ, Anderson F: *Two-Dimensional Anatomy of the Heart.* New York: John Wiley & Sons, 1982, pp 109–121.

73. Come PC, Riley MF: M mode and cross-sectional echocardiographic recognition of fibrosis and calcification of the mitral valve chordae and left ventricular papillary muscles. *Am J Cardiol.* 49:461–466, 1982.

74. Abascal VM, Wilkins GT, Choong CY, et al: Mitral regurgitation after percutaneous balloon mitral valvuloplasty in adults: evaluation by pulsed Doppler echocardiography. *J Am Coll Cardiol.* 11:257–263, 1988.

75. Wilkins GT, Weyman AE, Abascal VM, et al: Percutaneous balloon dilatation of the mitral valve: an analysis of echocardiographic variables related to outcome and the mechanism of dilatation. *Br Heart J.* 60:299–308, 1988.

76. Dennig K, Henneke KH, Dacian S: Are echocardiographic parameters predictive for the outcome of balloon catheter valvuloplasty in mitral stenosis? *Circulation.* 78(suppl II):II-1, 1988.

77. Brock RC: The surgical and pathological anatomy of the mitral valve. *Br Heart J.* 14:489–513, 1952.

78. Rusted IE, Scheifley CH, Edwards JE: Studies of the mitral valve, II: certain anatomic features of the mitral valve and associated structures in mitral stenosis. *Circulation.* 14:398–406, 1956.

79. Nichol PM, Boughner DR, Persaud JA: Noninvasive assessment of mitral insufficiency by transcutaneous Doppler ultrasound. *Circulation.* 54:656–661, 1976.

80. Abbasi AS, Allen MW, DeCristofaro D, et al: Detection and estimation of the degree of mitral regurgitation by range-gated pulsed Doppler echocardiography. *Circulation.* 61:143–147, 1980.

81. Areias JC, Goldberg SJ, de Villeneuve VH: Use and limitations of time interval histogram output from echo Doppler to detect mitral regurgitation. *Am Heart J.* 101:805–809, 1981.

82. Miyatake K, Kinoshita N, Nagata S, et al: Intracardiac flow pattern in mitral regurgitation

studied with combined use of the ultrasonic pulsed Doppler technique and cross-sectional echocardiography. *Am J Cardiol*. 45:155–162, 1980.

83. Quinones MA, Young JB, Waggoner AD, et al: Assessment of pulsed Doppler echocardiography in detection and quantification of aortic and mitral regurgitation. *Br Heart J*. 44:612–620, 1980.

84. Blanchard D, Diebold B, Peronneau P, et al: Non-invasive diagnosis of mitral regurgitation by Doppler echocardiography. *Br Heart J*. 45:589–593, 1981.

85. Veyrat C, Ameur A, Bas S, et al: Pulsed Doppler echocardiographic indices for assessing mitral regurgitation. *Br Heart J*. 51:130–138, 1984.

86. Omoto R, Yokote Y, Takamoto S, et al: The development of real-time two-dimensional Doppler echocardiography and its clinical significance in acquired valvular diseases. With special reference to the evaluation of valvular regurgitation. *Jpn Heart J*. 25:325–340, 1984.

87. Helmcke F, Nanda NC, Hsiung MC, et al: Color Doppler assessment of mitral regurgitation with orthogonal planes. *Circulation*. 75:175–183, 1987.

88. Miyatake K, Izumi S, Okamoto M, et al: Semiquantitative grading of severity of mitral regurgitation by real-time two-dimensional Doppler flow imaging technique. *J Am Coll Cardiol*. 7:82–88, 1986.

89. Zhang Y, Ihlen H, Myhre E, et al: Measurement of mitral regurgitation by Doppler echocardiography. *Br Heart J*. 54:384–391, 1985.

90. Chen C, Thomas JD, Anconina J, et al: Impact of impinging wall jet on color Doppler quantification of mitral regurgitation. Circulation 84:712–720, 1991.

91. Chen C, Flachskampf FA, Anconina J, et al: Three-dimensional shape of wall jets and free jets: implication for quantitation of valvular regurgitation by color Doppler imaging. *J Am Coll Cardiol*. 15:89A, 1990.

92. Chen C, Rodriguez L, Vlahakes GJ, et al: In vivo assessment of the effect of adjacent solid boundaries on the size of regurgitant jets by color Doppler flow mapping. *J Am Coll Cardiol*. 15:1458, 1990.

93. Rokey R, Sterling LL, Zoghbi WA, et al: Determination of regurgitant fraction in isolated mitral or aortic regurgitation by pulsed Doppler two-dimensional echocardiography. *J Am Coll Cardiol*. 7:1273–1278, 1986.

94. Blumlein S, Bouchard A, Schiller NB, et al: Quantitation of mitral regurgitation by Doppler echocardiography. *Circulation*. 74:306–314, 1986.

95. Spain MG, Smith MD, Grayburn PA et al: Quantitative assessment of mitral regurgitation by Doppler color flow imaging: angiographic and hemodynamic correlations. *J Am Coll Cardiol*. 13:585–590, 1989.

96. Mohr-Kahaly S, Lotter R, Brennecke R: Influence of color Doppler instrument set-up on the minimal encoded velocity—an in vitro study. *Circulation*. 78:II-12, 1988.

97. Thomas JD, Davidoff R, Wilkins GT, et al: The volume of a color flow jet varies directly with flow rate and inversely with orifice size: a hydrodynamic in vitro assessment. *J Am Coll Cardiol*. 11:19A, 1988.

98. Maurer G, Czer LSC, Chaux A, et al: Intraoperative Doppler color flow mapping for assessment of valve repair for mitral regurgitation. *Am J Cardiol*. 60:333–337, 1987.

99. Bolger AF, Eigler NL, Pfaff JM, et al: Computer analysis of Doppler color flow mapping images for quantitative assessment of in vitro fluid jets. *J Am Coll Cardiol*. 12:450–457, 1988.

100. Simpson IA, Valdes-Cruz LM, Sahn DJ, et al: Doppler color flow mapping of simulated in vitro regurgitant jets: evaluation of the effects of orifice size and hemodynamic variables. *J Am Coll Cardiol*. 13:1195–1207, 1989.

101. Sahn DJ: Instrumentation and physical factors related to visualization of stenotic and regurgitant jets by Doppler color flow mapping. *J Am Coll Cardiol.* 12:1354–1365, 1988.

102. Thomas JD, Liu CM, Flachskampf FA, et al: Quantification of jet flow by momentum analysis: an in vitro color Doppler flow study. *Circulation.* 81:247–259, 1990.

103. Switzer DF, Yoganathan AP, Nanda NC, et al: Calibration of color Doppler flow mapping during extreme hemodynamic conditions in vitro: a foundation for a reliable quantitative grading system for aortic incompetence. *Circulation.* 75:837–846, 1987.

104. Grantham RN, Daggett WM, Cosimi AB, et al: Transventricular mitral valvulotomy: analysis of factors influencing operative and late results. *Circulation.* 50(suppl II):II-200–II-211, 1974.

105. Ormiston JA, Shah PM, Tei C, et al: Size and motion of the mitral valve annulus in man, I: a two-dimensional echocardiographic method and findings in normal subjects. *Circulation.* 64:113–120, 1981.

106. Vijayaraghavan G, Boltwood CM, Tei C, et al: Simplified echocardiographic measurement of the mitral anulus. *Am Heart J.* 112:985–991, 1986.

107. Palacios IF, Tuzcu EM, Newell JB, et al: Four year clinical follow-up of patients undergoing percutaneous mitral balloon valvotomy. *Circulation.* 82:III-545, 1990.

108. Petit J, Vahanian A, Michel PL, et al: Percutaneous mitral valvotomy: French Cooperative Study: 114 patients. *Circulation.* 76(suppl IV):IV-496, 1987.

109. Babic UU, Dorros G, Pejcic P, et al: Mitral valvuloplasty: retrograde, transarterial double balloon technique. *J Am Coll Cardiol.* 11:14A, 1988.

110. Cunningham MJ, Diver DJ, Berman AD, et al: Acute hemodynamic results and clinical follow-up in patients undergoing balloon mitral valvuloplasty. *J Am Coll Cardiol.* 11:15A, 1988.

111. Vahanian A, Michel PL, Cormier B, et al: Results of percutaneous mitral commissurotomy in 200 patients. *Am J Cardiol.* 63:847–852, 1989.

112. Davidson CJ, Skelton TN, Kisslo KB, et al: A comprehensive evaluation of the risk of systemic embolization after percutaneous balloon valvuloplasty. *Circulation.* 76(suppl IV): IV-188, 1987.

113. Kronzon I, Tunick PA, Glassman E, et al: Transesophageal echocardiography to detect atrial clots in candidates for percutaneous transseptal mitral balloon valvuloplasty. *J Am Coll Cardiol.* 16:1320–1322, 1990.

114. Aschenberg W, Schlüter M, Kremer P, et al: Transesophageal two-dimensional echocardiography for the detection of left atrial appendage thrombus. *J Am Coll Cardiol.* 7:163–166, 1986.

115. Manning WJ, Reis GJ: Use of transesophageal echocardiography to detect left atrial thrombi prior to percutaneous mitral valvuloplasty: a prospective study. *Circulation.* 82(suppl III): III-546, 1990.

116. Chen C, Kremer P, Schroeder E, et al: Usefulness of anatomic parameters derived from two-dimensional echocardiography for estimating magnitude of left to right shunt in patients with atrial septal defect. *Clin Cardiol.* 10:316–321, 1987.

117. Radtke WE, Tajik AJ, Gau GT, et al: Atrial septal defect: echocardiographic observations. Studies in 120 patients. *Ann Intern Med.* 84:246–253, 1976.

118. Lieppe W, Scallion R, Behar VS, et al: Two-dimensional echocardiographic findings in atrial septal defect. *Circulation.* 56:447–456, 1977.

119. Patel AK, Rowe GG, Dhanani SP, et al: Pulsed Doppler echocardiography in diagnosis of pulmonary regurgitation: its value and limitations. *Am J Cardiol.* 49:1801–1805, 1982.

120. Kalmanson D, Veyrat C, Derai C, et al: Non-invasive technique for diagnosing atrial septal defect and assessing shunt volume using directional Doppler ultrasound. Correlations with phasic flow velocity patterns of the shunt. *Br Heart J.* 34:981–991, 1972.

122. Minagoe S, Tei C, Kisanuki A, et al: Noninvasive pulsed Doppler echocardiographic detection of the direction of shunt flow in patients with atrial septal defect: usefulness of the right parasternal approach. *Circulation*. 71:745–753, 1985.

123. Morimoto K, Matsuzaki M, Tohma Y, et al: Diagnosis and quantitative evaluation of atrial septal defect by transesophageal 2-D color Doppler echocardiography. *Circulation*. 76(suppl IV):IV-39, 1987.

124. Yoshida K, Yoshikawa J, Akasaka T, et al: Assessment of left-to-right atrial shunting after percutaneous mitral valvuloplasty by transesophageal color Doppler flow-mapping. *Circulation*. 80:1521–1526, 1989.

125. Come PC, Riley MF, Diver DJ, et al: Noninvasive assessment of mitral stenosis before and after percutaneous balloon mitral valvuloplasty. *Am J Cardiol*. 61, 817–825, 1988.

126. Reid CL, Kawanishi DT, Stellar W, et al: Long-term incidence of atrial septal defects after catheter balloon commissurotomy for mitral stenosis. *J Am Coll Cardiol*. 17:339A, 1991.

127. Griffen DL, Sheikh KH, Harrison JK, et al: Relationship of the echocardiographic score determined by transthoracic and transesophageal echocardiography to the success of balloon mitral valvuloplasty. *Circulation*. 82: III-44, 1990.

128. Tajik AJ, Seward JB, Khandheria BK: Transesophageal echocardiography: anatomic correlations. In: Erbel R, Khandheria BK, Brennecke R, et al: eds. *Transesophageal Echocardiography*. Berlin: Springer-Verlag, 1989, pp 27–43.

129. Wang X-F, Li Z-A, Cheng TO, et al: Biplane transesophageal echocardiography. An anatomic-ultrasonic-clinical correlative study. *Am Heart J*. in press for April, 1992.

130. Kronzon I, Tunick PA, Schwinger ME, et al: Transesophageal echocardiography during percutaneous mitral valvuloplasty. *J Am Soc Echocardiogr*. 2:380–385, 1989.

131. Visser CA, Jaarsma W, Haagen FDH, et al: Transesophageal echocardiographic observations during percutaneous balloon mitral valvuloplasty. In: Erbel R, Khandheria BK, Brennecke R, et al, eds. *Transesophageal Echocardiography*. Berlin: Springer-Verlag, 1989, pp 244–250.

132. Lababidi Z, Wu JR, Walls JT: Percutaneous balloon aortic valvuloplasty: results in 23 patients. *Am J Cardiol*. 53:194–197, 1984.

133. Cribier A, Savin T, Saoudi N, et al: Percutaneous transluminal valvuloplasty of acquired aortic stenosis in elderly patients: an alternative to valve replacement? *Lancet*. 1:63–67, 1986.

134. Hochberg MS, Morrow AG, Michaelis LL, et al: Aortic valve replacement in the elderly. *Arch Surg*. 112:1475–1480, 1977.

135. Quinlan R, Cohn LH, Collins JJ Jr: Determinants of survival following cardiac operations in elderly patients. *Chest*. 68:498–500, 1975.

136. Cabrol C, Gandjbakhch I, Pavie A: La chirurgie de remplacement valvulaires. In: Acar J, ed. *Les Cardiopathios Valvulaires*. acquises. Paris:Flammarion Médecine-Sciences, 1985, pp 513–546.

137. O'Keefe JH Jr, Vliestra RE, Bailey KR, et al: Natural history of candidates for balloon aortic valvuloplasty. *Mayo Clin Proc*. 62:986–991, 1987.

138. Cribier A, Savin T, Berland J, et al: Percutaneous transluminal balloon valvuloplasty of adult aortic stenosis: report of 92 cases. *J Am Coll Cardiol*. 9:381–386, 1987.

139. Safian RD, Berman AD, Diver DJ, et al: Balloon aortic valvuloplasty in 170 consecutive patients. *N Engl J Med*. 319:125–130, 1988.

140. Commeau P, Grollier G, Lamy E, et al: Percutaneous balloon dilatation of calcific aortic valve stenosis: anatomical and haemodynamic evaluation. *Br Heart J*. 59:227–238, 1988.

141. Sprigings DC, Jackson G, Chambers JB, et al: Balloon dilatation of the aortic valve for inoperable aortic stenosis. *Br Med J*. 297:1007–1011, 1988.

142. Serruys PW, Luijten HE, Beatt KJ, et al: Percutaneous balloon valvuloplasty for calcific aortic stenosis. A treatment 'sine cure'. *Eur Heart J.* 9:782–794, 1988.

143. Litvack F, Jakubowski AT, Buchbinder NA, et al: Lack of sustained clinical improvement in an elderly population after percutaneous aortic valvuloplasty. *Am J Cardiol.* 62:270–275, 1988.

144. Nishimura RA, Holmes DR, Michela MA, et al: Follow-up of patients with low output, low gradient hemodynamics after percutaneous balloon aortic valvuloplasty: the Mansfield Scientific Aortic Valvuloplasty Registry. *J Am Coll Cardiol.* 17:828–833, 1991.

145. McKay RG, for the Mansfield Scientific Aortic Valvuloplasty Registry Investigators: The Mansfield Scientific Aortic Valvuloplasty Registry: overview of acute hemodynamic results and procedural complications. *J Am Coll Cardiol.* 17:485–491, 1991.

146. Come PC, Riley MF, McKay RG, et al: Echocardiographic assessment of aortic valve area in elderly patients with aortic stenosis and of changes in valve area after percutaneous balloon valvuloplasty. *J Am Coll Cardiol.* 10:115–124, 1987.

147. Leo LR, Barrett MJ, Leddy CL, et al: Determination of aortic valve area by cross-sectional echocardiography. *Circulation.* 60(suppl II):II-203, 1979.

148. Godley RW, Green D, Dillon JC, et al: Reliability of two-dimensional echocardiography in assessing the severity of valvular aortic stenosis. *Chest.* 79:657–662, 1981.

149. Currie PJ, Seward JB, Reeder GS, et al: Continuous-wave Doppler echocardiographic assessment of severity of calcific aortic stenosis: a simultaneous Doppler-catheter correlative study in 100 adult patients. *Circulation.* 71:1162–1169, 1985.

150. Kosturakis D, Allen HD, Goldberg SJ, et al: Noninvasive quantification of stenotic semilunar valve areas by Doppler echocardiography. *J Am Coll Cardiol.* 3:1256–1262, 1984.

151. Myreng Y, Mølstad P, Endresen K, et al: Reproducibility of echocardiographic estimates of the area of stenosed aortic valves using the continuity equation. *Int J Cardiol.* 26:349–354, 1990.

152. Otto CM, Pearlman AS, Comess KA, et al: Determination of the stenotic aortic valve area in adults using Doppler echocardiography. *J Am Coll Cardiol.* 7:509–517, 1986.

153. Richards KL, Cannon SR, Miller JF, et al: Calculation of aortic valve area by Doppler echocardiography: a direct application of the continuity equation. *Circulation.* 73:964–969, 1986.

154. Zoghbi WA, Farmer KL, Soto JG, et al: Accurate noninvasive quantification of stenotic aortic valve area by Doppler echocardiography. *Circulation.* 73:452–459, 1986.

155. Simpson IA, Houston AB, Sheldon CD, et al: Clinical value of Doppler echocardiography in the assessment of adults with aortic stenosis. *Br Heart J.* 53:636–639, 1985.

156. Smith MD, Dawson PL, Elion JL, et al: Systematic correlation of continuous-wave Doppler and hemodynamic measurements in patients with aortic stenosis. *Am Heart J.* 111:245–252, 1986.

157. Otto CM, Janko C, Prestley R, et al: Measurements of peak flow velocity in adults with valvular aortic stenosis using high pulse repetition frequency duplex pulsed Doppler echocardiography. *J Am Coll Cardiol.* 3:494, 1984.

158. Stewart WJ, Galvin KA, Gillam LD, et al: Comparison of high pulse repetition frequency and continuous wave Doppler echocardiography in the assessment of high flow velocity in patients with valvular stenosis and regurgitation. *J Am Coll Cardiol.* 6:565–571, 1985.

159. Nishimura RA, Holmes DR Jr, Reeder GS, et al: Doppler evaluation of results of percutaneous aortic balloon valvuloplasty in calcific aortic stenosis. *Circulation.* 78:791–799, 1988.

160. Nishimura RA, Reeder GS, Holmes DR Jr, et al: Hemodynamic measurements immedi-

ately after percutaneous balloon valvuloplasty may underestimate the resultant valve area. *Circulation.* 76(suppl IV):IV-523, 1987.

161. Harpole DA, Jones RH, Bashore TM: Serial evaluation of left ventricular function after aortic valvuloplasty utilizing first-pass radionuclide angiography. *Circulation.* 76(suppl IV):IV-522, 1987.

162. Harpole DH, Davidson C, Skelton T, et al: Serial evaluation of ventricular function after percutaneous aortic balloon valvuloplasty. *Am Heart J.* 119:130–135, 1990.

163. Dormagen V, Chevalier B, Diebold B, et al: Is color Doppler useful to evaluate aortic stenosis? *Circulation.* 82(suppl III):III-46, 1990.

164. Hoffmann T, Kasper W, Meinertz T, et al: Determination of aortic valve orifice area in aortic valve stenosis by two-dimensional transesophageal echocardiography. *Am J Cardiol.* 59:330–335, 1987.

165. Stollberger C, Sehnal E, Karnik R, et al: Transesophageal echocardiography in the assessment of the severity of aortic stenosis. In: Erbel R, Khandheria BK, Brennecke R, et al, eds. *Transesophageal Echocardiography.* Berlin:Springer-Verlag, 1989, pp 66–71.

166. Grube E, Gerckens U, Cattelaens N: Is the quantification of mitral stenosis and aortic stenosis by transesophageal echocardiography feasible? In: Erbel R, Khandheria BK, Brennecke R, et al, *Transesophageal Echocardiography.* Berlin:Springer-Verlag, 1989, pp 58–65.

167. Pridie RB, Benham R, Oakley CM: Echocardiography of the mitral valve in aortic valve disease. *Br Heart J.* 33:296–304, 1971.

168. D'Cruz I, Cohen HC, Prabhu R, et al: Flutter of left ventricular structures in patients with aortic regurgitation, with special reference to patients with associated mitral stenosis. *Am Heart J.* 92:684–691, 1976.

169. Henzi M, Burckhardt D, Raeder EA, et al: Echocardiography as a method for the determination of the severity of aortic insufficiency. *Schweiz Med Wochenschr.* 106: 1557–1559, 1976.

170. Henry WL, Bonow RO, Borer JS, et al: Observations on the optimum time for operative intervention for aortic regurgitation, I: evaluation of the results of aortic valve replacement in symptomatic patients. *Circulation.* 61:471–483, 1980.

171. Henry WL, Bonow RO, Rosing DR, et al: Observations on the optimum time for operative intervention for aortic regurgitation, II: serial echocardiographic evaluation of asymptomatic patients. *Circulation.* 61:484–492, 1980.

172. Grayburn PA, Smith MD, Handshoe R, et al: Detection of aortic insufficiency by standard echocardiography, pulsed Doppler echocardiography, and auscultation. A comparison of accuracies. *Ann Intern Med.* 104:599–605, 1986.

173. Saal AK, Gross BW, Franklin DW, et al: Noninvasive detection of aortic insufficiency in patients with mitral stenosis by pulsed Doppler echocardiography. *J Am Coll Cardiol.* 5:176–181, 1985.

174. Esper RJ: Detection of mild aortic regurgitation by range-gated pulsed Doppler echocardiography. *Am J Cardiol.* 50, 1037–1043, 1982.

175. Ciobanu M, Abbasi AS, Allen M, et al: Pulsed Doppler echocardiography in the diagnosis and estimation of severity of aortic insufficiency. *Am J Cardiol.* 49:339–343, 1982.

176. Byard CE, Perry GJ, Roitman DI, et al: Quantitative assessment of aortic regurgitation by color Doppler. *Circulation.* 72(suppl III) III-146, 1985.

177. Veyrat C, Lessana A, Abitbol G, et al: New indexes for assessing aortic regurgitation with two-dimensional Doppler echocardiographic measurement of the regurgitant aortic valvular area. *Circulation.* 68:998–1005, 1983.

178. Kitabatake A, Ito H, Inoue M, et al: A new approach to noninvasive evaluation of aortic

regurgitant fraction by two-dimensional Doppler echocardiography. *Circulation.* 72: 523–529, 1985.

179. Rokey R, Sterling L, Zoghbi WA, et al: Determination of regurgitant fraction in isolated mitral or aortic regurgitation by pulsed Doppler two-dimensional echocardiography. *J Am Coll Cardiol.* 7:1273–1278, 1986.

180. Zhang Y, Nitter-Hauge S, Ihlen H, et al: Measurement of aortic regurgitation by Doppler echocardiography. *Br Heart J.* 55:32–38, 1986.

181. Masuyama T, Kodama K, Kitabatake A, et al: Noninvasive evaluation of aortic regurgitation by continuous-wave Doppler echocardiography. *Circulation.* 73:460–466, 1986.

182. Teague SM, Heinsimer JA, Anderson JL, et al: Quantification of aortic regurgitation utilizing continuous wave Doppler ultrasound. *J Am Coll Cardiol.* 8:592–599, 1986.

183. Hoffman A, Pfisterer M, Stulz P, et al: Non-invasive grading of aortic regurgitation by Doppler ultrasonography. *Br Heart J.* 55:283–285, 1986.

184. Diebold B, Peronneau P, Blanchard D, et al: Non-invasive quantification of aortic regurgitation by Doppler echocardiography. *Br Heart J.* 49:167–173, 1983.

185. Imaizumi T, Orita Y, Koiwaya Y, et al: Utility of two-dimensional echocardiography in the differential diagnosis of the etiology of aortic regurgitation. *Am Heart J.* 103:887–896, 1982.

186. Sequeira RF, Watt I: Assessment of aortic regurgitation by transcutaneous aortovelography. *Br Heart J.* 39:929–930, 1977.

187. Touche T, Prasquier R, Nitenberg A, et al: Assessment and follow-up of patients with aortic regurgitation by an updated Doppler echocardiographic measurement of the regurgitant fraction in the aortic arch. *Circulation.* 72:819–824, 1985.

188. Weintraub A, Pandian N, Salem D, et al: Realtime intracardiac two-dimensional echocardiography in the catheterization laboratory in humans. *J Am Coll Cardiol.* 15:16A, 1990.

189. Sherman W, Hershman R, Lazzam C, et al: Balloon valvuloplasty in adult aortic stenosis: determinants of clinical outcome. *Ann Intern Med.* 110:421–425, 1989.

190. Kan JS, White RI Jr, Mitchell SE, et al: Percutaneous balloon valvuloplasty: a new method for treating congenital pulmonary-valve stenosis. *N Engl J Med.* 307:540–542, 1982.

191. Kveselis DA, Rocchini AP, Snider AR, et al: Results of balloon valvuloplasty in the treatment of congenital valvar pulmonary stenosis in children. *Am J Cardiol.* 56:527–532, 1985.

192. Walls JT, Lababidi Z, Curtis JJ, et al: Assessment of percutaneous balloon pulmonary and aortic valvuloplasty. *J Thorac Cardiovasc Surg.* 88:352–356, 1984.

193. Kan JS, White RI Jr, Mitchell SE, et al: Percutaneous transluminal balloon valvuloplasty for pulmonary valve stenosis. *Circulation.* 69:554–560, 1984.

194. Tynan M, Baker EJ, Rohmer J, et al: Percutaneous balloon pulmonary valvuloplasty. *Br Heart J.* 53:520–524, 1985.

195. Van den Berg EJM, Niemeyer MG, Plokker TWM, et al: New triple-lumen balloon catheter for percutaneous (pulmonary) valvuloplasty. *Cathet Cardiovasc Diagn.* 12: 352–356, 1986.

196. DiSessa TG, Alpert BS, Chase NA, et al: Balloon valvuloplasty in children with dysplastic pulmonary valves. *Am J Cardiol.* 60:405–407, 1987.

197. Chen C, Nan Y, Wang Y, et al: Comparison of single- and double-balloon pulmonary valvotomy. *Z Kardiol.* 54(suppl I):122, 1988.

198. Stanger P, Cassidy SC, Girod DA, et al: Balloon pulmonary valvuloplasty: results of the Valvuloplasty and Angioplasty of Congenital Anomalies Registry. *Am J Cardiol.* 65:775–783, 1990.

199. Musewe NN, Robertson MA, Benson LN, et al: The dysplastic pulmonary valve: echocardiographic features and results of balloon dilatation. *Br Heart J.* 57:364–370, 1987.

200. Weyman AE, Hurwitz RA, Girod DA, et al: Cross-sectional echocardiographic visualization of the stenotic pulmonary valve. *Circulation.* 56:769–774, 1977.

201. Lima CO, Sahn DJ, Valdes-Cruz LM, et al: Noninvasive prediction of transvalvular pressure gradients in patients with pulmonary stenosis by quantitative two-dimensional echocardiographic Doppler studies. *Circulation.* 67:866–871, 1983.

202. Johnson GL, Kwan OL, Handshoe S, et al: Accuracy of combined two-dimensional echocardiography and continuous wave Doppler recordings in the estimation of pressure gradient in right ventricular outlet obstruction. *J Am Coll Cardiol.* 3:1013–1018, 1984.

203. Stevenson JG, Kawabori I: Noninvasive determination of pressure gradients in children: two methods employing pulsed Doppler echocardiography. *J Am Coll Cardiol.* 3:179–192, 1984.

204. Weyman AE, Dillon JC, Feigenbaum H, et al: Echocardiographic patterns of pulmonary valve motion in valvular pulmonary stenosis. *Am J Cardiol.* 34:644–651, 1974.

205. Sullivan ID, Robinson PJ, Macartney FJ, et al: Percutaneous balloon valvuloplasty for pulmonary valve stenosis in infants and children. *Br Heart J.* 54:435–441, 1985.

206. Rao PS, Fawzy ME, Solymar L, et al: Long-term results of balloon pulmonary valvuloplasty of valvar pulmonic stenosis. *Am Heart J.* 115:1291–1296, 1988.

207. Campbell M: Simple pulmonary stenosis. Pulmonary valvular stenosis with a closed ventricular septum. *Br Heart J.* 16:273–300, 1954.

208. Noonan JA: Hypertelorism with Turner phenotype. A new syndrome with associated congenital heart disease. *Am J Dis Child.* 116:373–380, 1968.

209. Linde LM, Turner SW, Sparkes RS. Pulmonary valvular dysplasia. A cardiofacial syndrome. *Br Heart J.* 35:301–304, 1973.

210. Koretzky ED, Moller JH, Korns ME, et al: Congenital pulmonary stenosis resulting from dysplasia of valve. *Circulation.* 40:43–53, 1969.

211. Vancini M, Roberts KD, Silove ED, et al: Surgical treatment of congenital pulmonary stenosis due to dysplastic leaflets and small valve anulus. *J Thorac Cardiovasc Surg.* 79:464–468, 1980.

212. Ockene IS: Tricuspid valve disease. In: Dalen JE, Alpert JS, eds. *Valvular Heart Disease.* Boston:Little Brown, 1987, 353–402.

213. Al Zaibag M, Ribeiro P, Al Kasab S: Percutaneous balloon valvotomy in tricuspid stenosis. *Br Heart J.* 57:51–53, 1987.

214. Guyer DE, Gillam LD, Foale RA, et al: Comparison of the echocardiographic and hemodynamic diagnosis of rheumatic tricuspid stenosis. *J Am Coll Cardiol.* 3:1135–1144, 1984.

215. Daniels SJ, Mintz GS, Kotler MN: Rheumatic tricuspid valve disease: two-dimensional echocardiographic, hemodynamic, and angiographic correlations. *Am J Cardiol.* 51:492–496, 1983.

216. Shimada R, Takeshita A, Nakumara M, et al: Diagnosis of tricuspid stenosis by M-mode and two-dimensional echocardiography. *Am J Cardiol.* 53:164–168, 1984.

217. Dennig K, Henneke KH, Rudolph W: Assessment of tricuspid stenosis by Doppler-echocardiography. *J Am Coll Cardiol.* 9:237A, 1987.

218. Parris TM, Panidis IP, Ross J, et al: Doppler echocardiographic findings in rheumatic tricuspid stenosis. *Am J Cardiol.* 60:1414–1416, 1987.

219. Veyrat C, Kalmanson D, Farjon H, et al: Non-invasive diagnosis and assessment of tricuspid regurgitation and stenosis using one and two dimensional echo-pulsed Doppler. *Br Heart J.* 47:596–605, 1982.

220. Sadee AS, Becker AE: In vitro balloon dilatation of mitral valve stenosis: the importance of subvalvular involvement as a cause of mitral insufficiency. *Br Heart J.* 65:277–279, 1991.

221. Parro A Jr, Helmcke F, Mahan EF III, et al: Value and limitations of color Doppler echocardiography in the evaluation of percutaneous balloon mitral valvuloplasty for isolated mitral stenosis. *Am J Cardiol.* 67:1261–1267, 1991.

222. Geibel A, Görnandt L, Kasper W, et al: Reproducibility of Doppler echocardiographic quantification of aortic and mitral valve stenoses: comparison between two echocardiography centers. *Am J Cardiol.* 67:1013–1021, 1991.

223. Galan A, Zoghbi WA, Quinones MA: Determination of severity of valvular aortic stenosis by Doppler echocardiography and relation of findings to clinical outcome and agreement with hemodynamic measurements determined at cardiac catheterization. *Am J Cardiol.* 67:1007–1012, 1991.

224. Dumesnil JG, Yoganathan AP: Theoretical and practical differences between the Gorlin formula and the continuity equation for calculating aortic and mitral valve areas. *Am J Cardiol.* 67:1268–1272, 1991.

CHAPTER 7

Magnetic Resonance Assessment

RAAD H. MOHIADDIN
DUDLEY J. PENNELL

Approximately two decades ago, the phrase **noninvasive imaging** was introduced to describe new methods for evaluation of cardiovascular anatomy and function that were based on external recordings. The term was chosen to differentiate these methods from methods based on cardiac catheterization, which was then the dominant diagnostic technique in cardiology. At first the contribution of new imaging techniques was small, but progress has been rapid and the balance has been profoundly altered, first by M-mode echocardiography, and then by two-dimensional, Doppler, and color flow echocardiography; nuclear medicine techniques; x-ray computed tomography; and most recently by magnetic resonance imaging (MRI). Over the same period, invasive investigation has changed little, so that with the conspicuous exception of the coronary artery anatomy, virtually every cardiac diagnosis previously made by cardiac catheterization can now be made noninvasively. In addition, noninvasive techniques are associated with lower levels of morbidity and mortality and with considerably lower x-ray exposure or none. These properties permit widespread application of noninvasive imaging to normal populations or to those considered at risk.

Magnetic resonance imaging (MRI) is recognized as an invaluable noninvasive technique for imaging the central nervous and musculoskeletal systems because of its excellent spatial resolution, the natural high contrast between different tissues, and the ability to acquire images in any orthogonal or oblique plane. Investigators are also studying variation of the magnetic resonance signal according to the local biochemical environment, which may allow discrimination between healthy and diseased tissues.

These investigations can be done at no known risk to the patient, because electromagnetic radiation instead of X-rays is used to form the images. Cardiovascular MRI has only recently begun to display its potential. Initially, there were technical difficulties associated with electrocardiographic gating and the dominant use of magnetic resonance scanners by radiologists, whose workload has not historically included the very specialized field of cardiac imaging. A few dedicated units have crossed this divide and demonstrated the feasibility of acquiring high resolution anatomic images and highly accurate functional information. With the recent development of subsecond and real-time magnetic resonance imaging (flash and echo-planar techniques), the application of this new imaging method to the cardiovascular system will expand rapidly, limited initially by availability.

PHYSICAL PRINCIPLES OF MRI

A basic understanding of the physics involved in magnetic resonance imaging is invaluable in appreciating the capabilities of the technique, and all the concepts involved are comprehensible to physicians. It is not necessary to grapple with the complex detail, although other more detailed descriptions are available.[1,2]

Nuclear Spin and Magnetism

All atomic nuclei contain charged protons which rotate at very high frequency. The combination of their spin and their electrical charge generates a small magnetic field so that the nucleus behaves like a small, spinning bar magnet. In addition to spinning on its axis, the proton also precesses at a far lower frequency in the same way that a spinning top precesses about a gravitational field. The resonant frequency of proton precession is directly proportional to the strength of the local magnetic field and can be brought into the radiofrequency range by means of magnets with a field strength in the order of 0.5 tesla (10,000 times the earth's magnetic field). Nuclei of different elements have different spins and charges and hence have different resonant frequencies. At 0.5 tesla, these frequencies are 21 MHz for the hydrogen nucleus and 9 MHz for the phosphorus nucleus.

The protons may exist with their nuclear magnetization vector parallel or opposite to the applied field. In a magnetic field of 0.5 tesla, of each million hydrogen nuclei, there are only two more in the lower energy state than in the higher. The transition from one state to the other can be caused by introducing energy at the resonant frequency.

Net Magnetization Vector

Magnetic resonance is most easily understood in terms of the net effect of all of the individual nuclear magnetization vectors; this sum is called the *net magnetization vector*. If the net magnetization vector is disturbed from equilibrium, it too will precess about the direction of the field, although it eventually spirals back to equilibrium because of the relaxation phenomena described in the next section. One means of disturbing the net magnetization vector is to add energy to the system from an alternating electromagnetic field. In order for energy to be transferred, the frequency of alternation must be equal to the resonant frequency. For clinical imaging, this frequency is usually a radiofrequency, and so the alternating field simply consists of radio waves. As the alternating field is applied, the magnetization vector spirals down with an increasing angle between itself and the static field. The angle of displacement depends on the amplitude and duration of the radio wave and is commonly chosen to be 90° or 180°.

Relaxation

When the net magnetization vector has been disturbed, processes occur that return the magnetization to equilibrium. These processes are called *spin-lattice* and *spin-spin relaxation*. After a 90° pulse, longitudinal magnetization is reduced from its equilibrium value to zero. It relaxes back at an exponential rate with a time constant T_1. This spin-lattice relaxation is caused by interaction with molecular oscillations in the surrounding lattice. T_1 tends to be long in solids and short in more mobile liquids, and in biologic tissues it ranges from hundreds of milliseconds to a few seconds. Conversely, a 90° pulse increases transverse magnetization from its equilibrium value of zero, and it then relaxes back at an exponential rate with a time constant T_2. This *spin-spin relaxation* is a result of neighboring nuclei altering the local magnetic environment and causing individual protons to spin out of phase so that their magnetization vectors begin to oppose each other and cancel. T_1 is always longer than T_2. Spin-spin relaxation is rapid in solids because the positions of nuclei are fixed, and it is slow in liquids when they are in motion and their magnetic effects are averaged. In biologic tissues T_2 ranges from tens to hundreds of milliseconds. It is possible to produce clinical images that highlight relaxation parameters in different tissues, thereby accentuating the natural contrast between them.

Free Induction Decay

If a 90° pulse is applied to a sample, the net magnetization vector is turned into the transverse plane, where it precesses and rapidly declines in intensity. This gives rise to a radio signal called the *free induction decay*, which can be detected by a receiving antenna. The free induction decay is not itself used for forming an image, but the signal can be reconstituted using further radiofrequency and magnetic pulses. Such pulse trains are known as sequences, and the reconstituted signal is known as an echo.

Pulse Sequences

There are innumerable pulse sequences, often known by acronyms for ease of recall. In cardiac imaging the most important are the spin echo, gradient echo, and velocity mapping sequences. In spin echo imaging the free induction decay signal is refocused into an echo using a second 180° radiopulse. The myocardium appears white and the blood black because protons in blood excited by the initial 90° pulse have flowed out of the imaging plane before echo formation. Spin echo imaging is particularly useful for high definition anatomic imaging. In gradient echo imaging the echo is refocused using short pulses of magnetic fields applied by additional coils around the main field. This has the advantage of producing fast echoes which freeze blood movement so that blood yields a high signal. The sequence can be rapidly repeated, allowing the acquisition of cine loops that are useful for the assessment of valves and the regional contractile function of the myocardium.[3] The gradient echo sequence can also be modified to include an extra magnetic gradient which alters the phase of protons that are moving in the imaging plane in direct proportion to their velocity. The phase shift can be resolved to yield velocity maps in which each point in the image reflects velocity at that point rather than water density.[4-6] These maps are invaluable in the calculation of flow in the heart and great vessels. A fuller description of the use of the sequences is given below.

Image Formation

An image is a map of the amplitude of a magnetic resonance signal point for point over a thin slice through the patient. After a simple excitation, the signal obtained contains no spatial information, and so different techniques are used to encode these data in the echoes. First, during the initial excitation a magnetic field gradient is applied from head to foot so that protons in different slices of the patient experience different magnetic fields and precess at different frequencies. The initial radiofrequency pulse of a single frequency will then excite only a single thin slice of the patient, and any resulting signal will come only from that slice. Second, during acquisition of the signal, another magnetic gradient is applied in the transverse direction which forces different lines within the plane to emit signals at different frequencies. The received signal is then complex, containing many different frequencies, each of an amplitude proportional to the proton density within the corresponding line. The amplitude at each frequency is resolved by a technique called Fourier transformation. Finally, a magnetic gradient is applied from front to back just before the signal acquisition. This alters the phase of precession of the protons by an amount dependent upon their position. By repeating the sequence of excitation and acquisition each time with an increasing phase-encoding gradient, the phase varies with a frequency dependent upon its position. A second Fourier transformation in this direction then extracts the amplitude information along this line, and amplitude can be assigned to individual points in the image.

Image Acquisition

All cardiac images are acquired using cardiac gating. The electrocardiogram is transmitted out of the magnetic field by means of a fiberoptic cable. The computer recognizes the R wave, and all images are acquired at a chosen time delay into the cardiac cycle. One phase-encoding step is applied in each cardiac cycle, so that a typical spin echo or gradient echo cardiac magnetic resonance scan is acquired over 256 heartbeats. This allows 128 lines of resolution in the phase-encoded direction, and each line is repeated twice to reduce the signal: noise ratio by averaging. The time required for acquisition is therefore related to the heart rate but is typically 4 minutes. Velocity encoding uses the system of subtracting a velocity-encoded image from a reference image, and this doubles the imaging time. However, in one imaging period of 4 minutes, the spin echo sequence may be used to obtain images at multiple levels, and the gradient echo sequence may be used to acquire multiple images at the same level. In the case of the gradient echo sequence, the multiple images can be viewed as a cine.

Instrumentation

An MRI machine consists of five major components. The magnet, which is usually superconducting, produces the static magnetic field, which has to be homogenous and stable with time and yet large enough to contain a human body. Resistive electromagnets are also required to alter the field for short periods, and these depend upon a large current circulating in coils to produce the magnetic field. The production of these fields is difficult and requires the use of magnetic field gradient amplifiers. The radiofrequency transmitter drives a radiofrequency alternating current through a transmitting coil over the body to produce the radiowave pulses, and the radiofrequency receiver amplifies the small signals from the receiver coil. Finally a computer plays a central role since it controls not only the magnetic field gradients but also the radiofrequency pulses. In addition it stores the received signal and transforms it into the image which it then displays. An array processor for the rapid handling of data is usual.

ASSESSMENT OF VALVULAR DISEASE

Anatomic Assessment

Valve Leaflets

It is difficult to image the valve leaflets by MRI. Their low water density results in a low signal, and respiratory motion averaged over the period of acquisition limits the spatial resolution of such fine structures. In addition, calcification of the leaflets leads to a low signal. Normal leaflets are only occasionally seen in spin echo images, but when thickened and immobile, their identification is more common. In cine gradient echo sequences, however, it is usual to identify the leaflets moving, a consequence of flow effects. As blood flows over the valve tips, eddies and mild turbulence occur, causing signal loss. Areas of turbulence associated with abnormal valves can be identified because of the greatly increased disturbance to normal laminar flow. Thus qualitative assessments of leaflet mobility may be made. Echocardiography has the advantages of real-time acquisition, which eliminates respiratory motion effects, and significant signal enhancement from abnormal leaflets, particularly those that are calcified. Thus, although the overall spatial resolution of echocardiography is inferior to that of MRI, it is currently the imaging technique of choice for assessment of the valve leaflets. It remains to be seen whether the implementation of real-time MRI using the echo planar technique, which has recently become commercially available, will improve leaflet definition.

Valve Annulus

The position of the valve annulus is clearly identifiable by means of spin echo and gradient echo sequences. Calcification is not detected. The size of the valve orifice cannot be directly assessed. Abnormalities in the appearance of the annulus occur when severe stenosis and thickening is present. The normal appearances of the mitral and aortic valves are shown in Figures 7.1 and 7.2.

Functional Assessment

Detection of Turbulence

The gradient echo sequence identifies areas of turbulent blood flow as areas of signal loss within the high blood signal.[7] This occurs because higher orders of motion, such as acceleration and jerk, cause dephasing of proton spins. The effect is highly dependent on the echo time of the sequence. As the echo time is reduced, signal loss from turbulence is reduced because of the shorter time before signal acquisition for

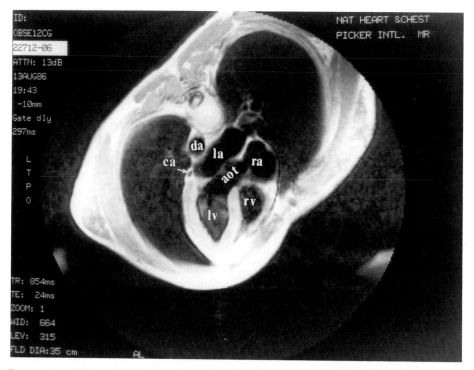

Figure 7.1 Horizontal long-axis spin echo image acquired with double oblique correction for the leftward and vertical rotation of the cardiac long axis. The left ventricle (*lv*), right ventricle (*rv*), left atrium (*la*), right atrium (*ra*), aortic outflow tract (*aot*), descending aorta (*da*), and coronary artery (*ca*) are marked.

spin dephasing takes effect. At an echo time of 14 ms, which is typically used for general cardiac studies, there is minor signal loss around the tips of the aortic and mitral valve cusps in normal subjects. In patients with valve abnormalities, the area of this turbulent signal loss is increased and immediately identifiable. The corollary to the ready detection of turbulence by signal loss is that functional measurements of blood flow velocity in the turbulent area are hindered by a lack of signal. This is overcome by repeating the image in the same plane with a reduced echo time of 6 ms or 3.6 ms.

Although signal loss and turbulence may not exactly correspond, the size of the signal loss has been used to provide a semiquantitative estimate of regurgitation through valves.[8-11] The extent of turbulence can be expressed by grading the size of the jet or, better, as an absolute volume.[9] Although color flow Doppler echocardiography is also capable of determining the site of turbulent flow,[12] volume measurements are not possible because of the inability to acquire contiguous parallel images of known thickness. A simple size grading system agrees well with the conventional grading system used in angiocardiography,[8] with grade 1 being signal loss close to the valve, grade 2 extending into the proximal chamber, grade 3 filling the whole of the proximal chamber, and grade 4 if the receiving chamber has signal loss throughout the whole of the relevant half of the cardiac cycle. The area of turbulence has also been used to assess semiquantitatively the severity of stenosis of a valve or great vessel,[13] but superior techniques using velocity mapping have replaced this unreliable method.

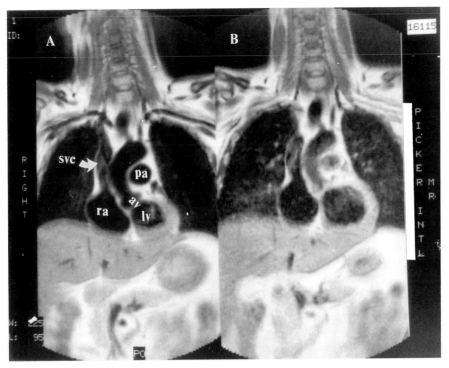

Figure 7.2 Coronal plane spin echo images, in systole (*A*) and diastole (*B*), through the left ventricle (*lv*) and aortic valve (*av*). The right atrium (*ra*), pulmonary artery (*pa*), and superior vena cava (*svc*) are also shown.

Velocity Mapping

Gradient echo cine imaging may be used in two ways to provide information about the cardiovascular system. The first has been described above: The amplitude of the signal at each point in the imaging plane is displayed, and the resulting magnitude images may be run in a cine loop allowing visual inspection of anatomy, contractile function, and blood flow turbulence. However, all waves bear a phase relationship to each other, and this information is not processed from the received radio signal for the magnitude images. The application of a short-lived magnetic gradient allows the phase of each point in the imaging plane to be encoded with a phase shift that is directly proportional to the velocity of that point. The amount of the phase shift depends on the strength and length of the applied magnetic gradient, and this can be chosen to suit the velocities expected on the basis of the clinical situation. Because of magnetic field inhomogeneities and eddy currents in the structure of the magnet, time- and position-varying phase shifts are normally present in an image, and for quantification of the technique, two studies must be acquired. The first is velocity encoded. The second is velocity compensated and acts as a control for the variable phase shifts. Subtraction then yields the actual phase relationship of the protons within the imaging plane. Stationary tissue of zero velocity is displayed as midgray and velocity is represented with shades of black or white. The depth of the gray shade is proportional to velocity and black and white indicate the direction of blood flow. The technique is sensitive and has an in vitro accuracy of approximately 4%. It allows both vessel area and mean velocity to be measured through the cardiac cycle with a minimum temporal resolution of 6 ms. In this way true blood flow can be calculated and velocities measured within jets of blood passing through vascular or valvular stenoses. Velocity maps acquired in a normal subject in the same plane as Figure 7.1 are shown in Figure 7.3.

The Modified Bernoulli Equation

A stenotic valve or vessel may be assessed by measuring the flow velocity in the jet of blood passing through a stenosis. In the case of a given flow, flow velocity increases as the orifice narrows. The relationship between the velocity of the jet and the difference in pressure on either side of the stenosis can be approximated by the modified Bernoulli equation, which in its simplest form is

$$\Delta P = 4V^2$$

where P = Pressure drop across the stenosis (mmHg) and V = Velocity (m/s).

This assumes that true velocity has been recorded and that the blood velocity before the stenosis was negligible. This calculation can be easily applied to determine the peak instantaneous gradient across the stenosis. It can also be used to calculate the mean gradient during the flow period and to determine the pressure differential between two chambers in the case of a regurgitant valve.

Velocity Mapping of Jets

The detection of turbulence in association with blood flow through a stenosed valve or vessel is the first step in assessing the velocity of blood in a jet. The magnitude image can be acquired with an echo time that clearly identifies the jet direction, and subsequent velocity mapping can then be accurately aligned. Accurate velocity mapping of jets through stenoses requires the use of very short echo times such as 3.6 ms. The signal loss associated with the turbulence is then regained, allowing accurate measurements in the vena contracta where peak velocities occur. The 3.6 ms velocity mapping sequence has been validated in vitro and shown to measure velocities accurately in jets up to 5.6 m/s. It has also been validated in vivo in comparison with Doppler echocardiography and hemodynamic measurements made during cardiac catheterization.[14,15] Acquisition of the velocity map may be *through-plane* with the jet passing perpendicularly through the chosen imaging plane, or *in-plane* with the imaging plane being chosen to encompass the length of the jet. In-plane imaging yields a greater number of pixels for analysis of velocity. In general it is preferable to acquire data in both planes, but if the jet is small, in-plane imaging is less reliable because of partial volume effects and movement of the jet out of the imaging plane. In cases of mitral and aortic stenosis, therefore, through-plane imaging is preferred. For the examination of a pulmonary conduit or coarctation in which a large jet is usually present, in-plane imaging often gives a clearer view of the anatomy.

Regurgitant Valves

Several methods are available for assessing the severity of valvular regurgitation. The first technique, described above, involves the identification of turbulent blood flow in the receiving chamber. This method has been validated as a semiquantitative measure of valvular regurgitation.[8,9,10,11] It suffers from problems that include a difficulty in separating the turbulent volumes when dual valve disease exists (such as mitral

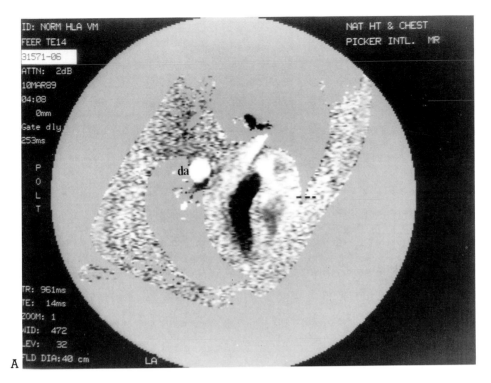

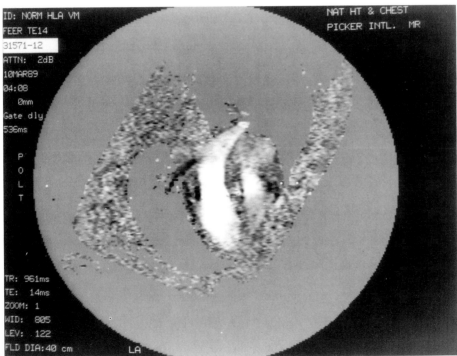

Figure 7.3 Velocity maps corresponding to Fig. 7.1 in a normal subject with vertical velocity encoding. Stationary tissue is depicted in midgray. Blood flowing up the image is depicted by black shades, whereas blood flowing down the plane is in white. *A* is in systole showing aortic ejection, and the descending aorta (*da*) is also seen. *B* is in diastole showing mitral and tricuspid flow.

stenosis and aortic regurgitation). Moreover, each center must calibrate the technique for its own equipment owing to the sensitivity of echo times and acquisition parameters. Other quantitative techniques are available, however. These depend on the ability of MRI to accurately determine both the stroke volume of the ventricles and the flow in the great vessels. A contiguous stack of spin echo images may be acquired in systole and diastole, thereby encompassing the entire heart. The endocardial outline in each image may be drawn and the volume computed in each slice from a knowledge of the slice thickness (usually 10 mm). The technique is accurate to approximately 2%.[16] The stroke volume ratio between right and left ventricles normally approaches 1:1 over an imaging period of minutes, and the extent of deviation from this ratio reflects the severity of regurgitant blood flow.[10,17] Radionuclide ventriculography yields a similar measurement,[18] but only isolated lesions can be assessed by this modality because one side of the heart must be normal for comparison. Likewise, it is not possible to distinguish the individual severity of valvular regurgitation when two valves on one side are affected.

A more robust technique to quantify the severity of valvular regurgitation involves the subtraction of flow in a great vessel as measured by velocity mapping from the stroke volume of the associated ventricle as calculated by the contiguous spin echo technique described above. This method allows true isolation of the left and right sides of the heart for assessment of regurgitant fraction and regurgitant volumes, but the technique cannot separate the regurgitant flow from two regurgitant valves on one side of the heart. Work is in progress, however, to assess whether aortic or pulmonary regurgitation may be quantified from the backflow of blood in the proximal great vessels as assessed by velocity mapping. If validated, such a measurement would allow accurate regurgitant volumes for each cardiac valve to be individually calculated in the presence of any mixture of valvular lesions.

Velocity mapping can be used to quantify the pulmonary:systemic flow ratio in patients with interatrial, interventricular, and aortopulmonary shunts.[19]

Other Techniques

As there are no atrial inflow valves, valvular disease of the tricuspid and mitral valves has characteristic effects on patterns of flow in the caval and pulmonary veins, and these have been assessed by velocity mapping.[20-22] Using spin echo anatomic imaging, valvular stenosis can be evaluated indirectly by studying the volume dimension and wall thickness of the loading and the receiving chambers.[23,24]

MRI ASSESSMENT OF INDIVIDUAL LESIONS

Mitral Valve

The mitral valve as well as left atrial and ventricular morphology can be studied in multilevel transverse planes or in oblique planes parallel to the horizontal and vertical long axes of the left ventricle. In mitral stenosis, the turbulence jet in the left ventricle during ventricular diastole can be visualized with the magnitude images of the cine gradient echo sequence with an echo time of 14 or 6 ms (Fig. 7.4A). During systole, a regurgitant jet in the left atrium can be seen in mitral regurgitation (Fig. 7.4B). The size of the signal loss can be used for semiquantitative assessment of mitral valve stenosis, but velocity mapping allows quantitative measurement of the blood flow

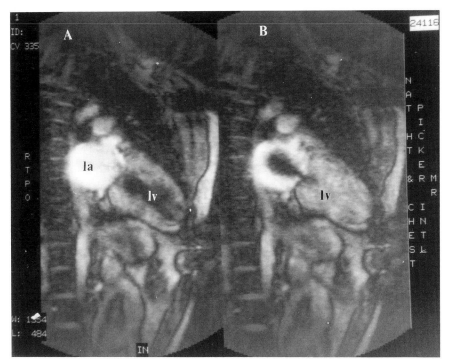

Figure 7.4 In mixed mitral valve disease, signal loss may be seen during diastole (*A*) in the left ventricle (*lv*), and during systole (B) in the left atrium (*la*). The gradient echo images were acquired in the vertical long-axis plane.

velocity in the valve jet. The technique has been validated against Doppler echocardiography for patients before and after percutaneous balloon valvuloplasty (Fig. 7.5). Using the velocity mapping technique, normal mitral flow shows two peaks, one during early ventricular diastole and the other during atrial contraction (Fig. 7.6). Peak mitral flow velocity (mean ± standard deviation) in early diastole was 68 ± 12 cm/sec, and during atrial contraction 39 ± 10 cm/sec. The ratio between the peak flow velocities was 1.9 ± 0.6. In mitral stenosis the pattern of flow velocity is abnormal, with persistent high velocities throughout diastole[14,15,22] (Fig. 7.7). The severity of mitral stenosis can be determined if a jet velocity measurement is aligned to the direction of flow through the valve. In most of the patient studies the stenotic jet had a complicated shape and direction which was misaligned with the horizontal long axis of the left ventricle, and appropriate oblique rotation of the imaging plane was essential to align the velocity encoding with the jet direction. In addition it was found that through-plane velocity measurements (short-axis tomogram at base of left ventricle with jet flow through the plane of the image; Fig. 7.8) were more reliable than the in-plane measurements (rotated horizontal long axis tomogram with jet flow vertically directed in the plane of the image; Fig. 7.9) because of movement of the narrow jet out of the imaging plane. The flow curve can be used to determine the mitral pressure half-time, which is the time taken for the pressure gradient to fall to half of the peak value. This has proved to be a useful echocardiographic indicator of the severity of mitral stenosis.

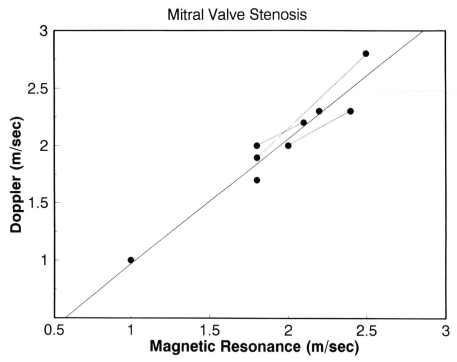

Figure 7.5 Comparison between peak mitral flow velocity measured by MRI and Doppler echocardiography. Points joined by *solid lines* indicate single patients with velocities measured before and after percutaneous balloon valvuloplasty.

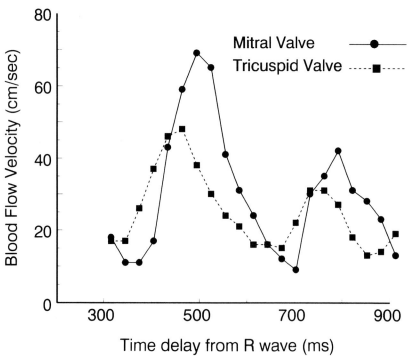

Figure 7.6 Time-velocity curves in diastole for mitral and tricuspid flow in a normal subject. Note the two velocity peaks of early ventricular diastole and atrial contraction.

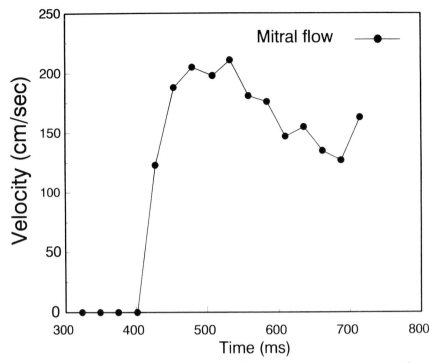

Figure 7.7 Time-velocity curve in diastole of mitral flow in a patient with mitral stenosis. Note the high peak velocity and its persistence when compared to the normal in Fig. 7.6.

The size of the left atrium and ventricle can be easily determined by MRI, and this measurement has been used as a marker of the success of percutaneous balloon mitral valvuloplasty.[23] Thrombosis in the left atrium associated with mitral stenosis is readily seen using a spin echo sequence. Any confusion between thrombus and slowly moving blood can be avoided by using a cine gradient echo sequence, where blood gives a high signal and the thrombus appears as a filling defect.[25]

Aortic Valve

The anatomy of aortic valve, the left ventricle, and part of the ascending aorta can be displayed in a single coronal plane in most subjects. The extent of aortic stenosis, regurgitation, or both can be evaluated semiquantitatively by using cine gradient echo imaging to measure the area of signal loss produced by the turbulent jet (Fig. 7.10). The gradient across the stenosis can be calculated by using a gradient echo sequence with a short echo time of 3.6 ms to measure the peak velocity in the aortic valve jet (Fig. 7.11). In vitro experiments have shown the technique with a 3.6 ms echo time to measure jet velocities accurately up to 5.6 m/s.[14] This allows the assessment of gradients up to 125 mmHg, which includes all physiologically relevant cardiovascular lesions. The use of the technique in vivo has been validated against Doppler echocardiography (Fig. 7.12) and hemodynamic measurements by catheterization.[14,15] The through-plane velocity map has generally been found more reliable than the in-plane map.

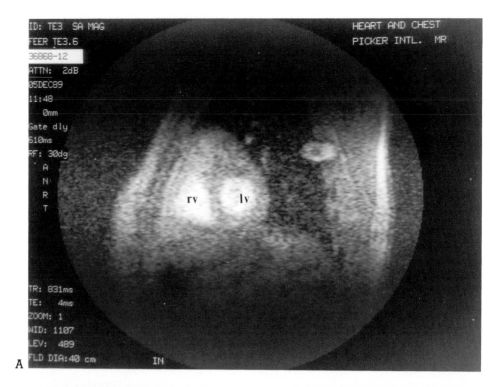

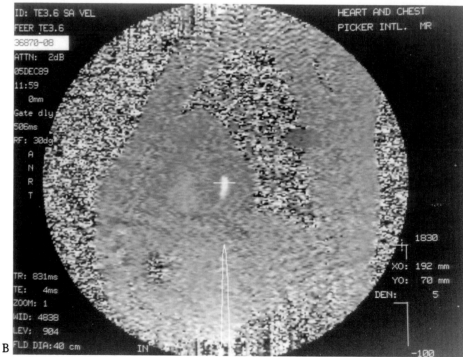

Figure 7.8 Short-axis gradient echo image (*A*) and corresponding velocity map (*B*) of mitral inflow jet, with through-plane velocity encoding. The left ventricle (*lv*) and right ventricle (*rv*) are marked. Note that by using the echo times (TE) of 3.6-ms sequence, there is no signal loss in the magnitude image. The velocity profile shows a peak velocity of 1.83 m/s (13 mmHg).

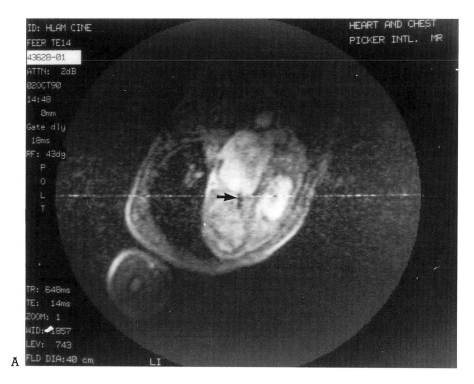

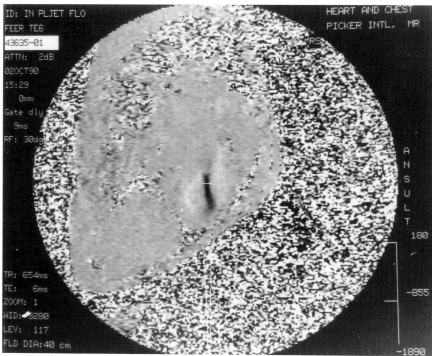

Figure 7.9 Rotated horizontal long-axis plane with in-plane (vertical) velocity encoding. The gradient echo image (*A*) with an echo time of 14 ms shows the stenotic jet (*arrow*). The corresponding velocity map (*B*) reveals a peak velocity of 1.89 m/s (14 mmHg).

199

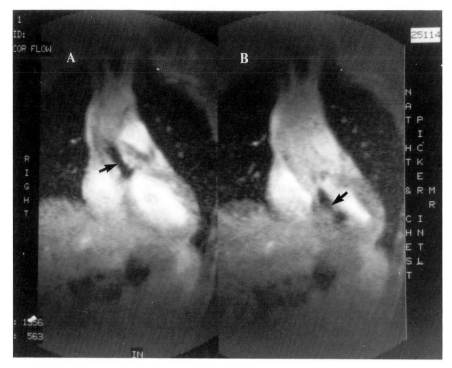

Figure 7.10 Gradient echo acquisition in the coronal plane showing turbulent signal loss in the ascending aorta (*arrow*) during systole (*A*), and in the left ventricle (*arrow*) during diastole (*B*), in a patient with mixed aortic valve disease.

Another area of MRI application is in suspected abscess in the heart or around the aortic root in postoperative patients with infection that is difficult to control (Fig. 7.13). Echocardiography is often equivocal in such patients, and spin echo images will usually provide a definitive answer.[26]

Pulmonary Valve

The pulmonary valve, right ventricular outflow tract, and main pulmonary artery may be assessed in the sagittal or oblique sagittal plane. Difficulties with acoustic windows and alignment of Doppler ultrasound have made magnetic resonance velocity mapping a useful tool in the assessment of pulmonary valve and pulmonary arterial blood flow[19,27] (Fig. 7.14).

Tricuspid Valve

The principles of examination of the tricuspid valve are essentially the same as those used for evaluation of the mitral valve. The tricuspid orifice is larger than the mitral orifice, and the pressure gradients associated with normal flow are lower in the right side of the heart than in the left (see Fig. 7.6). Thus magnetic resonance velocity mapping shows lower velocities than seen in the normal mitral valve. Tricuspid stenosis is relatively unusual in rheumatic heart disease but when present can be

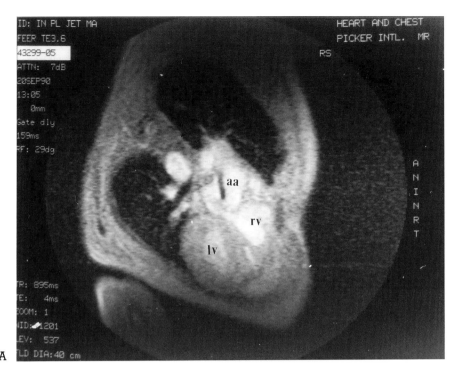

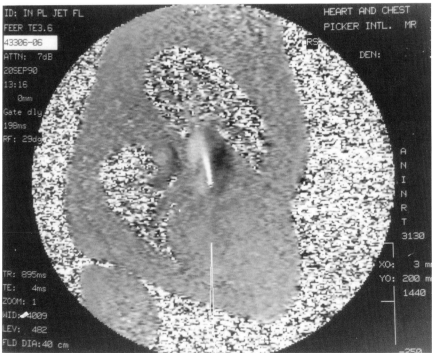

Figure 7.11 Gradient echo image (*A*) and corresponding velocity map (*B*) in a patient with aortic stenosis. The left ventricle (*lv*), right ventricle (*rv*), and ascending aorta (*aa*) are marked. The unusual oblique plane was necessary to orient the abnormal jet direction vertically for velocity encoding. The peak velocity was 3.13 m/s (39 mmHg).

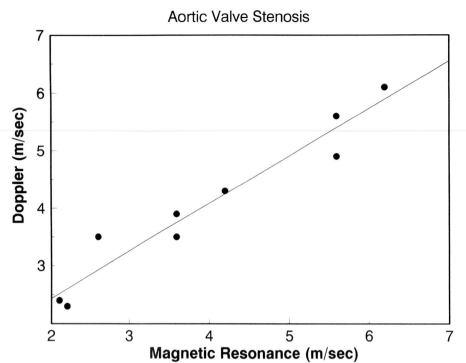

Figure 7.12 Comparison between peak aortic flow velocity measured by MRI and Doppler echocardiography.

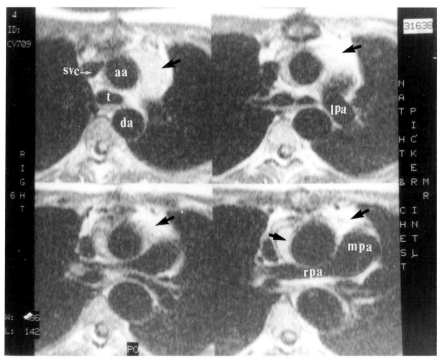

Figure 7.13 Spin echo images in the transverse plane at four contiguous levels in a patient with aortic valve replacement and postoperative pyrexia. The ascending aorta (*aa*), descending aorta (*da*), main pulmonary artery (*mpa*), right and left pulmonary arteries (*rpa, lpa*) superior vena cava (*svc*), and trachea (*t*) are shown. An abscess (*arrow*) is seen around the ascending aorta.

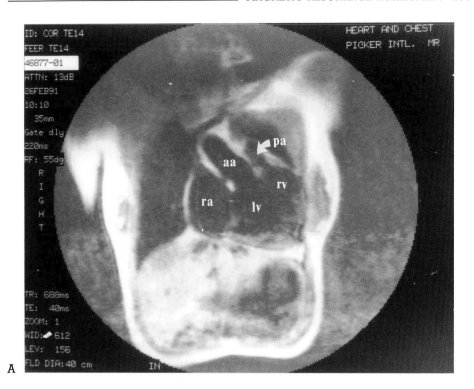

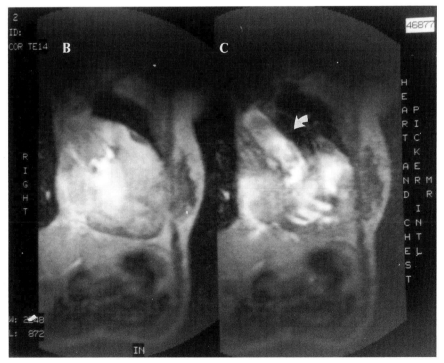

Figure 7.14 Spin echo image (A) and gradient echo images (B, C) in the coronal plane in a patient with Fallot's tetralogy. The left ventricle (*lv*), right ventricle (*rv*), right atrium (*ra*), pulmonary artery (*pa*), and ascending aorta (*aa*) are marked. The gradient echo images are in diastole (B) and systole (C). There is systolic signal loss in the pulmonary artery (*arrow*).

clearly diagnosed on cine gradient echo imaging. In addition, the pressure gradient, which is often difficult to assess by catheterization and Doppler echocardiography, can be estimated by velocity mapping. Tricuspid atresia is rare but is easily identified with spin echo imaging (Fig. 7.15). Tricuspid regurgitation is a much more common finding than stenosis (Fig. 7.16), and trivial tricuspid regurgitation can be found in many normal people.[28] In patients with significant left-sided disease there is often secondary tricuspid regurgitation due to right ventricular dilatation. If this is present it can be used to measure the peak jet velocity from right ventricle to right atrium and thus calculate the pressure differential between these two chambers in systole. These findings can be added to an evaluation of the right atrial pressure to estimate pulmonary artery pressure, providing there is no pulmonary artery stenosis. Right atrial size and the presence of thrombus can be assessed using spin echo and gradient echo imaging (Fig. 7.17).

Conduits

Valved conduits may be obstructed at the valve or within the tube, as when peel forms within Dacron tubes.[29,30] It is important to recognize significant obstruction early, before right ventricular dysfunction occurs. Noninvasive imaging techniques are preferable to repeated invasive measurements.[31] Conventional two-dimensional echocardiography has limited application in these instances, because the full extent of

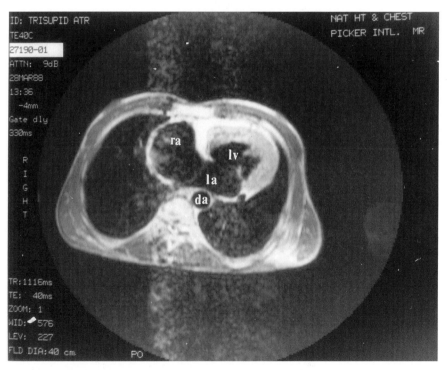

Figure 7.15 Spin echo image in a transverse plane in a patient with tricuspid atresia. The left ventricle (*lv*), left atrium (*la*), right atrium (*ra*), and descending aorta (*da*), are shown. There is no communication between the right atrium and the right ventricle, which was rudimentary.

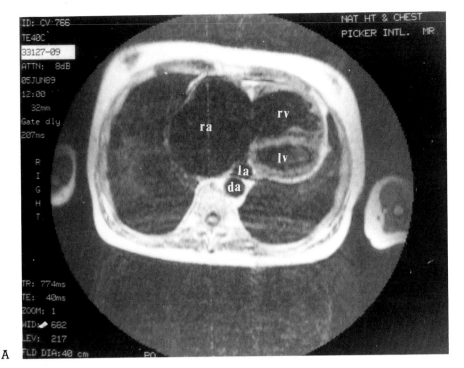

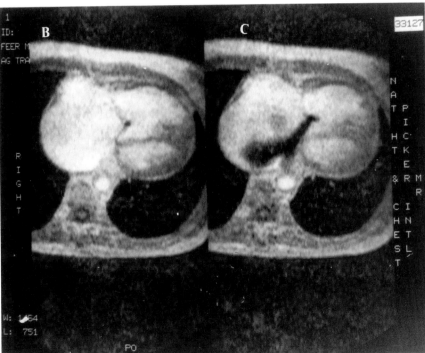

Figure 7.16 Spin echo (*A*) and gradient echo (*B*, *C*) images in the transverse plane in a patient with tricuspid regurgitation due to sarcoidosis. The left ventricle (*lv*), right ventricle (*rv*), left atrium (*la*), right atrium (*ra*), and descending aorta (*da*) are shown. The right atrium is very enlarged. In the gradient echo images in diastole (*B*) and systole (*C*), the jet of tricuspid regurgitation is clearly seen.

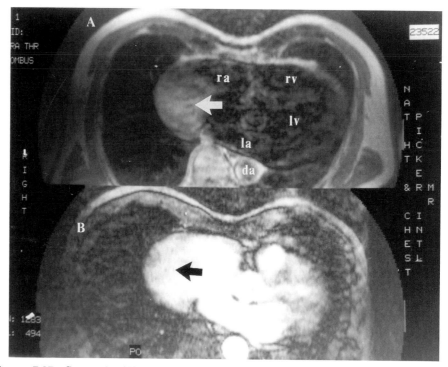

Figure 7.17 Spin echo (*A*) and gradient echo (*B*) images in the transverse plane in a patient with right atrial thrombus. The left ventricle (*lv*), right ventricle (*rv*), left atrium (*la*), right atrium (*ra*), and descending aorta (*da*) are shown. The thrombus (*arrow*) has a high intensity relative to blood in the spin echo image and a low intensity relative to the blood signal in the gradient echo image.

the conduit is not visualized in 83% of the cases.[32] The technique may detect proximal but not distal conduit lesions[33] and often fails to identify valvular obstruction. Continuous-wave Doppler has been useful in detecting the degree of obstruction when the conduit can be seen but gives little idea of the level, making further imaging necessary. In these patients, MRI obtains excellent images in 100%.[34] A correlation between definite obstruction and a conduit diameter of less than 18 mm has been found (Fig. 7.18). The use of velocity mapping increases the value of MRI, and measurement as well as localization and quantification of jet velocity have proved accurate when correlated with invasive hemodynamics (Fig. 7.19).[14]

Aortic Coarctation

Surgical treatment by a variety of techniques for the relief of coarctation of the aorta has been established for 40 years. Late complications, however, include restenosis, aneurysm in association with a Dacron patch,[35] and systolic hypertension. Careful long-term supervision is required. Chest radiography is not reliable for the recognition of restenosis, and an aneurysm may extend posteriorly and not be visible on the routine radiograph. Imaging by two-dimensional echocardiography is also unreliable

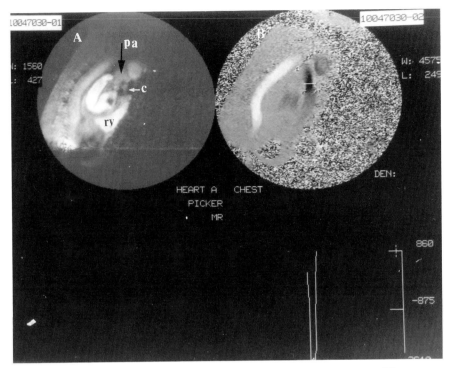

Figure 7.18 Gradient echo image (*A*) and corresponding velocity map (*B*) in a rotated sagittal plane in a patient with a conduit (*c*) from right ventricle (*rv*) to pulmonary artery (*pa*). There is narrowing of the conduit. The velocity profile shows a peak velocity in the conduit of 2.6 m/s (27 mmHg.)

because it may be difficult to obtain a good echo window.[36] However, continuous-wave Doppler measurements are useful for predicting the presence of a gradient.[37-39] When restenosis or aneurysm formation is suspected, catheterization and angiography would normally be performed to confirm the findings before reoperation. An alternative method of assessment is MRI, which can provide high resolution, dimensionally accurate images of the aorta and its lumen noninvasively and without administration of contrast agent.[40-43] Furthermore, cine magnetic resonance velocity mapping allows assessment of the hemodynamic significance of aortic coarctation[14] (Fig. 7.20).

Prosthetic Valves

Prosthetic valves with many different designs are now in widespread use. Evaluation of prosthetic valve function by catheter can be more difficult than with native valves and there is an increased potential morbidity for invasive investigation in these patients. The prostheses are not visible by MRI because they contain no mobile hydrogen atoms. The applied magnetic field is distorted by differences in the local magnetic field between the prosthesis and biologic tissue, and by the eddy current induced in the valve, and this leads to loss of signal from tissues for a variable distance

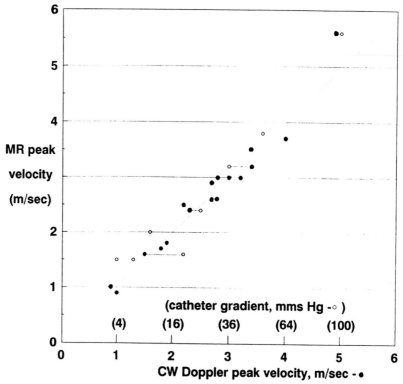

Figure 7.19 Validation of velocity mapping when compared to Doppler echocardiography (*solid dots*) and invasive hemodynamic measurement of cardiovascular stenoses (*open dots*).

around the prosthesis. This distance is small for spin echo images, and neighboring structures are seen normally (Fig. 7.21). In gradient echo images, however, the defect in the image is much larger, making it difficult to assess turbulent jets in the region of the valve (Fig. 7.22). Metal valves are not ferromagnetic, however, and at currently available magnetic field strengths the field does not affect their operation.[44-47]

VELOCITY MAPPING VERSUS DOPPLER ECHOCARDIOGRAPHY

The two techniques are complementary. Magnetic resonance velocity mapping is useful if the echo window is limited or alignment of the ultrasound is inadequate, because there is no limitation on velocity mapping for site or direction data acquisition. This advantage has proved particularly valuable in congenital heart diseases such as conduit stenosis and aortic coarctation. The other major advantage of velocity mapping is that true flow can be calculated with high accuracy because of the simultaneous acquisition of velocity and area of the vessel. Doppler echocardiography is accurate for measuring velocity, but poor at assessing true flow. The limitations of magnetic resonance velocity mapping include the relatively long acquisition times, and poor quality of cardiac-gated images in patients who have cardiac arrhythmias,

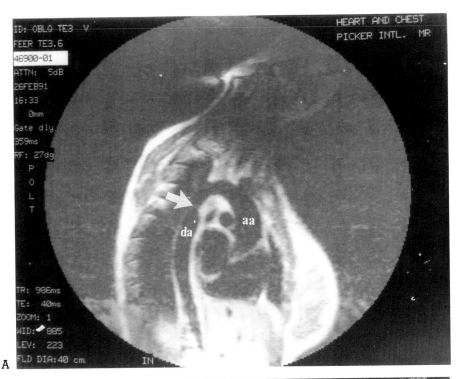

A

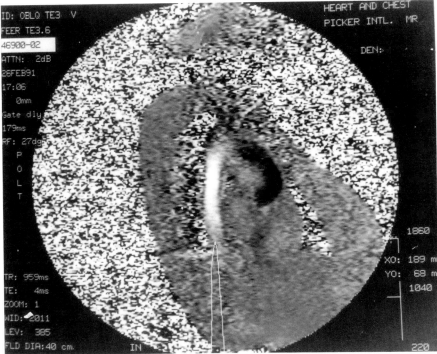

B

Figure 7.20 Spin echo image (*A*) and corresponding velocity map (*B*) in an oblique sagittal plane in a patient with aortic coarctation after percutaneous balloon dilatation. The ascending aorta (*aa*), descending aorta (*da*), and coarctation site (*arrow*) are shown. The peak velocity in the velocity map was 1.86 m/s (14 mmHg).

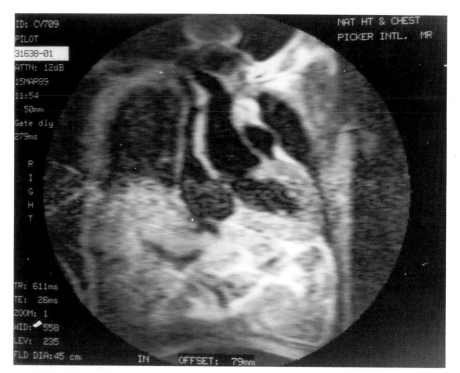

Figure 7.21 Spin echo image in the coronal plane in a patient with a Starr-Edwards aortic valve prosthesis. There is no signal from the metal valve and also little surrounding distortion.

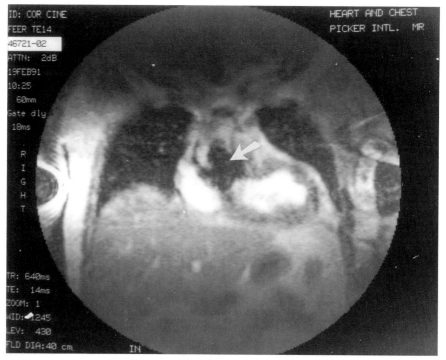

Figure 7.22 Diastolic gradient echo image in the coronal plane in a patient with a Starr-Edwards aortic valve prosthesis. Note the signal loss (*arrow*), which is greater than that seen with spin echo imaging (Fig. 7.21).

the confined bore of the magnet which may preclude use of the technique in patients with claustrophobia, and the high cost of the machine. These limitations may become less important with the development of real-time magnetic resonance velocity mapping using an echo planar technique,[48] open access magnets, and cheaper hardware.

REFERENCES

1. Longmore DB: The principles of magnetic resonance. *Br Med Bull.* 45:848–880, 1989.
2. Pykett IL, Newhouse JH, Buonanno FS, et al: Principles of nuclear magnetic resonance imaging. *Radiology.* 143:157–168, 1982.
3. Pennell DJ, Underwood SR, Ell PJ, et al: Dipyridamole magnetic resonance imaging: a comparison with thallium-201 emission tomography. *Br Heart J.* 64:362–369, 1990.
4. Moran PR: A flow velocity zeugmatographic interlace for NMR imaging in humans. *Magn Reson Imaging.* 1:197–203, 1982.
5. van Dijk P. Direct cardiac NMR imaging of heart wall and blood flow velocity. *J Comput Assist Tomogr.* 8:429–436, 1984.
6. Nayler GL, Firmin DN, Longmore DB. Blood flow imaging by cine magnetic resonance. *J Comput Assist Tomogr.* 10:715–722, 1986.
7. Evans AJ, Blinder RA, Herfkens RJ, et al: Effects of turbulence on signal intensity in gradient echo images. *Invest Radiol.* 23:512–518, 1988.
8. Underwood SR, Firmin DN, Mohiaddin RH, et al: Cine magnetic resonance imaging of valvular heart disease (abstr.). *Proc Soc Magn Reson Imaging.* 2:723, 1987.
9. Sechtem U, Pflugfelder PW, Cassidy MM, et al: Mitral or aortic regurgitation: quantification of regurgitant volumes with cine MR imaging. *Radiology.* 167:425–430, 1988.
10. Globits S, Mayr H, Frank H, et al: Quantification of regurgitant lesions by MRI. *Int J Card Imaging.* 6:109–116, 1991.
11. Wagner S, Auffermann W, Buser P, et al: Diagnostic accuracy and estimation of the severity of valvular regurgitation from the signal void on cine magnetic resonance images. *Am Heart J.* 118:760–767, 1989.
12. Helmcke F, Nanda NC, Hsiung MC, et al: Color Doppler assessment of mitral regurgitation with orthogonal planes. *Circulation.* 75:175–183, 1987.
13. de Roos A, Reicheck N, Axel L, et al: Cine MR imaging in aortic stenosis. *J Comput Assist Tomogr.* 13:421–425, 1989.
14. Kilner PJ, Firmin DN, Rees RSO, et al: Valve and great vessel stenosis: assessment with MR jet velocity mapping. *Radiology.* 178:229–235, 1991.
15. Manzara C, Pennell D, Kilner P, et al: Quantitative assessment of aortic and mitral stenosis by magnetic resonance velocity mapping (abstr.). *J Am Coll Cardiol.* 17:254A, 1991.
16. Longmore DB, Klipstein RH, Underwood SR, et al: Dimensional accuracy of magnetic resonance in studies of the heart. *Lancet.* 1:1360–1362, 1985.
17. Underwood SR, Klipstein RH, Firmin DN, et al: Magnetic resonance assessment of aortic and mitral regurgitation. *Br Heart J.* 56:455–462, 1986.
18. Sorenson SG, O'Rourke RA, Chaudhuri TK. Noninvasive quantitation of valvular regurgitation by gated equilibrium radionuclide angiography. *Circulation.* 62:1089–1098, 1980.
19. Bogren HG, Klipstein RH, Mohiaddin RH, et al: Pulmonary artery distensibility and blood flow patterns: a magnetic resonance study of normal subjects and of patients with pulmonary arterial hypertension. *Am Heart J.* 118:990–999, 1989.
20. Mohiaddin RH, Wann SL, Underwood SR, et al: Vena caval flow: assessment with cine MR velocity mapping. *Radiology.* 177:537–541, 1990.

21. Mohiaddin RH, Amanuma M, Longmore DB: Magnetic resonance measurement of pulmonary venous flow and distensibility. *Am J Noninvasive Cardiol.* 1991. (in press).

22. Mohiaddin RH, Amanuma M, Kilner PJ, et al: Magnetic resonance phase-shift velocity mapping of mitral and pulmonary venous flow. *J Comput Assist Tomogr.* 15:237–243, 1991.

23. Park JH, Han MC, Im J-G, et al: Mitral stenosis: evaluation with MR imaging after percutaneous balloon valvuloplasty. *Radiology.* 177:533–536, 1990.

24. Caputo GR, Suzuki JI, Kondo C, et al: Determination of left ventricular volume and mass with biphasic spin-echo MR imaging: comparison with cine MR. *Radiology.* 177:773–777, 1990.

25. Dinsmore RE, Wedeen V, Rosen B, et al: Phase-offset technique to distinguish slow blood flow and thrombus on MR images. *AJR.* 148:634–636, 1987.

26. Miller SW, Palmer EL, Dinsmore RE, et al: Gallium-67 and magnetic resonance imaging in aortic root abscess. *J Nucl Med.* 28:1616–1619, 1987.

27. Mohiaddin RH, Paz R, Theodoropolus S, et al: Magnetic resonance characterization of pulmonary arterial blood flow following single lung transplantation. *J Thorac Cardiovasc Surg.* 101:1016–1023, 1991.

28. Waggoner AD, Quinones MA, Young JB, et al: Pulsed Doppler echocardiographic detection of right-sided valve regurgitation. Experimental results and clinical significance. *Am J Cardiol.* 47:279–283, 1981.

29. Agarwal KC, Edwards WD, Feldt RH, et al: Clinicopathological correlates of obstructed right-sided porcine-valved extracardiac conduits. *J Thorac Cardiovasc Surg.* 81:591–601, 1981.

30. Agarwal KC, Edwards WD, Feldt RH, et al: Pathogenesis of nonobstructive fibrous peels in right-sided porcine-valved extracardiac conduits. *J Thorac Cardiovasc Surg.* 83:584–589, 1982.

31. Canter CE, Gutierrez FR, Molina P, et al: Noninvasive diagnosis of right-sided extracardiac conduit obstruction by combined magnetic resonance imaging and continuous-wave Doppler echocardiography. *J Thorac Cardiovasc Surg.* 101:724–731, 1991.

32. Khaw KT, Martinez JE, Somerville J, et al: Non-invasive MR and two-dimensional echocardiographic imaging of ventriculopulmonary conduits (abstr.). *Radiology.* 173(P):239, 1989.

33. Reeder GS, Currie PJ, Fyfe DA, et al: Extracardiac conduit obstruction: initial experience in the use of Doppler echocardiography for noninvasive estimation of pressure gradient. *J Am Coll Cardiol.* 4:1006–1011, 1984.

34. Khaw KT, Martinez JE, Somerville J, et al: Noninvasive MR and two-dimensional echocardiographic imaging of ventriculopulmonary conduits (abstr.). *Radiology.* 173(P):239, 1989.

35. Rheuban KS, Gutgesell HP, Carpenter MA, et al: Aortic aneurysm after patch angioplasty for aortic isthmic coarctation in childhood. *Am J Cardiol.* 58:178–180, 1986.

36. Sahn DJ, Allen HD, McDonald G, et al: Real-time cross-sectional echo-cardiographic diagnosis of coarctation of the aorta. A prospective study of echocardiographic–angiographic correlations. *Circulation.* 56:762–769, 1977.

37. Wyse RKH, Robinson PJ, Deanfield JE, et al: Use of continuous wave Doppler ultrasound velocimetry to assess the severity of coarctation of the aorta by measurement of aortic flow velocities. *Br Heart J.* 52:278–283, 1984.

38. Marx GR, Allen HD. Accuracy and pitfalls of Doppler evaluation of the pressure gradient in aortic coarctation. *J Am Coll Cardiol.* 7:1379–1385, 1986.

39. Hoadley SD, Duster MC, Miller JF, et al: Pulsed Doppler study of a case of coarctation of the aorta: demonstration of a continuous Doppler frequency shift. *Pediatr Cardiol.* 6:275–277, 1986.

40. Rees S, Somerville J, Ward C, et al: Coarctation of the aorta: MR imaging in late postoperative assessment. *Radiology.* 173:499–502, 1989.

41. Amparo EG, Higgins CB, Shafton EP: Demonstration of coarctation of the aorta by magnetic resonance imaging. *AJR.* 143:1192–1194, 1984.

42. von Schulthess GK, Higashino SM, Higgins SS, et al: Coarctation of the aorta: MR imaging. *Radiology.* 158:469–474, 1986.

43. Boxer RA, LaCorte MA, Singh S, et al: Nuclear magnetic resonance imaging in evaluation and follow-up of children treated for coarctation of the aorta. *J Am Coll Cardiol.* 7:1095–1098, 1986.

44. Soulen RL, Budinger TF, Higgins CB: Magnetic resonance imaging of prosthetic heart valves. *Radiology.* 154:705–707, 1985.

45. Randall PA, Kohman LJ, Scalzetti EM, et al: Magnetic resonance imaging of prosthetic cardiac valves in vitro and in vivo. *Am J Cardiol.* 62:973–976, 1988.

46. Shellock FG: MR imaging of metallic implants and materials: a compilation of the literature. *AJR.* 151:811–814, 1988.

47. Shellock FG, Crues JV. High-field-strength MR imaging and metallic biomedical implants: an ex vivo evaluation of deflection forces. *AJR.* 151:389–392, 1988.

48. Firmin DN, Klipstein RH, Hounsfield GL, et al: Echo-planar high-resolution flow velocity mapping. *Magn Reson Med.* 12:316–327, 1989.

CHAPTER **8**

Congenital Mitral Stenosis

ALBERT P. ROCCHINI

Childhood mitral stenosis is a rare but serious cardiac problem.[1] Even in children, rheumatic mitral disease is still the most common cause of mitral stenosis worldwide. With the recent decline in the incidence of rheumatic mitral disease, however, in many regions around the world congenital mitral abnormalities now represent the most common pediatric cause of mitral stenosis. Congenital mitral stenosis is usually categorized according to which component of the mitral apparatus is abnormal; it can be associated with a variable combination of mitral anomalies including thickened, rolled leaflet margins; thickened, shortened chordae tendineae; papillary muscle hypoplasia; decreased interpapillary muscle distance or fusion; abnormal chordal insertions; and fibrous obliteration of the interchordal spaces.[1-4] Because of the anatomic diversity of congenital mitral stenosis, surgical therapy has been difficult and at times impossible.[3,4] The success of balloon catheter in treating rheumatic mitral disease[5] and the frequent poor results of surgical therapy have led to attempts to use balloon valvuloplasty therapeutically in a few children with congenital mitral stenosis.[6-14] This chapter reviews experience with the use of balloon valvuloplasty for the treatment of children with mitral valve stenosis, placing special emphasis on the technique used to perform the valvuloplasty, on followup, and on complications associated with the procedure.

PROCEDURE

Children with symptomatic mitral stenosis are potential candidates for balloon valvuloplasty. *The only contraindications are severe mitral regurgitation and thrombus within the left atrium.*

Cardiac catheterization is performed from a percutaneous approach by way of the femoral artery and vein. To allow passage of one or two large valvuloplasty catheters the femoral vein should be entered as proximally as possible. Before the valvuloplasty is performed, the following hemodynamic and angiographic data should be obtained:

simultaneous left atrial and left ventricular end-diastolic pressures, cardiac output, and a left ventricular angiogram. The valvuloplasty procedure can be performed using one or two balloons.

The recommended method used to determine valvuloplasty balloon size is as follows:

1. If one balloon is used, the balloon diameter should equal or exceed by 1 to 2 mm the maximal mitral annulus diameter as estimated by two-dimensional echo-cardiography.
2. If two balloons are to be used, the combined balloon diameter should be 1.3 times the estimated mitral valve annulus.

The major advantage of using two balloons is that smaller catheters can be used and therefore it is unlikely that the atrial septum will have to be predilated.

Single-Balloon Method

The left atrium is entered with an 8- to 12-Fr. Mullins transseptal sheath. After the transseptal puncture is performed the patient should be systemically anticoagulated using 100 units of heparin per kilogram of body weight to a maximum of 3000 units. A 7-Fr. balloon end-hole catheter should then be advanced through the mitral and aortic valves into the descending aorta. At this point, a Teflon-coated 0.035 inch exchange guidewire is advanced into the descending aorta. The distal end of the guidewire is precurved with a 180° curve. The curve permits the wire to be well seated in the apex of the left ventricle when the valvuloplasty balloon is inflated, thereby reducing the chance of perforating the apex of the left ventricle. The sheath and end-hole balloon catheter are then removed, leaving the guidewire positioned in the descending aorta.

The valvuloplasty catheter is then advanced over the guidewire and across the atrial septum into the apex of the left ventricle. It is unlikely that the atrial septum will require predilatation to permit the valvuloplasty catheter to be advanced across the atrial septum if the transseptal sheath is at least 9 Fr. and the balloon valvuloplasty catheter is less than 20 mm. Otherwise, the atrial septum should be dilated with an 8-mm angioplasty catheter before trying to advance the valvuloplasty catheter across the atrial septum. Once the valvuloplasty catheter is positioned across the mitral valve the guidewire should be withdrawn into the left ventricle and the valvuloplasty balloon inflated with dilute contrast (to 3–4 atm) until the indentation in the balloon produced by the stenotic mitral valve disappears (Figs. 8.1 and 8.2). The total inflation time should be 8 to 15 seconds. After the valvuloplasty is performed, repeat the hemodynamic measurements and a left ventricular angiogram should be performed.

Double-Balloon Method

I preferred to perform balloon mitral valvuloplasty by using two balloon valvuloplasty catheters. There are two alternative techniques. The first approach is to perform two transseptal punctures. Both transseptal punctures can be performed from the right femoral vein. After two 8- to 12-Fr. Mullins transseptal sheaths have been advanced

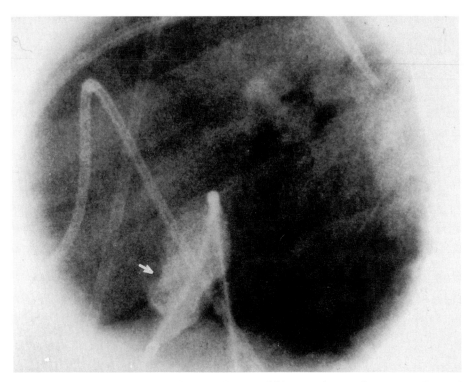

Figure 8.1 Lateral angiogram from an 8-year-old boy with mitral stenosis. A single 18-mm valvuloplasty balloon is positioned across the mitral valve. The *arrow* marks the small indentation produced by the stenotic valve.

into the left atrium, two 7-Fr. end-hole catheters can be advanced through the mitral and aortic valves into the descending aorta. Two exchange wires are then positioned in the aorta and two dilation balloons are advanced across the mitral valve (Fig. 8.3).

The second approach is to use only one transseptal catheter. Mansfield Scientific Inc. has recently developed a specially designed double-lumen catheter that permits two guidewires to be advanced into the left ventricle through a single transseptal sheath and dilator. If this specially designed catheter is used, two curved exchange guide wires are positioned in the apex of the left ventricle. The transseptal catheter is then removed and the balloon catheters are advanced one at a time through the same venous entry site and the same puncture in the atrial septum.

RESULTS

Clinical experience with balloon mitral valvuloplasty in children and young adults has not been extensive. Lock and associates[10] reported treating 8 patients (9 to 23 years of age) who had rheumatic mitral stenosis. After valvuloplasty there was an 84% mean increase in the mitral valve area and a 52% mean fall in the gradient, whereas cardiac output increased. Lock and associates performed postvalvuloplasty catheterizations 2 to 8 weeks later in 6 of the 8 patients. In 4 patients there was sustained hemodynamic improvement and 2 others experienced some degree of restenosis. Other investigators

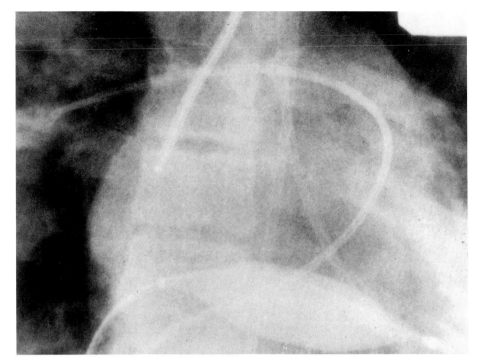

Figure 8.2 Posteroanterior angiogram from a 12-year-old girl with mitral stenosis. A single 25-mm valvuloplasty balloon is positioned, fully inflated, across the mitral valve.

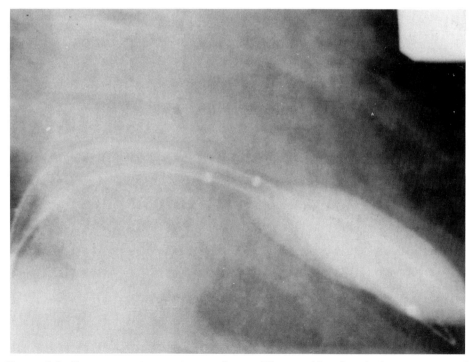

Figure 8.3 Posteroanterior angiogram from a 17-year-old girl with rheumatic mitral stenosis. Two 18-mm valvuloplasty balloons are positioned across the mitral valve.

have also reported good hemodynamic results with the use of balloon valvuloplasty to treat rheumatic mitral stenosis in children.[6,9,10,12-14] The combined hemodynamic results in these published cases document a mean reduction in the left atrial *a* wave to left ventricular end-diastolic pressure gradient from 23 mmHg to 8.2 mmHg, a mean increase in mitral valve area from 0.77 cm^2/m^2 to 1.29 cm^2/m^2, and a mean reduction in mean pulmonary artery pressure from 35 mmHg to 27 mmHg.

Kveselis and coworkers[6] first reported using balloon mitral valvuloplasty to treat a child with congenital mitral stenosis. Since that 1984 report the number of balloon mitral valvuloplasties performed at the University of Michigan has increased to a total of five children, three with congenital mitral stenosis and two with rheumatic mitral stenosis. In two of the patients with congenital mitral stenosis the valvuloplasty catheter could not be advanced across the mitral valve and balloon valvuloplasty could not be performed. In the other three children, balloon valvuloplasty acutely reduced the mean gradient between the left atrial *a* wave and left ventricular end-diastolic pressure from 28 mmHg to 12 mmHg, increased the mean mitral valve area from 0.87 cm^2/m^2 to 1.19 cm^2/m^2, and reduced the mean pulmonary artery pressure from 42 mmHg to 29 mmHg. The long-term followup of the three children who had successful balloon valvuloplasty documented the best outcome in the two children with rheumatic mitral stenosis. These two patients were followed for 3.5 and 2 years, and both reported persistent symptomatic relief. Repeat catheterization in one child 1.5 years after balloon valvuloplasty demonstrated sustained hemodynamic improvement. The one child who underwent balloon valvuloplasty for congenital mitral stenosis had symptomatic improvement for 6 months. Symptoms returned, however, and therefore surgery was performed. At surgery there was evidence of valvuloplasty-induced separation of the anterior but not the posterior commissure.

The Valvuloplasty and Angioplasty of Congenital Anomalies (VACA) Registry recently reported the results of 16 attempted dilatations of stenotic mitral valves.[9] The dilatation was classified a success in 10 and a failure in 1, and the results were unknown in 5. There was no information about the type of stenosis or the amount of mitral regurgitation present after dilatation. Alday and associates[7] reported an increase in mitral valve area with balloon valvuloplasty of congenital mitral stenosis in a single patient with no long-term followup. Spevak and associates[8] reported the results of a multicenter study on the use of balloon valvuloplasty in 9 children (ages 0.1 to 10 years) with congenital mitral stenosis. There was significant improvement of the transmitral gradient in 5, but 2 developed a recurrence of significant stenosis within 2 months. The failures or recurrences occurred in patients who had a "forme fruste" of parachute mitral valve with chordal attachments primarily to a single papillary muscle, severe shortening, and thickening of the chordae as in a mitral arcade, or in those with a very small mitral annulus. Perry and associates[11] reported the Boston experience with the use of balloon valvuloplasty to treat 10 children, 0.1 to 10 years of age, with congenital mitral stenosis. Perry reported a significant reduction in the transvalvular mitral gradient, which decreased from 15 ± 5 mmHg to 9 ± 7 mmHg. The valve area increased from 1.0 ± 0.4 cm^2/m^2 to 1.6 ± 0.7 cm^2/m^2. In 3 patients the balloon valvuloplasty did not bring about hemodynamic improvement. In the remaining 7 children who had initially successful balloon valvuloplasty, two valves restenosed within 3 months. Perry concluded that mitral valve morphology had a significant impact on whether or not balloon valvuloplasty would succeed, in that the most favorable results were observed in patients with classic mitral stenosis and the least favorable results were observed in children with parachute mitral valves or supravalvular mitral rings. Similar results and conclusions were reported by Grifka and coworkers[15] at the 32nd Annual Meeting of the American Academy of Pediatrics, Section on Cardiology, Boston, October 6, 1990.

Complications

Few complications have been reported with the use of balloon valvuloplasty to treat congenital mitral stenosis. Complications reported to the VACA registry include one each of the following: transient ventricular tachycardia, transient ST segment elevation, transient hypotension, and a 1.6 to 1 left to right atrial shunt.[9] Small left-to-right atrial shunts have also been reported by others.[8,10] Mitral regurgitation also can develop following balloon valvuloplasty. Spevak reported the development of moderate mitral regurgitation in 2 of 9 cases.[8] Similarly, Perry and associates[11] reported an increase in mitral regurgitation following balloon valvuloplasty in 4 of 10. Only one death has been reported in association with balloon mitral valvuloplasty for the treatment of congenital mitral stenosis.[11] Finally, there have been no reports of patients developing hemoptysis, pulmonary edema, or evidence of thromboembolic events.

SUMMARY

Balloon valvuloplasty is at present an experimental procedure for treating children with mitral stenosis. Based on the adult experience and the limited published experience in children it does appear that balloon mitral valvuloplasty has an important role in the management of children with rheumatic mitral stenosis. The role of balloon mitral valvuloplasty in the management of congenital mitral stenosis is more controversial. Although balloon valvuloplasty does bring a hemodynamic benefit to some children with congenital mitral stenosis, not enough information is available to predict which patients may benefit. On the basis of the available reports, however, it appears that success is more likely in patients with balanced chordal attachments, in whom chordal thickening and shortening are minimal, and in whom the annulus is not severely hypoplastic. Therefore, before balloon mitral valvuloplasty becomes the treatment of choice for the child with congenital mitral stenosis, we will need to know more about the extent and duration of clinical improvement produced by this technique.

REFERENCES

1. Baylen BG, Waldhausen JA: Diseases of the mitral valve. In: Adams FH, Emmanouilides GC, Riemenschneider TA, eds. *Moss' Heart Disease in Infants, Children and Adolescents.* Baltimore: Williams & Wilkins, 1989, pp 647–663.
2. Davachi F, Moller JH, Edwards JE: Diseases of the mitral valve in infancy: an anatomic analysis of 55 cases. *Circulation.* 43:565–579, 1971.
3. Ruckman RN, Van Praagh R: Anatomic types of congenital mitral stenosis: report of 49 autopsy cases with consideration of diagnosis and surgical implications. *Am J Cardiol.* 42:592–601, 1978.
4. Carpentier A, Branchini B, Cour JC, et al: Congenital malformations of the mitral valve in children. Pathology and surgical treatment. *J Thorac Cardiovasc Surg.* 72:854–866, 1976.

5. Inoue K, Owaki T, Nakamura T, et al: Clinical application of transvenous mitral commissurotomy by a new balloon catheter. *J Thorac Cardiovasc Surg.* 87:394–402, 1984.

6. Kveselis DA, Rocchini AP, Beekman R, et al: Balloon angioplasty for congenital and rheumatic mitral stenosis. *Am J Cardiol.* 57:348–350, 1986.

7. Alday LE, Juaneda E: Percutaneous balloon dilatation in congenital mitral stenosis. *Br Heart J.* 57:479–482, 1987.

8. Spevak PJ, Bass JL, Ben-Shachar G, et al: Balloon angioplasty for congenital mitral stenosis. *Am J Cardiol.* 66:472–476, 1990.

9. Mullins EC, Latson LA, Neches WH, et al: Balloon dilation of miscellaneous lesions: results of Valvuloplasty and Angioplasty of Congenital Anomalies Registry. *Am J Cardiol.* 65:802–803, 1990.

10. Lock JE, Khalilullah M, Shrivistava S, et al: Percutaneous catheter commissurotomy in rheumatic mitral stenosis. *N Engl J Med.* 313:1515–1518, 1985.

11. Perry SB, Spevak PJ, Keane JF, et al: Balloon valvuloplasty for congenital mitral stenosis. *Circulation.* 82(suppl III):III-584, 1990.

12. Palacios I, Block PC, Brandi S, et al: Percutaneous balloon valvotomy for patients with severe mitral stenosis. *Circulation.* 75:778–784, 1987.

13. Mullins CE, Nihill MR, Vick GW III, et al: Double balloon technique for dilation of valvular or vessel stenosis in congenital and acquired heart disease. *J Am Coll Cardiol.* 10:107–114, 1987.

14. Chen C, Lo Z, Huang Z, et al: Percutaneous transseptal balloon mitral valvuloplasty: the Chinese experience in 30 patients. *Am Heart J.* 115:937–947, 1988.

15. Grifka RG, Nihill MR, Mullins CE: Percutaneous transseptal double balloon valvuloplasty for congenital mitral stenosis. *Am J Cardiol.* 66:522, 1990.

CHAPTER 9

Acquired Mitral Stenosis: Double Balloon Catheter Technique

IGOR F. PALACIOS
PETER C. BLOCK

Since its introduction by Inoue and associates[1] in 1984, percutaneous balloon mitral valvuloplasty has become an efficacious nonsurgical technique for the treatment of patients with symptomatic mitral stenosis.[1-8] There is no unique technique of balloon mitral valvuloplasty, but most of the techniques employed require transseptal left heart catheterization and use of the antegrade approach. Antegrade percutaneous balloon mitral valvuloplasty can be accomplished using a single or a double balloon catheter technique.[2,3] In this latter approach the two balloon catheters may be placed through a single femoral venous puncture and a single transseptal puncture[3] or through two separate femoral venous punctures and two separate atrial septal punctures.[4] In the retrograde technique of balloon mitral valvuloplasty[9] the dilating catheters are advanced percutaneously through the right and left femoral arteries over guidewires that have been snared from the descending aorta. These guidewires have been advanced transseptally from the right femoral vein into the left atrium, the left ventricle, and the ascending aorta.

This chapter reviews patient selection, technique, immediate outcome, complications and midterm followup results of the double balloon catheter technique of percutaneous balloon mitral valvuloplasty.

TECHNIQUE

Selection of patients for percutaneous balloon mitral valvuloplasty should be based on symptoms, physical examination, and two-dimensional and Doppler echocardiographic findings. The criteria required for patients to be considered for such a procedure include: (1) symptomatic mitral stenosis, (2) no recent embolic event, (3) mitral regurgitation of less than grade 2 as established by contrast ventriculography, and (4) no evidence of left atrial thrombus on two-dimensional echocardiography. Transesophageal echocardiography should be performed whenever the transthoracic echocardiogram is not conclusive and in all patients with a history of embolic events. Patients in atrial fibrillation and patients with previous embolic episodes should be anticoagulated with warfarin to achieve a therapeutic prothrombin time for at least 3 months before percutaneous balloon mitral valvuloplasty. Patients with thrombus in the left atrium on two-dimensional echocardiography should be excluded. Percutaneous balloon mitral valvuloplasty should be performed with the patient in the fasting state under mild sedation. Antibiotic therapy (dicloxacillin 500 mg p.o. every 6 hours for 4 doses) is started before the procedure. Patients allergic to penicillin should receive vancomycin 1 gram intravenously at the time of the procedure.

All patients carefully chosen as candidates for balloon mitral valvuloplasty should undergo right and transseptal left heart catheterization. Right heart catheterization is generally performed percutaneously from the right internal jugular vein with a thermodilution Swan-Ganz catheter. Transseptal left heart catheterization is then performed from the right femoral vein using a Mullins transseptal sheath and a modified Brockenbrough needle. Following transseptal left heart catheterization, systemic anticoagulation is achieved by the intravenous administration of 100 units of heparin per kg body weight. In patients older than 40 years, coronary arteriography should also be performed.

Hemodynamic measurements, cardiac output and cine left ventriculography are performed before and after percutaneous balloon mitral valvuloplasty. Cardiac output is measured by the thermodilution and Fick method techniques. Mitral valve calcification and severity of mitral regurgitation are graded qualitatively from 0+ to 4+ as previously described.[3] An oxygen diagnostic run is performed before and after the procedure to determine the presence of left-to-right shunting across the atrial septal puncture.

After transseptal catheterization, a 7-Fr. flow-directed balloon catheter is advanced through the Mullins sheath across the mitral valve into the left ventricle. The catheter is then advanced through the aortic valve into the ascending and then the descending aorta. A 0.038-inch, 260-cm long Teflon-coated exchange wire is then passed through the catheter. The sheath and the catheter are removed, leaving the wire behind. A 5-mm balloon dilating catheter is used to dilate the atrial septum. A second exchange guidewire is passed parallel to the first guidewire through the same femoral vein and atrial septum punctures using a double-lumen catheter. The double-lumen catheter is then removed leaving the two guidewires across the mitral valve in the ascending and descending aorta (Fig. 9.1 *Left*). During these maneuvers care should be taken to maintain large and smooth loops of the guidewires in the left ventricular cavity to allow appropriate placement of the dilating balloons. If the guidewires' loops become short, it is impossible to place the dilating balloons in a position adequate for a successful percutaneous balloon mitral valvuloplasty. If a second guidewire cannot be placed into the ascending and descending aorta, a 0.038-inch Amplatz-type transfer guidewire with a preformed curled at its tip can be placed at the left ventricular apex. In patients with an aortic valve prosthesis both guidewires with preformed curled tips should be placed at the left ventricular apex. When one or both guidewires have been placed in the left ventricular apex, the balloons should be inflated sequentially. Care should be taken to avoid forward movement of the balloons and guidewires to prevent left ventricular perforation.

Two balloon dilating catheters, chosen according to the patients' body surface area, are then advanced, one over each of the guidewires, and positioned across the mitral valve parallel to the longitudinal axis of the left ventricle (Fig. 9.1 *Middle*). Care should be taken to keep the guidewires and the balloon dilating catheters closely

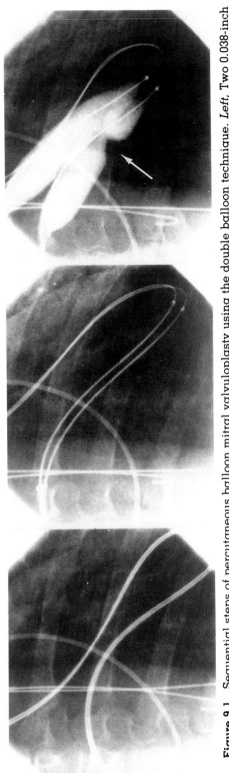

Figure 9.1 Sequential steps of percutaneous balloon mitral valvuloplasty using the double balloon technique. *Left.* Two 0.038-inch guidewires are placed parallel to each other through the atrial septum, across the mitral valve into the left ventricle, then the ascending and descending aorta with their tips at the level of diaphragm. *Middle.* Two balloon catheters are placed straddling the stenotic mitral valve. Markers identifying the proximal ends of the balloons are well beyond the atrial septum; markers identifying the distal ends of the balloons are at the left ventricular apex. *Right.* The balloons are inflated (*arrow* points to the waist produced by the stenotic valve) until the waist disappears.

parallel to each other and the proximal portion of the balloons distal to the atrial septum to minimize the possibility of left-to-right shunting through the atrial septum. The balloon valvuloplasty catheters are then inflated by hand until the indentation produced by the stenotic mitral valve is no longer seen (Fig. 9.1 *Right*). Generally one, but occasionally two or three, inflations are performed. After complete deflation the balloon catheters are removed sequentially.

MECHANISM OF PERCUTANEOUS BALLOON MITRAL VALVULOPLASTY

Successful percutaneous balloon mitral valvuloplasty splits the fused commissures toward the mitral annulus, thereby widening the commissure.[10] This mechanism has been demonstrated by pathologic,[10] surgical,[10] and echocardiographic[11] studies. In patients with calcific mitral stenosis, the balloons also may increase mitral valve flexibility by fracturing the calcified deposits in the mitral valve leaflets.[7] Although rare, undesirable complications such as leaflet tears, left ventricular perforation, tearing of the atrial septum, and rupture of chordae, mitral annulus, and papillary muscle could also occur.

IMMEDIATE OUTCOME

In most series percutaneous balloon mitral valvuloplasty has been reported to increase mitral valve area from less than 1.0 cm^2 to $\geq$ 2.0 cm^2. Table 9.1 shows the changes in mitral valve area reported by several investigators using the double-balloon technique of balloon mitral valvuloplasty. From July 1986 until March 1991, 432 patients with mitral stenosis have undergone percutaneous balloon mitral valvuloplasty at the Massachusetts General Hospital. There were 351 females and 81 males with a mean age of 54 ± 1 (range 14–87) years. Before the procedure 55 patients were in New York Heart Association (NYHA) functional class IV, 268 patients in class III, 107 in class II, and 2 in class I. Eighty-five patients had previously undergone surgical mitral commissurotomy and had presented with mitral restenosis; 217 patients were in normal sinus rhythm and 215 had atrial fibrillation. Evidence of mitral valve calcification under fluoroscopy was present in 195 patients. A mild degree of mitral valve regurgitation ($\leq$ grade 2) was demonstrated by cine left ventriculography in 151 patients before balloon mitral valvuloplasty.

Table 9.1 CHANGES IN MITRAL VALVE AREA PRODUCED BY PERCUTANEOUS BALLOON MITRAL VALVULOPLASTY (PBMV)

Institution	Mitral Valve Area, cm^2	
	Pre-PBMV	Post-PBMV[a]
Massachusetts General Hospital (n = 432)	0.9 ± 0.1	2.0 ± 0.1
Loma Linda University (n = 320)	0.9 ± 0.1	2.4 ± 0.1
Beth Israel Hospital (n = 120)	1.0 ± 0.1	2.0 ± 0.1
Tennon Hospital, France (n = 300)	1.1 ± 0.1	2.2 ± 0.1

[a] p < 0.001.

The hemodynamic changes produced by percutaneous balloon mitral valvuloplasty in the 432 patients who underwent such a procedure at the Massachusetts General Hospital are shown in Table 9.2. Percutaneous balloon mitral valvuloplasty resulted in a significant decrease in mitral gradient from 15 ± 1 to 5 ± 1 mm Hg (p<.0001). The mean cardiac output increased from 3.9 ± 0.1 to 4.5 L/min (p<.0001) and the calculated mitral valve area from 0.9 ± 0.1 to 2.0 ± 0.1 cm^2 (p<.0001). Mean pulmonary artery pressure decreased from 37 ± 1 to 28 ± 1 mm Hg (p<.0001). The mean left atrial pressure decreased from 25 ± 1 to 16 ± 1 mm Hg (p<.0001) and the calculated pulmonary vascular resistance decreased significantly following the procedure. Figure 9.2 shows an example of the hemodynamic changes produced by percutaneous balloon mitral valvuloplasty in one patient. We had previously reported that pulmonary vascular resistance continues to decrease during the 24 hours following balloon mitral valvuloplasty.[12] A good hemodynamic outcome (defined as a post-balloon mitral valvuloplasty mitral valve area ≥ 1.5 cm^2) was obtained in 79% of the patients. Although a suboptimal result occurred in 21% of the patients, a post-balloon mitral valvuloplasty mitral valve area ≤ 1.0 cm^2 (critical mitral valve area) was present in only 7% (Fig. 9.3).

Univariate analysis demonstrated that the increase in mitral valve area with percutaneous balloon mitral valvuloplasty is directly related to the balloon size employed, as they reflect the effective balloon dilating area and are inversely related to the echocardiographic score, the presence of atrial fibrillation, the presence of calcification on fluoroscopy, the presence of previous surgical commissurotomy, older age, high pre-procedure NYHA class, and presence of mitral regurgitation before balloon mitral valvuloplasty. Multiple stepwise regression analysis demonstrated that the increase in mitral valve area with percutaneous balloon mitral valvuloplasty is directly related to balloon size (p < .02) and inversely related to the echocardiographic score (p < .0001), presence of atrial fibrillation (p < .009), and mitral regurgitation before the procedure (p < .03).

A more important predictor of the immediate and long-term results of percutaneous balloon mitral valvuloplasty is a morphologic **echocardiographic score** developed at the Massachusetts General Hospial.[11,13] In this score system, leaflet rigidity, leaflet thickening, valvular calcification, and subvalvular disease are each scored from 0 to 4 (Table 9.3). A higher score would represent a heavily calcified, thickened, and immobile valve with extensive thickening and calcification of the

Table 9.2 CHANGES IN HEMODYNAMIC VARIABLES PRODUCED BY PERCUTANEOUS BALLOON MITRAL VALVULOPLASTY (MASSACHUSETTS GENERAL HOSPITAL, N = 432)

	Pre-PBMV	Post-PBMV[a]
Mitral gradient, mmHg	15 ± 1	5 ± 1*
Cardiac output, L/min	3.9 ± 0.1	4.5 ± 0.1*
Mitral valve area, cm^2	0.9 ± 0.1	2.0 ± 0.1*
Mean pulmonary arterial pressure, mmHg	37 ± 1	28 ± 1*
Mean left atrial pressure, mmHg	25 ± 1	15 ± 1*
Pulmonary arteriolar resistance, (dynes-s-cm^{-5})	316 ± 15	268 ± 12*

[a] p < 0.0001.

PBMV—percutaneous balloon mitral valvuloplasty.

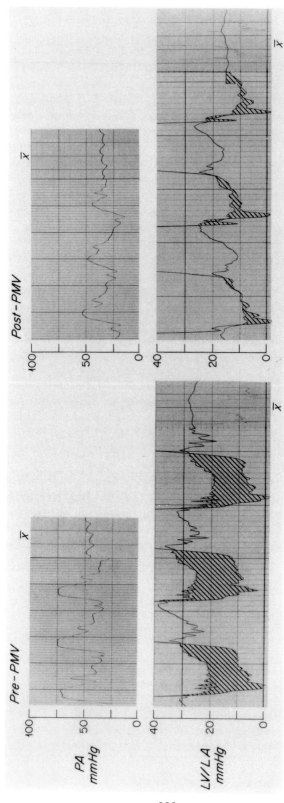

Figure 9.2 Simultaneous pulmonary artery (top) and left atrial and left ventricular (bottom) pressures before (left) and after (right) successful percutaneous mitral valvuloplasty. LA—left atrium. PA—pulmonary artery. PMV—percutaneous mitral valvuloplasty.

POST-PMV MITRAL VALVE AREA

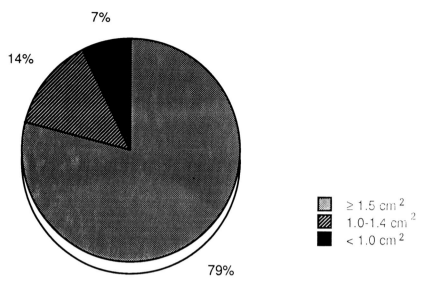

Figure 9.3 Distribution of the mitral valve areas immediately after percutaneous mitral valvuloplasty (PMV) in 432 consecutive patients at the Massachusetts General Hospital.

Table 9.3 THE ECHOCARDIOGRAPHIC SCORE

Grade	Mobility	Subvalvar Thickening	Thickening	Calcification
1	Highly mobile valve with only leaflet tips restricted	Minimal thickening just below the mitral leaflets	Leaflets near normal in thickness (4–5 mm)	A single area of increased echo brightness
2	Leaflet mid and base portions have normal mobility	Thickening of chordal structures extending up to one third of the chordal length	Mid-leaflets normal, considerable thickening of margins (5–8 mm)	Scattered areas of brightness confined to leaflet margins
3	Valve continues to move forward in diastole, mainly from the base	Thickening extending to the distal third of the chords	Thickening extending through the entire leaflet (5–8 mm)	Brightness extending into the midportion of the leaflets
4	No or minimal forward movement of the leaflets in diastole	Extensive thickening and shortening of all chordal structures extending down to the papillary muscles	Considerable thickening of all leaflet tissue (>8–10 mm)	Extensive brightness throughout much of the leaflet tissue

From Wilkins GT, Weyman AE, Abascal VM, et al. Percutaneous balloon dilatation of the mitral valve — an analysis of echocardiographic variables related to outcome and the mechanism of dilatation. *Br Heart J.* 60:299, 1988. With permission.

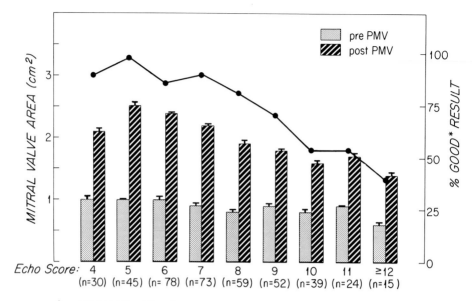

*post PMV MVA ≥ 1.5 cm²

Figure 9.4 Relationship between the echocardiographic score (*x* axis), the increase in the mitral valve area (MVA) produced by percutaneous mitral valvuloplasty (PMV) (*left* axis), and the percentage of patients having a good result (post-PMV MVA ≥ 1.5cm²) (*right* axis).

subvalvular apparatus. Among the four components of the echocardiographic score, valve leaflet thickening and subvalvular disease correlate the best with the increase in mitral valve area produced by percutaneous balloon mitral valvuloplasty.[14] Multiple stepwise logistic regression analysis demonstrated that suboptimal results with percutaneous balloon mitral valvuloplasty are more likely to occur in patients with valves more rigid and thickened and in those with more subvalvular fibrosis and calcification.[11] The increase in mitral valve area with percutaneous balloon mitral valvuloplasty is inversely related to the echocardiographic score (Fig. 9.4). The best outcomes with balloon mitral valvuloplasty occur in those patients with echocardiographic scores ≤ 8 (91% of good results). The increase in mitral valve area is significantly greater in patients with echocardiographic scores ≤ 8 than in those with echocardiographic score > 8 (p < .01).

The increase in mitral valve area with percutaneous balloon mitral valvuloplasty is directly related to **balloon size.** The effect of balloon size was first evaluated in a subgroup of patients who underwent repeat balloon valvuloplasty.[15] They had initially undergone balloon mitral valvuloplasty with a single balloon catheter resulting in a mean mitral valve area of 1.2 ± 0.2 cm². They underwent repeat balloon valvuloplasty using the double-balloon catheter technique, which increased the effective balloon dilating area (EBDA) normalized by body surface area (EBDA/BSA) from 3.41 ± 0.2 to 4.51 ± 0.2 cm²/m². The mean mitral valve area in this group after repeat balloon valvuloplasty was 1.8 cm² ± 0.2 cm². As can be seen in Table 9.4, the increase in mitral valve area in 405 patients who underwent balloon valvuloplasty using the double-balloon catheter technique (EBDA of 6.4 ± 0.03 cm²) was significantly greater

Table 9.4 IMPACT OF THE EFFECTIVE BALLOON DILATING AREA (EBDA) ON IMMEDIATE OUTCOME

	Mitral Valve Area, cm^2	
	Pre-PBMV	Post-PBMV
Single balloon (EBDA = 4.4 ± 0.2 cm^2) (n = 27)	0.7 ± 0.1	1.4 ± 0.1
Double balloon (EBDA = 6.4 ± 0.03 cm^2) (n = 405)	0.9 ± 0.1	2.0 ± 0.1[a]

[a] $p < 0.0001$. (post-PBMV).

PBMV — percutaneous balloon mitral valvuloplasty.

than the increase in mitral valve area achieved in 27 patients who underwent balloon valvuloplasty using the single-balloon catheter technique (EBDA of 4.4 ± 0.02 cm^2): 2.0 ± 0.1 cm^2 vs. 1.4 ± 0.1 cm^2 ($p < 0.0001$).

Care should be taken in the selection of dilating balloon catheters so as to obtain an adequate final mitral valve area and no change or a minimal increase in mitral regurgitation. We have demonstrated that the ratio of the effective balloon dilating area to body surface area (EBDA/BSA) is the only predictor of increased mitral regurgitation after percutaneous balloon mitral valvuloplasty.[16] The EBDA is calculated using standard geometric formulas (Fig. 9.5). The incidence of mitral regurgitation is lower if balloon sizes are chosen so that EBDA/BSA is ≤4.0 cm^2/m^2. The single-balloon catheter technique results in a lower incidence of mitral regurgitation but provides less relief of mitral stenosis than the double-balloon catheter technique. Thus, there is an optimal balloon size between 3.1 and 4.0 cm^2/m^2 which achieves a maximal mitral valve area with a minimal increase in mitral regurgitation.

The immediate outcome of patients undergoing percutaneous balloon mitral valvuloplasty is also related to the **severity of valvular calcification seen by fluoroscopy.** Patients without fluoroscopic evidence of calcification have a greater increase in mitral valve area after balloon valvuloplasty than patients with calcified valves. Patients with either no or 1 + fluoroscopic calcification have a greater increase in mitral valve area after balloon valvuloplasty than those patients with 2 +, 3 +, or 4 + calcification (Fig. 9.6).

The increase in mitral valve area with percutaneous balloon mitral valvuloplasty is inversely related to the presence of **atrial fibrillation** (Table 9.5); the post-balloon valvuloplasty mitral valve area of 217 patients in normal sinus rhythm was 2.2 ± 0.1 cm^2 as compared with a valve area of 1.8 ± 0.1 cm^2 of 215 patients in atrial fibrillation ($p < 0.001$).

Although the increase in mitral valve area following balloon dilation is inversely related to the presence of **previous surgical mitral commissurotomy** (Table 9.6), percutaneous balloon mitral valvuloplasty can produce a good outcome in this group of patients.[17] The mean mitral valve area in 85 patients with previous surgical commissurotomy was 1.8 ± 0.1 cm^2 compared with a valve area of 2.0 ± 0.1 cm^2 in patients without previous surgical commissurotomy ($p < 0.01$). In this group of pa-

Effective Balloon Dilating Area
(cm^2)

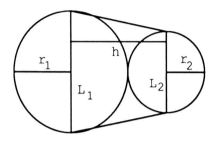

$$EBDA = h \left(\frac{L_1 + L_2}{2} \right) + \frac{\pi (r_1^2 + r_2^2)}{2}$$

EFFECTIVE BALLOON DILATING AREA
(cm2)

	0	15	18	20
15	1.77	4.02	4.89	5.55
18	2.54	4.89	5.78	6.46
20	3.14	5.55	6.46	7.14
23	4.15	6.57	7.55	8.27
25	4.91	7.46	8.41	9.11

Figure 9.5 Normogram used to calculate the effective balloon dilating area (EBDA) of any two balloon size combinations (*top*) and diagramatic representation of the effective balloon dilating area (EBDA) for any two-balloon combination (*bottom*). (From: Roth RB et al: Predictors of increased mitral regurgitation after percutaneous mitral balloon valvotomy. *Cathet Cardiovasc Diagn.* 20:17–21 1990. With permission.)

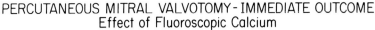

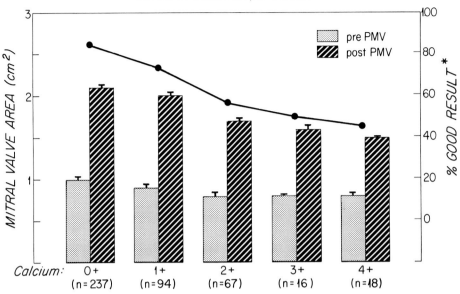

PERCUTANEOUS MITRAL VALVOTOMY - IMMEDIATE OUTCOME
Effect of Fluoroscopic Calcium

Figure 9.6 Relationship between the degree of calcification identified under fluoroscopy (*x* axis), the increase in mitral valve area (**MVA**) produced by percutaneous mitral valvuloplasty (**PMV**) (*left* axis), and the percentage of patients having a good result (post-PMV MVA $\geq$ 1.5 cm^2) (right axis).

Table 9.5   EFFECT OF THE PRESENCE OF ATRIAL FIBRILLATION ON IMMEDIATE OUTCOME

	Mitral Valve Area, cm^2	
	Pre-PBMV	Post-PBMV
Normal sinus rhythm (n = 217)	1.0 ± 0.1	2.2 ± 0.1
Atrial fibrillation (n = 215)	0.9 ± 0.1	1.8 ± 0.1[a]

[a] $p < 0.001$. (post-PBMV)

PBMV — percutaneous balloon mitral valvuloplasty.

tients an echocardiographic score ≤ 8 was again the most important predictor of a good immediate outcome.[17]

The immediate outcome of percutaneous balloon mitral valvuloplasty is also directly related to the **age** of the patients. Elderly patients more frequently have atrial fibrillation, calcified valves, and higher echocardiographic scores. Table 9.7 shows the relationship between the age of the patients and the increase in mitral valve area produced by percutaneous balloon mitral valvuloplasty as well as the percentage of patients obtaining a good result with this procedure. A successful outcome from

Table 9.6 EFFECT OF PREVIOUS SURGICAL COMMISSUROTOMY ON IMMEDIATE OUTCOME

	Mitral Valve Area, cm²	
	Pre-PBMV	Post-PBMV
Previous surgical commissurotomy (n = 85)	0.9 ± 0.1	1.8 ± 0.1
No previous surgical commissurotomy (n = 347)	0.9 ± 0.1	2.0 ± 0.1[a]

[a] p < 0.01. (post-PBMV)

PBMV — percutaneous balloon mitral valvuloplasty.

Table 9.7 EFFECT OF AGE ON IMMEDIATE OUTCOME

Age, yr	n	Calcification, %	Atrial Fibrillation, %	Echo Score >8, %	Mitral Valve Area		Good[a], %
					Pre-PBMV	Post-PBMV	
≤30	29	24	0	3	0.8 ± 0.1	2.3 ± 0.1	97
31–40	44	14	16	11	0.9 ± 0.1	2.2 ± 0.1	84
41–50	60	28	32	12	1.0 ± 0.1	2.2 ± 0.1	90
51–60	70	53	59	39	0.9 ± 0.1	2.0 ± 0.1	84
61–70	73	63	77	51	0.9 ± 0.1	1.7 ± 0.1	63
71–80	35	77	71	71	0.9 ± 0.1	1.8 ± 0.1	60
>80	9	100	67	89	0.6 ± 0.1	1.5 ± 0.1	33

[a] Good: post-PBMV MVA ≥ 1.5 cm².

PBMV — percutaneous balloon mitral valvuloplasty

MVA — mitral valve area

balloon mitral valvuloplasty (defined as post-balloon valvuloplasty mitral valve area ≥ 1.5 cm², < 2 grade increase in mitral regurgitation, and ≤ 1.5:1 left- to-right shunting through the iatrogenic interatrial communication) was obtained in less than 50% of patients ≥ 65 years old.[18] The percentage of patients obtaining a good result with this technique decreases as age increases.

Percutaneous balloon mitral valvuloplasty has been shown to be safe and effective in controlling the symptoms of mitral stenosis in **pregnant women** after the 20th week.[19-21] Patients with low echocardiographic scores can have percutaneous balloon mitral valvuloplasty performed quickly with minimal radiation to the fetus.[22] The risks of anesthesia and heart surgery for the mother and the fetus can thus be avoided. Of course, the ideal situation would be to perform balloon mitral valvuloplasty in these young women with hemodynamically significant mitral stenosis before they become pregnant.

The presence and severity of **mitral regurgitation before percutaneous balloon mitral valvuloplasty** is an independent predictor of unfavorable outcome. As can be seen in Table 9.8, the increase in mitral valve area after the procedure is inversely related to the severity of mitral regurgitation determined by angiography before the procedure. This negative relationship between the presence of mitral regurgitation and immediate outcome occurs because patients with mitral regurgitation are more

**Table 9.8 IMPACT OF THE PRESENCE AND SEVERITY OF
MITRAL REGURGITATION ON IMMEDIATE
OUTCOME**

Mitral Regurgitation	Mitral Valve Area, cm^2	
	Pre-PBMV	Post-PBMV
Zero (n = 260)	1.0 ± 0.1	2.1 ± 0.1
Grade one (n = 131)	0.9 ± 0.1	1.8 ± 0.1
Grade two (n = 20)	0.9 ± 0.1	1.6 ± 0.1

PBMV = percutaneous balloon mitral valvuloplasty.

frequently older and more frequently have atrial fibrillation, a higher echocardiographic score, and evidence of mitral valve calcification under fluoroscopy.

COMPLICATIONS

Mortality and morbidity with percutaneous balloon mitral valvuloplasty is low and similar to those seen in surgical commissurotomy. In the series from the Massachusetts General Hospital there was a 0.7% mortality. No death has occurred in the last 300 patients undergoing this procedure. There was a 1.1% incidence of thromboembolic episodes and stroke. Severe mitral regurgitation (4+) occurred in 2% of the patients. Four of these patients required in-hospital mitral valve replacement. Transient heart block (< 24 h duration) occurred in 0.4% of the patients. Pericardial tamponade occurred in six patients (1.3%) in this series: from ventricular perforation in two patients and from transseptal catheterization in the other four. Percutaneous balloon mitral valvuloplasty was associated with a 16% incidence of left-to-right atrial shunt immediately after the procedure. The pulmonary to systemic flow ratio was ≥ 2:1 in 9 patients.

We have demonstrated that severe mitral regurgitation (4+) occurred in about 2% of patients undergoing percutaneous balloon mitral valvuloplasty. An undesirable increase in mitral regurgitation (≥ 2+) occurred in 12.5% of patients. Most patients tolerated it well. More than half have less mitral regurgitation at followup cardiac catheterization. The single-balloon catheter technique is associated with less incidence of increased mitral regurgitation but affords less relief of mitral stenosis than the double-balloon catheter technique. The effective balloon dilating area is the only predictor of increased mitral regurgitation with percutaneous balloon mitral valvuloplasty (p < .02). A balloon combination should be chosen so that EBDA/BSA is < 4.0 cm^2/m^2.

Left-to-right shunting through the created atrial communication occurred in 20% of the patients undergoing percutaneous balloon mitral valvuloplasty. The size of the defect is small, as reflected in a pulmonary to systemic flow ratio of < 2:1 in the majority of patients. Older age, fluoroscopic evidence of mitral valve calcification, a higher echocardiographic score, lower pre-prodecure cardiac output, and higher NYHA class are the factors that predispose patients to developing a left-to-right shunt post-balloon mitral valvuloplasty.[19] Clinical, echocardiographic, surgical, and hemodynamic followup of patients with post-balloon valvuloplasty left-to-right shunt demonstrated that the defect closed in 59%. Persistent left-to-right shunt at followup is small (QP/QS < 2:1) and clinically well tolerated. From the series from the Massachusetts General Hospital there was one patient in whom the shunt remained significant at followup with evidence of hemodynamic compromise. This patient's atrial defect was closed with a clamshell device placed percutaneously using transcatheter technique.

FOLLOWUP

At the Massachusetts General Hospital 320 patients were followed for 20 ± 1 (range 0–49) months after percutaneous balloon mitral valvuloplasty. Endpoints of followup were death, mitral valve replacement, and clinical evaluation in accordance with the New York Heart Association functional classification.[20] The survivorship of patients at 1, 2, 3, and 4 years after percutaneous balloon mitral valvuloplasty was 96%, 94%, 91%, and 92% respectively. The predictors of death at followup were higher echocardiographic score, a calcified mitral valve under fluoroscopy, and a smaller EBDA employed during balloon mitral valvuloplasty.

At 4-year followup, 87% of the patients had not required mitral valve replacement. Patients more likely to require mitral valve replacement at followup are those with post-balloon valvuloplasty mitral regurgitation or a larger post-balloon valvuloplasty mitral gradient, those in atrial fibrillation, and those with a history of surgical mitral commissurotomy.

Of the surviving patients, 83% were NYHA classes I or II and without reintervention at 4-year followup. Patients with a higher left atrial pressure and a larger residual mitral gradient post-balloon valvuloplasty are more likely to be symptomatic (NYHA class III or IV) at followup.

Sixty-seven percent of the patients were free of all events (death, mitral valve replacement, and NYHA classes III or IV) at 4 years. Predictors of unfavorable long-term outcome were calcified mitral valve as seen by fluoroscopy, higher pre-balloon valvuloplasty NYHA class, smaller change in mitral gradient with balloon valvuloplasty, presence of atrial fibrillation, lower pre-balloon valvuloplasty cardiac output, and smaller EBDA and post-balloon valvuloplasty mitral valve area.

Patients with echocardiographic scores ≤ 8 have a significantly greater survival and freedom from events (death, mitral valve replacement, and NYHA class III or IV) than those patients with echocardiographic scores > 8. Patients with echocardiographic scores ≤ 8 have a 99% 4-year survival. At 4-year followup 93% of them had not required mitral valve replacement; 87% of the surviving patients were NYHA classes I or II; and 80% of the patients were free of events (death, mitral valve replacement, and NYHA classes III or IV). In contrast, patients with echocardiographic scores > 8 have a 75% 4-year survival. At 4-year followup 78% of them were free of mitral valve replacement; 69% of the surviving patients were NYHA classes I or II and only 40% were free of events. In addition, in patients with echocardiographic scores > 8, restenosis (loss $\geq 50\%$ of the gain in mitral valve area produced by balloon valvuloplasty) is frequently demonstrated by followup cardiac catheterization (70%) and two-dimensional echocardiography (25%).[6,21]

Survival after percutaneous balloon mitral valvuloplasty is similar to that reported after surgical mitral commissurotomy. Freedom from mitral valve replacement and freedom from all events are lower than those reported after surgical commissurotomy. However, freedom from both mitral valve replacement and all events in patients with echocardiographic scores ≤ 8 is similar to that reported after surgical mitral commissurotomy.

CONCLUSIONS

Percutaneous balloon mitral valvuloplasty results in a good clinical and hemodynamic outcome in most patients with mitral stenosis. Morbidity and mortality with percutaneous balloon mitral valvuloplasty are low and similar to that of surgical mitral commissurotomy. Younger patients with low echocardiographic scores, particularly those ≤ 8, are the best candidates for percutaneous balloon mitral valvuloplasty; 93% of them have a good immediate result from balloon valvuloplasty and their followup shows ongoing clinical, hemodynamic, and echocardiographic stability. Patients with higher echocardiographic scores have only a 50% chance of obtaining a good result with percutaneous balloon mitral valvuloplasty. In these patients restenosis can frequently be demonstrated at followup by cardiac catheterization or two-dimensional echocardiography. In patients with echocardiographic scores ≥ 12 it is unlikely that percutaneous balloon mitral valvuloplasty could produce a good immediate or long-term result. They preferably should undergo open heart surgery. However, percutaneous balloon mitral valvuloplasty could be performed in these patients if they are high-risk surgical candidates.

REFERENCES

1. Inoue K, Owaki T, Nakamura T, et al: Clinical application of transvenous mitral commissurotomy by a new balloon catheter. *J Thorac Cardiovasc Surg.* 87:394–402, 1984.
2. Lock JE, Kalilullah M, Shrivastava S, et al: Percutaneous catheter commissurotomy in rheumatic mitral stenosis. *N Engl J Med.* 313:1515–1518, 1985.
3. Palacios I, Block PC, Brandi S, et al: Percutaneous balloon valvotomy for patients with severe mitral stenosis. *Circulation.* 75:778–784, 1987.
4. Zaibag MA, Ribeiro PA, Al Kasab SA, et al: Percutaneous double-balloon mitral valvotomy for rheumatic mitral-valve stenosis. *Lancet.* 1:757–761, 1986.
5. Vahanian A, Michel PL, Cormier B, et al: Results of percutaneous mitral commissurotomy in 200 patients. *Am J Cardiol.* 63:847–852, 1989.
6. Palacios IF, Block PC, Wilkins GT, et al: Follow-up of patients undergoing percutaneous mitral balloon valvotomy. Analysis of factors determining restenosis. *Circulation.* 79:573–579, 1989.
7. McKay RG, Lock JE, Safian RD, et al: Balloon dilation of mitral stenosis in adult patients: postmortem and percutaneous mitral valvuloplasty studies. *J Am Coll Cardiol.* 9:723–731, 1987.
8. McKay CR, Kawanishi DT, Rahimtoola SH: Catheter balloon valvuloplasty of the mitral valve in adults using a double-balloon technique. Early hemodynamic results. *JAMA.* 257:1753–1761, 1987.
9. Babic UU, Pejcic P, Djurisic Z, et al: Percutaneous transarterial balloon valvuloplasty for mitral valve stenosis. *Am J Cardiol.* 57:1101–1104, 1986.

10. Block PC, Palacios IF, Jacobs M, et al: Mechanism of percutaneous mitral valvotomy. *Am J Cardiol.* 59:178–179, 1987.

11. Wilkins GT, Weyman AE, Abascal VM, et al: Percutaneous balloon dilatation of the mitral valve: an analysis of echocardiographic variables related to outcome and the mechanism of dilatation. *Br Heart J.* 60:299–308, 1988.

12. Block PC, Palacios IF: Pulmonary vascular dynamics after percutaneous mitral valvotomy. *J Thorac Cardiovasc Surg.* 96:39–43, 1988.

13. Abascal VM, Wilkins GT, Choong CY, et al: Mitral regurgitation after percutaneous balloon mitral valvuloplasty in adults: evaluation by pulsed Doppler echocardiography. *J Am Coll Cardiol.* 11:257–263, 1988.

14. Abascal VM, Wilkins GT, O'Shea JP, et al: Prediction of successful outcome in 130 patients undergoing percutaneous balloon mitral valvotomy. *Circulation.* 82:448–456, 1990.

15. Herrmann HC, Wilkins GT, Abascal VM, et al: Percutaneous balloon mitral valvotomy for patients with mitral stenosis: analysis of factors influencing early results. *J Thorac Cardiovasc Surg.* 96:33–38, 1988.

16. Roth RB, Block PC, Palacios IF: Predictors of increased mitral regurgitation after percutaneous mitral balloon valvotomy. *Cathet Cardiovasc Diagn.* 20:17–21, 1990.

17. Rediker DE, Block PC, Abascal VM, et al: Mitral balloon valvuloplasty for mitral restenosis after surgical commissurotomy. *J Am Coll Cardiol.* 11:252–256, 1988.

18. Tuzcu EM, Block PC, Griffen BP, et al: Immediate and long term outcome of percutaneous mitral valvotomy in patients 65 years and older. *Circulation.* 1992 (in press).

19. Safian RD, Berman AD, Sachs B, et al: Percutaneous balloon mitral valvuloplasty in a pregnant woman with mitral stenosis. *Cathet Cardiovasc Diagn.* 15:103–108, 1988.

20. Palacios IF, Block PC, Wilkins GT, et al: Percutaneous mitral balloon valvotomy during pregnancy in a patient with severe mitral stenosis. *Cathet Cardiovasc Diagn.* 15:109–111, 1988.

21. Mangione JA, Zuliani MF, Del Castillo JM, et al: Percutaneous double balloon mitral valvuloplasty in pregnant women. *Am J Cardiol.* 64:99–102, 1989.

22. Block PC, Tuzcu EM, Palacios IF: Percutaneous mitral balloon valvotomy. *Cardiol Clin* 9:271–287, 1991.

23. Casale P, Block PC, O'Shea JP, et al: Atrial septal defect after percutaneous mitral balloon valvuloplasty: immediate results and follow-up. *J Am Coll Cardiol.* 15:1300–1304, 1990.

24. Palacios IF, Tuzcu EM, Newell JB, et al: Four year clinical follow-up of patients undergoing percutaneous mitral balloon valvotomy. *Circulation.* 82(suppl III):III-545, 1990.

25. Abascal VM, Wilkins GT, Choong CY, et al: Echocardiographic evaluation of mitral valve structure and function in patients followed for at least 6 months after percutaneous balloon mitral valvuloplasty. *J Am Coll Cardiol.* 12:606–615, 1988.

CHAPTER **10**

Mitral Stenosis: Inoue Balloon Catheter Technique

KANJI INOUE
JUI-SUNG HUNG
CHUAN-RONG CHEN
TSUNG O. CHENG

In 1984, a novel nonsurgical mitral commissurotomy technique using a size-adjustable, self-positioning balloon catheter was introduced by Inoue and associates[1] as a promising therapeutic alternative to surgical treatment of patients with severe mitral stenosis. The fused mitral commissures are split with a balloon catheter inserted percutaneously via the femoral vein after transseptal catheterization, and the method was therefore termed percutaneous transvenous mitral commisssurotomy (PTMC). Extensive clinical experience in the Far East have established the effectiveness and safety of the procedure in well selected patients.[2-17] The PTMC—percutaneous balloon mitral valvuloplasty using the Inoue balloon catheter—has flourished beyond the region and has been adopted in North America,[18-21] Europe,[22,23] and South Africa.[24] It is estimated that the procedure has been performed in more than 15,000 patients worldwide. Since a state-of-art review of the procedure a few years ago,[7] its long-term results have begun to unfold, technical refinements have developed, and case selection and countermeasures against complications have evolved. This chapter incorporates recent developments regarding PTMC and presents a comprehensive review of the procedure.

INSTRUMENTATION

The Inoue balloon catheter system consists of a balloon catheter and its accessories (Fig. 10.1). Before performing the PTMC procedure, the surgeon and assistants should thoroughly familiarize themselves with the structure and function of this system.

Inoue Balloon Catheter

The coaxial, double-lumen catheter has a 12F polyvinyl chloride tube shaft (Figs. 10.1*A* and 10.2). As shown in Figure 10.3, the inner lumen of the catheter (*a*) permits pressure measurements, blood sampling, or insertion of a metal tube, a guidewire, or

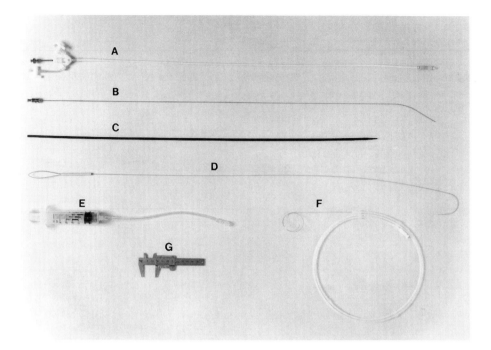

Figure 10.1 Inoue balloon catheter and its auxiliary instruments (see text for discussions).

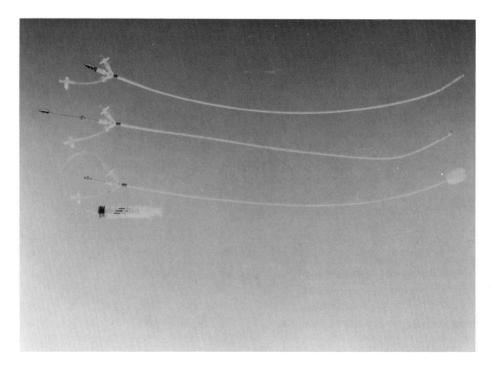

Figure 10.2 Profile of the Inoue balloon catheter.

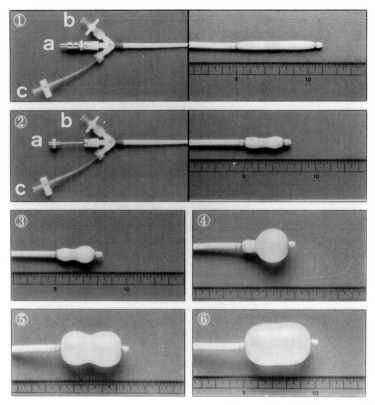

Figure 10.3 Versatility of the Inoue balloon catheter. The balloon can be transformed to various forms to serve different functions.

a stylet. The outer lumen connects proximally with a two-way stopcock (*b*), used to connect the catheter to an inflation/deflation syringe and a vent (*c*), and distally with a balloon mounted at the end of the shaft. The balloon is made of double layers of latex tubing and one layer of nylon micromesh between the latex layers. There are four types of balloon catheter, each designated by a symbol followed by its maximally inflatable balloon diameter (in mm): PTMC-30, PTMC-28, PTMC-26, and PTMC-24. The second-generation catheter balloons now in use (manufactured after September 1989) are less compliant and thus more pressure resistant than the first-generation ones. The pressure-volume curves of the present catheter balloons are shown in Figure 10.4.

The balloon (Fig. 10.3) can be transformed to various shapes from its natural form (②) to serve different functions. The balloon section is stiffened and slenderized when the latex balloon is stretched (①) by inserting a metal tube, as will be described later. The slenderized balloon allows a smooth entry of the balloon catheter into the femoral vein without the use of an introducer set. It also permits an easy passage of the catheter across the atrial septum after the septum has been dilated with a dilator. The synthetic mesh of the balloon is wound in such a way that the balloon changes its shape in three stages, depending on the extent of inflation. Initially, only the distal half inflates (③ and ④); then the proximal half inflates (⑤), with a constriction remaining in the middle. Finally, at full inflation, the constriction disappears (⑥) and

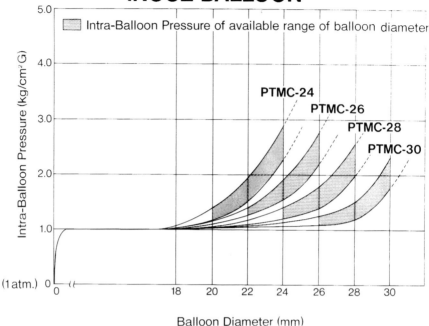

Figure 10.4 Intra-balloon pressure of Inoue balloon catheters. (Reproduced by kind permission of Toray Industries, Inc.)

the balloon assumes a more barrel-like shape with a maximal length of 45 mm. The entire inflation/deflation cycle takes about 5 seconds.

Auxiliary Instruments (Fig. 10.1)

1. An 80-cm *18-gauge metal tube* (Fig. 10.1*B*): The tube is inserted to lock with the inner lumen tube, thereby stiffening the catheter tip. The catheter tip is slenderized further by pushing the metal hub of the inner tube to a locked position (Fig. 10.1*B*). In this way, the balloon segment is stretched and made slender (diameter of 4.5 mm and length of 60 mm).

2. A 70-cm **14F** *polyethylene dilator* (Fig. 10.1*C*): The dilator has a tapering tip. It is used to dilate the puncture openings of the atrial septum and the femoral vein at the same time.

3. An 80-cm 0.038-inch high-torque *J-tipped spring wire stylet* (Fig. 10.1*D*): The stylet has a preformed J-shaped tip with a waist length of about 4.5 cm. It is inserted into the balloon catheter after its entry in the left atrium to provide the catheter with excellent steerability. Axial movement of the catheter is achieved by 1:1 torque control of the stylet. When the stylet is withdrawn from the catheter, the catheter tip advances forward, and vice versa.

4. An 180-cm **0.025-inch** *stainless steel guidewire* with coiled floppy tip (Fig.

10.1*F*): The guidewire is inserted through the transseptal catheter to the left atrium to guide the balloon catheter to the left atrium.

5. A **30-mL** *plastic syringe and a connecting tube* (Fig. 10.1*E*): The extent of balloon inflation is controlled by adjusting the volume of diluted contrast material in the syringe, which is injected manually into the catheter through a two-way stopcock (*b* in Fig. 10.3).

6. A *ruler* (Fig. 10.1*G*): The ruler is used to measure the diameter of inflated balloons in pretestings before insertion of the catheter into the patient.

PREOPERATIVE AND POSTOPERATIVE MANAGEMENT

Preoperative Evaluation

Candidates for PTMC should be carefully evaluated by history taking, physical examination, and laboratory tests including electrocardiography, chest x-rays, and echocardiography. Two-dimensional echocardiography is essential to evaluate the mitral valve morphologies and the presence or absence of left atrial thrombus. Color Doppler examination, when available, is helpful in assessing the degree of mitral regurgitation. However, exclusion of patients from PTMC is usually based on angiographic findings of $> 2 +$ mitral regurgitation.

Medications

1. **Antiarrhythmic drugs**: Drugs such as digitalis and beta-adrenergic blockers are maintained to control ventricular rates in patients with atrial fibrillation. These drugs are also given to patients in sinus rhythm to prevent rapid ventricular rates during paroxysmal atrial fibrillation, which infrequently occurs during PTMC.

2. **Premedication**: A mild sedative such as diazepam is used as in ordinary cardiac catheterization.

3. **Warfarin**: Patients with atrial fibrillation are treated with warfarin for at least 4 weeks before the procedure. Warfarin pretreatment is usually not necessary in patients with sinus rhythm. Patients with a history of systemic embolism are treated with warfarin for at least 6 weeks. Sudden discontinuation of warfarin may cause a rebound phenomenon with formation of new thrombus. Therefore, one of the authors (KI) maintains warfarin treatment before the procedure.

4. **Heparin during PTMC**: The total dose of heparin given by Inoue is 100 U/Kg body weight in patients maintained on warfarin and 150 U/Kg body weight in patients not receiving warfarin. Half of the dose is given at the beginning of cardiac catheterization. To reduce the risk of cardiac tamponade in case the needle or catheter erroneously perforates the heart, the other half is reserved until confirmation of successful atrial septal puncture. In aged patients (over 75 years) or patients with reduced clotting function due to complications such as hepatic dysfunction, the warfarin and heparin doses need to be reduced to avoid serious hemorrhagic tendencies from their combined use. Hemostasis at the groin puncture sites is usually achieved by manual compression. If necessary, protamine can be given to facilitate the hemostasis.

Postoperative Management

Patients are kept in bed rest after the procedure as in ordinary cardiac catheterization. They are allowed to ambulate several hours after complete hemostasis in the groin is ensured. When cardiac tamponade is suspected, echocardiography should be performed immediately. Otherwise, it is performed electively to evaluate the results of PTMC. The patients are usually discharged from the hospital in 2 to 3 days to resume their usual work. In patients with atrial fibrillation, digitalis or a beta-adrenergic blocker is maintained to control the ventricular rate. In patients with suboptimal results from PTMC, diuretics are continued. Warfarin treatment is maintained in patients with atrial fibrillation.

ATRIAL SEPTAL PUNCTURE

Transseptal catheterization is a prerequisite to the introduction of guidewires and balloon catheters into the left atrium. Two major problems in atrial septal puncture are cardiac perforation and an inappropriate atrial puncture site. The former may lead to the serious complication of cardiac tamponade, and the latter to a difficulty in inserting the Inoue balloon catheter across the mitral orifice. Therefore, a well-executed transseptal catheterization is the key to a successful PTMC. Atrial septal puncture not only has to be made safely but also at an optimal site.

In the standard transseptal technique, the site for puncture is the fossa ovalis of the atrial septum. Under fluoroscopy, a needle-fitted transseptal catheter is moved in a downward direction from the superior vena cava and to detect the subtle movement of the catheter tip when it enters the fossa ovalis.[25-27] However, in cases of mitral stenosis, the movement of the needle tip is often difficult to detect because the bulging of the atrial septum toward the right atrium makes the fossa ovalis more shallow. Based on a review of personal experience, Inoue has made a modification to the standard transseptal technique. Applied in many cases, the modified method with the aid of right atrial angiography ensures safe and optimal atrial transseptal puncture. This method is particularly useful for those who are less than maximally proficient in transseptal catheterization. It is also very helpful in cases in which atrial septal puncture is difficult, such as in patients with a large left atrium.

Landmarks for Atrial Septal Puncture

Right atrial angiography is performed under normal respiration until the aorta is visualized (Fig. 10.5). The position of the upper end of the tricuspid valve at systole on a stopped-frame frontal right atrial image is regarded as point A. The point is translated to the left atrial stopped-frame image. On the latter image, a horizontal line is drawn from point A, and the point where it intersects with the right lateral edge of the left atrium is regarded as point B. A vertical line is drawn at the midpoint between A and B, and its intersection with the caudal edge of the left atrium is regarded as point C. The puncture site is determined on this vertical line at a point about one vertebral body height above point C. This position is then translated to an equivalent point in relation to the fluoroscopic image of the vertebral bodies for performing the atrial septal puncture. After right atrial angiography, one should keep the fluoroscopic device stand unmoved because the positional relationship between the vertebral body

A

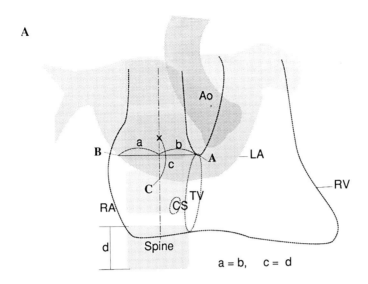

B Giant LA

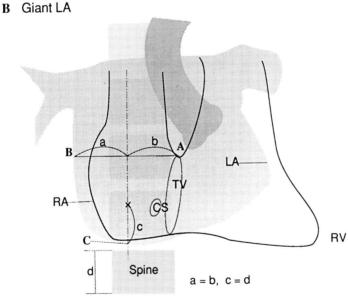

Figure 10.5 Schematic illustration showing choosing of a landmark for atrial septal puncture from frontal-plane right atrial angiography: A, in moderately enlarged left atrium and B, in giant left atrium. A horizontal line from the upper end of the tricuspid valve at systole (point A) intersects the right border of the left atrium at point B. A vertical line from the mid point of line AB intersects the lower border of the left atrium at point C. A puncture point (X) is chosen on the vertical line about a vertebral body height (d) cephalad to point C. *Ao:* aorta, *LA:* left atrium, *RA:* right atrium, *RV:* right ventricle, *TV:* tricuspid valve, *CS:* coronary sinus.

and cardiac shadow on the fluoroscopic image may be shifted by changes in the angle of irradiation.

The above means of targeting the puncture site is also applicable to cases of large left atrium (Fig. 10.5B). In such cases, the site for puncture is closer to the lower part of the cardiac shadow. In cases of giant left atrium the center of the atrial septum projects markedly toward the right atrium (Fig. 10.6); hence, it is difficult to place the puncture close to the center of the septum (Fig. 10.6, 2). Even when puncture can be done at the center of the atrial septum in such cases, subsequent insertion of a balloon catheter into the mitral orifice is difficult, because the tip of the balloon catheter tends to be directed toward the posterior wall of the left atrium (Fig. 10.6, 4). Therefore, if such cases are encountered clinically, it is better to make a second puncture in an area of the designated point that is lower than the first puncture attempt. When a biplane device is available, the lateral view assists in spatial orientation of the catheter tip direction. In extremely difficult cases, it may be necessary to perform biplane right angiography to delineate atrial septal orientation and relative anatomic relationships among the right atrium, the left atrium, the tricuspid valve, and the aorta, thus facilitating safe and accurate puncture of the septum.

Procedure of Atrial Septal Puncture

The puncture is performed using a 7F Mullins transseptal catheter (with or without its sheath) and a Brockenbrough needle. Use of the sheath is recommended for inexperienced operators to prevent inadvertent perforation of the catheter during insertion of the needle. Under local anesthesia, a J-shaped 0.032-inch guidewire is inserted via the right femoral vein into the superior vena cava. The transseptal catheter is inserted over the guidewire into the cava and the guidewire is removed. Then, the transseptal needle is inserted into the catheter and carefully advanced under fluoroscopic view. The operator should place the right index finger on the needle in front of the direction indicator as a stop. The needle is advanced until its tip is slightly (2 to 3 mm) proximal to the tip of the catheter. Extreme care should be taken not to let the needle slip further. The stop-finger is firmly kept between the catheter hub and the direction indicator of the needle to keep the needle from protruding from the catheter tip. A catheter/needle fitting exercise is recommended before insertion of the catheter/needle into the patient.

To direct the needle tip perpendicular to the atrial septum, the direction indicator is rotated clockwise so that the direction arrow points leftward and posteriorly. The arrow direction varies according to left atrial size. In general, it is in 4 o'clock direction in a relatively small left atrium (<4 cm), between 4 and 5 o'clock direction in the usual-sized left atrium, and in 6 o'clock direction in a large left atrium (>5 cm). However, it should be noted that the division lines along small, usual, and large left atrium as determined by M-mode echocardiograms are arbitrary, and the needle direction may vary considerably among patients with similarly sized left atria. If the atrial septum projects sharply toward the right atrium, as in cases of giant left atrium, it is difficult to apply the needle tip perpendicular to the septal surface. More concretely, the needle faces strong resistance at the 4 o'clock direction when the needle tip touches the bulged septal surface. If the needle is rotated farther clockwise despite the resistance, the septal surface will give away suddenly as the needle tip flips toward the right side of the patient with the direction arrow to 9 o'clock. To prevent this from occurring, the needle tip should be maintained at the point of resistance and

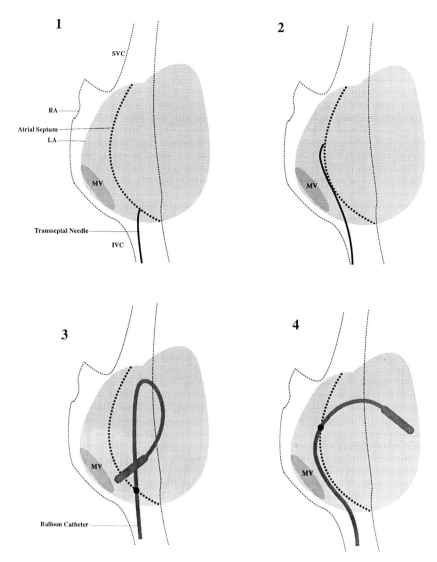

Figure 10.6 Technique of transseptal puncture and balloon insertion in case of giant left atrium in the lateral view. The needle tip is placed at the optimal point (1), and the balloon is easily placed across the mitral valve (3). When the needle tip is placed at a site cephalad to the predesignated target (2), it is difficult to puncture the septum. Even if the puncture is successful, subsequent insertion of the balloon across the mitral valve is quite difficult (4). *SVC:* superior vena cava, *IVC:* inferior vena cava, *RA:* right atrium, *LA:* left atrium, *MV:* mitral valve.

the direction indicator is gently rotated clockwise to maintain its arrow at 6 to 7 o'clock. During the process a slight counterclockwise twist to the transseptal catheter by the left hand will counterbalance excessive clockwise rotation of the needle.

After the needle tip has been applied perpendicular to the septum, the catheter with its concealed needle is pulled downward (caudally) to the target point. In this process, the catheter tip sometimes shows a movement, as if falling into the left side near the target position. This movement indicates that the needle tip has entered the fossa ovalis; this movement occurs more easily if the direction arrow is rotated slightly counterclockwise. However, as stated before, the movement of the needle tip is often difficult to detect in patients with severe mitral stenosis because the atrial septal bulging toward the right atrium makes the fossa ovalis more shallow.

Once the catheter tip is at the target position of the fossa ovalis, the catheter and the concealed needle are pushed slightly forward until a resistance is felt. As the catheter is held firm against the septum, cardiac pulsation is usually felt by the right hand holding the catheter and the needle. The next step is to release the fingerstop and push the needle forward with the right hand, while fixing the catheter firmly against the septum with the left hand to keep it from slipping away from the target site. After blood is aspirated from the needle for oximetry, contrast material is injected into the needle and needle entry to the left atrium is confirmed by opacification of the left atrium. If contrast material stains the atrial septum, the puncture is repeated at another site. If contrast material enters the pericardial cavity, the needle is withdrawn, and contrast material is injected again via the catheter to determine whether the catheter has perforated through the heart into the pericardial cavity. If only the needle has perforated the heart, cardiac tamponade usually does not occur. When the absence of tamponade is confirmed by echocardiography 10 minutes after contrast material injection, atrial septal puncture can be resumed. If the catheter has perforated through the heart, the catheter should be withdrawn only after preparations to cope with cardiac tamponade have been made. In such cases, the procedure is discontinued, and protamine is used to neutralize heparin if the latter has been previously given. Patients with cardiac perforation by the catheter are followed by echocardiography. Usually, catheter perforation causes only pericardial pooling of small amounts of blood, and PTMC can be performed again 2 to 3 days later.

After needle entry to the left atrium is confirmed by contrast material injection, oximetry, and pressure recording, the indicator arrow is set toward 3 o'clock and both the needle and catheter are advanced 2 cm farther into the left atrium. Then, the catheter alone is advanced another 2 cm while the needle is being withdrawn. It is important not to push the catheter carelessly because its sharp tip may perforate the superior wall of the left atrium. Once the catheter is in the left atrium, heparin should be given through the catheter immediately upon removing the needle.

Inappropriate Puncture Sites

High Septum

If the puncture site is markedly deviated in the upper (cephalad) direction from the predetermined target point, the thick muscular wall of the upper edge of the fossa ovalis will be punctured (Fig. 10.7). If this occurs, strong resistance is faced during the passage of the balloon catheter through the muscular wall, and subsequent manipulation of the catheter will be limited. In addition, because the balloon catheter tip tends to point toward the posterior wall of the left atrium, catheter insertion across the more ventrally located mitral orifice is difficult.

Anterior Septum

If the puncture site is unusually deviated to the left of the target point (Fig. 10.8), it is made in the anterior atrial septum. The site is too close to the mitral orifice and the

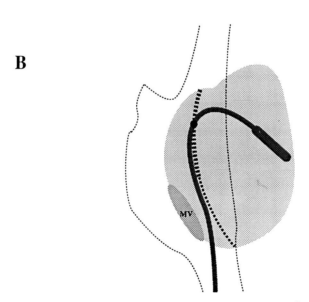

Figure 10.7 PTMC procedure and atrial septal puncture site in the lateral view. **A,** The balloon catheter inserted through the optimal puncture site is easily directed toward the mitral orifice. **B,** The balloon catheter tends to be directed toward the posterior wall of the left atrium when septal puncture site is cephalad to the optimal target. *SVC:* superior vena cava, *IVC:* inferior vena cava, *RA:* right atrium, *LA:* left atrium, *MV:* mitral valve.

A

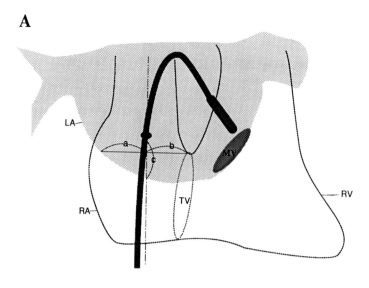

B

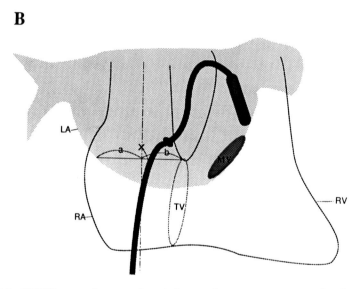

Figure 10.8 PTMC procedure and atrial septal puncture site in the frontal view. **A,** The balloon catheter inserted through the optimal puncture point is easily directed toward the mitral orifice. **B,** When the septal puncture site is deviated leftward from the optimal target, it is difficult to direct the balloon catheter toward the mitral orifice because the balloon catheter curves in steps at the septum. *LA:* left atrium, *RA:* right atrium, *RV:* right ventricle, *TV:* tricuspid valve, *MV:* mitral valve.

catheter curves in steps at the punctured region, resulting in marked restriction of catheter movement and difficulty in advancing the catheter across the mitral orifice.

Sites Associated with Risk of Cardiac Tamponade

Besides the tricuspid valve, the following sites should not be punctured, lest cardiac tamponade may ensue.

Coronary Sinus:
The coronary sinus opens near the lower end of the tricuspid valve. If the catheter tip has entered this sinus, the operator may erroneously assume that the tip has entered the fossa ovalis. Puncture of the coronary sinus leads to obstinate hemorrhage which frequently requires surgical intervention.

Vicinity of the Lateral Edge of the Left Atrial Shadow:
In the region near the right lateral border of the left atrial shadow, there is no atrial septum. If this region is punctured, the needle perforates through the right atrial wall and then through the left atrial wall into the left atrial cavity (the so-called "stitching" phenomenon). If the operator continues the procedure under the assumption that the left atrium has been entered through a normal route, tamponade occurs after withdrawal of the catheter.

Aorta:
When the needle has punctured the aorta, as confirmed by contrast injection or pressure recording, the catheter should not be advanced and the needle should be withdrawn immediately. The result is usually uneventful. Should the catheter be inadvertently advanced into the aorta, it should not be withdrawn. The patient is then sent for emergency surgery with the catheter left in place.

Treatment of Cardiac Tamponade

Although cardiac tamponade is a serious complication, the life of the patient can always be saved without any sequela if tamponade is promptly diagnosed and treated. In this sense, adequate preparations for swift countermeasures are essential. During PTMC, an echocardiographic device should stand ready for diagnosing tamponade. Preparation for rapid pericardial puncture and drainage is also necessary. Tamponade with severe symptoms usually shows a massive pericardial blood pool, thus usually allowing for safe and simple pericardical drainage. If the pooled blood is eliminated by pericardiocentesis, symptoms improve rapidly. By this time, hemorrhage usually ceases. If hemorrhage persists, immediate surgical intervention is required. Neutralization of heparin and warfarin by intravenous protamine and vitamin K, respectively, promotes hemostasis.

PERCUTANEOUS TRANSVENOUS MITRAL COMMISSUROTOMY PROCEDURE

PTMC is usually performed as a one-stage procedure immediately after diagnostic catheterization. Standard right- and left-heart catheterization using a 7F flow-directed thermodilution catheter and a 7F pigtail catheter is performed to confirm the severity of mitral stenosis. Left ventriculograms are performed to exclude those patients with severe mitral regurgitation (3+ and 4+) from the procedure, and also to provide useful landmarks for transseptal puncture and the mitral orifice.

Baseline Hemodynamic Measurements

After atrial septal puncture and placement of the transseptal catheter in the left atrium, baseline hemodynamic measurements are obtained. The mitral valve gradient is measured by simultaneous recordings of the left atrial pressure through the transseptal catheter and left ventricular pressure through a pigtail catheter retrogradely inserted by way of the femoral artery. Cardiac output is determined by the thermodilution technique using a flow-directed thermodilution catheter placed by way of the femoral vein, and the mitral valve area is calculated by the Gorlin formula.

Preparation of the Balloon Catheter

During baseline hemodynamic measurements, the balloon catheter is prepared for its insertion into the patient.

Pretesting of Balloon Size:

Air in the balloon is purged by injecting diluted contrast material (1:3 dilution with 5% dextrose or saline solution) in a 10-mL syringe from the vent port. The inflation/deflation syringe containing diluted contrast material is connected to the injection port for pretesting of balloon sizes. The volume and its corresponding balloon size at full inflation have been tested by the manufacturer and marked on the syringe with red print. However, before insertion of the balloon catheter into the patient, they should be confirmed in a two-step test: first, of the balloon size to be used in the first dilatation procedure, and second, of the maximal diameter of the balloon (eg, 26 mm for PTMC-26 catheter). For the second testing additional volume is supplied to the injection syringe from the reservoir 10-mL syringe attached to the vent port.

Stretching of the Balloon Segment:

After the tests the balloon is deflated by releasing both stopcocks in the injection and the vent ports. The metal cannula is inserted all the way into the balloon catheter and Luer-locked with the inner tube of the balloon catheter. The balloon segment is stretched by pushing the inner tube with the metal tube locked in place until the pin of the inner tube is locked in the slot. The inner tube should not be pushed to stretch the balloon without the metal tube being locked in place. Otherwise, the balloon segment will be bent and damaged.

Guidewire Insertion

The transseptal catheter is carefully pulled back 1 to 2 cm so that its tip does not touch the left atrial wall. A stainless steel guidewire is inserted into the catheter and advanced until its coiled loop touches the superior wall (or roof) of the left atrium. The catheter is then withdrawn entirely for insertion of the dilator.

Dilation of the Catheter Entry Site and the Atrial Septum

A dilator is inserted over the guidewire to dilate the groin entry site and the puncture in the femoral vein. It is advanced until its tip is near the roof of the left atrium to dilate the atrial septal puncture site. The dilator is then removed.

Insertion of Balloon Catheter Into the Femoral Vein

The prepared balloon catheter with its balloon segment stretched is inserted into the femoral vein over the guidewire. Usually the insertion is smooth (Fig. 10.9*A, 1*). However, because the entering catheter tip is thicker than the guidewire, a resistance is occasionally encountered by the catheter tip at the venous wall (Fig. 10.9*A, 2*). To solve this problem, the balloon catheter is inserted into the vein at an angle of about 90° (Fig. 10.9*B, 1*). The catheter tip enters the vein and touches its posterior wall (Fig. 10.9*B, 2*). Then, the catheter is tilted more horizontally and is advanced along the vein (Fig. 10.9*B, 3*). If insertion of the catheter is not feasible by this method, a 14F sheath is used.

Insertion of Balloon Catheter Into the Left Atrium (Fig. 10.10)

Passage of the Catheter Tip Across the Atrial Septum (Fig. 10.10A, 1):
The balloon catheter is advanced over the guide until a slight resistance is met at the atrial septum. Usually the catheter tip passes across the septum easily. If its passage is difficult, a slight twist to the catheter (usually clockwise) will facilitate its passage. After its passage across the atrial septum, the catheter is further advanced until its tip approaches the roof of the left atrium, leaving part of the balloon's proximal portion within the right atrium. In cases of large left atrium, however, there is enough room for the entire balloon segment to be placed in the left atrium. It is important to avoid pushing the catheter tip against the roof of the left atrium because the guidewire could be bent into an acute angle, making subsequent manipulation of the catheter system difficult (Fig. 10.10*B*).

Placement of the Entire Balloon Segment in the Left Atrium:
When the balloon tip is advanced near the roof of the left atrium, the metal tube is released and withdrawn for 2 to 3 cm from the inner tube (Fig. 10.10*A, 2*). This makes the balloon tip flexible because the balloon is no longer stretched by the metal tube. The balloon catheter with the metal tube is advanced to place the entire balloon within the left atrium (Fig. 10.10*A, 3*). Next, the inner tube is released from its locked position and pulled back to its marked limit, reducing the stretched balloon to its original length and shape (Fig. 10.10*A, 4*). With the metal tube held fixed, only the balloon catheter is further advanced over the coiled guidewire to place the catheter tip near the mitral valve (Fig. 10.10*A, 5*). Finally, the guidewire and metal tube are removed simultaneously in toto. It is important to note that the guidewire must not be pulled back with the balloon segment still stretched: otherwise, the balloon and the inner tube might be bent into angles, making subsequent manipulation difficult.

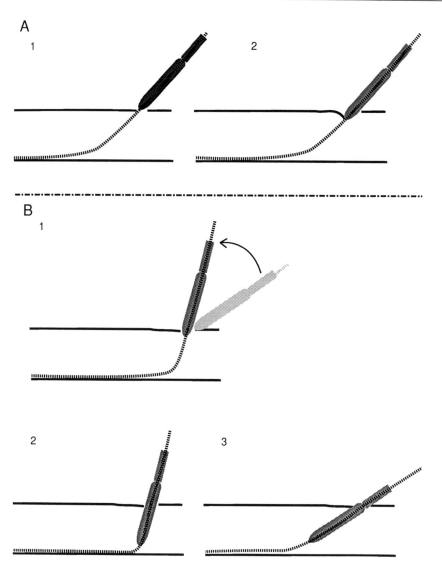

Figure 10.9 Balloon catheter insertion into the femoral vein (see text for discussions).

Crossing of the Mitral Orifice

1. Fluoroscopic 30° Right Anterior Oblique Projection:

After placement of the balloon catheter in the left atrium, the fluoroscopic projection is changed from the frontal to the 30° right anterior oblique view. In this view, the left ventricular long axis is better aligned with the fluoroscopic plane. This allows easier orientation for manipulating the balloon catheter toward and across the mitral orifice and profiling the balloon during its inflation process. When a biplane fluoroscopic unit is available, a left anterior oblique view adds a clearer view of the positional relationship between the balloon catheter and the heart.

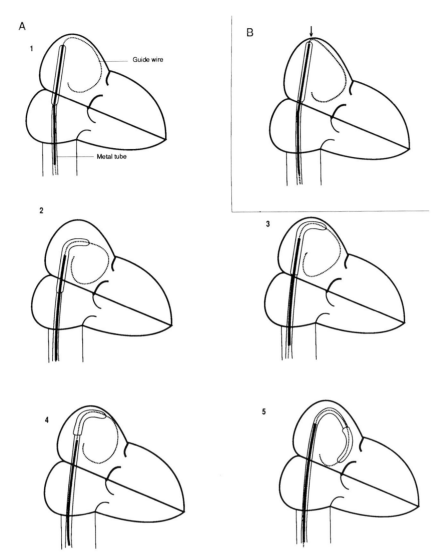

Figure 10.10 Insertion of the balloon catheter into the left atrium through the atrial septum. A-1. The tip of the stretched balloon catheter reaches the upper border of the left atrium, while the proximal part of the balloon remains in the right atrium. B. If the balloon is pushed too forcefully, the guide wire is kinked at the tip of the balloon catheter (arrow). A-2. The metal tube inserted is pulled back about 3 cm through the balloon catheter, so that the balloon tip curves along the guide wire. A-3. The catheter is advanced further to place the entire balloon segment in the left atrium. A-4. The stretched balloon is reduced to its original length and shape. A-5. The balloon catheter is advanced further to place the catheter tip near the mitral orifice.

2. Inflation of Distal Balloon:

The distal balloon is partially inflated to a diameter of 10 to 15 mm with 1 to 2 mL of diluted contrast material to allow the catheter to flow across the stenosed mitral orifice into the left ventricle. Inflating the distal balloon also prevents the catheter tip from straying between tendinous cords in the left ventricle.

In some cases of tight mitral stenosis, engagement of the balloon at the mitral orifice may cause dampening of the systolic blood pressure. Sudden deflation of the balloon allows entry of the catheter tip into the left ventricle and rapid restoration of the systolic pressure. In other cases of very tight mitral stenosis, the mitral valve may have to be crossed with the balloon deflated and the catheter tip stretched by pushing the inner tube of the catheter forward after the stylet is inserted and advanced to the balloon tip. It is important to note that when the mitral valve is crossed with the deflated balloon the operator has to be certain that the catheter has not strayed between tendinous cords before the inflation process.

Insertion of the balloon across the mitral orifice may be made easier if its tip is inflated with carbon dioxide instead of diluted contrast material as was done in the early experience.[7]

3. Directing the Balloon Tip Toward the Mitral Orifice (Fig. 10.11):

When a spring-wire stylet is inserted all the way to the end of the balloon catheter, the distal segment of the catheter forms a J shape with its tip directed downward (Fig. 10.11A, 1). Then, with a counterclockwise twisting of the stylet, the balloon catheter is directed anteriorly (ventrally) toward the mitral orifice. At this time, the distal segment of the balloon catheter is aligned with the long axis of the left ventricle by adjusting the loop of the catheter with the left hand. When the catheter tip is near the mitral orifice, one sees the balloon move back and forth along the long axis of the left ventricle with each cardiac cycle.

4. Advancing the Balloon Catheter Across the Orifice (Fig. 10.11A, 2 and 3):

While the balloon catheter is being fixed, the stylet is withdrawn 4 to 5 cm while being twisted (usually with 180° rotation). This maneuver usually allows the balloon to pass across the stenotic mitral valve and enter the left ventricle during diastole. It is also possible to advance the balloon catheter while fixing the stylet. Fixing the balloon is more effective if the balloon has been inserted deeply in the left atrium, whereas fixing the stylet is more effective if the balloon has been inserted less deeply. Insertion is easier when both manipulations are done simultaneously: the stylet is kept twisted counterclockwise and pulled back 4 to 5 cm and the balloon is advanced forward 4 to 5 cm at the same time. This continuation of movements places the balloon deep in the ventricular apex.

Reshaping of the Stylet:

Reshaping of the original curvature of the spring-wire stylet is usually not necessary. However, when the balloon tip cannot be directed toward the orifice with the stylet, it should be withdrawn from the catheter and its tip reshaped according to the positional relationship between the atrial puncture site and the mitral orifice. For example, in patients with a large left atrium, its tip is shaped to a larger smooth curve.

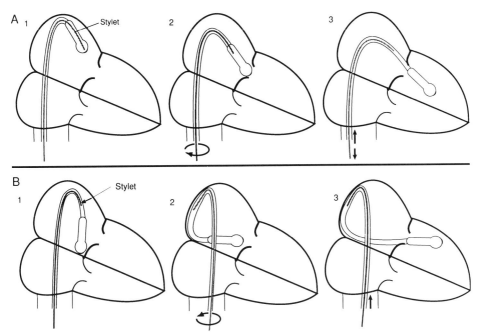

Figure 10.11 Two different techniques of balloon insertion into the mitral orifice: the direct method (top) and the alternative loop method (bottom). In the direct method, a stylet is inserted completely into the balloon catheter. While rotating the stylet counterclockwise about 180 degree, the balloon catheter and the stylet is moved together to direct its tip toward the mitral orifice (A-1). The balloon catheter is advanced toward the mitral orifice while the stylet is held in place, or the stylet is pulled back while the catheter is held still (A-2 &3). In the loop method, the balloon catheter is inserted deeply in the left atrium, and the stylet is inserted into the balloon catheter to a point 2 to 3 cm from the balloon base (B-1). The stylet is rotated clockwise about 360 degree to form a catheter loop (B-2). With the stylet held firm, only the catheter is advanced, allowing the balloon to cross the mitral valve into the left ventricle (B-3).

Alternative Method (Loop Method) for Crossing of the Mitral Orifice (Fig. 10.11*B*)

The conventional method described above is called the direct method, whereas the modified alternative method described here is called the loop method.[28] The conventional method is affected by the position of the septal puncture. Inserting the balloon catheter across the mitral orifice is particularly difficult when the transseptal puncture is made further upward (cephalad) or to the left (closer to the mitral valve) than the appropriate site. The loop method is useful in such cases.

First, the balloon catheter is inserted far into the left atrium to a site near the mitral valve to make a large catheter loop. Then, the stylet is inserted to a point 2 to 3 cm proximal to the balloon base. With the stylet twisted clockwise, the balloon tip is brought toward the posterior and inferior wall of the left atrium. The catheter then forms a loop in the left atrium (Fig. 10.11*B, 1*). With the stylet held firm, only the

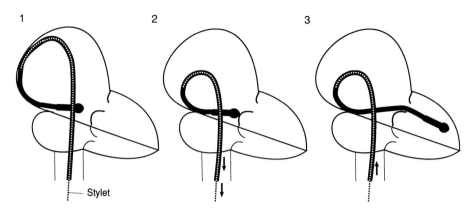

Figure 10.12 Loop formation technique in case of giant left atrium. 1. The length of the balloon catheter limits the balloon to reach the left ventricle, because of a large catheter loop in the left atrium. 2. The balloon catheter and the stylet are pulled back to reduce the loop diameter. 3. The balloon catheter is advanced while the stylet is held in place.

balloon catheter is advanced, allowing the balloon to move forward and leftward to the mitral orifice (Fig. 10.11*B*, 2). In this way, the balloon catheter can be easily inserted across the mitral orifice (Fig. 10.11*B*, 3). If the loop diameter is too large and the remainder of the catheter is not sufficiently long, the balloon catheter or the stylet or both are pulled back 3 or 4 cm to reduce the loop diameter, and only the balloon catheter is advanced again (Fig. 10.12).

When the balloon enters the left ventricle by this alternative method, its tip may point upward. The loop is then carefully reduced and the balloon is aligned with the long axis of the left ventricle to be certain that the balloon tip has not strayed among tendinous chords.

Dilation of the Mitral Orifice

1. Inflation of the Distal Balloon and Its Fixation in the Orifice (Fig. 10.13):

Once the balloon is in the left ventricle, the 10-mL syringe containing diluted contrast medium (1:3 dilution with 5% dextrose or saline solution) is connected to the vent port. When air is being purged out the system, the injection syringe containing a predetermined amount of diluted contrast for the initial balloon size for valve dilation is connected to the injection port. The two-way stopcock of the vent is closed. With the distal portion of the balloon partially inflated with diluted contrast, the balloon is moved back and forth two to three times inside the left ventricle to be certain that it is free in the left ventricular cavity and has not strayed among the chordal structures. The catheter is then pulled until a resistance is felt. In this way, the balloon is fixed at the mitral valve (Fig. 10.13*A*, *1* and 2). However, if the orifice is too narrow or if there is a severe mitral subvalvular lesion, the inflated distal balloon lodges at the stenosed portion of the valve or subvalvular structures, and a greater portion of the balloon remains in the left ventricle while it is being further inflated (Fig. 10.13*B,1*). If the balloon is then fully inflated, it inflates within the left ventricle and not at the orifice (Fig. 10.13*B,2*). Although inflation of the balloon within the left ventricle is usually

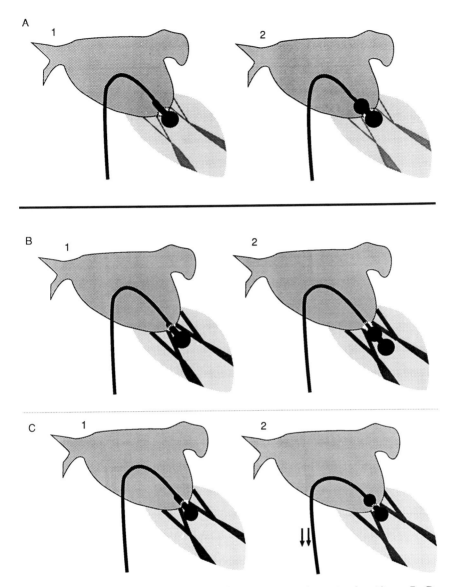

Figure 10.13 Positioning of balloon catheter across the mitral orifice. **A,** Proper position of the balloon during inflation. **B,** In cases of severe stenosis and/or severe subvalvular stenosis, the tip-inflated balloon tends to be trapped in the subvalvular region and slips down in the left ventricle during inflation. **C,** Countermeasure against forward slippage of balloon during inflation. The size of the tip-inflated balloon is reduced to a smaller size.

harmless, the balloon should be quickly deflated in this situation. The diameter of the distal balloon is reduced at the next attempt (Fig. 10.13 *C,1*), and the catheter is pulled firmly to anchor the balloon at the mitral orifice (Fig. 10.13*C,2*).

After the mitral orifice is widened by the first dilation procedure, slippage of the balloon may occur during subsequent inflations with larger balloons (Fig. 10.14). To avoid this, the stylet is inserted far into the balloon segment to stiffen the catheter,

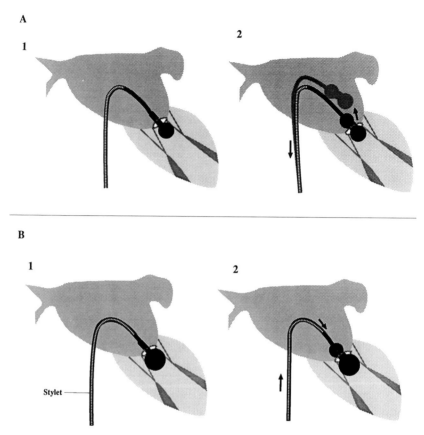

Figure 10.14 A, Slippage of the balloon to the left atrium during subsequent infla-tions after the mitral orifice is widened by the first dilation procedure. B, Counter-measure against the slippage of balloon. Size of the tip-inflated balloon should be as large as possible to anchor the balloon at the mitral orifice (1), and balloon catheter is pushed forward when the balloon assumes an hour-glass shape. (2).

and the distal balloon is inflated to a slightly larger diameter than the previous size before the catheter is pulled to anchor the balloon at the orifice. As soon as the balloon being inflated assumes an hourglass shape, the balloon catheter is advanced slightly to prevent it from slipping back into the left atrium. (Fig. 10.14B,2).

2. Straying of The Catheter Among the Tendinous Cords:

If the balloon catheter has strayed among the tendinous cords in the left ventricle, these cords may be torn during the balloon inflation (Fig. 10.15A). This is one of the reasons why the balloon catheter is inserted into the left ventricle with its distal balloon slightly inflated. However, if the orifice is very narrow, it may become necessary to insert the catheter across the orifice with its balloon segment completely deflated, as previously discussed. In this case, the catheter may stray among the tendinous cords when it enters the left ventricle.

Whether or not the balloon catheter has strayed among the tendinous cords can be easily determined by viewing the positional relationship of the catheter and the

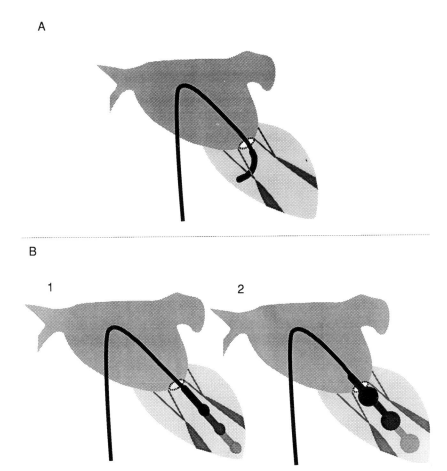

Figure 10.15 Confirmation of proper balloon position in the left ventricle under fluoroscopy in the right anterior oblique projection. **A,** When entangled among the chordae, the balloon is curved toward the lateral wall of the left ventricle and does not move freely. **B,** When placed properly, the balloon directs toward the apex of the left ventricle and moves freely.

cardiac shadow under fluoroscopic right anterior oblique projection. If it has strayed, the catheter will be curved within the left ventricle and will not advance (Fig. 10.15*A*). If properly inserted, the catheter can be advanced straight toward the cardiac apex. The motion of the inflated distal balloon synchronizes with cardiac pulsations, or the balloon can be moved freely within the left ventricle between the apex and the mitral valve according to the operator's intent (Fig. 10.15*B, 1* and *2*).

3. Full Inflation of the Balloon at The Orifice:
Inflation of the balloon at the orifice is performed under fluoroscopy by two individuals: the operator manipulating the catheter system and an assistant handling the syringe. First, after the assistant has inflated the distal balloon, the operator pulls the catheter back until a resistance is felt when the balloon catheter is stopped after it moves slightly from the apex toward the cardiac base.

When the foregoing procedure is repeated by advancing and pulling the catheter several times, the operator can more definitely feel and confirm the mitral orifice site. Then, after gently pulling the catheter and maintaining the balloon's contact with the orifice, the operator immediately instructs the assistant to inflate the balloon fully. The operator instructs the assistant to rapidly inject all the predetermined amount of diluted contrast material in the syringe. Subsequent to the distal balloon, the proximal balloon inflates, resulting in a hourglass shape with a constriction in the middle. At full inflation, the middle constriction disappears, resulting in a barrellike shape. To shorten the balloon inflation time, as soon as the balloon attains its full inflation, the assistant applies a negative pressure to the syringe to deflate the balloon rapidly. The inflation/deflation process takes about 5 seconds. Left ventricular pressure is monitored constantly during the procedure with a pigtail catheter. Systolic blood pressure is maintained above 50 to 60 mmHg during occlusion of the mitral valve.[7]

4. Minimizing Injury to the Atrial Septum:
If the catheter is pulled too forcefully during inflation of the balloon, an avulsion of the atrial septum may occur, leading to a significant atrial shunt after the procedure (Fig. 10.16). This tends to occur with inexperienced operators or in aged or cachectic patients in whom atrial tissues tend to be fragile. To avoid avulsion of the atrial septum during the balloon inflation, the operator should release his or her hand to set the catheter free when the balloon takes an hourglass shape. Once the balloon assumes this shape, it will remain at the orifice even without a pulling force.

5. Assessment of Efficacy Based on Degree of Constriction:
The narrower the mitral orifice, the more marked is the degree of constriction observed in the middle of the inflated balloon. If the balloon slips off the mitral orifice into the left ventricle during its inflation, the constriction is least pronounced and unclear. Experienced operators can recognize the balloon being inflated in the left ventricle and immediately discontinue the inflation procedure. If the valvular commissures are severely fused, the constriction may remain even after injection of all the diluted contrast material in the syringe. In such cases, inflation should be repeated by upsizing the balloon by adding an additional quantity of diluted contrast, as discussed in the stepwise dilation technique below. Or one may choose a smaller catheter (eg,

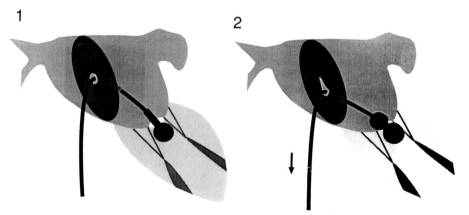

Figure 10.16 Laceration of the atrial septum caused by undue traction of balloon catheter during inflation (see text for discussions).

change from size PTMC-26 to size PTMC-24), which is less compliant, to inflate the balloon to the same diameter as that of the balloon in the previous inflation procedure.

Assessment of Efficacy

After each dilation procedure, the balloon catheter is withdrawn to the left atrium. It is important not to pull the catheter excessively, lest the balloon base be trapped at the transseptal puncture site. If the balloon is advanced after the balloon base is trapped, the catheter will become curved within the right atrium and be unable to advance further (Fig. 10.17, 1). In this case, the guidewire is inserted again into the left atrium to lead the balloon catheter deeply into the left atrium (Fig. 10.17, 2 and 3).

Once the stylet is removed from the catheter, left atrial pressures are readily measured with the catheter. The efficacy of the dilation is assessed by means of mitral transvalvular gradient measurement, auscultation, and two-dimensional color Doppler echocardiography. Creation of significant mitral regurgitation is also judged by these means and, if necessary, with left ventricular angiography. When the effects are determined to be inadequate, the dilation procedures are repeated according to the stepwise dilation method described in the next section until satisfactory results are attained or a significant increase in mitral regurgitation develops.

At the conclusion of the dilation procedure hemodynamic measurements are repeated, including determinations of the transvalvular gradient and cardiac output. A right-heart oximetry series is repeated to search for evidence of a new left-to-right shunt after removal of the catheter from the left atrium. Left ventriculograms are repeated to assess the degree of mitral regurgitation after PTMC.

Removal of the Balloon Catheter

1. Balloon Catheter Stretching:

Upon completion of the dilation procedure, the balloon catheter is stretched to avoid injury to the atrial septum and the right femoral vein when the catheter is being

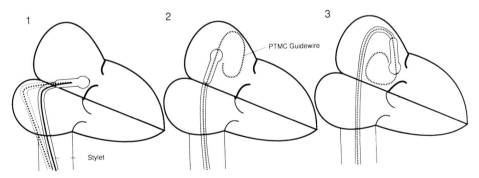

Figure 10.17 Countermeasure against the catheter being trapped in the atrial septum. 1. If the balloon is placed near the atrial septum, it is difficult to advance the balloon in the left atrium because the balloon is trapped at the atrial septal puncture site. 2. The guide wire is inserted again into the balloon catheter, and 3. The balloon catheter is advanced deeply into the left atrium over the guide wire.

withdrawn. First, the catheter is pulled gently until a resistance is felt at the atrial septal puncture site. With the balloon catheter fixed at this point, the metal tube and guidewire are inserted. Before insertion, the guidewire is inserted into the metal tube until its tip is protruding from the tube for about 10 cm. Once the tube and guidewire have been inserted into the catheter, the guidewire tip is made to coil in the left atrium. The metal tube is advanced all the way to the tip of the balloon to stretch the balloon segment as is done at its original insertion. Then, the stretched catheter is withdrawn through the atrial septum and from the femoral vein.

2. Difficulty in Guidewire Insertion:

After the dilation procedures, the balloon segment may bend in an acute angle preventing passage of the guidewire or the metal tube. This results from curving of the elastic inner rubber tube. To solve this problem, the balloon catheter is slightly advanced and inflated within the left atrium. As the curved inner tube is stretched in the process, the guidewire and the metal tube can be advanced.

SELECTION OF THE BALLOON CATHETER (TABLE 10.1)

It is important to use a balloon catheter size appropriate to the individual case. If the balloon diameter is too small, inadequate dilation of the mitral valve may result after PTMC, reflected in suboptimal improvement of symptoms and posing a high risk for future restenosis. If the balloon diameter is too large, excessive avulsion of the commissures may cause significant mitral regurgitation. The following factors should be considered in determining the appropriate size of the balloon catheter for a given patient: (1) height, (2) sex, (3) age, (4) occupation, and (5) valve condition. Four sizes of balloon catheters are available: PTMC-30, PTMC-28, PTMC-26, and PTMC-24.

In the early experience, the patient's body surface area was used as a reference in choosing the catheter size. Hung and associates[15] retrospectively correlated the final balloon size used for PTMC with the patient's height, body weight, and body surface area in the first 59 patients with pliable, noncalcified valves who did not develop significant mitral regurgitation after PTMC. It was found that height correlated best with the final balloon size. Therefore, we now use height as the first criterion in choosing the balloon catheter size. The size is then modified according to the other factors mentioned above.

For example, because most **aged patients** (over 70 years) engage in less strenuous physical activities, the mitral orifice need not be dilated as much as younger patients'. In addition, because their tolerance to surgical stress is reduced, creation of severe mitral regurgitation after PTMC should be avoided as much as possible. For these reasons, a PTMC-24 catheter is usually appropriate for these patients.

Another example is the case of **severe valvular lesions.** It is usually difficult to predict resultant mitral regurgitation on the basis of mitral valve morphologies assessed by two-dimensional echocardiography. However, certain valvular characteristics bear a high risk for development of mitral regurgitation. Two-dimensional echocardiography may identify regional valve leaflet fragility such as cleftlike lesions, or an uneven echo density may create a mosaic appearance of the leaflet. When these features are accompanied by markedly thickened and fused commissures, as well as severe subvalvular lesions, balloon dilation may cause tearing of the fragile leaflet or

Table 10.1 SELECTION OF BALLOON SIZE FOR PERCUTANEOUS TRANSVENOUS MITRAL COMMISSUROTOMY

Catheter selection guide by patient's height

Catheter	Diameter Range, (mm)	Height, (cm)
PTMC-30	26–30	>180
PTMC-28	24–28	>160
PTMC-26	22–26	>147
PTMC-24	20–24	≤147

Other determinants
Sex
Age
Working conditions
Severity of valve pathology
High surgical risk

Stepwise dilation technique
Diameter at initial dilation: 4 mm less than maximal diameter
  (eg, 22 mm in PTMC-26)
Diameter at subsequent dilations: increased by 1 or 2 mm

Decision criteria for further dilation
Resultant mitral regurgitation
Increase in mitral valve area
Degree of commissure separation
Disappearance of balloon waist

excessive avulsion of the contralateral commissure, resulting in severe mitral regurgitation. To avoid this, a balloon catheter one size smaller than otherwise indicated should be chosen. If such risk seems to be particularly high, even when a PTMC-24 size catheter is indicated, the initial dilation should be started at a diameter of 20 mm.

STEPWISE DILATION TECHNIQUE

In the initial balloon dilation procedure, the balloon is inflated to a diameter equal to the maximal diameter less 4 mm. If the effects of the dilation are suboptimal or there is no significant mitral regurgitation, repeat inflations are made with stepwise increments in the balloon size. In each subsequent dilation, the diameter is increased by 2 mm. However, in patients at high risk for developing mitral regurgitation, to be discussed later, an increment of 1 mm is often used in the high pressure range of the balloon (2 mm within the maximal balloon size): for example, a 24 to 26 mm range in PTMC-26.

In assessing the need for further dilation, the following factors are important.

1. *Presence or absence, severity, and location of regurgitation:* Immediately after each dilation, Doppler echocardiography is performed to determine the severity and location of mitral regurgitation, if any. If regurgitation is caused by excessive splitting of the commissures, the regurgitant flow is frequently directed along

the left atrial wall and tends to be overlooked or underestimated by the Doppler method. Therefore, regurgitant signals should be carefully sought not only on the left ventricular long-axis view but also on the short-axis view. If the severity of regurgitation is difficult to assess by Doppler technique, left ventricular angiography is needed. If the degree of mitral regurgitation increases by one or more grade by Sellers' criteria,[29] the dilation procedure is terminated.

2. *Increase in orifice area:* The efficacy of PTMC is best determined by comparing the mitral valve area before and after the procedure. There are three methods for measurement of the valve area, each with its own merits and shortcomings: the hemodynamic method using Gorlin's equation, planimetry of the mitral orifice by two-dimensional echocardiography, and the valve area derived from flow velocity as determined by the Doppler method. The Gorlin equation is the standard one. Because it is affected by the accuracy of cardiac output determination, however, it is not always reliable. Therefore, we recommend that one of the other two methods be used in combination with the Gorlin method. The mean post-PTMC increase in orifice area, as determined by the Gorlin equation, is 0.85 cm^2 for pliable valves and 0.6 cm^2 for rigid valves in Inoue's experience. This can be used as a rough criterion in assessing the need for further dilations.

3. *Commissure avulsion:* It is important to estimate the degree of commissure splitting by two-dimensional echocardiography in the short-axis view. If both commissures are sufficiently split to a point near the annulus, further dilation will cause significant mitral regurgitation. If only one commissure is adequately split, further dilation requires extra care because of the risk of excessive avulsion of that commissure to the mitral annulus, resulting in severe mitral regurgitation.

4. *Constriction in the inflated balloon:* During the dilation procedure, a marked decrease in or disappearance of constriction in the inflated balloon should be checked under fluoroscopy. Persistence of marked constriction indicates intense fusion of the commissures and indicates that the inner pressure of the inflated balloon is insufficient. In such cases, the balloon is upsized by increasing the amount of diluted contrast medium injected to increase its inner pressure. Alternatively, a catheter one size smaller can be substituted and inflated to its full extent to produce sufficient inner pressure.

In some cases, the mitral orifice area does not increase sufficiently despite the complete disappearance of the constriction. This is frequently seen in valves with reduced leaflet mobility. Such valves open like a slit at diastole even though the commissures have been adequately dilated. In such cases, further dilation is useless.

PATIENT SELECTION (TABLE 10.2)

Valvular Morphology

Patients who have pliable valves without severe subvalvular lesions are ideal candidates for PTMC. The results of the procedure are comparable to those of surgical commissurotomy. If valvular mobility is poor, the commissures are severely fused, and severe subvalvular lesions are present, the orifice area after PTMC is markedly

**Table 10.2   PATIENT SELECTION FOR PERCUTANEOUS
TRANSVENOUS MITRAL COMMISSUROTOMY**

A: First choice	
B: Conditional choice	
C: Contraindicated	
Valve with marked sclerosis or calcification	B
Orifice area	
Narrow (<0.7 cm²)	A
Relatively wide (>1.5 cm²)	B
Left atrial thrombus	B
Fresh thrombus	C
Thrombus on atrial septum	C
Embolic history	A
Presence of mitral regurgitation	
Mild (Sellers 1+)	A
Moderate (Sellers 2+)	B
Severe (Sellers 3+ and 4+)	C
Presence of other valvular diseases	A
End-stage mitral stenosis	A
Associated diseases of other organs	A

smaller and the incidence of mitral regurgitation is higher than in the ideal cases.[15] Even in such cases, however, improvement of clinical symptoms is usually seen and it is rare that PTMC is totally useless. PTMC in these cases is also valuable considering that it is very safe and that its physical burden as well as the time required for the procedure are comparable to those for diagnostic cardiac catheterization. Obviously, it is essential to explain in advance to the patient the possibility of unfavorable results and the possible necessity for post-PTMC valve replacement, and to obtain his or her consent.

Mitral Orifice Size

Lower Limit:
Because the balloon catheter can be inserted into the orifice irrespective of the size of the orifice, there is no lower limit of mitral orifice size for performing PTMC. Patients with a very narrow orifice frequently have severe clinical symptoms. The procedure should therefore be done expeditiously to minimize the time that the orifice is obstructed by the balloon catheter, even in the deflated position and thereby avoid exacerbating their symptoms. Operator experience is vital to speed.

Upper Limit:
If patients with mild to moderate mitral stenosis present with clinical symptoms, they are suitable candidates for PTMC. This is especially true for individuals with strenuous occupations who are disabled by their symptoms. In these patients, PTMC is indicated even when the orifice is relatively wide or there is no mitral valve gradient at rest. Analyses of PTMC results show that the incidence of mitral regurgitation is relatively low in patients who have wide orifices before the procedure. This finding further endorses the application of PTMC to patients with moderate mitral stenosis who are symptomatic.

Left Atrial Thrombus

Atrial thrombi are discussed in Chapter 11. Percutaneous transvenous mitral commissurotomy is contraindicated for patients with a left atrial thrombus that is fresh or attached to the atrial septum. Because an old left atrial thrombus is unlikely to be detached during the procedure, such thrombi are not a contraindication. Although the distinction between fresh and old thrombi is not easy, PTMC is performed in patients with left atrial thrombi after warfarin treatment for 1 month or longer. This is based on the assumption that the fresh thrombus has organized and none have newly formed.

Embolic History

Patients with a history of systemic embolism may be candidates for PTMC, because findings at open heart surgery have indicated that a history of embolism is not always related to left atrial thrombi.

Associated Mitral Regurgitation

Mitral regurgitation $\geq 3+$ by Sellers' criteria is a contraindication for PTMC. In patients with $2+$ regurgitation, PTMC is indicated only if the degree of stenosis is severe and clinical symptoms are chiefly due to the stenosis.

Other Associated Valvular Diseases

Other valvular diseases, even though severe, do not hamper PTMC. In addition, post-PTMC hemodynamic changes (ie, increased inflow to the left ventricle) do not aggravate such valvular diseases. If other valves are also stenosed, they should be concurrently dilated (also see Chapter 19).

End-stage Mitral Stenosis

Percutaneous transvenous mitral commissurotomy is also applicable to patients with end-stage mitral stenosis. For example, PTMC can be applied in Fowler's position in orthopneic patients. For patients at the terminal stage, PTMC is the only possible treatment because they are frequently not suitable for open heart surgery. If its effects are suboptimal in patients with an unfavorable valvular status, PTMC may be considered as a bridge to cardiac surgery after impovement and stabilization of the patients.

Associated Illness

Percutaneous transvenous mitral commissurotomy is the only possible treatment in cases where serious complications prohibit open heart surgery. These complications include renal and hepatic diseases and respiratory diseases such as chronic obstructive lung disease and kyphoscoliosis.[15] In cases where urgent noncardiac surgery such as resection of a malignant tumor is needed, PTMC can be performed to improve the patients' hemodynamic status and thus lessen the risk of subsequent noncardiac surgery. In pregnant women in whom the delivery is expected to be complicated

Table 10.3   FAILURE AND COMPLICATION RATES OF PERCUTANEOUS TRANSVENOUS MITRAL COMMISSUROTOMY

	Inoue[7] n = 527	Hung n = 366	Chen n = 149	Nobuyoshi[9] n = 106
Failure	12(2.3%)	3(0.8%)	3(2.0%)	2(1.9%)
Mortality	0	1(0.3%)	0	0
Mitral regurgitation				
Increase	97(18.8%)	136(37.4%)	20(13.7%)	20(19.2%)
Severe	10(1.9%)	19(5.2%)	2(1.7%)	5(4.8%)
Cardiac tamponade	8(1.5%)	0	1(0.7%)	2(1.9%)
Emergency surgery	7(1.3%)	0	0	0
Thromboembolism	3(0.6%)	9(2.5%)	2(1.3%)	0
Atrial septal defect	66(12.5%)[a]	41(11.2%)[a]	1(0.7%)[a]	
			4(2.7%)[b]	5(4.5%)[b]

[a] By oximetry. [b] By Doppler echocardiography.

because of severe mitral stenosis, it is recommended that PTMC be performed after 5 months of gestation when the impact of the X-ray irradiation on the fetus has decreased.

TECHNICAL FAILURES AND COMPLICATIONS

Extensive experience with PTMC has yielded high technical success rates and an encouraging safety record. Table 10.3 lists technical failure and complication rates of PTMC in the multicenter study previously reported by Inoue and Hung[7] and in three other single-institution/single-operator studies by Hung in Taiwan, Chen in Guangzhou, China, and Nobuyoshi in Japan. The multicenter study[7] consisted of 527 patients who underwent PTMC between June 1982 and March 1988 performed by 8 operators in 48 institutions (45 in Japan, 1 in Taiwan, and 2 in mainland China). Therefore, it also includes early experiences of Hung, Chen, and Nobuyoshi.

Patient characteristics including age, sex, cardiac rhythm, embolic history, mitral regurgitation (1+ and 2+), associated aortic regurgitation, and postsurgical mitral restenosis are shown in Table 10.4. In regard to mitral valvular status, 66 of Chen's 149 patients (44%) had valvular calcification as identified by chest film and two-dimensional echocardiography. On the basis of echocardiographic characteristics of the mitral apparatus, Nobuyoshi and associates[9] categorized their 106 patients as follows: 37 patients with pliable, 59 patients with semipliable, and 10 patients with rigid mitral valves. Of Hung's 366 patients, 237 (65%) had pliable, noncalcified valves, 93 (25%) had calcified mitral valves (as seen under fluoroscopy), and 74 (20%) had severe subvalvular lesions. The latter were determined by two-dimensional echocardiographic findings of severe thickening and shortening of chordal structures and by angiographic compression signs on the inflated balloon.[15] Hung's cases also included patients at increased mitral surgical risk: 12 patients with chronic obstructive pulmonary disease, 2 patients with severe kyphoscoliosis, 3 patients with uremia, and 1 each with pneumoconiosis, systemic lupus erythematosus, and liver cirrhosis.

Table 10.4 PATIENT CHARACTERISTICS

	Inoue[7] n = 527	Hung n = 366	Chen n = 149	Nobuyoshi[9] n = 106
Age (mean)	16–78(50)	19–80(43)	15–56(35)	24–75(53)
Female	374(71%)	257(70%)	103(69%)	81(76%)
Atrial fibrillation	306(58%)	237(65%)	27(18%)	40(38%)
Embolic history	69(13%)	54(15%)	0	not reported
Mitral regurgitation (1+ & 2+)	149(28%)	103(28%)	21(14%)	
Aortic regurgitation (1+ & 2+)			50 (33%)	
Aortic regurgitation (3+)		22(6%)	0	not reported
Postsurgical mitral restenosis	53(10%)	4(1%)	0	8(8%)

Technical Failures

As shown in Table 10.3, the technical success rate of PTMC ranged from 99.2 to 97.7%. All the failures occurred in each operator's early experience.[7,9,10,15] The common causes of technical failure were transseptal puncture failure, terminated procedure because of cardiac tamponade related to transseptal puncture, and failure in crossing the mitral valve with the balloon catheter. In the multicenter study of 527 cases,[7] technical failures occurred in 12 patients (2.3%) owing to transseptal puncture failure in 6 patients, inability to traverse the mitral valve with the balloon catheter in 5 patients, and instrument failure of a prototype balloon catheter in 1 patient. In both of Nobuyoshi's failed cases, the procedure was aborted because of transseptal puncture complicated by cardiac tamponade.[9] In Chen's 3 cases, the causes of technical failure were procedure termination because of tamponade following transseptal puncture, atrial wall injury without tamponade, and failure to cross a tight mitral valve with a mitral valve area of 0.5 cm². Although Hung has not experienced any failure or complications related to transseptal puncture, 3 technical failures occurred among the first 15 attempts: 2 due to failure in manipulating the balloon across the valve and the other due to instrument failure of a prototype balloon catheter.[15]

The major differences between the Inoue balloon catheter technique and other prevailing balloon catheter techniques have been described in detail.[7] The Inoue double-lumen coaxial, self-positioning balloon catheter system is very versatile, and it has safety features and excellent steerability not offered by the other catheter techniques. As compared with percutaneous balloon mitral valvuloplasty using the double polyethylene balloon technique, PTMC using the Inoue balloon catheter technique achieves a better success rate,[11] lower complication rates,[11] and a shorter procedure time.[11,21,23] PTMC using the Inoue balloon catheter technique has been reported successful in cases of failed percutaneous balloon mitral valvuloplasty using the double polyethylene balloon technique.[11,30]

In-hospital Mortality

In the authors' experience there has been no PTMC procedure–related mortality. The only in-hospital death in Hung's study occurred in a premoribund patient in whom last-resort emergency PTMC created 3+ mitral regurgitation of the densely calcified valve. This patient died 3 days later of multiple organ failure.[15]

Systemic Embolism

Embolic complication rates ranged from 0 to 2.5%. When this complication occurs, it is usually manifested by cerebral embolism. In the multicenter study reported by Inoue and Hung,[7] systemic embolization manifesting as cerebrovascular accidents occurred in three patients (0.6%). Cerebral embolism occurred in two of Chen's patients (1.3%). Embolic complication resulted in nine of Hung's cases (2.5%), manifested by cerebrovascular accidents in five patients during the procedure, delayed transient cerebral ischemic attacks 6 to 20 hours after the procedure in three patients, and popliteal artery occlusion in one patient.

Atrial Left-to-right Shunt

New atrial septal defects after PTMC detected by oximetry occurred in about 11 to 12% of patients. In most of these patients, the magnitude of the shunt was small, with a pulmonary-to-systemic flow ratio ≤ 1.5, and it posed no hemodynamic or clinical consequences.[7,15] Color Doppler echocardiographic studies have shown that the defect usually diminishes over time.[8,31] Rarely, the left-to-right shunt may increase and lead to development of right ventricular failure and severe tricuspid regurgitation, necessitating surgical repair of the shunt, mitral valve surgery, and tricuspid annuloplasty. This is exemplified in a case reported by Chen and associates[32] and one of Hung's cases.

Forceful traction of the balloon catheter during the dilation process tends to injure the atrial septum and create an atrial shunt.[7] Therefore, the catheter should be pulled gently to anchor the balloon at the mitral valve. In addition, as soon as the balloon being inflated assumes an hourglass shape, tension applied to the catheter should be released.

Cardiac Tamponade

In PTMC, almost all cases of cardiac tamponade occurred as a complication of transseptal puncture.[7,9] In the multicenter study,[7] cardiac tamponade occurred in eight patients (1.5%): as a complication of transseptal puncture in seven and of diagnostic catheterization in one. In two patients (1.9%) of Nobuyoshi, and associates[9] the tamponade was related to transseptal puncture. In our experience, there has been no instance of cardiac tamponade resulting from left ventricular perforation by the balloon catheters, as has been reported to occur with percutaneous balloon mitral valvuloplasty using other techniques.[11,33-35]

Emergency Surgery

In the multicenter study,[7] emergency surgery was required in seven patients (1.3%), in five for cardiac tamponade and in two for severe mitral regurgitation. The latter occurrence can be minimized by avoiding creation of severe mitral regurgitation with careful execution of the stepwise dilation technique, especially in patients with non-pliable, calcified valves, severe mitral subvalvular lesions, or both.

Mitral Regurgitation

Mitral regurgitation either appeared or increased after PTMC in 14 to 37% of patients (Table 10.3). Rarely the degree of mitral regurgitation may decrease, as occurred in 2 of 216 patients reported by Hung and associates[15] and in 2 of Chen's 149 patients.

In most of the patients with the resultant mitral regurgitation, its degree was mild to moderate and posed no significant impact on the patients' hemodynamic results or clinical outcome. In a minority of the patients (1.7 to 5.2%), severe (3 + and 4 +) mitral regurgitation resulted after PTMC. However, in most of the patients with 3 + mitral regurgitation clinical improvements were also observed. The other patients may require elective mitral replacement surgery.[7,15] Creation of 4 + mitral regurgitation mandates emergency or urgent mitral valve surgery.[7,9]

Development of mitral regurgitation is closely related to the morphologic status of the diseased mitral valve.[7,9,15] In the multicenter study,[7] the incidence of resultant mitral regurgitation was significantly higher in patients with thickened mitral commissures and severely restricted mitral valves (mitral valve area < 1 cm^2). Nobuyoshi and associates[9] found a higher incidence of resultant mitral regurgitation after PTMC in patients with rigid valves than in those with pliable valves: 33% in rigid valves, 20% in semipliable valves, and 14% in pliable valves. Hung and associates[15] observed that patients with calcified valves, severe subvalvular lesions, or both were at higher risk of developing mitral regurgitation than those with pliable, noncalcified valves. Increases in the degree of mitral regurgitation were more frequent in patients with nonpliable, calcified valves or severe mitral subvalvular lesions than in patients with pliable, noncalcified valves (38% vs 31%). Multivariate analysis identified oversizing of the balloon to be the sole predictor for increase in mitral regurgitation $\geq 2 +$ in patients with pliable, noncalcified valves. In contrast, preexisting mitral regurgitation — but not balloon size — was a predictor for the increase $\geq 2 +$ in patients with nonpliable calcified valves, severe mitral subvalvular lesions, or both. In other words, in the latter patients, significant mitral regurgitation may develop with any balloon size. Therefore, the stepwise dilation technique should be executed with extra care.

Intraoperative findings in patients with severe mitral regurgitation created as a result of PTMC showed thickened commissures and severe subvalvular fusions to be usual. Mitral regurgitation in these valves was caused by rupture or tearing of the mitral leaflets,[7,9,15] tearing of the unilateral commissure associated with avulsion of papillary muscle,[9] or rupture of the chordae tendineae in one of Hung's recent cases. However, severe mitral regurgitation necessitating mitral valve surgery may be created in patients with lesser pathologic changes in the mitral valve, as experienced by Nobuyoshi and associates in two patients.[9] Severe mitral regurgitation resulted from separation of the unilateral commissure not only to but through the valve ring in one patient with a mildly calcified mitral valve, and from tearing of the posterior mitral leaflet in the other patient with a pliable mitral valve.

EFFECTS OF PERCUTANEOUS TRANSVENOUS MITRAL COMMISSUROTOMY

Immediate Hemodynamic results

Supine Examination
Hemodynamic effects of PTMC in several studies of large numbers of patients are shown in Table 10.5. The studies have consistently shown that PTMC brings about immediate hemodynamic improvements in patients with severe rheumatic mitral stenosis. The average mitral valve area is doubled, or increased by 1.0 cm^2. The

Table 10.5 HEMODYNAMIC DATA BEFORE AND AFTER PERCUTANEOUS TRANSVENOUS MITRAL COMMISSUROTOMY

	Inoue[7] n = 527	Hung[15] n = 204	Chen n = 149	Nobuyoshi[9] n = 104
LA, mmHg				
Before	not reported	24.2 ± 5.6	22.1 ± 8.2	18 ± 8
After	not reported	15.1 ± 5.1	10.0 ± 5.7	11 ± 8
MV gradient, mmHg				
Before	11.9 ± 0.27	13.0 ± 5.1	17.4 ± 7.6	12 ± 7
After	5.5 ± 0.14	5.7 ± 2.6	2.7 ± 3.1	7 ± 6
Mean PA pressure, mmHg				
Before	not reported	39.7 ± 13.0	34.1 ± 13.3	not reported
After	not reported	30.6 ± 10.9	22.7 ± 9.8	not reported
MV area (cm²)				
Before	1.13 ± 0.02	1.0 ± 0.3	1.06 ± 0.21	not reported
After	1.97 ± 0.04	2.0 ± 0.7	2.04 ± 0.32	not reported
CO (L/min) or CI[a] (L/min/m²)				
Before	4.15 ± 0.05	4.4 ± 1.4	3.2 ± 0.7[a]	not reported
After	4.55 ± 0.06	4.7 ± 1.2	3.9 ± 0.5[a]	not reported

CO — cardiac output. *CI* — cardiac index. *LA* — left atrial. *MV* — mitral valve. *PA* — pulmonary artery.

increase in the valve area is also comparable with that of double-balloon mitral valvuloplasty using conventional Mansfield balloon catheters[22,23,34,36] or combinations of a Mansfield and a trefoil balloon catheter.[36] As a result of the increase in the valve area, the mitral valve gradient, left atrial pressure, and mean pulmonary artery pressure are immediately reduced.

Response to Exercise

Effects of PTMC on hemodynamic response to supine ergometer exercise testing were examined by Nobuyoshi and associates[9] in 80 patients. The exercise testing revealed a significant decrease in peak pulmonary artery pressure (systolic, from 68 ± 17 to 57 ± 14 mmHg, $p < 0.0001$; diastolic, from 30 ± 9 to 23 ± 8 mmHg, $p < 0.00001$), and a significant increase in cardiac index (from 5.28 ± 1.12 to 6.16 ± 1.45 L/min/m², $p < 0.0001$) after PTMC.

Predictors for Hemodynamic Results

As in percutaneous balloon mitral valvuloplasty using the double-balloon technique,[36,37] results of PTMC are related to the morphology of the diseased mitral valve.[7,9,12,15]

In the multicenter study,[7] Inoue and Hung analyzed the following variables to determine the factors that influence the immediate hemodynamic results of PTMC: pliability of the mitral valve leaflet, thickened mitral commissures, subvalvular lesions, mitral valve calcification (on fluoroscopy), preexisting mitral regurgitation, previous mitral commissurotomy, cardiac rhythm, patient age, and mitral valve area before PTMC. Among the variables, nonpliability of the valve predicted a suboptimal result from PTMC in terms of the percentage of increase in the mitral valve area attained.

The percentage of increase in the mitral valve area was lower in less severe mitral stenosis (mitral valve area more than 1 cm^2). Hung and associates[15] compared several clinical and hemodynamic variables in 167 patients with good hemodynamic results after PTMC with those in 37 patients with suboptimal results (arbitrarily defined as a gain in the mitral valvular area of <50%). Univariate analysis showed older age, atrial fibrillation, larger left atrial size and cardiothoracic ratio on chest x-ray, an echocardiographic score of > 8 using the system proposed by Wilkins and associates,[37] valvular calcification, and severe subvalvular lesions as predictors for suboptimal results. Multivariate analysis identified an echocardiographic score > 8, valvular calcification, and severe subvalvular lesions as being independent predictors for suboptimal hemodynamic results.

The majority of patients with suboptimal hemodynamic results do show clinical improvement.[15] This finding suggests that symptomatic improvements can be achieved when a certain mitral valve orifice beyond a critical area is attained by PTMC. Therefore, in patients at higher risk for development of significant mitral regurgitation, namely, those with calcified valves, severe subvalvular lesions, or both, the operator should not be too aggressive in upsizing the balloon diameter in the stepwise dilation technique.

Echocardiographic Results

The mean mitral valve area as determined by echocardiographic planimetry increased from 1.19 ± 0.01 before to 1.91 ± 0.02 cm^2 after PTMC in the multicenter study of 527 patients,[7] and from 0.99 ± 0.49 before to 1.78 ± 0.65 cm^2 after PTMC in 204 patients reported by Hung and associates.[15] The mean mitral valve area as determined by the Doppler pressure half-time method increased from 1.4 ± 0.4 before to 2.0 ± 0.5 cm^2 after PTMC in 104 patients of Nobuyoshi and associates,[9] and from 1.06 ± 0.21 before to 2.04 ± 0.32 cm^2 after PTMC in 146 patients studied by Chen and Cheng.

Chen and Cheng also studied the effects of PTMC on the mitral valve gradient determined by the Doppler method and on the left atrial and left ventricular dimensions measured by M-mode echocardiography. The mitral valve gradient decreased significantly from 17.4 ± 7.6 before to 5.0 ± 4.4 mmHg after PTMC and the left atrial dimension from 43.6 ± 6.3 before to 38.4 ± 5.6 mm after PTMC. The left ventricular end-diastolic dimension did not change significantly before and after PTMC (43.3 ± 5.2 before vs 44.8 ± 4.6 mm after, $p > 0.05$).

Clinical Results

After PTMC, clinical improvements in symptoms and exercise tolerance can be expected in the majority of patients. The improvements mirror hemodynamic benefits that result from PTMC. In the study of Nobuyoshi and associates,[9] significant symptomatic improvement defined as reclassification by one or more NYHA functional classes was achieved in 97 of 106 patients (92%): 36 of 37 patients (97%) with pliable valves, 55 of 59 patients (93%) with semipliable valves, and 6 of 10 patients (60%) with rigid valves. Two patients were reclassified from class IV to class I, 9 from class III to class I, 64 from class II to class I, 2 from class IV to class II, and 20 from class III to class II. Hung and associates[15] reported improvement in symptoms and in NYHA functional class by at least one class in 209 of 215 patients (97%) at followup visits 1 to 2 weeks after successful PTMC. The improvements were obtained in all 136 patients who had pliable, noncalcified mitral valves and 73 of 79 patients (92%) who had calcified mitral valves with or without severe mitral subvalvular lesions. Relatively lower rates of clinical improvement after PTMC in the latter group reflect suboptimal hemodynamic results obtained in these patients. As stated previously, hemodynamic results of PTMC are closely related to morphology of the diseased mitral valve.

Treadmill Exercise Tests

Hung and associates[15] objectively documented improved exercise tolerance after PTMC by noting increases in treadmill exercise duration. A symptom-limited treadmill exercise test using Naughton's protocol[38] was performed in 159 patients before and 3 months after PTMC. The duration increased in all patients, and the group mean exercise duration increased from 8.9 ± 4.9 to 14.7 ± 4.3 minutes (p = 0.0001).

LATE OUTCOMES

Recently Chen and associates[12] and Hung and associates[15] began to unravel the long-term results of PTMC by investigating and reporting PTMC followup results. We have further expanded the followup studies to more extended periods of observation in large numbers of patients. And the results as discussed below are most reassuring.

Chen and Cheng have performed a comprehensive followup study of the first 146 patients who successfully underwent PTMC from November 1985 to December 1990 at Guangdong Provincial Cardiovascular Institute. Seven of the patients were lost to followup. The other 139 patients were followed for a mean period of 29.4 ± 7.2 months (range 2–61 mo). The hemodynamic and clinical improvements were significant immediately after PTMC and also at followup. Noninvasive studies including echocardiography, electrocardiography, phonocardiography, and cardiopulmonary exercise testing also substantiated sustained benefits of PTMC at followup.

Clinical Followup

Figure 10.18 illustrates the cardiac functional status of the patients before and after PTMC and at followup. In the 149 patients who underwent PTMC, functional status before PTMC was NYHA functional class IV in 3, class III in 82, and class II in 64. The status after successful PTMC in 146 patients was functional class III in 2, class II in 15, and class I in 129. At followup the NYHA functional class in 139 patients was class I in 123 patients, class II in 13, and class III in 3 patients.

In the three class III patients, mitral restenosis occurred. The first patient developed severe mitral calcification and mitral restenosis after 36 months; the restenosis was amenable to repeat PTMC with restoration to NYHA functional class I. The second patient developed severe mitral calcification and mitral restenosis after 18 months and underwent mitral valve replacement surgery, but died 3 days after the surgery. The third patient had echocardiographic evidence of mitral restenosis. The patient declined further invasive investigations and interventions.

Late death occurred 6 months after PTMC in one patient with atrial fibrillation who underwent direct current cardioversion. After the cardioversion restored sinus

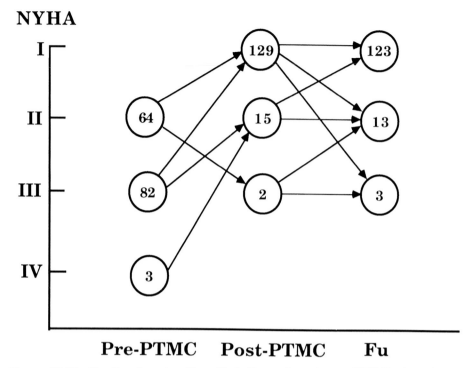

Figure 10.18 Cardiac function New York Heart Association (NYHA) classification indicating significant improvement following percutaneous transvenous mitral commissurotomy (PTMC) and at followup. (Fu).

rhythm, the patient developed ventricular fibrillation which was then converted to sinus rhythm by the second DC countershock. The patient was found dead the day after the cardioversion presumably from quinidine overdose. The plasma level of quinidine was found to be 36 mg/L, which was 6 times the therapeutic level. Pericardial effusion with cardiac tamponade occurred in one patient 12 months after PTMC. The effusion resolved after five weekly pericardiocenteses with a total recovery of over 1 L of clear fluid. Etiology of the effusion remained unknown.

Hemodynamic and Echocardiographic Results

Pre-, post PTMC and follow-up mean diastolic mitral gradients by catheter method were 17.4 ± 7.6, 2.7 ± 3.1, and 3.8 ± 2.7 mmHg, respectively ($p < 0.001$ pre versus post PTMC and pre PTMC versus follow-up; and $p > 0.05$ post PTMC versus follow-up). By 2D echo and Doppler method the mean diastolic gradient was 17.4 ± 7.6, 5.0 ± 4.4, and 6.5 ± 3.8 mmHg, respectively ($p < 0.001$ pre versus post PTMC; and $p > 0.05$ post PTMC versus follow-up). Mitral valve area was 1.06 ± 0.21, 2.04 ± 0.32 and 1.93 ± 0.56 cm^2, respectively ($p < 0.001$ pre versus post PTMC; and $p > 0.05$ post PTMC versus follow-up). By M-mode echocardiograms, the left atrial dimension was 43.6 ± 6.3, 38.4 ± 5.6, and 38.3 ± 6.2 mm, respectively ($p < 0.001$ pre versus post PTMC; and $p > 0.05$ post PTMC versus follow-up). The left ventricular end-diastolic dimension was 43.3 ± 5.2, 44.8 ± 4.6 and 43.9 ± 4.8 mm, respectively ($p > 0.05$ pre versus post PTMC; and $p > 0.05$ post PTMC versus follow-up).

Phonocardiographic, Electrocardiographic, and Vectorcardiographic Results

The phonocardiographic, electrocardiographic, and vectorcardiographic studies showed significant improvements immediately after PTMC and at followup. The phonocardiographic interval between the Q wave and the mitral component of the first heart sound (Q–S_1 interval) decreased from 84.1 ± 13.6 to 73.8 ± 12.4 ms after PTMC ($p < 0.001$) and to 72.4 ± 13.7 ms at followup ($p > 0.05$ post vs followup). The phonocardiographic interval between the aortic second sound and the opening snap (A_2–OS) increased from 72.3 ± 18.2 to 87.9 ± 10.6 ms after PTMC ($p < 0.001$) and to 92.0 ± 144.9 ms at followup ($p < 0.001$ pre vs post PTMC and pre vs followup; and $p > 0.05$ post vs followup).

On electrocardiography the amplitude of the P wave in lead II was 2.23 ± 0.60 mV pre PTMC, 1.65 ± 0.67 mV post PTMC, and 1.53 ± 0.72 mV at followup ($p < 0.001$ pre vs post PTMC and $p > 0.05$ post vs followup). The P wave terminal force in lead V_1 was -0.08 ± 0.05 mm-sec pre PTMC, -0.04 ± 0.03 mm-sec post PTMC, and -0.04 ± 0.03 mm-sec at followup ($p < 0.001$ pre vs post PTMC and $p > 0.05$ post vs followup).

The vectorcardiogram showed a marked decrease of the voltage of the P-loop: 0.19 ± 0.05 mV pre PTMC, 0.16 ± 0.04 mV post PTMC, and 0.15 ± 0.03 mV at followup in the horizontal plane; and 0.24 ± 0.03 mV pre PTMC, 0.20 ± 0.04 mV post PTMC, and 0.19 ± 0.03 mV at followup in the frontal plane ($p < 0.001$ pre vs post PTMC and $p > 0.05$ post vs followup). The frontal plane QRS axis was $88.7 \pm 21.6°$ pre PTMC, $81.3 \pm 18.8°$ post PTMC, and $78.7 \pm 26.2°$ at followup ($p < 0.01$ pre vs post PTMC and $p > 0.05$ post vs followup).

Cardiopulmonary Exercise Testing

Although cardiopulmonary exercise testing showed no significant improvement within 30 days after PTMC, very good results were seen in the maximal oxygen pulse, the maximal oxygen consumption, and the anaerobic threshold (AT) during the followup period (Table 10.6). The maximal oxygen pulse was 5.8 ± 1.3 mL per beat before PTMC, 6.7 ± 1.5 mL per beat after PTMC, and 9.1 ± 2.1 mL per beat at followup ($p > 0.05$ before vs after; $p < 0.001$ before vs followup, and $p < 0.05$ after vs followup). The maximal oxygen consumption was 19.8 ± 4.3 mL per minute per kilogram before PTMC, 22.4 ± 5.1 mL per minute per killogram after PTMC,

Table 10.6 CARDIOPULMONARY EXERCISE TESTING BEFORE AND AFTER PERCUTANEOUS TRANSVENOUS MITRAL COMMISSUROTOMY

	Pre-PTMC	Post-PTMC	Followup
O_2 pulse $_{max}$ (mL/beat)	5.8 ± 1.3	[a] 6.7 ± 1.5	[b] 9.1 ± 2.1[c]
$\dot{V}O_{2max}$/kg (mL/min/kg)	19.8 ± 4.3	[a]22.4 ± 5.1	[b]27.0 ± 4.1[c]
$\dot{V}O_2$AT/kg (mL/min/kg)	14.7 ± 1.5	[a]16.0 ± 4.5	[b]19.9 ± 4.5[d]

PTMC – Percutaneous transvenous mitral commissurotomy.

[a] $p > 0.05$, pre vs post.

[b] $p < 0.001$, pre vs followup.

[c] $p < 0.05$, post vs followup.

[d] $p < 0.001$, post vs followup.

and 27.0 ± 4.1 mL per minute per kilogram at followup ($p > 0.05$ before vs after; $p < 0.001$ before vs followup, and $p < 0.05$ after vs followup). The anaerobic threshold (AT) was 14.7 ± 1.5 mL per minute per kilogram before PTMC; and 16.0 ± 4.5 mL per minute per kilogram after PTMC; and 19.9 ± 4.5 mL per minute per kilogram at followup ($p > 0.05$ before vs after; $p < 0.001$ before vs followup and after vs followup).

Cardiovascular Event Free Survival

Hung obtained followup data for at least 3 months in all 361 patients discharged from the hospital after successful PTMC performed at Chang Gung Memorial Hospital between January 1987 and December 1990. The patients consisted of 205 group 1 patients with pliable noncalcified valves followed for up to 52 months and 156 group 2 patients with calcified valves and/or severe subvalvular lesions followed for up to 47 months. The cumulative cardiovascular event-free rates by the Kaplan-Meir method are shown in Figure 10.19. The rate for group 1 was 100% for the entire followup period. That for group 2 was 95% and 93% at 6 and 12 months, respectively, and it held at 84% at 24 months and beyond. Nine group 2 patients underwent elective mitral valve surgery: in 1 patient because of recurrent symptoms in 22 months resulting from mitral restenosis which was not amenable to repeat PTMC and in 8 patients within 1 to 20 months after PTMC because of lack of clinical improvement. Of the 8 patients, 5 had severe subvalvular lesions despite separation of one or both commissures, 1 patient had a large atrial septal defect (as mentioned previously), and 2 patients had severe mitral regurgitation resulting from a tear in the anterior mitral leaflet in one and ruptured anterior leaflet chordae tendineae in the other.

Late deaths occurred in seven group 2 patients: five cardiac deaths and two noncardiac deaths (traffic accidents). Of the five cardiac deaths, two were sudden at

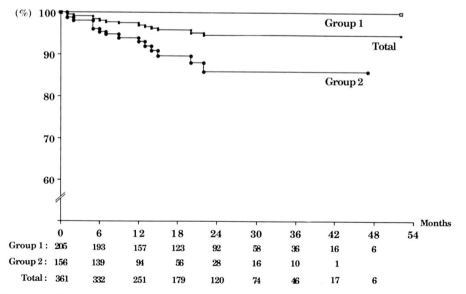

Figure 10.19 Cumulative cardiovascular event-free survival rates for group 1 (with pliable, non-calcified mitral valves) and group 2 patients (with calcified valves or severe mitral subvalvular lesions, or both).

7 and 12 months, two as a result of cerebral embolism after 4 and 6 months, and the other because of uremia and heart failure 7 months after PTMC. There were continued clinical improvements in the other 140 group 2 patients and in all group 1 patients at their last followup examinations. None of these patients had clinical evidence of mitral restenosis.

Late outcomes of this study are most encouraging. Patients with pliable non-calcified valves, usually young and in sinus rhythm, were free of cardiovascular events for as long as 51 months. The long-term effects of PTMC in this group of patients are expected to be excellent. Thus, such patients are ideal candidates for PTMC.

When restenosis of the mitral valve occurs in these patients, it is likely that repeat PTMC can still be performed. This is suggested by the limited experience of Inoue[7] as well as that of Chen and Cheng described above. It is also suggested by earlier reports of successful PTMC for restenosed mitral valves following surgical commissurotomy[7,9,15,34,36,39] (also see Chapter 12). Although the late outcomes in patients with calcified valves and/or severe subvalvular lesions are less favorable, the procedure may yet be a desirable palliative option. PTMC is safe and it is worthwhile even if clinical improvement is sustained for only several years. When mitral restenosis occurs in these patients, PTMC may be repeated with an equally successful result. In all these patients, mitral valve surgery can still be performed at a later date without difficulties that might be encountered in patients with previous thoracotomy.

CONCLUSIONS

At present, results of surgery on the mitral valve are excellent, and operative mortality is low. The use of PTMC would be limited if it were not as safe as, or safer than, surgery. In fact, the safety of this procedure has been well demonstrated: no deaths directly attributable to PTMC have occurred. Therefore, attention should now be directed to indications for this procedure. Patients with pliable mitral valves are ideal candidates for PTMC. In contrast, patients with severely thickened or even calcified valves and severe subvalvular lesions are problematic. Although the efficacy of PTMC is evidently less optimal in patients with such conditions than in those with pliable valves, the more severe the valvular lesions, the more marked are the post-PTMC improvements in symptoms. In the past, these patients were treated with valve replacement surgery, but the problems of durability and thrombosis associated with the long-term use of artificial valves are far from being resolved. Bearing this in mind, we have not excluded patients from PTMC on the basis of valvular pathology. In the future, however, this factor should also be scrutinized.

The safety of PTMC should be backed up by the availability of cardiac surgery.[40] Although PTMC is the only available life-saving procedure for patients not suitable for surgery, on the other hand its risk is increased without surgical backup. In applying PTMC to inoperable cases, the procedure should be done carefully with its safety as top priority.

REFERENCES

1. Inoue K, Owaki T, Nakamura T, et al: Clinical application of transvenous mitral commissurotomy by a new balloon catheter. *J Thorac Cardiovasc Surg.* 87:394–402, 1984.

2. Inoue K, Nakamura T, Kitamura F, et al: Transvenous mitral commissurotomy by a new balloon catheter. *Eur Heart J.* 5(suppl I):111, 1984.

3. Inoue K, Owaki T, Nakamura T, et al: Transvenous mitral commissurotomy: long-term follow-up and recent modification. *Circulation.* 74(supple II):II-208, 1986.

4. Inoue K, Nobuyoshi M, Chen CR, et al: Advantage of Inoue-balloon (self-positioning balloon) in percutaneous transvenous mitral commissurotomy and aortic valvuloplasty (abstr). *Eur Heart J.* 9(suppl I):110, 1988.

5. Inoue K, Nobuyoshi M, Chen C, et al: Advantages of Inoue-balloon (self-positioning balloon) in percutaneous transvenous mitral commissurotomy (PTMC) and aortic valvuloplasty (PTAV) (abstr). *J Am Coll Cardiol.* 13:18A, 1989.

6. Inoue K, Chen C: Percutaneous transvenous mitral commissurotomy guided and assessed by echocardiography. In: Cikes I, ed. *Echocardiography in Cardiac Interventions.* Netherlands: Kluwer Academic Publishers, 1989, pp 67–76.

7. Inoue K, Hung JS: Percutaneous transvenous mitral commissurotomy (PTMC): the Far East experience. In: Topol EJ. *Textbook of Interventional Cardiology.* 1st ed. Philadelphia: WB Saunders Co, 1990, pp 887–899.

8. Yoshida K, Yoshikawa J, Akasaka T, et al: Assessment of left-to-right atrial shunting after percutaneous mitral valvuloplasty by transesophageal color Doppler flow-mapping. *Circulation.* 80:1521–1526, 1989.

9. Nobuyoshi M, Hamasaki N, Kimura T, et al: Indications, complications, and short-term clinical outcome of percutaneous transvenous mitral commissurotomy. *Circulation.* 80:782–792, 1989.

10. Chen C, Lo Z, Huang Z, et al: Percutaneous transseptal balloon mitral valvuloplasty: the Chinese experience in 30 patients. *Am Heart J.* 115:937–947, 1988.

11. Chen CR, Huang ZD, Lo ZX, et al: Comparison of single rubber-nylon balloon and double polyethylene balloon valvuloplasty in 94 patients with rheumatic mitral stenosis. *Am Heart J.* 119:102–111, 1990.

12. Chen CR, Hu SW, Chen JY, et al: Percutaneous mitral valvuloplasty with a single rubber-nylon balloon (Inoue balloon). Long-term results in 71 patients. *Am Heart J.* 120:561–568, 1990.

13. Hung JS, Fu M, Cherng WJ, et al: Rapid fall in elevated plasma atrial natriuretic peptide levels after successful catheter balloon valvuloplasty of mitral stenosis. *Am Heart J.* 117:381–385, 1989.

14. Hung JS, Fu M, Yeh SJ, et al: Hemodynamic and clinical efficacies of catheter balloon percutaneous transvenous mitral commissurotomy: experience of 100 patients with rheumatic mitral stenosis. *J Formosan Med Assoc.* 89:182–189, 1990.

15. Hung JS, Chern MS, Wu JJ, et al: Short- and long-term results of catheter balloon percutaneous transvenous mitral commissurotomy. *Am J Cardiol.* 67:854–862, 1991.

16. Ongtengco IV Jr, Del Moro MV, Esposo EA, et al: Percutaneous transvenous mitral commissurotomy using a single balloon technique in patients with calcific rheumatic mitral stenosis. *Philippines J Cardiovasc Med.* 2:22–26, 1988.

17. Shim WH, Jang YS, Cho SY, et al: Comparison of outcome between double and Inoue balloon techniques for percutaneous mitral valvuloplasty — single blind randomized prospective study. *J Am Coll Cardiol.* 17(suppl A):83A, 1991.

18. Feldman T, Carroll JD: Valve deformity and balloon mechanics in percutaneous transvenous mitral commissurotomy. *Am Heart J.* 121:1628–1633, 1991.

19. Nishimura RA, Holmes DR Jr, Reeder GS: Efficacy of percutaneous mitral balloon valvuloplasty with the Inoue balloon. *Mayo Clin Proc.* 66:276–282, 1991.

20. Dietz WA, Waters JB, Ramaswamy K, et al: Use of Inoue balloon catheter to perform staged balloon inflations in combination with serial evaluation by color-flow Doppler minimizes mitral regurgitation as a complication of percutaneous mitral valvuloplasty. (abstr) *J Am Coll Cardiol.* 17(suppl A):82A, 1991.

21. Ramaswamy K, Losordo DW, Rosenfield K, et al: Inoue balloon mitral valvuloplasty vs. double balloon technique: procedure duration and radiation exposure (abstr). *J Am Coll Cardiol.* 17(suppl A):253A, 1991.

22. Fernández-Ortiz A, Macaya C, Cortés J, et al: Percutaneous mitral valvotomy: single balloon versus double-balloon technique. *J Am Coll Cardiol.* 17(suppl A):82A, 1991.

23. Bassand J-P, Schiele F, Bernard Y, et al: Comparative results of the double balloon technique and the Inoue's technique in percutaneous mitral valvulotomy. *J Am Coll Cardiol.* 17(suppl A):83A, 1991.

24. Patel JJ, Mitha AS, Hassen F, et al: Balloon mitral valvuloplasty: single catheter technique comparing bifoil/trefoil and Inoue balloons. *J Am Coll Cardiol.* 17(suppl A):82A, 1991.

25. Ross J Jr, Braunwald E, Morrow AG: Transseptal left atrial puncture. New technique for the measurement of left atrial pressure in man. *Am J Cardiol.* 3:653–655, 1959.

26. Cope C: Newer techniques of transseptal left-heart catheterization. *Circulation.* 27:758–761, 1963.

27. Bloomfield DA, Sinclair-Smith BC: The limbic ledge: a landmark for transseptal left heart catheterization. *Circulation.* 31:103–107, 1965.

28. Hosokawa H, Suzuki T, Itoh F, et al: Insertion of Inoue balloon catheter in percutaneous transvenous mitral commissurotomy. *Shin Kekkan.* 5:118–123, 1990.

29. Sellers RD, Levy MJ, Amplatz K, et al: Left retrograde cardioangiography in acquired cardiac disease. Technic, indications and interpretations in 700 cases. *Am J Cardiol.* 14:437–447, 1964.

30. Benit E, Rocha P, de Geest H, et al: Successful mitral valvuloplasty using the Inoue balloon in a patient with mitral stenosis associated with subvalvular fibrosis and reduced left ventricular inflow cavity: a case report. *Cathet Cardiovasc Diagn.* 22:35–38, 1991.

31. Ishikura F, Nagata S, Yasuda S, et al: Residual atrial septal perforation after percutaneous transvenous mitral commissurotomy with Inoue balloon catheter. *Am Heart J.* 120:873–878, 1990.

32. Chen CH, Lin SL, Hsu TL, et al: Iatrogenic Lutembacher's syndrome after percutaneous transluminal mitral valvotomy. *Am Heart J.* 119:209–211, 1990.

33. Babic UU, Dorros G, Pejcic P, et al: Percutaneous mitral valvuloplasty: retrograde, transarterial double-balloon technique utilizing the transseptal approach. *Cathet Cardiovasc Diagn.* 14:229–237, 1988.

34. Ruiz CE, Allen JW, Lau FYK: Percutaneous double balloon valvotomy for severe rheumatic mitral stenosis. *Am J Cardiol.* 65:473–477, 1990.

35. Robertson JM, de Virgilio C, French W, et al: Fatal left ventricular perforation during mitral balloon valvoplasty. *Ann Thorac Surg.* 49:819–821, 1990.

36. Vahanian A, Michel PL, Cormier B, et al: Results of percutaneous mitral commissurotomy in 200 patients. *Am J Cardiol.* 63:847–852, 1989.

37. Wilkins GT, Weyman AE, Abascal VM, et al: Percutaneous balloon dilatation of the mitral valve: an analysis of echocardiographic variables related to outcome and the mechanism of dilatation. *Br Heart J.* 60:299–308, 1988.

38. Patterson JA, Naughton J, Pietras RJ, et al: Treadmill exercise in assessment of the functional capacity of patients with cardiac disease. *Am J Cardiol.* 30:757–762, 1972.

39. Medina A, Suarez de Lezo J, Hernandez E, et al: Balloon valvuloplasty for mitral restenosis after previous surgery: a comparative study. *Am Heart J.* 120:568–571, 1990.

40. Cheng TO: Left ventricular perforation following percutaneous balloon mitral valvuloplasty. *Can J Cardiol.* 7(4):XI, 1991.

CHAPTER **11**

Mitral Stenosis with Left Atrial Thrombi: Inoue Balloon Catheter Technique

JUI-SUNG HUNG

Since 1984, when Inoue and associates[1] introduced percutaneous transvenous mitral commissurotomy (PTMC) using a single rubber balloon catheter for the non-surgical treatment of mitral stenosis, this procedure has become an effective, safe alternative to surgical treatment in well-selected patients with symptomatic mitral stenosis.[2-9] Although the long-term results of the procedure are yet to be determined, so far its late outcomes have been encouraging.[5,6]

The presence of left atrial thrombus is generally considered to be a contraindication for percutaneous balloon mitral valvuloplasty[3-9] because embolic complications may result from inadvertent dislodgement of left atrial thrombi during manipulation of guidewires and catheters in the left atrium. If this contraindication is adhered to, a significant proportion of potential candidates for percutaneous balloon mitral valvuloplasty will be denied the benefits of the procedure, as left atrial thrombus is a frequent complication in mitral stenosis.[10-15] In the past, candidates for percutaneous balloon mitral valvuloplasty have been screened for the presence of left atrial thrombus using only transthoracic two-dimensional echocardiography.[2-9] Since this modality is insensitive in detecting left atrial thrombi,[12-15] the balloon catheter intervention has undoubtedly been performed in some patients with unsuspected left atrial thrombi. With the recent advent of transesophageal echocardiography, more patients are expected to be denied the procedure because this highly sensitive and specific diagnostic method, especially with the biplane technique, will detect even more left atrial and auricular thrombi.[16-18]

Our preliminary observations indicate that percutaneous balloon mitral valvuloplasty using the Inoue balloon catheter technique (PTMC) may be performed safely in selected patients with left atrial thrombi. In this chapter, the author will review, on the basis of personal experience, the feasibility and safety of the procedure in patients with left atrial thrombi. It is important to note that the discussions herein do not apply to the other percutaneous balloon mitral valvuloplasty techniques such as the transvenous or transarterial double-balloon technique using conventional Mansfield balloon catheters or combinations of a Mansfield and a trefoil balloon catheter.[7-9]

LEFT ATRIAL THROMBI IN MITRAL STENOSIS

Scope and Magnitude of the Issue

Left atrial thrombus is a frequent complication of rheumatic mitral stenosis.[10-15] The presence of a left atrial thrombus in patients with rheumatic mitral stenosis is clinically significant in several ways, and it may dictate or alter therapeutic approaches in these patients. First, although left atrial thrombus infrequently takes a mobile or pedunculated form, patients with this type of thrombus are at high risk for systemic embolism[13] and sudden cardiac death,[19] and they require urgent surgical intervention. Second, although in patients with a history of systemic embolism, left atrial thrombus is more frequently found than not,[13] little information is available regarding whether or not patients with left atrial thrombus are at higher risk for future systemic embolism. Nevertheless it is a common practice to treat patients having left atrial thrombi with long-term warfarin anticoagulant therapy in an attempt to prevent this complication. Third, and most significant for the subject under discussion in this chapter, the presence of left atrial thrombus is considered to be a contraindication for percutaneous balloon mitral valvuloplasty and surgical closed mitral commissurotomy.

Incidence

Left atrial thrombi are found at surgery in 15 to 44% (mean 18%) of patients with predominant mitral stenosis (Table 11.1). The wide variations in the reported incidences of left atrial thrombus are largely due to differences in patient selection. Atrial fibrillation and large left atrial size are positive predictors and coexistent mitral regurgitation is a negative predictor for the presence of left atrial thrombi in patients with mitral stenosis. In our study, all patients with left atrial thrombi had atrial fibrillation.[15] Left atrial thrombi have been reported to occur infrequently in patients with sinus rhythm — in 1 of 76 patients (1.3%) by Colman and associates[11] and in 2 of 192 cases (1.0%) by Beppu and associates.[13] In the study by the Beppu group, the incidence of left atrial thrombi decreased with increasing severity of mitral regurgitation, and no thrombi were found at surgery in patients with grade 3 or 4 mitral regurgitation. When the subjects were limited to those patients with atrial fibrillation

Table 11.1 **INCIDENCE OF LEFT ATRIAL THROMBUS IN SURGICAL PATIENTS WITH MITRAL STENOSIS**

Series	Incidence	
Nichols et al[10]	44/200	(22%)
Colman et al[11]	76/507	(15%)
Shrestha et al[12]	51/293	(17%)
Beppu et al[13]	43/246	(18%)
Bansal et al[14]	12/84	(14%)
Fu et al[15]	33/75	(44%)
	259/1405	(18%)

and an enlarged left atrium (> 60 mm) but without grade 3 or 4 mitral regurgitation, the thrombi were observed in 50% of such patients.

Diagnosis of Left Atrial Thrombus

Noninvasive diagnostic methods for left atrial thrombi include chest x-ray, computed tomography, and echocardiography. However, detection of left atrial thrombus by a chest x-ray finding of calcification is rare. Although computed tomography has high sensitivity and specificity in evaluation of left atrial thrombi,[20] its cost is prohibitive for routine application. Echocardiography is safe and allows serial followup examinations of patients. It is therefore the diagnostic technique of choice for detecting left atrial thrombi.

Invasive methods for the diagnosis of left atrial thrombi depend on demonstration of filling defects in the angiographically opacified left atrium. In the past, these methods included intravenous angiocardiography, left atrial angiography following direct percutaneous puncture of the left atrium or atrial transseptal catheterization, and pulmonary angiography. Because it provides better resolution than intravenous angiocardiography and is safer than direct left atrial angiography,[21] pulmonary angiography had been the preferred diagnostic method until it was replaced by echocardiography. Recently, coronary angiographic demonstration of coronary neovascularization has been recognized as a specific sign for the presence of left atrial appendage thrombi in patients with mitral stenosis.[15] Coronary angiography is an established and safe invasive procedure. Its use in patients with mitral stenosis can not only delineate their coronary anatomy but also aid in detecting thrombi in the left atrial appendage area.

Currently used noninvasive and invasive diagnostic methods for detection of left atrial thrombi are elaborated below.

Transthoracic Two-dimensional Echocardiography

Transthoracic two-dimensional echocardiography, a safe noninvasive test, allows serial followup examinations of patients and is therefore the diagnostic technique of choice for detecting left atrial thrombi. However, the diagnostic sensitivity of transthoracic two-dimensional echocardiography for detecting left atrial thrombi depends on the size and the location of the thrombi. The majority of left atrial thrombi cannot be detected by this technique because most of the thrombi are confined within and around the left atrial appendage,[12] which is not well visualized by transthoracic two-dimensional echocardiography. The technique is also insensitive in detecting small thrombi with a diameter < 1 cm in the left atrial cavity.[12] The overall reported sensitivity of transthoracic two-dimensional echocardiography for detecting left atrial thrombi found at mitral valve surgery is 50 to 59% and its specificity is 98 to 100%. For thrombi in the left atrial cavity, Shrestha and associates[12] reported a sensitivity of 75%, Beppu and associates[13] 78%, and Bansal and associates[14] 71%. For detecting left atrial appendage thrombi, Beppu and associates reported a sensitivity of 35% and Bansal and associates a sensitivity of 17%. Shrestha and associates missed all the left atrial appendage thrombi found at surgery.

Transesophageal Echocardiography

The recently introduced transesophageal echocardiographic method readily visualizes the left atrium because of its close proximity to the esophageal transducer. Therefore, transesophageal echocardiography is very useful in detecting thrombi in the left atrial appendage, and it complements the traditional transthoracic two-dimensional echocardiographic examination. In studies of limited numbers of patients,[16-18] diagnostic sensitivity of transesophageal echocardiography for left atrial appendage thrombi confirmed at surgery was reported to be 90 to 100% and the specificity to be 98 to 100%.

Coronary Angiography

In 1975 Standen, using selective coronary angiography, described "tumor vascularity" with abnormal vessels arising from the left circumflex artery to the left atrium in a patient with severe mitral stenosis.[22] A left atrial thrombus was found at surgery. Since then, sporadic case reports have also described abnormal vessels from the circumflex arteries or coronary neovascularization with fistula formation to the left atrium in patients with severe mitral stenosis who had left atrial appendage thrombi.[23-26] Colman and associates,[11] on the other hand, in a retrospective study of a large number of patients with mitral valve disease, have shown coronary neovascularization with fistula formation to be a specific sign for the presence of left atrial thrombi.

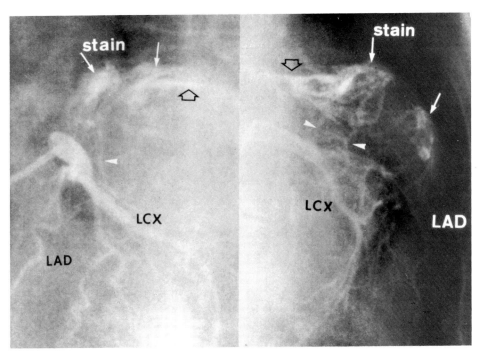

Figure 11.1 Coronary angiograms in left anterior oblique (*left*) and right anterior oblique (*right*) views showing neovascularizations (*white arrowheads*) arising from the left circumflex (*LCX*) artery with fistula formation manifested by a dense mass stain (*white arrows*) and squirting of contrast material into the left atrial cavity (*wide hollow arrows*). LAD—left anterior descending artery. (From: Fu et al: Coronary neovascularization as a specific sign for left atrial appendage thrombus in mitral stenosis. *Am J Cardiol.* 67:1158–1160, 1991. With permission.)

Combined Coronary Angiography and Transthoracic Two-dimensional Echocardiography

To study their diagnostic values for detecting left atrial thrombi in severe rheumatic mitral stenosis, we correlated coronary angiographic findings of neovascularization (Fig. 11.1) and transthoracic two-dimensional echocardiographic findings of left atrial thrombi with the presence or absence of thrombi at surgery in 75 consecutive patients.[15] This prospective study was conducted before the era of percutaneous balloon mitral valvuloplasty at our institution. The diagnostic sensitivity and specificity and the positive predictive accuracy of coronary neovascularization for detecting left atrial thrombi were respectively 58%, 98%, and 95%. The diagnostic sensitivity and specificity, and the positive predictive accuracy of positive transthoracic two-dimensional echocardiographic findings in detecting left atrial thrombi were respectively 45%, 86%, and 71%. When these methods were combined, the diagnostic sensitivity increased to 73%. Our study also showed that coronary neovascularization with fistula formation is specific for left atrial thrombi in the appendage area, and coronary angiographic findings of neovascularization with fistula formation also complements transthoracic two-dimensional echocardiography's 98 to 100% specificity[13-15] in detecting cavity thrombi in the left atrium. When transesophageal echocardiography is not available or when the patient cannot tolerate it, coronary angiography, though having a sensitivity of only 58%, may be used as a next best alternative for detection of left atrial appendage thrombi.

PERCUTANEOUS BALLOON MITRAL VALVULOPLASTY AND LEFT ATRIAL THROMBUS

Unsuspected Left Atrial Thrombi

Prior to the advent of transesophageal echocardiography, candidates for the percutaneous balloon mitral valvuloplasty procedure were screened by the insensitive transthoracic two-dimensional echocardiographic method for the presence of left atrial thrombus. Since transthoracic two-dimensional echocardiography is insensitive in detecting left atrial thrombi, it is estimated that 9 to 10% of the patients who underwent percutaneous balloon mitral valvuloplasty had unsuspected left thrombi, particularly in the appendage area. This estimate is derived with an assumed average incidence of left atrial thrombi of 18% (Table 11.1) and a transthoracic two-dimensional echocardiographic sensitivity of 50 to 58%.

The reported incidence of embolic complications in percutaneous balloon mitral valvuloplasty has ranged from 1.4 to 4% in large series of patients.[6-8] Whether the complication resulted from dislodgement of unsuspected left atrial thrombi is difficult to ascertain. In our experience with percutaneous balloon mitral valvuloplasty using the Inoue balloon catheter technique performed between January 1987 and December 1989 in 219 patients,[6] systemic embolism occurred in three patients (1.4%): two overly prolonged procedures in our early experience and one patient in whom heparin administration after transseptal catheterization was delayed. The embolism appeared to be related to inadequate heparinization rather than dislodgement of unsuspected left atrial thrombi. Embolization has not occurred in any of 36 patients with a history of systemic embolism nor in the 9 patients in whom percutaneous balloon mitral valvuloplasty was performed after resolution of left atrial cavity thrombi.[6]

Detected Left Atrial Cavity Thrombi

Although anecdotal evidences suggest that percutaneous balloon mitral valvuloplasty using the Inoue balloon catheter technique is safe in selected patients with left atrial cavity thrombi detected by transthoracic two-dimensional echocardiography, the feasibility and safety of the procedure in such patients deserve careful future study. Inoue has performed uncomplicated percutaneous balloon mitral valvuloplasty in a limited number of patients with left atrial thrombi treated with warfarin for 4 to 6 weeks before the procedure. These thrombi were thus regarded as old and organized.

By transthoracic two-dimensional echocardiographic studies, we recently observed incidental resolution of thrombi in the left atrial cavity in two patients with severe rheumatic mitral stenosis — one after 1 year of warfarin treatment (Fig. 11.2) and the other after 8 months of treatment. Percutaneous balloon mitral valvuloplasty using the Inoue balloon catheter technique was performed successfully and without complication in both patients.[27] Despite the likely presence of residual left atrial appendage thrombi in the patients, we felt it safe to proceed with the procedure on the

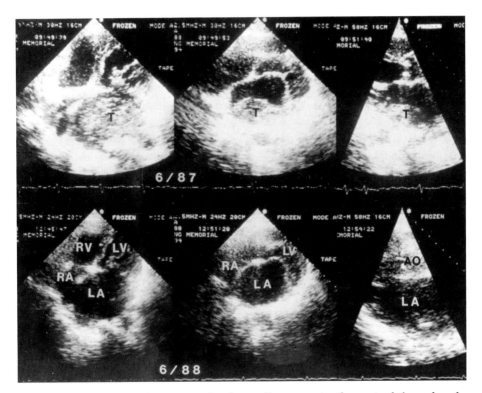

Figure 11.2 *Top,* Two-dimensional echocardiograms in the apical four-chamber (*left*), the modified parasternal short-axis (*middle*), and the parasternal long-axis (*right*) views show a large thrombus attached to the posterolateral and the superior walls of the left atrium. Bottom, The thrombus is not seen 1 year later in comparable views. *AO*—aorta. *LA*—left atrium. *LV*—left ventricle. *RA*—right atrium. *RV*—right ventricle. *T*—thrombus. (From: Hung et al: Successful percutaneous transvenous catheter balloon mitral commissurotomy after warfarin therapy and resolution of left atrial thrombus. *Am J Cardiol.* 64: 126–128, 1989.)

following two premises. First, the thrombi, if any, were well organized since the patients had received long-term warfarin treatment. Second, as we have become proficient in the procedure, potential contact between the Inoue balloon catheter and the appendage area of the left atrium could be minimized or avoided. This was later proved by intraoperative transesophageal echocardiographic monitoring of percutaneous balloon mitral valvuloplasty using the Inoue balloon catheter technique to be discussed later. This unprecedented observation has prompted us to design a prospective study investigating the natural history of left atrial thrombi in patients under long-term warfarin therapy by performing serial transthoracic two-dimensional echocardiography at 3-month intervals. In this ongoing prospective study, we have further observed resolution of left atrial cavity thrombi after 3 to 12 months (mean 8) of warfarin treatment in 11 patients with mitral stenosis — 5 men and 6 women, aged 36 to 65 years. All 11 patients had atrial fibrillation. Before percutaneous balloon mitral valvuloplasty, 9 of the 11 patients were examined by transesophageal echocardiography after the latter became available. All 9 patients were found to have left atrial appendage thrombi.

This limited experience indicates that it is feasible to manage patients with severe mitral stenosis and left atrial cavity thrombi under warfarin treatment if their clinical and hemodynamic status does not warrant immediate surgery. If the thrombus resolves, percutaneous balloon mitral valvuloplasty using the Inoue balloon catheter technique can then be performed safely. Further documentation awaits completion of our ongoing study of left atrial thrombus resolution in patients with mitral stenosis under warfarin treatment.

Left Atrial Appendage Thrombi

Prior to the advent of transesophageal echocardiography, detection of left atrial thrombi in candidates for the procedure was solely dependent on the use of transthoracic two-dimensional echocardiography, as transesophageal echocardiography improves accuracy in diagnosing left atrial appendage thrombi, a new issue arises: should patients with thrombi confined in the left atrial appendage, as detected by transesophageal echocardiography, be denied the potential benefits of percutaneous balloon mitral valvuloplasty and instead be subjected to mitral valve surgery? In a series of staged studies, we systematically investigated the feasibility and safety of percutaneous balloon mitral valvuloplasty using the Inoue balloon catheter technique in patients with left atrial appendage thrombi.

Appendage Thrombi Detected by Coronary Angiography

Between January 1989 and December 1989, in a prospective study of 116 consecutive patients, coronary angiography was performed after the completion of percutaneous balloon mitral valvuloplasty rather than before, to detect coronary neovascularization and fistula formation. The patients were 27 men and 89 women, aged 20 to 76 (mean 43). Forty-eight patients were in sinus rhythm, including 3 with a history of paroxysmal atrial fibrillation. The other 68 had atrial fibrillation. Percutaneous balloon mitral valvuloplasty was successful and uncomplicated in all patients. Coronary neovascularization and fistula formation were demonstrated in 23 patients (20%). All of these patients had atrial fibrillation, representing 34% of those patients with atrial fibrillation. One patient with atrial fibrillation and coronary neovascularization had a cerebral artery embolism manifested by hemiparesis which resolved over several months. Whether the embolism was caused by dislodgement of the thrombus is not known. Assuming a sensitivity of 58% and a positive predictive accuracy of 95% for diagnosis of left atrial appendage thrombi by coronary angiographic findings of neovascularization,[15] the estimated number of patients with left atrial appendage thrombi unsuspected by transthoracic two-dimensional echocardiography would have been 23 × 0.95/0.58, or 38. Therefore, the estimated embolic risk of percutaneous balloon mitral valvuloplasty using the Inoue balloon catheter technique in patients with left atrial appendage thrombi was 1/38 or 2.6%, which is comparable to the embolic rates of 1.4 to 4.0% in percutaneous balloon mitral valvuloplasty performed in large numbers of patients.[6-8]

Intraoperative Biplane Transesophageal Echocardiography during Percutaneous Balloon Mitral Valvuloplasty

To investigate whether the left atrial appendage area would be trespassed by the guidewire and the balloon catheter during percutaneous balloon mitral valvuloplasty using the Inoue balloon catheter technique, the entire procedure was monitored by biplane transesophageal echocardiography (Aloka SSD 870 CFM system) performed at our institution by Dr. Shunei Kyo of Saitama Medical College, Japan. The patients were two men and five women, aged 28 to 65. All had atrial fibrillation. Left atrial appendage thrombi undetected by transthoracic two-dimensional echocardiography was identified by transesophageal echocardiographic in five patients. The intraoperative transesophageal echocardiographic findings were blind to the author who performed percutaneous balloon mitral valvuloplasty.

After atrial transseptal puncture, an Inoue balloon catheter was introduced to the left atrium over a floppy-tipped guidewire coiled in the left atrium, and the catheter tip was placed near the mitral orifice (Fig. 11.3). A high-torque spring-wire stylet with a preformed J tip was inserted into the balloon catheter to direct the balloon tip toward the mitral valve so that it crossed the stenosed valve and passed into the left ventricle (Fig. 11.4). The balloon inflation procedure is shown in Figure 11.5. The transesophageal echocardiographic examinations did not detect any contact between the guidewire/catheter and the left atrial appendage area or thrombi within the appendage. Percutaneous balloon mitral valvuloplasty was successful and uncomplicated in all seven patients.

The study confirmed that contact of the balloon catheter with the left atrial appendage can be avoided when percutaneous balloon mitral valvuloplasty is properly executed using the Inoue balloon catheter technique. Use of a coiled tipped guidewire and a high-torque spring-wire stylet enables the operator to steer the balloon catheter away from the left atrial appendage area. This ability to "steer" the Inoue device is a critical advantage of its use when atrial appendage thrombi are present.[28]

Left Atrial Appendage Thrombi Diagnosed by Transesophageal Echocardiography

Kronzon and associates[9] reported uncomplicated percutaneous balloon mitral valvuloplasty in a patient with metastatic cancer having transesophageal echocardiographic findings of a 3-cm thrombus that filled the left atrial appendage,

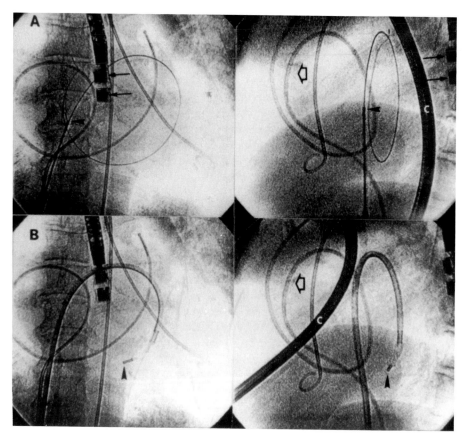

Figure 11.3 Angiographic frontal (*left*) and lateral (*right*) views showing the guidewire and the Inoue balloon catheter remaining clear of the left appendage area (*wide hollow arrows*). *A,* After atrial transseptal puncture, a floppy-tipped guidewire is introduced and coiled in the left atrium. An Inoue balloon catheter with its balloon segment stretched is advanced over the guidewire to the atrial septum (*arrowheads*). *B,* After its entry into the left atrium, the balloon segment is de-stretched, the catheter tip (*arrowheads*) is placed near the mitral orifice, and the guidewire is removed. Biplane transesophageal tranducers (*arrows*), a Swan-Ganz balloon catheter in the pulmonary artery, and a pigtail catheter in the left ventricle are also seen in all frames. *C*—Cord of the transducer.

extended into the adjacent portion of the left atrium, and exhibited some independent motion during the cardiac cycle. The technique of the valvuloplasty was not specified, but we assumed it to be the double-balloon technique.

Since transesophageal echocardiography became available at our institution in mid-1990, 24 patients with left atrial appendage thrombi documented by transesophageal echocardiography have undergone percutaneous balloon mitral valvuloplasty using the Inoue balloon catheter technique — successfully and without complications. They were 7 men and 17 women, aged 26 to 66 years. All had atrial fibrillation. The group included 9 patients who had left atrial cavity thrombi resolved after warfarin therapy, as stated previously.

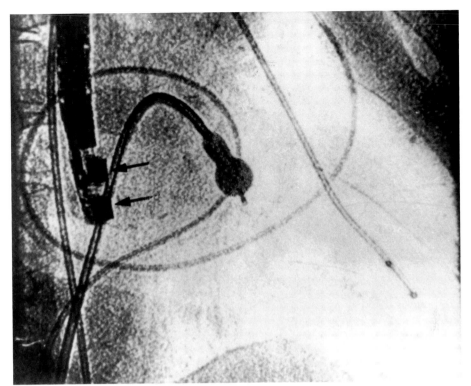

Figure 11.4 Angiographic right anterior oblique view of the Inoue balloon catheter after insertion of a J-tipped spring-wire stylet. The high-torque stylet provides the catheter with an excellent steerability. *Arrows* indicate the biplane transesophageal tranducers.

On the basis of the foregoing circumstantial and direct evidence, the author feels it safe to perform percutaneous balloon mitral valvuloplasty using the Inoue balloon catheter technique in patients with left atrial appendage thrombi. However, the view may be disputed by others, especially by those who perform percutaneous balloon mitral valvuloplasty with other techniques. For those who disagree, our preliminary finding of resolution of left atrial appendage thrombus after warfarin treatment in patients with mitral stenosis[30] may provide an alternative in management of such patients. One may elect to administer warfarin to the patients with mitral stenosis and left atrial appendage thrombus if their clinical and hemodynamic status does not warrant immediate surgery. If the thrombus resolves, percutaneous balloon mitral valvuloplasty can then be performed safely.

ANTICOAGULATION

The policy of routine warfarin therapy pretreatment for all percutaneous balloon mitral valvuloplasty patients was modified after the first 70 cases.[6] Our current policy is to treat patients with a history of systemic embolism with warfarin for 4 to 6 weeks

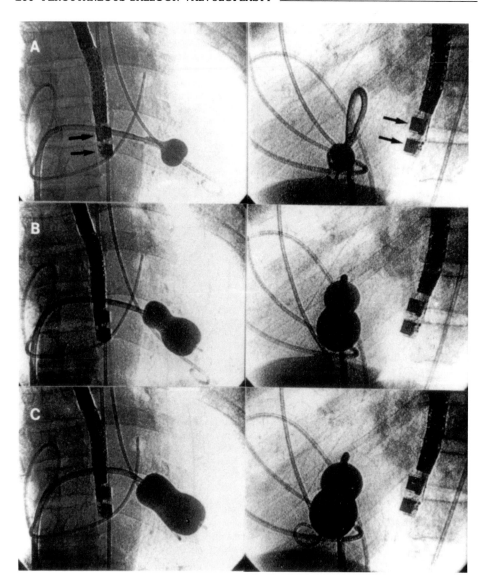

Figure 11.5 Sequence of mitral valve dilation using Inoue size-adjustable balloon catheter in angiographic frontal (*left*) and lateral (*right*) views. *A*, The catheter with its more compliant distal half partially inflated is pulled back to anchor the balloon at the mitral valve. *B*, As the proximal balloon is inflated, a waist is created by the stenosed valve. *C*, at full inflation, the waist disappears as the commissures are split. Repeat inflations with larger balloon diameters may be performed (stepwise dilation technique) until satisfactory hemodynamic results are obtained. Biplane transephageal transducers (*arrows*), a Swan-Ganz balloon catheter in the pulmonary artery, and a pigtail catheter in the left ventricle are also seen in all frames.

before percutaneous balloon mitral valvuloplasty. In addition, patients with left atrial cavity thrombi are given long-term warfarin therapy so that we can study the natural history of the thrombus under warfarin therapy. In patients treated with warfarin, the drug is discontinued several days before percutaneous balloon mitral valvuloplasty, and intravenous heparin is given until several hours before the procedure. Heparin, 1 mg per kg body weight, is given immediately following the transseptal puncture of the interatrial septum as in every percutaneous balloon mitral valvuloplasty procedure to prevent thromboembolic complications. It cannot be overemphasized that intravenous heparin must be given immediately after confirming entry of the transseptal catheter into the left atrium, and should be supplemented if the procedure is prolonged.

CONCLUSIONS

At present, the presence of a left atrial thrombus is generally considered to be a contraindication for balloon catheter intervention procedures for mitral stenosis. However, it is feasible and safe to perform percutaneous balloon mitral valvuloplasty using the Inoue balloon catheter technique in selected patients with left atrial thrombi, provided that the procedure is executed with proper care. Although the risk of embolization is nominal, it must be carefully considered by the individual operator in relation to the anticipated benefit from percutaneous balloon mitral valvuloplasty.

Patients with left atrial cavity thrombi can be managed under long-term warfarin treatment if their clinical and hemodynamic status does not warrant immediate surgery. When the thrombus resolves, percutaneous balloon mitral valvuloplasty using the Inoue balloon catheter technique can then be applied safely. However, a mobile thrombus in the left atrium is a high risk for systemic embolization, and it deserves urgent surgical intervention.

Uncomplicated percutaneous balloon mitral valvuloplasty using the Inoue balloon catheter technique after 4 to 6 weeks of warfarin treatment in a limited number of patients with left atrial thrombus who were thought to be at high risk for mitral valve surgery suggests that the procedure is safe in selected patients with organized left atrial cavity thrombi. However, the feasibility and safety of percutaneous balloon mitral valvuloplasty in such patients deserve careful future study.

Mounting evidence, both direct and indirect, indicates that it is safe to perform percutaneous balloon mitral valvuloplasty using the Inoue balloon catheter technique in patients with left atrial appendage thrombi. In the rare instances of left atrial thrombi situated in the atrial septum and of thrombi that obstruct the mitral orifice or the pulmonary veins, percutaneous balloon mitral valvuloplasty is considered absolutely contraindicated.

REFERENCES

1. Inoue K, Owaki T, Nakamura T, et al: Clinical application of transvenous mitral commissurotomy by a new balloon catheter. *J Thorac Cardiovasc Surg.* 87:394–402, 1984.

2. Inoue K, Hung JS: Percutaneous transvenous mitral commissurotomy (PTMC): the Far East experience. In: Topol EJ: *Textbook of Interventional Cardiology.* 1st ed. Philadelphia: WB Saunders Co., 1990, pp 887–899.

3. Nobuyoshi M, Hamasaki N, Kimura T, et al: Indications, complications, and short-term clinical outcome of percutaneous transvenous mitral commissurotomy. *Circulation.* 80:782–792, 1989.

4. Hung JS, Fu M, Yeh SJ, et al: Hemodynamic and clinical efficacies of catheter balloon percutaneous transvenous mitral commissurotomy: experience of 100 patients with rheumatic mitral stenosis. *J Formosan Med Assoc* 89:182–189, 1990.

5. Chen CR, Hu SW, Chen JY, et al: Percutaneous mitral valvuloplasty with a single rubber-nylon balloon (Inoue balloon): long-term results in 71 patients. *Am Heart J.* 120:561–568, 1990.

6. Hung JS, Chern MS, Wu JJ, et al: Short- and long-term results of catheter balloon percutaneous transvenous mitral commissurotomy. *Am J Cardiol.* 67:854–862, 1991.

7. Vahanian A, Michel PL, Cormier B, et al: Results of percutaneous mitral commissurotomy in 200 patients. *Am J Cardiol.* 63:847–852, 1989.

8. Ruiz CE, Allen JW, Lau FYK: Percutaneous double balloon valvotomy for severe rheumatic mitral stenosis. *Am J Cardiol.* 65:473–477, 1990.

9. Babic UU, Dorros G, Pejcic P, et al: Percutaneous mitral valvuloplasty: retrograde, transarterial double-balloon technique utilizing the transseptal approach. *Cathet Cardiovasc Diagn.* 14:229–237, 1988.

10. Nichols HT, Blanco G, Morse DP, et al: Open mitral commissurotomy. Experience with 200 consecutive cases. *JAMA.* 182:268–270, 1962.

11. Colman T, de Ubago JLM, Figueroa A, et al: Coronary arteriography and atrial thrombosis in mitral valve disease. *Am J Cardiol.* 47:973–977, 1981.

12. Shrestha NK, Morena FL, Narciso FV, et al: Two-dimensional echocardiographic diagnosis of left atrial thrombus in rheumatic heart disease. A clinicopathologic study. *Circulation.* 67:341–347, 1983.

13. Beppu S, Park YD, Sakakibara H, et al: Clinical features of intracardiac thrombosis based on echocardiographic observation. *Jpn Circ J.* 48:75–82, 1984.

14. Bansal RC, Heywood JT, Applegate PM, et al: Detection of left atrial thrombi by two-dimensional echocardiography and surgical correlation in 148 patients with mitral valve disease. *Am J Cardiol.* 64:243–246, 1989.

15. Fu M, Hung JS, Lee CB, et al: Coronary neovascularization as a specific sign for left atrial appendage thrombus in mitral stenosis. *Am J Cardiol.* 67:1158–1160, 1991.

16. Aschenberg W, Schlüter M, Kremer P, et al: Transesophageal two-dimensional echocardiography for the detection of left atrial appendage thrombus. *J Am Coll Cardiol.* 7:163–166, 1986.

17. Mügge A, Daniel WG, Hausmann D, et al: Diagnosis of left atrial appendage thrombi by transesophageal echocardiography: clinical implications and follow-up. *Am J Cardiac Imaging.* 4:173–179, 1990.

18. Wang, XF, Li ZA, Cheng TO, et al: Biplane transesophageal echocardiography. An anatomic-ultrasonic-clinical correlative study. *Am Heart J.* in press for April, 1992.

19. Lie JT, Entman ML: "Hole-in-one" sudden death: mitral stenosis and left atrial ball thrombus. *Am Heart J.* 91:798–804, 1976.

20. Tomoda H, Hoshiai M, Furuya H, et al: Evaluation of intracardiac thrombus with computed tomography. *Am J Cardiol.* 51:843–852, 1983.

21. Parker BM, Friedenberg MJ, Templeton AW, et al: Preoperative angiocardiographic diagnosis of left atrial thrombi in mitral stenosis. *N Engl J Med.* 273:136–140, 1965.

22. Standen JR: "Tumor vascularity" in left atrial thrombus demonstrated by selective coronary arteriography. *Radiology.* 116:549–550, 1975.

23. Soulen RL, Grollman JH Jr, Paglia D, et al: Coronary neovascularity and fistula formation. A sign of mural thrombus. *Circulation.* 56:663–666, 1977.

24. Bochna AJ, Falicov RE: Diagnosis of intracardiac thrombi in mitral stenosis and left ventricular dysfunction. Use of selective coronary arteriography. *Arch Intern Med.* 140:759–762, 1980.

25. Cipriano PR, Guthaner DF: Organized left atrial mural thrombus demonstrated by coronary angiography. *Am Heart J.* 96:166–169, 1978.

26. Hubbard WN, Hine AL, Rubens M, et al: Visualization of left atrial thrombi by coronary arteriography. *Cathet Cardiovasc Diagn.* 13:22–25, 1987.

27. Hung JS, Lin FC, Chiang CW: Successful percutaneous transvenous catheter balloon mitral commissurotomy after warfarin therapy and resolution of left atrial thrombus. *Am J Cardiol.* 64:126–128, 1989.

28. Nishimura RA, Holmes DR Jr, Reeder GS: Efficacy of percutaneous mitral balloon valvuloplasty with the Inoue balloon. *Mayo Clin Proc.* 66:276–282, 1991.

29. Kronzon I, Tunick PA, Glassman E, et al: Transesophageal echocardiography to detect atrial clots in candidates for percutaneous transseptal mitral balloon valvuloplasty. *J Am Coll Cardiol.* 16:1320–1322, 1990.

30. Tsai LM, Hung JS, Chen JH, et al: Resolution of left atrial appendage thrombus in mitral stenosis after warfarin therapy. *Am Heart J.* 121:1232–1234, 1991.

Mitral Restenosis: The Cordoba–Las Palmas Experience

ALFONSO MEDINA
JOSÉ SUÁREZ DE LEZO
ENRIQUE HERNÁNDEZ
MANUEL PAN
MIGUEL ROMERO
FRANCISCO MELIAN
EVA LARAUDOGOITIA
DJORDJE PAVLOVIC

Percutaneous balloon mitral valvuloplasty was originally described in 1984[1] after the initial success of separating fused commissures of the mitral valve under direct vision as an auxiliary means of open mitral commissurotomy.[2] It has become established as a nonsurgical alternative in the treatment of isolated mitral stenosis.[3-10] An optimal palliation is more frequently obtained in valves with a preserved anatomy in which stenosis is based mainly on the presence of commissural fusion.[6] Intraoperative and postmortem studies have clearly shown that in valves that are not heavily calcified, successful percutaneous balloon mitral valvuloplasty is associated with splitting of fused commissures toward the mitral annulus.[11] On the other hand, in valves with an advanced degree of calcification, immediate and mid-term results are poorer[7,12] and consequently these patients are treated with surgery unless they are poor surgical candidates.

This chapter reports the experience of the universities of Cordoba and Las Palmas, Spain, with percutaneous balloon mitral valvuloplasty. From May 1986 to January 1991 we studied 300 patients with mitral stenosis from our two institutions who were treated by this procedure.

METHODS

Patients were chosen as candidates on the basis of the following criteria: no evidence of left atrial thrombus (in the last 90 patients transesophageal echocardiography was performed), no recent history of systemic embolism, and no greater than grade 2 of pre-existing mitral regurgitation. Sixty-two patients experienced restenosis after surgical commissurotomy and will be discussed later. All patients underwent clinical and noninvasive studies before and after balloon valvuloplasty. At cardiac catheterization, the diagnostic phase included simultaneous pressure measurements, cardiac output determination, and left ventricular angiography before and after balloon valvuloplasty. The left ventriculogram was carefully analyzed and quantified for volume, ejection fraction, and the degree of subvalvular fibrosis. The subvalvular fibrosis was quantified by the distance ratio (DR), which has been described as an indicator of the degree of subvalvular disease and a useful parameter in predicting the need for valve replacement in patients with mitral stenosis.[13] Patients over 40 years of age also underwent coronary angiography. In 260 patients, clinical and echocardiographic followup studies were performed 21 ± 11 months (range 1–60 mo) after the balloon valvuloplasty. In 62 patients, hemodynamic evaluation was performed 21 ± 8 months later after the balloon valvuloplasty. We used two different techniques of balloon valvuloplasty. In 260 patients we performed the transarterial single trefoil or bifoil balloon technique, as described by Babic and associates[14]; the transvenous Inoue technique was performed in 40 patients.

Transarterial Trefoil or Bifoil Technique

A long guidewire was introduced into the right femoral vein through a flow-directed balloon catheter and advanced transseptally to the left ventricle and aorta; there, it was caught using an intravascular retrieval set. The guidewire was subsequently drawn out of the body through the left femoral artery to establish a long guidewire-exteriorized circuit. At this point, a single trefoil or bifoil balloon catheter was inserted from the left femoral artery over the guidewire and advanced to the level of the mitral valve. Once the catheter was stabilized within the mitral valve, the balloon was inflated. A trefoil balloon (3×15 mm) was used in 18 patients and a bifoil (2×15 or 2×19 mm) was used in 242 patients (Fig. 12.1A). Balloon size was selected on the basis of echocardiographic and angiographic measurements of the mitral annulus. After the transseptal puncture all patients were given an intravenous infusion of heparin.

Inoue Balloon Technique

The procedure was performed using the Inoue balloon catheter (Fig. 12.1B) introduced through the femoral vein after the vascular access and atrial septum had been dilated by means of a special guidewire previously positioned in the left atrium after a conventional transseptal puncture.[1] The Inoue balloon catheter was passed to the left atrium with the aid of a metal tube that stiffens and slenderizes the balloon. Once in the left atrium the metal tube and guidewire were removed and the balloon was inflated with CO_2 to become a flow-directed catheter. With a preshaped J-tipped spring-wire stylet the crossing of the mitral valve can be accomplished without much difficulty. In the left ventricle the balloon was inflated with diluted contrast medium until the CO_2 was flushed out through a vent. After the vent was closed a syringe containing a predetermined amount of diluted contrast medium was connected to the two-way stopcock of the outer lumen. With the distal portion of the balloon partially inflated the balloon was moved back and forth two or three times inside the left

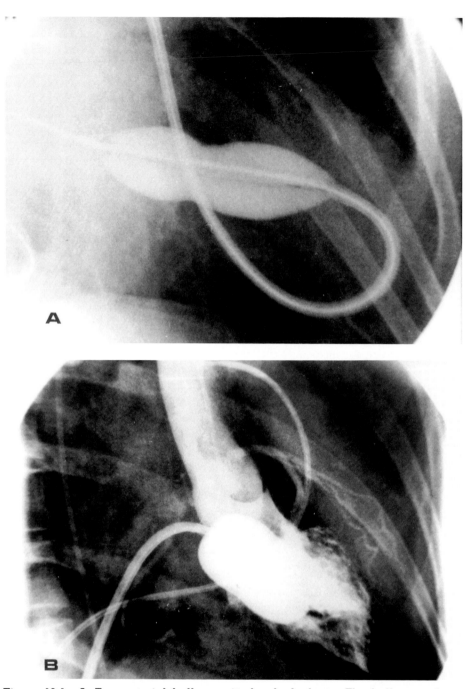

Figure 12.1 *A*, Transarterial balloon mitral valvuloplasty. The balloon catheter (bifoil 2×17) is inflated across the mitral valve. *B*, The transseptal Inoue balloon catheter is clearly visible across the mitral valve with the aid of contrast injected into the left ventricle.

ventricle to ascertain that it was free in the left ventricular cavity. The catheter was then pulled until resistance was felt at the level of the mitral valve, and the balloon was quickly inflated until the waist disappeared. At the conclusion of the dilation procedure the balloon was removed by means of the guidewire and metal tube.

IMMEDIATE RESULTS

The immediate results in our series of 300 patients showed a significant increase in mitral valve area (1 ± 0.3 to 2 ± 0.7 cm$_2$) and a significant decrease in mitral gradient (18 ± 8 to 6 ± 4 mmHg) and mean pulmonary artery pressure (33 ± 12 to 23 ± 12 mmHg).

COMPLICATIONS

Complications included an overall in-hospital mortality of 2.7%. Early mitral surgery was required in 2.3% of patients. Cerebral embolic accident occurred in three patients (1%), two of whom had a partial recovery. Cardiac tamponade was detected and treated in eight patients. Three patients with cardiac tamponade needed emergency surgery, and two with ventricular perforation died. The remaining six did well without surgery after a successful dilation.

VALVULOPLASTY IN ACUTE PULMONARY EDEMA

Seven patients developed acute pulmonary edema[15] during the diagnostic period. In all of them the acute pulmonary edema disappeared immediately after an emergency balloon mitral valvuloplasty was successfully accomplished.

MILD MITRAL STENOSIS

Although balloon mitral valvuloplasty is generally recommended for moderate to severe mitral stenosis, we have studied a small group of patients (n = 21) with mild mitral stenosis (baseline area >1.5 cm^2).[16] Immediate and followup results were excellent. There were no major complications in this group.

FACTORS INFLUENCING AN OPTIMAL RESULT

We studied factors determining an optimal result, defined as a final mitral valve area of >1.5 cm^2, an increase of at least 75%, and a postvalvuloplasty mitral regurgitation less than grade 2.[17] The univariate analysis identified the presence of sinus rhythm, a younger age, the presence of a pliable valve, and the absence of pre-procedure mitral regurgitation as clinical predictors of optimal results. However, other clinical factors such as functional class, a history of previous surgical commissurotomy, or sex did not significantly influence the final result. The multivariate analysis identified the presence of a pliable valve and the absence of pre-procedure mitral regurgitation as independent predictors of an optimal result.

DETERMINANTS OF PROGRESSION OF MITRAL REGURGITATION

We also studied factors determining progression of mitral regurgitation, which was defined as the increase in mitral regurgitation to grade 2 or more after balloon mitral valvuloplasty.[18] Progression of mitral regurgitation occurred in 18% of our patients. The univariate analysis indicated an older age, a smaller mitral valve area, the presence of atrial fibrillation, the presence of mild mitral regurgitation, a larger left atrium, a larger left ventricular end-diastolic volume, and a lower ejection fraction as significant factors influencing progression. In the multivariate analysis the independent predictor factors were an older age, a higher baseline left ventricular end-diastolic volume, and a lower ejection fraction.

COMBINED PROCEDURES

Combined procedures were performed in 27 patients. In 25 a sequential dilation of both mitral and aortic valves was performed.[19] In all of them we used a transarterial retrograde technique, dilating the aortic valve first. In one patient dilation of the mitral and tricuspid valves was performed[20] in the same procedure. In another patient a concurrent angioplasty of the proximal right coronary artery was also performed in the same procedure.

MITRAL RESTENOSIS AFTER SURGICAL COMMISSUROTOMY

In western nations, where the incidence of rheumatic fever has decreased dramatically in the last few decades, new cases of isolated mitral stenosis are relatively rare. However, there is an increasing number of patients who have already undergone surgical commissurotomy, frequently more than 10 years before presentation. The morphology of the mitral valve in most cases is not essentially different from that observed in unoperated mitral stenosis, mainly in the same age groups.[21,22] Thus, as surgery in mitral restenosis is associated with a higher risk and patients are frequently treated with mitral valve replacement, percutaneous balloon mitral valvuloplasty seems to be a very attractive therapeutic alternative.[23-25] Since the initial report,[21] several series have been published showing encouraging initial and midterm followup results.[22,26]

THE CORDOBA-LAS PALMAS EXPERIENCE: A COMPARATIVE STUDY

Of 300 patients, 62 (group A) had undergone closed (n = 42) or open (n = 20) surgical commissurotomy, 16 ± 7 years before. Four of them had undergone two previous closed mitral valve operations. The remaining 238 patients had not undergone previous surgery (group B). Our comparative study focuses on baseline clinical profile, immediate results including complication rate, and a 5-year followup analysis.

Data are expressed as mean ± standard deviation (SD). Differences in group means were analyzed with use of the unpaired t-test. The paired t-test was used for comparing the changes after balloon valvuloplasty. Differences between categorical data were estimated by means of the chi-square test. Five-year event-free probability curves were constructed using the Kaplan-Meier methods. Differences between curves were analyzed by the log-rank test. Significance was established at the level of $p < 0.05$.

Immediate Results

Table 12.1 summarizes the clinical, echocardiographic, and hemodynamic profiles of both groups before percutaneous balloon mitral valvuloplasty. Age, sex, incidence of sinus rhythm, functional class, history of embolism, and frequency of associated balloon aortic valvuloplasty were similar in both groups. In group A there was a greater frequency of associated mild aortic regurgitation. M-mode echocardiographic findings showed a similar EF slope in both groups, but the DE amplitude was lower in group A. Two-dimensional echocardiographic findings showed a significant difference in the morphology of the mitral valve. The incidence of pliable valves was

Table 12.1   BASELINE DATA FOR PATIENTS IN CORDOBA–LAS PALMAS STUDY

	Group A: Restenosis n = 62	Group B: Unoperated n = 238	p value
Clinical Findings			
Age, yr	45 ± 12	46 ± 13	ns
Sex, % *female*	83%	77%	ns
Sinus rhythm	40%	51%	ns
Functional class			ns
II	21%	38%	
III–IV	79%	62%	
Previous embolism	8%	7%	ns
Mild aortic regurgitation	26%	47%	<0.01
Associated aortic dilation	3%	10%	ns
Echocardiographic Findings			
"DE" amplitude, *mm*	16 ± 5	18 ± 5	<0.05
"EF" slope, *mm/s*	14 ± 6	14 ± 8	ns
Left atrium, *mm*	52 ± 9	50 ± 9	ns
Flexibility			<0.01
Flexible	27%	49%	
Fibrocalcified	73%	51%	
Hemodynamic Findings			
Mild mitral regurgitation	31%	33%	ns
Subvalvular fibrosis (DR)	0.15 ± 0.06	0.17 ± 0.05	ns
Fluoroscopic calcium	29%	24%	ns

DR – distance-ratio.[13]

Table 12.2 RESULTS IN BALLOON VALVULOPLASTY FOR RESTENOSIS. CORDOBA-LAS PALMAS STUDY

		Group A: Restenosis n = 62	Group B: Unoperated n = 238	p value
Gradient, *mmHg*	Pre	19 ± 7	18 ± 8	ns
		p<0.001	p<0.001	
	Post	7 ± 4	7 ± 4	ns
Area, *cm²*	Pre	1.00 ± 0.3	1.02 ± 0.3	ns
		p<0.001	p<0.001	
	Post	2.00 ± 0.7	2.10 ± 0.7	ns
Cardiac output, *L/min*	Pre	4.5 ± 1.2	4.4 ± 1.2	ns
		ns	*ns*	
	Post	4.6 ± 1.3	4.6 ± 1.3	ns
APR, *(Wood U.)*	Pre	2.3 ± 2.5	2.4 ± 2.5	ns
		ns	*ns*	
	Post	2.3 ± 2.0	2.5 ± 2.7	ns
Ejection fraction, %	Pre	57 ± 8	57 ± 9	ns
		ns	*ns*	
	Post	58 ± 6	57 ± 10	ns
Optimal result		55%	51%	ns
Severe mitral regurgitation		8%	6%	ns
Annulus: balloon ratio		1.12 ± 0.2:1	1.17 ± 0.2:1	ns
Mortality		3.2%	2.4%	ns

APR – arteriolar pulmonary resistance.

higher in patients who had not undergone surgery. The hemodynamic and angiographic findings were similar in both groups.

There were no significant differences between the two groups in mitral valve area, grade of mitral regurgitation, or ejection fraction. The DR index[14] was similar in both groups.

Table 12.2 shows the changes induced by balloon valvuloplasty in both groups. There was a similar decrease in mitral gradient and a similar increase in mitral valve area. Cardiac output, pulmonary arteriolar resistance, and ejection fraction did not change significantly after balloon valvuloplasty in either group. Mitral regurgitation (Table 12.2) progressed to grade 2 or more in 12 patients (19%) from group A and in 35 patients (15%) from group B. The development of severe (grade 3 or 4) mitral regurgitation was similar in both groups (8% vs 6%), as was the mortality (3.2% vs 2.4%)

In the group of 300 as a whole, an optimal immediate result, as defined earlier, was obtained in 156 patients (52%), whereas 144 (48%) had a suboptimal result. A similar percentage of patients from both groups had an optimal result (55% vs 51%).

Followup Results

The mean clinical followup for the total series was 21 ± 11 months. At that time, most patients (85%) are event free and have a functional class (NYHA) grade I or II. Restenosis after balloon valvuloplasty was defined as the loss of 50% or more of the initial gain, as determined by echo-Doppler studies and confirmed by hemodynamic

Table 12.3 5-YEAR CUMULATIVE EVENT-FRE PROBABILITY (KAPLAN-MEIER)

	Restenosis	Unoperated	p value
Mortality, %	87 ± 5[a]	93 ± 2	ns
Surgery, %	63 ± 18	93 ± 2	$= 0.07$
Restenosis, %	79 ± 8	98 ± 2	< 0.001

[a] Data are expressed as % $\pm$ SE.

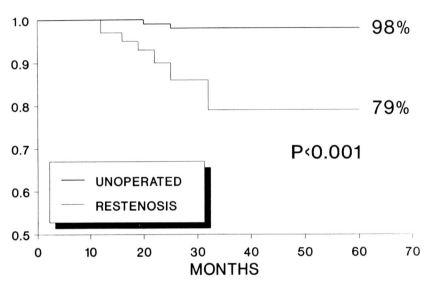

Figure 12.2 Actuarial probability that patient will be free of restenosis.

studies. Based on these criteria restenosis after valvuloplasty was detected in 8 patients, at a mean followup period of 21 ± 6 months (range: 12–32 months). This possibility occurred more frequently in older patients ($p < 0.05$), those with calcified valves ($p < 0.001$), and those who had had a previous surgical commissurotomy ($p < 0.01$). However regarding the comparative study, there were no other differences, in terms of immediate and followup results, between groups A and B. Table 12.3 shows the actuarial probability of an event-free course (no restenosis, need for surgery, or late mortality) in both groups of patients. Figure 12.2 shows a graphical representation of the actuarial probability that the patient will be free of restenosis.

DISCUSSION

Restenosis after surgical commissurotomy is a well-known possibility although its incidence varies according to the series.[23-25,27-29] It has been reported after both open and closed mitral commissurotomy. Investigators at one institution[29] reported that surgical technique (closed vs open) is not a risk factor influencing late death, the need for further surgery, or poor functional status in patients undergoing mitral commissurotomy, and that most cases of clinical recurrence are due to restenosis. In addition, restenosis is probably time related, as other studies suggest.[21,22,26]

The mechanism of restenosis is thought to be fusion of the leaflets, with or without the appearance of degenerative changes (fibrosis and calcification) in the leaflets and the subvalvular apparatus. Additional reasons for clinical deterioration after mitral surgical commissurotomy are operatively induced mitral regurgitation and the presence of cardiac abnormalities unrelated to the mitral valve.[22,25]

The morphology of the mitral valve in patients who have undergone commissurotomy suggests a more advanced degree of disease than that seen in patients who have not been operated on.[21,26] In our series the incidence of pliable valves, as defined by echocardiography, was not so frequent as unoperated patients. However, other baseline characteristics related to the morphology of the mitral valve (calcification on fluorscopy and status of the subvalvular apparatus) were similar in both groups. This might explain the similar proportion of optimal results found in this study. Nevertheless our comparative midterm followup after percutaneous balloon mitral valvuloplasty has shown a significantly higher rate of early restenosis in patients with previous surgery, although numbers are still low. This could be related to the slight difference in the anatomy of the mitral valve at the time of balloon dilation and, at least theoretically, to an individual tendency to recurrence.

However, the 79% 5-year restenosis free probability is an encouraging result and favors percutaneous treatment for this condition in valves with a suitable anatomy. Longer-term followup data are still needed to define more precisely the role of this technique as an alternative to surgery in these patients.

In contrast, there is no information so far regarding the role of percutaneous balloon mitral valvuloplasty in patients with true restenosis after a good immediate result following balloon valvuloplasty. Most of the reported patients with "early" restenosis after balloon valvuloplasty belong to the group with a suboptimal immediate result. These patients frequently have a poorer mitral valve anatomy and therefore should be treated by mitral valve replacement. Perhaps in future reevaluation, patients who currently have an optimal immediate result after percutaneous balloon mitral valvuloplasty and then develop restenosis could be treated with repeated percutaneous balloon mitral valvuloplasty if the mitral valve anatomy is suitable.

REFERENCES

1. Inoue K, Owaki T, Nakamura T, et al: Clinical application of transvenous mitral commissurotomy by a new balloon catheter. *J Thorac Cardiovasc Surg.* 87:394–402, 1984.

2. Inoue K, Hung JS: Percutaneous transvenous mitral commissurotomy (PTMC): the Far East experience. In: Topol EJ: *Textbook of Interventional Cardiology.* Philadelphia:Saunders, Co, 1990, pp 887–899.

3. Herrmann HC, Wilkins GT, Abascal VM, et al: Percutaneous balloon mitral valvotomy for patients with mitral stenosis. Analysis of factors influencing early results. *J Thorac Cardiovasc Surg.* 96:33–38, 1988.

4. Al Zaibag M, Ribeiro PA, Al Kasab S, et al: Percutaneous double-balloon mitral valvotomy for rheumatic mitral-valve stenosis. *Lancet.* 1:757–761, 1986.

5. Medina A, Suarez de Lezo J, Pan M, et al: Papel de la valvuloplastia percutanea en la

estenosis mitral reumatica. Estudio cooperativo Cordoba–Las Palmas. *Rev Esp Cardiol.* 43:640–647, 1990.

6. Smucker ML: Percutaneous mitral balloon valvulotomy or balloon valvuloplasty? It's not just semantics anymore. *Circulation.* 82:643–645, 1990.

7. Palacios IF, Block PC, Wilkins GT, et al: Follow-up of patients undergoing percutaneous mitral balloon valvotomy. Analysis of factors determining restenosis. *Circulation.* 79:573–579, 1989.

8. Vahanian A, Michel PL, Cormier B, et al: Results of percutaneous mitral commissurotomy in 200 patients. *Am J Cardiol.* 63:847–852, 1989.

9. Abascal VM, Wilkins GT, O'Shea JP, et al: Prediction of successful outcome in 130 patients undergoing percutaneous balloon mitral valvotomy. *Circulation.* 82:448–456, 1990.

10. McKay CR, Tawanishi DT, Kotlewsky A, et al: Improvement in exercise capacity and exercise hemodynamics 3 months after double-balloon, catheter balloon valvuloplasty treatment of patients with symptomatic mitral stenosis. *Circulation.* 77:1013–1021, 1988.

11. McKay RG, Lock JE, Safian RD, et al: Balloon dilation of mitral stenosis in adult patients: postmortem and percutaneous mitral valvuloplasty studies. *J Am Coll Cardiol.* 9:723–731, 1987.

12. Vahanian A, Michel PL, Iung B, et al: Should balloon valvotomy be performed for severely calcified mitral stenosis? *Circulation.* 82(suppl III):III–79, 1990.

13. Akins CW, Kirklin JK, Block PC, et al: Preoperative evaluation of subvalvular fibrosis in mitral stenosis. A predictive factor in conservative vs replacement surgical therapy. *Circulation.* 60:I71–I76, 1979.

14. Babic UU, Pejcic P, Djurisic Z, et al: Percutaneous transarterial balloon valvuloplasty for mitral valve stenosis. *Am J Cardiol.* 57:1101–1104, 1986.

15. Romero M, Melian F, Suarez de Lezo J, et al: Transarterial mitral valvuloplasty in conditions of acute pulmonary edema. *Am Heart J.* 119:1416–1419, 1990.

16. Pan M, Medina A, Suarez de Lezo J, et al: Balloon valvuloplasty for mild mitral stenosis. *Cathet Cardiovasc Diagn.* 24:1–5, 1991.

17. Suarez de Lezo J, Medina A, Bethencourt A, et al: Transarterial mitral valvuloplasty: factors determining an optimal result (abstr.). *Eur Heart J.* 10(Abstract Supplement):339, 1989.

18. Sancho M, Medina A, Suarez de Lezo J, et al: Factors influencing progression of mitral regurgitation after transarterial balloon valvuloplasty for mitral stenosis. *Am J Cardiol.* 66:737–740, 1990.

19. Medina A, Bethencourt A, Coello I, et al: Combined percutaneous mitral and aortic balloon valvuloplasty. *Am J Cardiol.* 64:620–624, 1989.

20. Bethencourt A, Medina A, Hernandez E, et al: Combined percutaneous balloon valvuloplasty of mitral and tricuspid valves. *Am Heart J.* 119:416–418, 1990.

21. Rediker DE, Block PC, Abascal VM, et al: Mitral balloon valvuloplasty for mitral restenosis after surgical commissurotomy. *J Am Coll Cardiol.* 11:252–256, 1988.

22. Medina A, Suarez de Lezo J, Hernández E, et al: Balloon valvuloplasty for mitral restenosis after previous surgery: a comparative study. *Am Heart J.* 120:568–571, 1990.

23. Higgs LM, Glancy DL, O'Brien KP, et al: Mitral restenosis: an uncommon cause of recurrent symptoms following mitral commissurotomy. *Am J Cardiol.* 26:34–37, 1970.

24. Rutledge R, McIntosh CL, Morrow AG, et al: Mitral valve replacement after closed mitral commissurotomy. *Circulation.* 66(suppl I):I-162–I-166, 1982.

25. John S, Bashi VV, Jairaj PS, et al: Closed mitral valvotomy: early results and long-term follow-up of 3724 consecutive patients. *Circulation.* 68:891–896, 1983.

26. Vahanian A, Michel PL, Cormier B, et al: Mid-term results of mitral balloon valvotomy for re-stenosis after surgical commissurotomy. *Circulation.* 82(suppl III):III-80, 1990.

27. Al Zaibag M, Ribeiro PA, Al Kasab, et al: One-year follow-up after percutaneous double balloon mitral valvotomy. *Am J Cardiol.* 63:126–127, 1989.

28. Glover RP, Davila JC, O'Neill TJE, et al: Does mitral stenosis recur after commissurotomy? *Circulation.* 11:14–28, 1955.

29. Kirklin JW, Hickey MSJ, Blackstone EH, et al: Outcome after closed and open surgical mitral commissurotomy: implications for balloon valvuloplasty. *Circulation.* 80(suppl II):II-359, 1989.

CHAPTER **13**

Congenital Obstruction of the Left Ventricular Outflow Tract

Zuhdi Lababidi

Obstruction to the left ventricular outflow is estimated to occur in 5 to 7% of patients with congenital heart disease.[1,2] Of these obstructions, about 75% occur at the aortic valve level (aortic valve stenosis), 23% just below the aortic valve (discrete subvalvular aortic stenosis), and 1 to 2% just above the aortic valve (supravalvular aortic stenosis).[3] Obstruction may also be caused by hypertrophic obstructive cardiomyopathy, but the following discussion relates only to the first three groups.

Balloon aortic valvuloplasty for congenital valvular aortic stenosis was a logical development in the growing field of interventional cardiology. Our group introduced its use in the treatment of congenital valvular aortic stenosis in November 1982.[4,5] In 1986 Cribier and coworkers[6] reported that the technique was also effective in lowering the gradient across acquired calcific aortic stenoses. The balloon dilatation technique has also been applied to several other forms of left ventricular outflow obstruction and was found by our group to be effective in treating thin discrete subaortic stenoses.[7]

CONGENITAL AORTIC VALVE STENOSIS

Aortic valve stenosis without associated mitral valve disease very rarely occurs on a rheumatic basis but is usually either congenital or degenerative in origin.[8,9] Congenital aortic valve stenosis accounts for three fourths of patients with congenital left ventricular outflow obstructions and is much more common among males than females, in a 3:1 ratio.[10,11] Most commonly the aortic valve is biscupid with two commissures, one or both of which are fused to varying degrees; a third rudimentary commissure or raphe often is present in the larger of the two leaflets. Less frequently encountered is the unicommissural or noncommissural valve, in which the orifice is often slitlike. Rarely, the valve is tricuspid with fusion of one or more of the three commissures.[12] The bicuspid aortic valve is the most frequent congenital malformation of the heart, with a prevalence of 1 to 2% of the population.[13] Its occasional association with coarctation of the aorta, patent ductus arteriosus, ventricular septal defect, and isolated pulmonary stenosis is well established.[14]

Natural History

Unicuspid valves produce severe obstruction in early infancy. Bicuspid valves may be stenotic with commissural fusion at birth, but more commonly they develop progressive stenosis due to fibrosis secondary to turbulent blood flow.[9,15] Fenoglio and coworkers[16] have suggested that about one third of the children with nonstenotic bicuspid aortic valves will go on to develop aortic stenosis by the age of 20 years, one third will develop aortic regurgitation, and the last third will remain free of any significant hemodynamic problems. Tricuspid valves with unequal cusps and commissural fusion also develop progressive stenosis owing to turbulence.

In individuals who survive to adulthood, varying degrees of calcification may appear in the valvular tissue, leading to rigidity of the valve leaflets. The minimum age at which calcification occurs is not clear, although it has been reported occasionally in adolescents.[10,17] The frequency with which calcification occurs increases with age[16] and to encounter stenosis without calcification after age 40 years is uncommon. The reported incidence of sudden death from aortic stenosis has varied from 1 to 19%, with an accepted average incidence of 7.5%.[3,10,13] Infective endocarditis on the aortic valve poses a serious threat in the form of systemic emboli, aortic regurgitation, congestive heart failure, shock, and death. Bacterial endocarditis occurs in 4% of patients with congenital aortic valve stenosis.[12] In adults, the mean survival after the onset of angina, syncope, and congestive heart failure is 5 years, 3 years, and 2 years, respectively.[18,19]

Clinical Features

Although the systolic ejection murmur of congenital aortic stenosis may be heard during the neonatal period, it is detected in only half the patients during the first year of life.[1] Growth and development usually are normal and the vast majority are asymptomatic. Easy fatigue, dyspnea, syncope, angina, and (rarely) sudden death may occur and suggest severe obstruction, but severe obstruction may also exist in the absence of any symptoms.[3,20] In infants and children with valvular aortic stenosis, the aortic valve orifice may not enlarge much with time, thus making the obstruction more severe as the child and the heart grow while the size of the orifice remains fixed.[21] The cardiac output is maintained by hypertrophy of the left ventricle, which sustains a high pressure gradient for many years without reduction in cardiac output, enlargement of the left ventricle, or development of symptoms.[12] The gradient across the aortic valve rises with exertion, and the cardiac output which may be normal at rest fails to rise during exertion in the majority of patients with severe aortic stenosis. Syncope is often orthostatic and is most commonly due to a reduction in cerebral perfusion during exertion related to peripheral vasodilatation. Syncope at rest may be caused by transient ventricular tachyarrhythmia or atrial fibrillation.

Exertional dyspnea, orthopnea, and pulmonary edema are late symptoms of severe aortic stenosis. In advanced stages, systolic and pulse pressures are both reduced. In mild stenosis however, especially with associated aortic regurgitation, both systolic and pulse pressures may be normal or even elevated. The absence of left ventricular hypertrophy does not exclude the presence of severe aortic stenosis.[22] T-wave inversion and ST-segment depressions greater than 0.3 mV suggest that severe ventricular hypertrophy is present.[14] In the presence of a normal cardiac output, a gradient of 75 mmHg or greater or a valve area of less than 0.5 cm² per m² of body surface area (BSA) is considered severe[14]; a gradient between 50 and 74 mmHg or a valve area between 0.5 and 0.8 cm² per m² BSA is considered moderate; a gradient of less than 50 mmHg or a valve area greater than 0.9 cm² per m² BSA is considered mild. Friedman and associates[20] have encouraged the general acceptance of 0.7 cm² per m² BSA as a marker for a clinically severe obstruction. They have also demonstrated progression of the gradient on follow-up.

Continuous-wave Doppler echocardiography guided by two-dimensional echocardiographic imaging appears to predict very accurately the systolic pressure gradient across discrete forms of left ventricular outflow tract obstruction.[23,24] Two-dimensional echocardiography can distinguish valvular from supravalvular and subvalvular obstructions. Normally, aortic valve leaflets are barely visible in systole. In patients with severe aortic stenosis, thickened leaflets and eccentric closure are often recognized on the M-mode echocardiogram. A reduced valve opening is usually seen in aortic stenosis, but it also occurs in congestive heart failure with a low cardiac output.[25,26]

Infantile Critical Aortic Stenosis

Infants with critical valvular aortic stenosis present with severe congestive heart failure manifested by tachypnea, tachycardia, hepatomegaly, low urine output, cool extremities, and acidosis.[27] Associated cardiac anomalies are common in these infants[28]; patent ductus arteriosus occurs in 60%, a small left ventricular cavity in 47%, endocardial fibroelastosis in 27%, coarctation of the aorta in 23%, and a hypoplastic aortic arch in 20%. As the severity of valvular stenosis increases, the incidence of associated endocardial fibroelastosis increases and the presenting age of the patient decreases. The hemodynamics of neonatal congenital valvular aortic stenosis are similar to those of acquired aortic stenosis except that left atrial pressure is reduced owing to the persistence of the ductus arteriosus and the patent foramen ovale. Consequently, the pulmonary venous pressure is lower, and there is less pulmonary edema. Infants with critical aortic stenosis present with congestive heart failure within the first week or two of life, and they represent true medical emergencies. Patients with critical aortic stenosis in the neonatal period make up less than 10% of children with valvular aortic stenosis.[1]

Surgical Treatment

In children and adolescents with congenital valvular aortic stenosis, who most commonly have bicuspid aortic valves, simple commissurotomy under direct vision usually leads to hemodynamic improvement. Surgery is generally recommended for any patient with a peak systolic pressure gradient exceeding 75 mmHg or a calculated effective orifice less than 0.5 cm² per m² BSA. In the presence of symptoms, a left ventricular strain pattern on the electrocardiogram (ECG), or an abnormal exercise ECG, surgery may be recommended with a gradient of greater than 50 mmHg or an orifice area of less than 0.75 cm² per m² BSA. When the operation is performed in childhood, a mortality of less than 2% can be expected.[14,29] The subsequent development of regurgitation and restenosis after 10 to 20 years may necessitate reoperation and valve replacement. When surgery is carried out in patients with frank left ventricular failure or a depressed ejection fraction, the operative risk is higher, and the mortality in the first 3 postoperative days ranges from 10 to 25%.[30] Complications of aortic commissurotomy include aortic regurgitation, residual stenosis, endocarditis, and possibly restenosis and calcification later in life. In 42 patients studied by Jack and Kelly,[31] aortic regurgitation was present in 80% postoperatively, and in 25% the regurgitation was moderate to severe. Among 179 patients operated on in the Joint Study, [32] 6% of the survivors developed serious aortic regurgitation. One third of the survivors had systolic pressure gradients of less than 25 mmHg, while another third had residual gradients ranging from 25 to 50 mmHg. The final third were found to have either recurrent or residual gradients above 50 mmHg, and 11 of those were in the severe range. Surgery was palliative in most if not all instances.

Despite medical therapy, as many as 30% of infants under one month of age with critical aortic stenosis die before operation.[27] The goal of surgery for critical aortic stenosis in the neonate is acute relief of the obstruction and interruption of the rapidly fatal course. More definitive procedures on the aortic valve are reserved for older, larger patients with less valvular dysplasia. Critical aortic stenosis of the newborn is life-threatening and must be treated promptly. Of infants who had aortic valvotomy, 45% had endocardial fibroelastosis, which is seen in 14% of infants with bicuspid valves, and in 76% with unicuspid valves.[3] Newborns with symptomatic aortic stenosis require urgent or emergency valvotomy, which carries a high risk. In infants 1 month of age or younger, the mortality has ranged from 29 to 86%, with most reports showing a mortality of at least 30%.[33-36] Aortic valvotomy has been performed by an open method with and without cardiopulmonary bypass, by a closed method with a transventricular blunt dilator through an incision in the left ventricular apex, and, more recently, by a transventricular balloon catheter after thoracotomy. The high incidence (40–75%) of associated anomalies in these infants has contributed to the high mortality.[33-36]

Balloon Aortic Valvuloplasty in Infants, Children and Young Adults

Although the past three decades have witnessed outstanding technical changes in catheter usage and design, the 1980s introduced a new meaning to cardiac catheterization. The catheterization laboratory is no longer just a diagnostic laboratory but a sophisticated and elaborate theater for the treatment of simple as well as complex congenital cardiac anomalies at any age. Of all interventional cardiac procedures, balloon dilatation has become the most popular. It has offered palliative as well as definitive therapy for most congenital and acquired stenotic cardiac anomalies. Since balloon aortic valvuloplasty requires temporary obstruction of the left ventricular outflow tract, it must be performed only by experienced interventional cardiologists.

Indications for Balloon Dilatation
The indications for balloon aortic valvuloplasty have changed slightly in the past few years. Originally, standards for surgical intervention were used for balloon intervention: a peak systolic gradient exceeding 75 mmHg, a calculated effective aortic valve orifice less than 0.5 cm^2 per m^2 BSA, or presence of symptoms and T-wave changes.[14] Because of the low morbidity and mortality in children and young adults, most

cardiologists are now performing the procedure with gradients exceeding 50 mmHg or a valve area less than 0.7 cm^2 per m^2 BSA, even in the absence of symptoms and ECG changes, hoping that it will prevent deterioration in left ventricular function over time.[5,37] The dilatation seems to work equally well in native and postoperative aortic restenosis.[38]

Neonates with critical aortic stenosis often benefit from balloon aortic valvuloplasty.[39-43] However, if the valve annulus is very small or if endocardial fibroelastosis is present, they do not tolerate left ventricular outflow obstruction in the catheterization laboratory; in such cases, surgical valvotomy, open or by intraoperative balloon dilatation, may be advisable.[44-46] Balloon aortic valvuloplasty should not be performed in the presence of severe aortic regurgitation or in patients who are candidates for valve replacement.[5] Surgical aortic valvotomy and balloon aortic valvuloplasty are both palliative procedures.[37] Since balloon valvuloplasty does not cause intrathoracic adhesions, it makes future aortic valve replacement technically less difficult. Therefore, if the risks and complications of the two procedures are comparable, balloon dilatation should be offered to patients with congenital valvular aortic stenosis, as an alternative to open aortic valvotomy.

Dilatation Technique

The diagnosis and the assessment of the degree of valvular aortic stenosis are made by clinical, roentgenographic, electrocardiographic and Doppler echocardiographic studies. Once a moderate to severe stenosis has been diagnosed, percutaneous cardiac catheterization and cineangiography are performed to confirm the clinical and noninvasive diagnosis and to consider balloon dilatation.[47] The technique and the risks involved should be carefully explained to the patient and family by the interventional cardiologist.

Percutaneous right and left heart catheterization is performed in the usual manner with measurements of resting cardiac output. The left ventricle is entered retrogradely and a resting pullback pressure gradient is measured across the aortic valve. Aortic root biplane cineangiography is then performed to determine the degree of aortic regurgitation, the size of the valve orifice, and the number and shape of the aortic leaflets. The left ventricle is again entered retrogradely and biplane left ventricular cineangiography is performed to determine the size of the left ventricle, the diameter of the aortic root, the size of the valve orifice, and left ventricular function (Fig. 13.1). To avoid the pullback and reentering of the left ventricle, especially in eccentric and severely stenotic aortic valves, the cardiologist may elect to place an extra catheter in the left ventricle via the transseptal technique and a third catheter, retrogradely, in the aorta, thereby providing continuous measurement of the left ventricular to aortic pressure gradient throughout the procedure without the necessity to pull back and reenter across the stenotic aortic valve. The left ventricle, however, needs to be entered with a single end-hole or end-and-side-hole catheter over a long exchange guidewire which is used to manipulate the balloon catheter across the aortic valve.

After the aortic root and left ventricular cineangiograms are performed, the left ventricle is allowed to rest for a few minutes until the left ventricular end-diastolic pressure returns to normal. The balloon catheter, which is chosen with a balloon equal to or 2 mm less than the diameter of the aortic valve annulus, is introduced over a stiff 0.038 exchange guidewire with a 15-mm curved flexible tip. The stiff guidewire

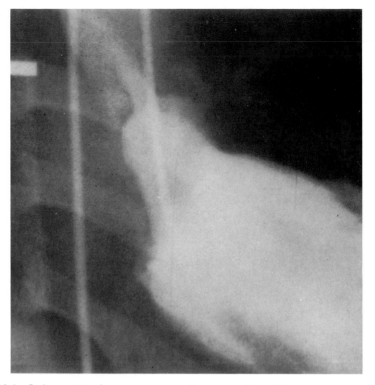

Figure 13.1 Left ventricular angiogram demonstrating diameters of aortic valve annulus and stenotic valve orifice.

is used to anchor the balloon across the aortic valve and prevent its recoil into the aorta during systole while being inflated. The curved flexible tip protruding from the end is used to minimize ventricular ectopy and to prevent left ventricular perforation by the sharp tip of the balloon catheter (Fig 13.2). The two radioopaque markers at both ends of the balloon are used to guide centering of the middle of the balloon across the stenotic valve opening with a slight forward push so that the catheter's shaft at the level of the brachiocephalic arteries is touching the greater curvature of the aortic arch. If the balloon is inflated while the catheter's shaft is touching the lesser curvature of the aortic arch, there is a good chance that the balloon will be ejected out of the left ventricle during systole.

Once the hourglass shape of the balloon disappears and the balloon is fully inflated there is no need to add extra volume or extra pressure to the balloon and there is no need to repeat the procedure with the same balloon size (Fig. 13.3). In contrast to calcific aortic stenosis, multiple inflations are not necessary in congenital valvular aortic stenosis. Once the balloon is fully inflated, the valve orifice opens to equal the balloon diameter. Further inflation will only cause balloon rupture and repeating the inflation will only add to the time and complications of the procedure.

One trick to prevent the ejection of the balloon into the aorta is to "tickle" the left ventricle with the guidewire during inflation (Fig. 13.2). This maneuver causes short runs of ventricular premature beats that decrease the left ventricular ejection force for

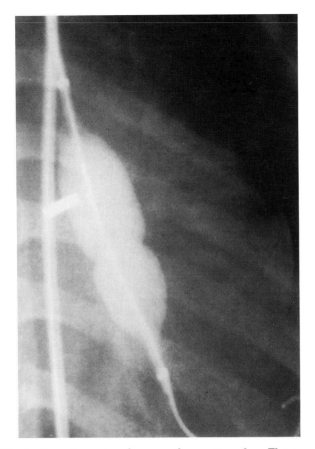

Figure 13.2 The balloon is centered across the aortic valve. The curved flexible tip of the guidewire protrudes from the catheter tip to prevent left ventricular perforation and to minimize ectopy.

the 3 to 5 seconds of balloon inflation. The balloon catheter is then deflated and removed, leaving the guidewire in the left ventricle.

The left ventricle is again allowed to rest for a few minutes. Cardiac output and the pressure gradients across the aortic valve are measured again (Fig. 13.4). An aortic root cineangiogram is then performed to determine the degree of aortic regurgitation and the relief of the aortic obstruction (Fig. 13.5). Although the small femoral artery in the neonate limits the use of larger balloons, 5- to 6-mm balloons on 5-Fr. catheters create an adequate valve opening for that age (Fig. 13.6). Larger balloons may be used during repeat valvuloplasty when the patient is older, larger, and past the critical period. The catheterization and dilatation procedures can be performed percutaneously, transumbilically, or through an open femoral arteriotomy. Balloons 6 to 8 mm in diameter are now available on 5.3 Fr. catheters (Proflex 5) that follow the umbilical artery course with ease.[43]

Balloon aortic valvuloplasty is technically relatively simple in the hands of an experienced catheterization team. Performed as an immediate continuation of the diagnostic catheterization, it prolongs the procedure by only 15 to 30 minutes.

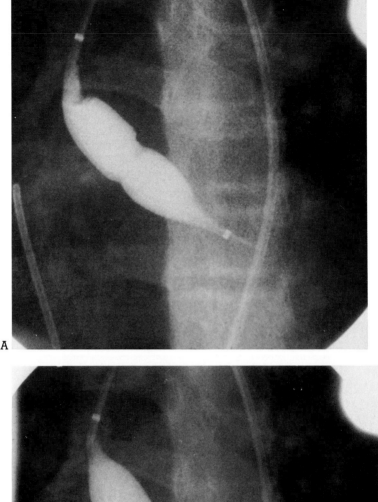

A

B

Figure 13.3 *A*, Hourglass balloon shape at beginning of inflation. *B*, Fully inflated balloon across the aortic valve.

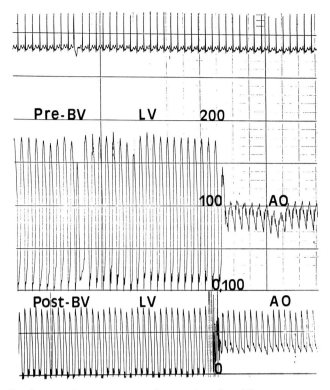

Figure 13.4 Gradient reduction across the aortic valve: The *top* tracing is a pullback across the aortic valve before dilatation. The *lower* tracing is a pullback soon after the dilatation showing no residual gradient. *AO*—aorta. *BV*—balloon valvuloplasty. *LV*—left ventricle.

Balloon Preparation

There are several approaches to balloon preparation. Some cardiologists do not flush the balloon before insertion and aortic valve dilatation. Instead, the balloon is aspirated and put on full suction to attain the smallest profile to make the entry easier. Care should be taken to avoid balloon rupture if this approach is chosen.[48] Other cardiologists purge the balloon with saline or contrast solution initially. We recommend purging repeatedly with carbon dioxide followed by saline solution (Fig. 13.7). The carbon dioxide removes any air and thereby decrease the chance of air embolism if balloon rupture occurs. The saline is used instead of a contrast medium because it is easier to purge with, since its viscosity is less than that of any contrast medium. The balloon is inflated with a dilute contrast mixture to keep the inflation and deflation time to a minimum yet provide adequate opacification.

Balloon Inflation

The balloon can be inflated with a hand-held syringe. The balloon inflation is monitored either by using a manometer to measure the inflation pressure or by observing the balloon configuration on fluoroscopy. We originally depended on the manometer to avoid excessive inflation and balloon rupture, but more recently we found that observing the balloon configuration on fluoroscopy was more reliable. The

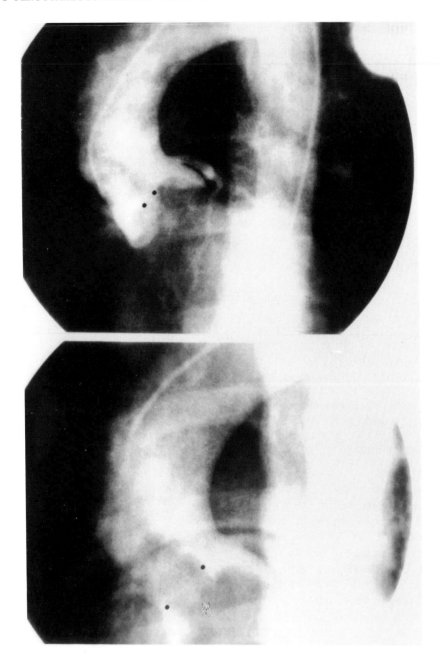

Figure 13.5 Aortic angiograms. The *top* tracing demonstrates the small aortic valve opening before dilatation. The *lower* tracing demonstrates the enlarged opening after dilatation. The valve opening in each tracing is indicated by the *black dots*.

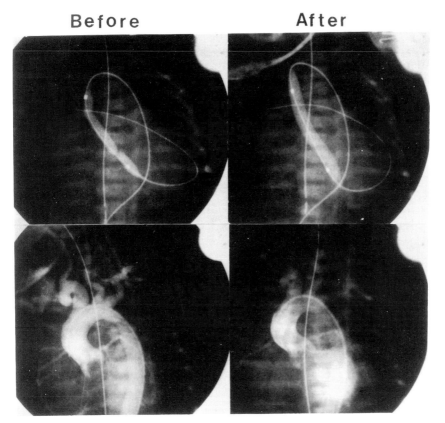

Figure 13.6 Balloon dilatation of critical aortic stenosis in a neonate. The guidewire extends out of the tip of the catheter into the left ventricle and through the mitral valve into the left atrium. Balloon dilatation relieved the obstruction but caused moderate aortic regurgitation. *Before*—before balloon dilatation. *After*—after balloon dilatation.

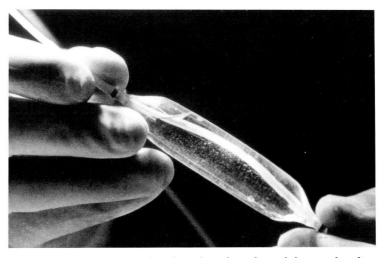

Figure 13.7 The balloon is purged with carbon dioxide and then with saline solution before the balloon catheter is introduced into the femoral artery.

balloon is deflated as soon as the hourglass shape of the balloon disappears, indicating full inflation. A few mechanical devices have been used for inflation; we use the Medrad injector, employing its manual button for inflation and deflation without programming.

Selection of Balloon Size

In balloon pulmonary valvuloplasty, the inflated balloon can be 20 to 40% larger than the pulmonary annulus.[49] In aortic valvuloplasty, however, it is important not to exceed the aortic annulus diameter by more than 10% so as to avoid excessive aortic regurgitation.[5,37] Because of the higher systemic pressure, aortic regurgitation is clinically much more significant than pulmonary regurgitation. Disruption of the aortic annulus during balloon inflation can be fatal. For a single-catheter technique, a balloon equal to or 2 mm less than the valve annulus is chosen. If the dilatation is inadequate, a balloon 2 mm larger than the annulus may be used. The aortic valve annulus is measured by echocardiography[50,51] and can be confirmed on cineangiography after the aortic root injection. Sequential sizing[52] that is often used in calcific aortic stenosis is not necessary in congenital aortic stenosis. The fewer the manipulations and catheter exchanges, the fewer the arterial complications at the entry site. When the double-balloon technique is used, the following formula is used to calculate the effective balloon size:

$$\frac{D_1 + D_2 + \pi (0.5 \, D_1 + 0.5 \, D_2)}{\pi}$$

where D_1 and D_2 are diameters of the balloons used.[47] When both balloons are equal in diameter, neither should exceed 60% of the annulus. Although the double-balloon technique is recommended by others,[53,54] we have always advocated the use of a single balloon to avoid trauma to two sites of arterial access instead of one. As the balloon profile becomes smaller with improved technology, larger single balloons can be used with minimal peripheral arterial trauma; these developments may obviate the need for the bilateral femoral double-balloon technique. Balloon length is also important. Short balloons are often ejected out of the left ventricle before they are fully inflated. Larger balloons (5.5 cm) are less likely to be ejected (Fig. 13.8).

Left Ventricular Decompression

Our initial work[4,5] in 1982 in attempting to decompress the left ventricle via a connecting catheter in the right atrium during balloon inflation (Fig. 13.9) was followed by pulmonary artery occlusion in 1985,[55] transluminal venous balloon inflow occlusion in 1986,[56] the use of trefoil balloon catheters also in 1986,[57] and double balloons in 1987.[53] As more clinical trials were attempted, the need for left ventricular decompression became less significant. In the presence of a normal ejection fraction the left ventricle seems to tolerate total outflow occlusion for a few seconds without the need for decompression.

Catheterization Approaches

The percutaneous retrograde transfemoral approach is most widely used, although a brachial cutdown may be used if the femoral artery is obstructed or tortuous. An arterial sheath may be used, but with the new tapered low profile balloon catheters there is no need for a sheath since it adds to the diameter of the hole in the arterial

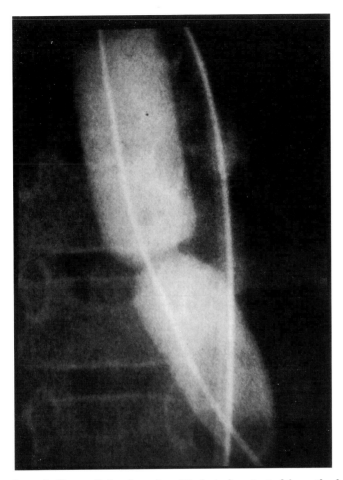

Figure 13.8 Long balloons (5.5cm) are less likely to be ejected from the left ventricle during balloon inflation.

entry site. Arterial access should be obtained as high as possible in the femoral artery but always below the inguinal ligament to decrease the size of the hematoma and to provide a larger artery for entry. A transvenous, transseptal[58] approach can be used utilizing the Mullins sheath and a Brockenbrough needle. An end-hole balloon flotation catheter is advanced through the sheath into the left ventricle and antegradely into the ascending and then the descending aorta. An exchange guidewire is then used to manipulate the balloon catheter across the aortic valve. Care must be taken, in this technique, not to pass the balloon behind the mitral chordae which can rupture during the balloon inflation resulting in mitral regurgitation as well as aortic regurgitation.[37]

Mechanism of Dilatation

For balloon embolectomies and septostomies, the operator uses an axial force to perform the procedure. In balloon dilatations the balloon is placed across the obstruction, and when it is inflated a radial force is exerted against the obstruction.[59,60] The

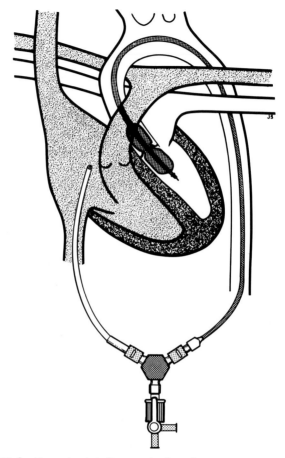

Figure 13.9 Initial attempt at left ventricular decompression via a connecting catheter in the right atrium. When the balloon obstructs the aortic valve, the blood is ejected from the left ventricle through the catheters into the right atrium.

obstruction initially resists the radial force, and consequently the balloon has an hourglass shape at the beginning of the inflation. When the balloon's radial force supersedes that of the obstruction, the balloon attains a cylindrical shape with no indentations indicating that the obstruction has been dilated to the maximum diameter of the balloon. Since most balloons are made of nonstretchable polyethylene material, overinflating the balloon will rupture it. In valvular stenosis, the mechanism of dilatation is a tearing and stretching of the obstruction at the area of least resistance. Care should be taken not to push the balloon into the left ventricle, which would cause prolapse and avulsion of the aortic leaflets. The larger the balloon diameter, the greater the dilating force on the stenotic area. Also, the larger the balloon, the less inflating pressure is needed to exert high balloon wall tension. Since balloons can be inflated more easily with small syringes, it is advisable not to use syringes much bigger than the balloon capacity.

The probable modes of action of balloon valvuloplasty are stretching of the leaflets, rupture of commissural fusion, splitting of the unicuspid dome, annular dilatation, and tearing and avulsion of the leaflets. Cracking of calcium deposits was also reported in elderly patients.[61] The mechanism of the aortic balloon valvuloplasty in children was assessed by Walls and associates[62] by inspection under direct vision at surgical open valvotomy. Tearing of the valve raphae, tearing of the valve leaflets, and avulsion of the valve leaflets can occur. In adults with congenital aortic stenosis, Waller and associates[63] found commissural splitting with and without cuspal cracks. In most patients, it seems that there is no real damage to the leaflets, and in particular no tearing of the leaflet tissue: Preexisting aortic regurgitation does not increase and. no regurgitation is created.[5,37] Even more, in some patients there was a *decrease* in the preexisting aortic regurgitation, confirming that the leaflets have been stretched and their coaption has been improved.

Results of Balloon Aortic Valvuloplasty

Balloon aortic valvuloplasty reduces the pressure gradient across the aortic valve and increases the aortic valve area. Our first patient[4] was an 11-year-old boy who had valvular aortic stenosis with an 85-mmHg peak systolic gradient. The valvuloplasty was surprisingly well tolerated; the patient had an excellent hemodynamic response with a gradient reduction from 85 to 28 mmHg and was able to go to school the next day. Within a span of a few months, the procedure was applied to several other children.[5] The goal of the procedure was to reduce the gradient to 20 to 25 mmHg with little aortic regurgitation. Confirmation of our initial results was reported by other centers.[53,64,65]

The following are the results of balloon aortic valvuloplasty performed at the University of Missouri – Columbia between 1982 and 1991. These results are based on 93 patients with congenital valvular aortic stenosis whose mean age was 10 ± 6 years (range of 2 days to 23 years). Other than the infants, who were in congestive heart failure, these children and young adults were asymptomatic. Signs of left ventricular hypertrophy were present in all patients by ECG, echocardiography, or both. A moderate to severe gradient was confirmed by Doppler echocardiography or by a previous cardiac catheterization.

Tolerance of the procedure was excellent, and balloon inflation with left ventricular outflow occlusion for 3 to 6 seconds was surprisingly well tolerated. A period of disorientation lasting 20 to 30 seconds occurred after balloon deflation in 42 patients. There were no residual neurologic signs or symptoms, such as cerebrovascular accidents or abnormal behavior on followup.

The mean peak systolic left ventricular-aortic gradient was decreased from 93 ± 37 to 25 ± 14 mmHg, and on 1 to 8 year's followup in 32 patients the gradient remained low (30 ± 18 mmHg). The results demonstrated that percutaneous balloon aortic valvuloplasty in congenital valvular aortic stenosis is feasible and can produce an appreciable decrease in the left ventricular-aortic peak systolic gradient despite variability in valvular deformities. In general the gradient reduction was acceptable and spared the patient open valvotomy. In the early part of the study 3 patients required open valvotomy because the gradient had been inadequately reduced by the balloon dilation. However, in retrospect, those patients might have benefited from dilatation with a larger balloon.

In all 93 patients, a supravalvular angiogram was performed before and soon after the dilatation. Of these, 81 patients had a preexisting aortic insufficiency (74 grade 1, 6 grade 2, 1 grade 3). The regurgitation did not change in 72 patients and increased slightly in 21 patients. Only three patients had moderate increase in regurgitation (from grade 1 to grade 3). None of the patients, however, had aortic regurgitation severe enough to require valve replacement. Although aortic regurgitation was an anticipated complication, the number and severity were comparable to patients who had open valvotomy. No deaths related to the procedure occurred in the hospital or on followup. No patient had embolization, internal hemorrhage, infarction, rupture of the mitral apparatus, or rupture of the aorta. There were 22 patients who developed femoral arterial complications with transient pulse loss, hematoma, or thrombosis, but surgery to relieve the obstruction was required in only 3 patients. The complications were probably due to the large size of the balloon catheter. The procedure has a higher risk than simple diagnostic cardiac catheterization.

It is difficult at present, owing to insufficient long-term followup, to evaluate the restenosis rate after percutaneous balloon aortic valvuloplasty. The definition of a good result is arbitrary and includes hemodynamic success, an absence of complications, and improvement in symptoms. Some cardiologists define hemodynamic success as a reduction of 50% in the peak systolic gradient.[37,53,64,65] We, on the other hand, define it as a residual gradient of less than 30 mmHg.

Complications of Balloon Aortic Valvuloplasty

Arterial access problems due to the large balloon size are the most common complication of balloon aortic valvuloplasty. The use of a sheath adds to the dimension of the balloon and increases the chances of arterial trauma. The development and use of smaller, tapered catheters with low profile balloons should greatly decrease these problems. Thrombosis is also a potential problem. Most cardiologists believe that systemic heparinization can minimize thrombosis, but we do not heparinize so long as the procedure from the time of balloon insertion to its removal does not last more than 30 minutes. Heparinization increases the chances of bleeding at the entry site and therefore prolongs the time of squeezing the groin for hemostasis. Squeezing causes further trauma to the entry site and leads to the formation of a hematoma that may compress the artery and occlude it or may form a pseudoaneurysm. Local dissection and perforation are possible and have been reported to result in fatal hemorrhage.[37]

Care must be taken in catheter and balloon insertion and removal from the groin to avoid arterial severing. If there is any doubt that this has happened, a cutdown should be performed and the artery repaired. Balloon rupture due to overinflation occurs frequently and is usually longitudinal but can occasionally be transverse (Fig. 13.10). On one occasion we had a transverse catheter rupture inside the balloon which also had a longitudinal tear (Fig. 13.11). If the balloon does not come out easily from the artery in the groin after rupture, a cutdown should be performed to avoid severing the artery. Fibrinolytic agents, either steptokinese or urokinese, may be used if the leg remains pulseless 24 to 48 hours after the procedure.[66]

There is a concern about the risk of femoral artery injury when percutaneous valvuloplasty is performed during the neonatal period.[43] To avoid this problem, some pediatric cardiologists find the transumbilical route easier. Embolization may result from prolonged catheter use. Frequent wire exchanges, arterial flushing with a heparinized solution, and speeding up the procedure will minimize these problems.

In most patients the degree of aortic regurgitation present after balloon valvuloplasty is the same or only mildly greater than that present before dilatation (Fig. 13.12). Significant regurgitation can result from balloon oversizing with excessive

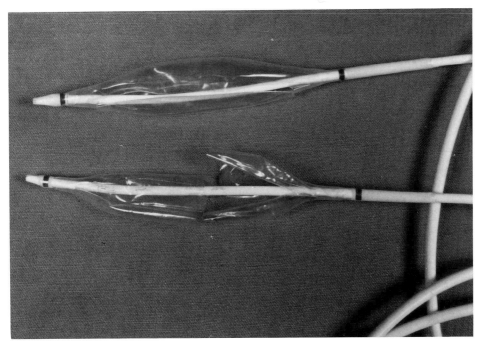

Figure 13.10 Balloon rupture. *Top,* common longitudinal tear. *Bottom,* Balloon with rare transverse tear is more difficult to remove from the femoral artery.

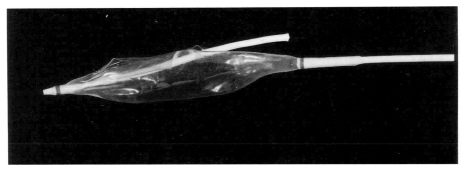

Figure 13.11 Catheter rupture within a longitudinal balloon rupture. A rare complication.

commissural splitting or leaflet tearing, especially in unicuspid valves. Early fears of severe congestive heart failure due to a sudden increase in aortic regurgitation and fears of cardiac arrest due to obstruction of left ventricular outflow by the inflated balloon have not been realized (Fig. 13.13). The balloon may obstruct the coronary ostia during inflation. This, combined with the decrease in systemic pressure, may explain why in 9 of our patients there was marked transient ST depression and transient left bundle branch block. These alarming phenomena are expected to be more pronounced when there is associated coronary artery disease or a prolonged inflation period. Ventricular ectopy and nonsustained ventricular tachycardia are very

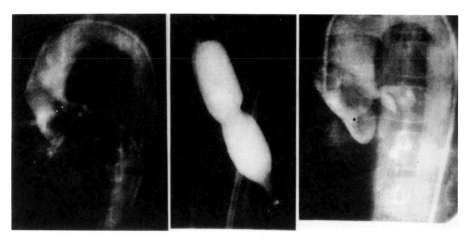

Figure 13.12 Balloon aortic valvuloplasty. Notice the improvement in valve opening (*dots*) without the development of aortic regurgitation.

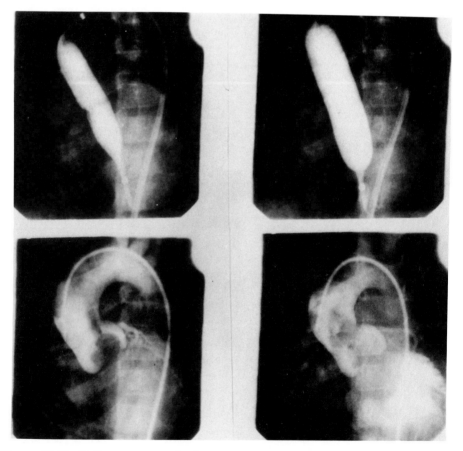

Figure 13.13 Balloon aortic valvuloplasty with impressive increase in the aortic valve opening. The complicating aortic regurgitation was well tolerated by the patient.

common and transient. They are due to catheter and guidewire manipulation. Bradycardia may occur during occlusion of the valve during the inflation procedure but resolves as soon as the balloon is deflated. Most of the complications occur in infants.

The Valvuloplasty and Angioplasty of Congenital Anomalies Registry[37] reports only 2 of 166 children over 1 year of age with major complications. One was a catheter malfunction and one had mitral valve tearing requiring open heart surgery. Aortic regurgitation developed or increased in severity in 15 of 166 patients. Loss of femoral pulses due to femoral thrombosis occurred in 13 of 166. The ratio of balloon:annulus diameter was significantly larger in those children who developed arterial thrombosis or aortic regurgitation. Since the development of femoral artery damage was significantly related to both patient age and balloon:annulus diameter ratio, the incidence of this complication was significantly reduced by the development of new low profile balloon catheters with a smaller shaft size.

Finally, we must be cautious concerning the oversizing of the balloon as compared with the size of the aortic annulus. Although ruptures of the annulus and the myocardium are certainly rare, they undoubtedly can occur, and the use of over-sized balloons must be avoided whenever possible.[37,67]

DISCRETE SUBAORTIC STENOSIS

Discrete subaortic stenosis accounts for approximately 8 to 20% of all cases of congenital left ventricular outflow tract obstructions, and it occurs more frequently in males than in females by a 2:1 ratio.[68] Although discrete subaortic stenosis, fixed subaortic stenosis, subaortic shelf, subaortic ridge, and diaphragmatic subaortic stenosis are used as synonyms, they may represent a spectrum of lesions obstructing the left ventricular outflow tract. The following discussion of pathogenesis, pathology, and clinical features of discrete subaortic stenosis should explain why balloon dilatation works only in certain types of fixed subaortic obstructions.

Pathogenesis

The etiology of discrete subaortic stenosis is still incompletely understood. In 1970 Van Praagh and associates[69] speculated that it may be caused by maldevelopment of the endocardial cushion tissue of the atrioventricular canal that usually forms the anterior leaflet of the mitral valve. Van Mierop[70] noted that it may be associated with malformation of the proximal extremity of the truncus septum where it joins the conus septum. In 1971 Roberts[71] postulated that fibrous plaques in the left ventricular outflow tract can be attributed to trauma associated with the impact of septal hypertrophy and the mitral valve during systole. In 1976 Pyle and associates[72] pointed out that in Newfoundland dogs, discrete subaortic stenosis is caused by polygenic influences that manifest after birth because persistent embryonic tissue proliferates in the left ventricular outflow tract. The acquired nature of the obstruction in humans has been documented by serial cardiac catheterizations.[68,73-75] Important genetic inheritance has not been demonstrated in humans, and Ferrans and colleagues[76] demonstrated significant histologic differences between the Newfoundland dog's and the human's discrete subaortic stenosis.

Pathology

Although the spectrum of presentation is broad there are three types of fixed discrete subaortic stenosis with a substantial overlap between them.[68,75,77-81] It is not known whether the three types share the same pathogenesis. In type I, a thin discrete fibrous membrane is situated immediately subjacent to the aortic valve. It is 1 to 2 mm thick and is located 1 to 20 mm below the aortic valve annulus. (ie, anywhere at the level of the aortic-mitral annulus). It usually forms a crescent or complete ring of fibroelastic tissue. It is attached to the interventricular septum and extends to the superior part of the anterior leaflet of the mitral valve with a structurally normal mitral valve movement. It may or may not have continuity with the aortic cusps. The excised diaphragm or ring is described as a thin pliable white fibrous and muscular tissue. When attached to the septum and mitral valve annulus, it forms the floor of a small subaortic chamber, and when severe it is associated with concentric left ventricular hypertrophy.

Type II is a fibromuscular ridge with a muscular base that forms a collarlike left ventricular outflow tract obstruction. Compared to type I, it is thicker, situated lower and is often attached to the anterior leaflet of the mitral valve. It is associated with a septal myocardial bulging with considerable muscular hypertrophy and narrowing of the left ventricular outflow tract. Usually the ridge is 2 to 3 mm thick and is more prominent anteriorly and laterally than posteriorly on the mitral-aortic annulus. It may be present as a complete fibrous diaphragm, and the stenotic orifice may be central, eccentric, or slitlike. Severe left ventricular hypertrophy is usually present. The aortic valve cusps are thickened and regurgitant, particularly after 5 years of age, and mitral valve abnormalities occur in about 10% of the patients. Type I and type II have been reported to occur in the same patient.[82]

Type III is a diffuse subaortic tunnel obstruction and is considered the extreme form of fibromuscular stenosis. It is a circumferential irregular stenosis commencing close to the aortic valve annulus and extending downward for 10 to 30 mm. The mitral-aortic annulus is longer than normal and the diameter of the aortic valve annulus, on the average, is smaller than normal. The left ventricular outflow tract appears hypoplastic with fibrous, thickened endocardium and muscular narrowing. Type III occurs less commonly than type I and type II obstructions.

Clinical Features

Infants with discrete subaortic stenosis are asymptomatic. Symptoms are uncommon in children even when stenosis is severe, and they present as effort syncope. Middle-aged adults may present with angina, dyspnea, endocarditis, or occasionally with congestive heart failure.[73] Exertional dyspnea occurs in 17% of children[68] as compared with 80% of adults.[79] The obstruction is usually severe. An outflow gradient of more than 60 mmHg is common.[83] Although the systolic murmur in discrete subaortic stenosis is similar to that of valvular aortic stenosis, the absence of a systolic ejection click and the presence of an aortic regurgitant murmur are suggestive of discrete subaortic stenosis. Trivial or mild aortic regurgitant murmur is found in 30 to 55% of children[68,77] and 66% of adults[79] with discrete subaortic stenosis. Aortic regurgitation murmur is rare in infants and is reported to increase with age.

There are several possible reasons for the aortic regurgitation in discrete subaortic stenosis. In 1973 Roberts[71] emphasized aortic valve problems due to jet lesions from the stenotic subvalvular orifice causing thickening and fibrosis of the valve leaflets.[71,78] The aortic valve may be damaged by endocarditis, a not uncommon complication of discrete subaortic stenosis.[79] Fontana and Edwards reported a 45% incidence of endocarditis in 29 postmortem subjects with discrete subaortic stenosis.[84] Resection of the lesion minimizes but does not completely prevent the occurrence of endocarditis.[79] Discrete subaortic stenosis is not a static lesion. It is progressive in nature. Obstruction which is not present at birth begins to be evident after the first year of life. Isolated fixed subaortic stenosis becomes severe after 10 years. Recurrence after surgical resection is also in favor of it being acquired and progressive in nature. The progression may be caused by proliferation of the fibrous tissue or, with growth of the patient, the fixed narrowing may become significant.[83] Echocardiography[85] may be useful in distinguishing valvular from subvalvular stenosis. The subaortic lesion is best appreciated through the left parasternal long-axis view of the left ventricular outflow tract by two-dimensional echocardiography. The subaortic thin membrane domes toward the aortic valve with systole. Most patients exhibit systolic flutter and brisk partial closure of the aortic leaflets with subsequent reopening and gradual closure of the aortic valve.

Surgical Treatment

In type I the membrane is easily excised in toto, and resection of the adjacent tissue in the outflow tract may not be necessary. In type II the fibromuscular ring is resected with some muscle tissue. Without the myotomy, significant residual obstruction may remain. Because of the likelihood of developing progressive obstruction and aortic regurgitation, the presence of mild to moderate subaortic stenosis has warranted elective surgery. Most authors[68,81] agree that a gradient of 40 to 50 mmHg or more is a reasonable indication for surgery, especially if there is a thin membrane below the valve. It is still debatable whether early surgery prevents progressive aortic valve disease, including aortic regurgitation.[79] There is a tendency for the stenosis to recur or progress postoperatively, especially in the fibromuscular and tunnel obstructions. Newfeld and colleagues[68] reported 17 of 40 patients who had surgical resection and cardiac catheterization 1 to 8 years postoperatively. In 9 patients the residual gradient was 50 mmHg or greater and 3 had repeat surgical resection. Somerville[73] found that patients who had a good long-term result without restenosis were those operated on when under 8 years of age, with less than 20 mmHg residual gradient after excision, and with normal aortic root size.

Balloon Dilatation

Percutaneous balloon dilatation is slowly being accepted as a nonsurgical technique to dilate thin subaortic fixed obstructions.[7,86-90] From 1982 to 1990, 32 patients with clinical, echocardiographic, and hemodynamic diagnosis of discrete subaortic stenosis underwent percutaneous balloon dilatation at the University of Missouri – Columbia hospital and clinics. There were 28 patients with type I stenosis. Their mean age was 8.7 ± 4.7 years; the youngest was 10 weeks and the oldest 18 years. The mean predilatation gradient was 73 ± 34 mmHg, which was reduced to 17 ± 10 mmHg after dilatation. Followup gradients were obtained by repeat cardiac catheterization in 4 patients and continuous-wave Doppler in 15 patients. The mean followup gradient was 13 ± 7 mmHg over a followup period of 4.5 years. There were 4 patients with type II stenosis that had a mean gradient of 155 ± 15 mmHg, which was reduced to 84 ± 37 mmHg. Because of their high residual gradients they all had subsequent surgical myotomy. Before 1984 balloon dilatation was attempted on both type I (Fig. 13.14) and type II (Fig. 13.15) subaortic obstructions at our center. Because all four patients with type II obstruction subsequently required open surgical resection and myotomy, only patients with type I obstruction have been treated by balloon dilatation since 1984. We now believe that both echocardiography and cineangiography must show a subaortic membrane less than 2 mm in thickness before balloon dilatation is attempted.

The technique of balloon dilatation for discrete subaortic stenosis is similar to that of balloon aortic valvuloplasty. Originally the balloon was chosen to be equal to or 1 mm less than the diameter of the aortic valve annulus. If there is no associated valvular aortic stenosis, we now use balloons equal to or 2 mm larger than the annulus diameter. Balloons of this size seem to reduce the gradients adequately without increasing aortic regurgitation. The balloons should be 55 mm long with low profile to lessen the chance of being ejected from the left ventricle or causing femoral complications. The gradient is reduced by tearing of subaortic membrane, as documented by cineangiography (Fig. 13.16) and echocardiography (Fig. 13.17). When the membrane is intact, it bulges slightly toward the aortic valve during systole. After balloon dilatation, the edges of the torn membrane open widely, flutter, and extend toward the aortic valve during systole, sometimes protruding through it. On followup

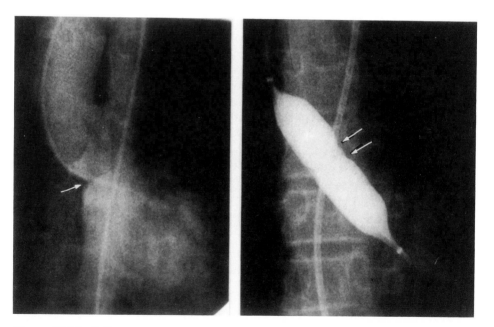

Figure 13.14 Balloon dilatation of thin discrete subaortic stenosis. *Left,* The subaortic membrane (*arrow*) must be 2 mm or less in thickness. *Right,* The balloon demonstrates the indentations formed by the valve annulus (*upper arrow*) as well as the subaortic membrane (*lower arrow*).

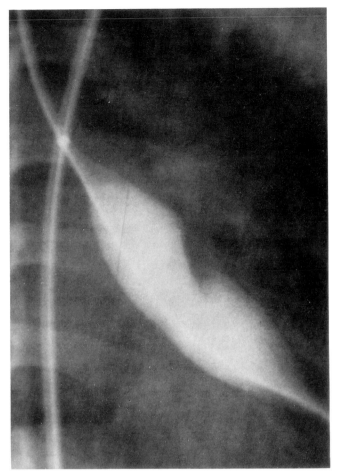

Figure 13.15 Balloon dilatation of fibromuscular subaortic stenosis is not successful owing to the thick muscular ridge indenting the balloon.

echocardiography, the obstruction changes to a small globular ridge on the interventricular septal surface.

The complications of percutaneous balloon dilatation for discrete subaortic stenosis are similar to the complications of percutaneous balloon aortic valvuloplasty. Femoral arterial complications have been reduced by the use of low profile balloons, and aortic regurgitation is less frequently seen when there is no associated valvular aortic stenosis.

SUPRAVALVULAR AORTIC STENOSIS

Congenital supravalvular aortic stenosis may be localized or diffuse, originating at the superior margin of the sinuses of Valsalva just above the level of the coronary arteries.[14] Obstruction of the left ventricular outflow tract by a ridge of tissue just

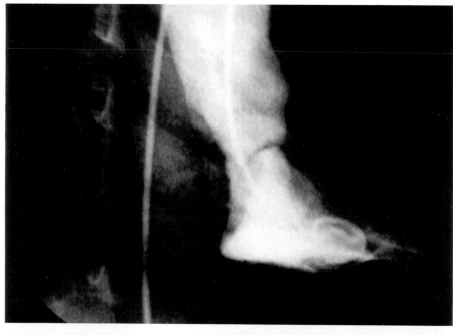

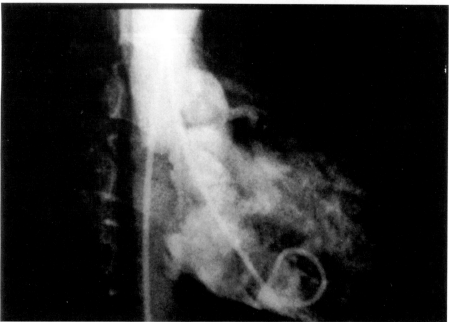

Figure 13.16 *A*, Subaortic membrane angiography. Before balloon dilatation, the membrane is taut. *B*, After balloon dilatation, the membrane is torn and moves toward the aortic valve during systole.

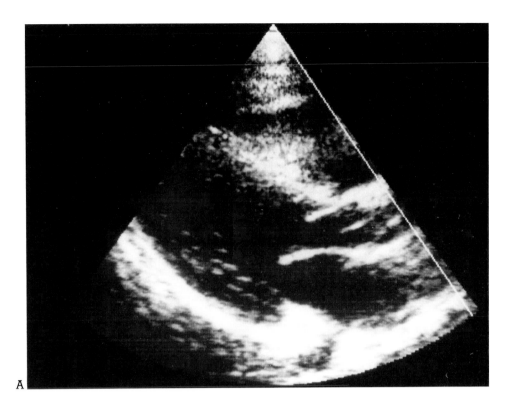

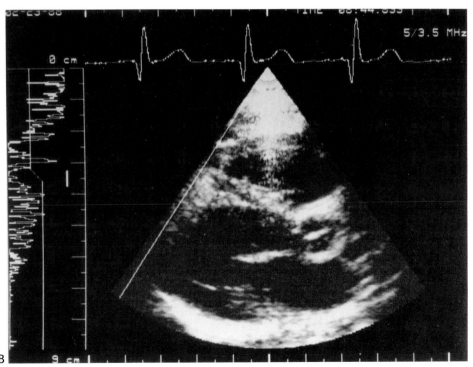

Figure 13.17 *A,* Two-dimensional echocardiography soon after the balloon dilatation. Long-axis view demonstrates the torn membrane moving away from the aortic valve in the diastole. *B,* Long-axis view 6 months after the balloon dilatation demonstrates shrinking of the torn subaortic membrane.

distal to the sinuses of Valsalva was first described by Chevers[91] in 1842. However, it was not until the report of Denie and Verheugt[92] in 1958 that the clinical differentiation between supravalvular and other types of left ventricular outflow tract obstruction was emphasized.

Clinical Features

There are three anatomic types of supravalvular stenosis. The most common type is the hourglass deformity, which is characterized by thickening of the medial layer of the ascending aorta. The media is thickened by fibrous and elastic tissue that is in disarray.[93,94] The other two types, the fibromuscular diaphragm and uniform hypoplasia of the ascending aorta, are less common. The coronary vessels are often dilated and tortuous owing to the elevated aortic pressure proximal to the obstruction.[95] In 1961 Williams[96] and his colleagues reported four cases of supravalvular aortic stenosis in patients with mental retardation and "elfin-like" facies. Genetic studies suggest that when the anomaly is familial, it is transmitted as an autosomal dominant trait with variable expression.[97] The supravalvular aortic stenosis in Williams syndrome may be progressive,[21,98] and careful monitoring of the supravalvular obstruction is indicated. The high incidence of associated cardiac anomalies, including coarctation of the aorta and abnormalities of the aortic valve, coronary arteries, renal arteries, brachiocephalic vessels, pulmonary valve, and pulmonary artery branches, has been well documented.[99-101]

Clinical assessment of the severity can be difficult. In contrast to valvular stenosis, there is rarely an ejection click. Echocardiography and Doppler assessment of supravalvular stenosis are somewhat reliable, but cardiac catheterization remains the most reliable diagnostic technique for this lesion. Patch aortoplasty has been the surgical procedure of choice for supravalvular aortic stenosis. Rastelli and associates[102] observed that gradients persisted after patch aortoplasty in 14 of 16 patients. Keane and associates[103] found residual gradients in 5 postoperative patients, 2 of which occurred at the valvular level. Doty and coworkers[104] pointed out that patch aortoplasty leads to an asymmetrical surgical repair and occasionally does not relieve outflow tract obstruction. Therefore, they divided the supravalvular stenosing ring, allowing lengthening of the aortic leaflets with better valve function. This type of repair may be needed in some patients in whom the coronary leaflets have fused to the supravalvular tissue. Abnormalities of the aortic leaflets can accompany supravalvular aortic stenosis and may contribute to the postoperative residual gradients.

Balloon Dilatation of Supravalvular Aortic Stenosis

As an extension of balloon aortic valvuloplasty and balloon subaortic dilatation, our group attempted, in 1983, balloon dilatation in three patients with supravalvular aortic stenosis. Their ages were 4, 13, and 14 years. The mean predilatation gradient of 64 mmHg decreased to 40 mmHg immediately after the procedure. At 2 to 3 months' followup examination the Doppler gradients were back to the original predilatation level, indicating that the dilatation had occurred by temporary stretching of the thickened media of the narrow portion of the aorta. All three patients had the hourglass deformity (Fig. 13.18). On the other hand Tyagi and associates[105] reported successful balloon dilatation in 2 out of 3 patients; one had a membranous

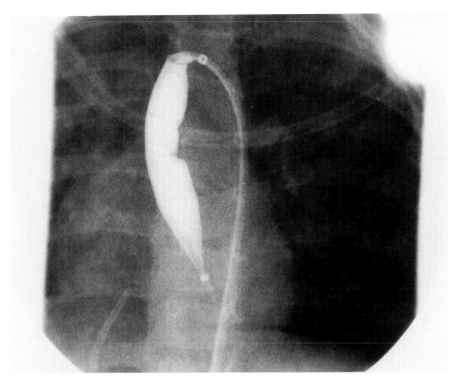

Figure 13.18 Unsuccessful balloon dilatation of supravalvular aortic stenosis demonstrating the hourglass deformity of the stenosis impinging on the balloon.

and the other had an hourglass obstruction. We strongly believe that supravalvular aortic stenosis should be treated surgically. Dilatation achieves only temporary stretching or reduces the gradient by dilatation of an associated valvular stenosis.

CONCLUSIONS

Balloon aortic valvuloplasty for congenital valvular aortic stenosis was developed and applied in attempts to overcome the potential problems of aortic valve surgery. Balloon aortic valvuloplasty was shown to provide effective gradient relief in congenital aortic valve stenosis, with minimal restenosis on followup. It is justifiable as an alternative procedure because the sponataneous course of severe aortic stenosis is disastrous. Surgical valvotomy should be reserved for those patients in whom balloon dilatation is unsuccessful or impossible. Complications of balloon aortic valvuloplasty are not uncommonly encountered. Most are transient. The incidence and degree of aortic regurgitation is comparable to that associated with surgical open valvotomy.

Balloon dilatation of discrete subaortic stenosis seems to work well when the subaortic membrane is less than 2 mm thick. Its complications, like those of balloon aortic valvuloplasty, are mostly related to femoral arterial access.

Supravalvular aortic stenosis, in our opinion, is not amenable to balloon dilatation. The latter merely induces a gradient reduction by either temporary stretching of the thickened aortic media or dilatation of an associated aortic valvular stenosis.

Critical aortic stenosis in neonates is an emergency. In these infants balloon dilatations as well as open valvotomies are undertaken to interrupt an immediately life-threatening process. At present both techniques carry high morbidity and mortality when the aortic annulus is small or if there is associated endocardial fibroelastosis. Dramatic improvement in survival may depend on future advances in fetal diagnosis and intervention.

REFERENCES

1. Keane JF, Berhard WF, Nadas AS. Aortic stenosis surgery in infancy. *Circulation* 52:1138–1143, 1975.

2. Samanek M, Slavik Z, Zborilova B, et al. Prevalence, treatment, and outcome of heart disease in live-born children: A prospective analysis of 91, 823 live-born children. *Pediatr Cardiol* 10:205–211, 1989.

3. Braunwald E, Goldblatt A, Aygen MM, et al. Congenital aortic stenosis. *Circulation* 27:426–462, 1963.

4. Lababidi Z. Aortic balloon valvuloplasty. *Am Heart J* 106:751–752, 1983.

5. Lababidi Z, Wu J, Walls JT. Percutaneous balloon aortic valvuloplasty: Results in 23 Patients. *Am J Cardiol* 53:194–197, 1984.

6. Cribier A, Savin T, Saoudi N, et al. Percutaneous transluminal valvuloplasty of acquired aortic stenosis in elderly patients: an alternative to valve replacement. *Lancet* 1:63–67, 1986.

7. Lababidi Z, Weinhaus L, Stoeckle H Jr., et al. Transluminal balloon dilatation for discrete subaortic stenosis. *Am J Cardiol* 58:423–425, 1987.

8. Waller BF. Rheumatic and nonrheumatic conditions producing valvular heart disease. In: Frankl, WS and Brest AN (eds). Valvular Heart Disease: Comprehensive Evaluation and Management. *Cardiovascular Clinics*. Philadelphia, FA Davis P. 1986. Vol 16, No. 2, 1986. pp. 3–104.

9. Roberts WC. Anatomically isolated aortic valvular disease. The case against its being of rheumatic etiology. *Am J Med* 49:151–159, 1970.

10. Campbell M. The natural history of congenital aortic stenosis. *Br Heart J* 30:514–526, 1968.

11. Hossack KF, Neutze JM, Lowe JB, et al. Congenital valvar aortic stenosis. Natural history and assessment for operation. *Br Heart J* 43:561–573, 1980.

12. Friedman WF. Congenital heart disease in infancy and childhood. In: Braunwald E (ed). *Heart Disease*, Philadelphia, WB Saunders, pp 932–933.

13. Friedman WF, Johnson AD. Congenital aortic stenosis. In: Roberts, WC (ed). *Adult Congenital Heart Disease*. Philadelphia, FA Davis Co., 1987. pp 357–374.

14. Friedman WF Aortic stenosis. In: Adams FH, Emmanouilides GC, Riemenschneider TA (eds). *Moss' Heart Disease in Infants, Children, and Adolescents*. 4th ed. Baltimore, Williams and Wilkins, 1989. pp 224–243.

15. Stein PD, Sabbah HN, Pitha JV. Continuing disease process of calcific aortic stenosis — Role of microthrombi and turbulent flow. *Am J Cardiol* 39:159–163, 1977.

16. Fenoglio JJ Jr, McAllister HA Jr., DeCastro CM, et al. Congenital bicuspid aortic valve after age 20. *Am J Cardiol* 39:164–169, 1977.

17. Bernhard WF, Keane JF, Fellows KE, et al. Progress and problems in the surgical management of congenital aortic stenosis. *J Thorac Cardiovasc Surg* 66:404–419, 1973.

18. Frank S, Johnson A, Ross J Jr. Natural history of valvular aortic stenosis. *Br Heart J* 35:41–46, 1973.

19. Rapaport E. Natural history of aortic and mitral valve disease. *Am J Cardiol* 35:221–227, 1975.

20. Friedman WF, Modlinger J. Morgan JR. Serial hemodynamic obstructions in asymptomatic children with valvar aortic stenosis. *Circulation* 43:91–97, 1971.

21. El-Said G, Galiato FM Jr., Mullins CE, et al. Natural hemodynamic history of congenital aortic stenosis in childhood. *Am J Cardiol* 30:6–12, 1972.

22. Wagner HR, Weidman WH, Ellison RC, et al. Indirect assessment of severity in aortic stenosis. *Circulation* 56 (suppl I):I-20–I-23, 1977.

23. Snider AR, Stevenson JG, French JW, et al. Comparison of high pulse repetition frequency and continuous wave Doppler echocardiography for velocity measurement and gradient prediction in children with valvar and congenital heart disease. *J Am Coll Cardiol* 7:873–879, 1986.

24. Richards KL, Cannon SR, Miller JF, et al. Calculation of aortic valve area by Doppler echocardiography: a direct application of the continuity equation. *Circulation* 73:964–969, 1986.

25. Robinson PJ, Wyse RKH, Dearfield JE, et al. Continuous wave Doppler velocimetry as an adjunct to cross sectional echocardiography in the diagnosis of critical left heart obstructions in neonates. *Br Heart J* 52:552–556, 1984.

26. Ohlsson J, Wranne B. Noninvasive assessment of valve area in patients with aortic stenosis. *J Am Coll Cardiol* 7:501–508, 1986.

27. Lakier JB, Lewis AB, Heymann MA, et al. Isolated aortic stenosis in the neonate. Natural history and hemodynamic considerations. *Circulation* 50:801–808, 1974.

28. Brown JW, Stevens LS, Holly S, et al. Surgical spectrum of aortic stenosis in children: A thirty-year experience with 257 children. *Ann Thorac Surg* 45:393–403, 1988.

29. Kirklin JW, Barratt-Boyes BG. Congenital valvar aortic stenosis. In: *Cardiac Surgery*. New York. John Wiley and Sons, 1986. pp 972–988.

30. O'Toole JD, Geiser EA, Reddy S, et al. Effect of preoperative ejection fraction on survival and hemodynamic improvement following aortic valve replacement. *Circulation* 58:1175–1184, 1978.

31. Jack WD III, Kelly DT. Long-term follow-up of valvulotomy for congenital aortic stenosis. *Am J Cardiol* 38:231–234, 1976.

32. Wagner HR, Ellison RC, Keane JF, et al. Clinical course in aortic stenosis. In: Nadas AS (ed), Pulmonary Stenosis, Aortic Stenosis, Ventricular Septal Defect: Clinical Course and Indirect Assessment (Report from the Joint Study on the Natural History of Congenital Heart Defects). *Circulation* 55 (suppl I):I-47–I-56, 1977.

33. Sink JD, Smallhorn JF, Macartney FJ, et al. Management of critical aortic stenosis in infancy. *J Thorac Cardiovasc Surg* 87:82–86, 1984.

34. Messina LM, Turley K, Stanger P, et al. Successful aortic valvotomy for severe congenital valvular aortic stenosis in the newborn infant. *J Thorac Cardiovasc Surg* 88:92–96, 1984.

35. Gundry SR, Behrendt DM. Prognostic factors in valvotomy for critical aortic stenosis in infancy. *J Thorac Cardiovasc Surg* 92:747–754, 1986.

36. Hammon JW Jr, Lupinetti FM, Maples MD, et al. Predictors of operative mortality in critical valvular aortic stenosis presenting in infancy. *Ann Thorac Surg* 45:537–540, 1988.

37. Rocchini AP, Beekman RH, Shachar GB, et al. Balloon aortic valvuloplasty: results of the Valvuloplasty and Angioplasty of Congenital Anomalies Registry. *Am J Cardiol* 65:784–789, 1990.

38. Meliones JN, Beekman RH, Rocchini AP, et al. Balloon valvuloplasty for recurrent aortic

stenosis after surgical valvotomy in childhood: immediate and follow-up studies. *J Am Coll Cardiol* 13:1106–1110, 1989.

39. Lababidi Z, Weinhaus L. Successful balloon valvuloplasty for neonatal critical aortic stenosis. *Am Heart J* 112:913–916, 1986.

40. Rupprath G, Neuhaus K-L. Percutaneous balloon valvuloplasty for aortic valve stenosis in infancy. *Am J Cardiol* 55:1655–1656, 1985.

41. Kasten-Sportes CH, Piechaud J-F, Sidi D, et al. Percutaneous balloon valvuloplasty in neonates with critical aortic stenosis. *J Am Coll Cardiol* 13:1101–1105, 1989.

42. Zeevi B, Keane JF, Castaneda AR, et al. Neonatal critical valvar aortic stenosis. A comparison of surgical and balloon dilation therapy. *Circulation* 80:831–839, 1989.

43. Beekman RH, Rocchini AP, Andes A. Balloon valvuloplasty for critical aortic stenosis in the newborn: influence of new catheter technology. *J Am Coll Cardiol* 17:1172–1176, 1991.

44. Freedom RM. Balloon therapy of critical aortic stenosis in the neonate. The therapeutic conundrum resolved? *Circulation* 80:1087–1088, 1989.

45. Turley K, Bove EL, Amato JJ, et al. Neonatal aortic stenosis. *J Thorac Cardiovasc Surg* 99:679–684, 1990.

46. Brown JW, Robinson RJ, Waller BF. Transventricular balloon catheter aortic valvotomy in neonates. *Ann Thorac Surg* 39:376–378, 1985.

47. Rao PS. Percutaneous balloon valvotomy/angioplasty in congenital heart disease. In: Bashore TM and Davidson CJ (eds). *Percutaneous Balloon Valvuloplasty and Related Techniques*, Baltimore, Williams & Wilkins 1991. pp. 251–277.

48. Holmes DR Jr, Nishimura RA, Reeder GS. Aortic valvuloplasty in the adult. In: Holmes DR Jr and Vliestra RE (eds). *Interventional Cardiology*, Philadelphia, F.A. Davis Company, 1989. pp 120–137.

49. Radtke W, Keane JF, Fellows KE, et al. Percutaneous balloon valvotomy of congenital pulmonary stenosis using over-sized balloons. *J Am Coll Cardiol* 8:909–915, 1986.

50. Nishimura RA, Holmes DR Jr, Reeder GS, et al. Doppler echocardiographic observations during percutaneous aortic balloon valvuloplasty. *J Am Coll Cardiol* 11:1219–1226, 1988.

51. Cyran SE, Kimball TR, Schwartz DC, et al. Evaluation of balloon aortic valvuloplasty with transesopheageal echocardiography. *Am Heart J* 115:460–462, 1988.

52. Letac B, Cribier A. Balloon aortic valvuloplasty. In: Kapoor AS (ed). *Interventional Cardiology*, New York/Berlin: Springer-Verlag, 1989. pp. 239–253.

53. Mullins CE, Nihill MR, Vick GW III, et al. Double balloon technique for dilation of valvular or vessel stenosis in congenital and acquired heart disease. *J Am Coll Cardiol* 10:107–114, 1987.

54. Beekman RH, Rocchini AP, Crowley DC, et al. Comparison of single and double balloon valvuloplasty in children with aortic stenosis. *J Am Coll Cardiol* 12:480–485, 1988.

55. Macaya C, Santalla A, Perez de la Cruz JM, et al. Valvuloplastia transluminal percutánea con catéter-balón en la estenosis congénita de la válvula aórtica. *Rev Esp Cardiol* 38:396–399, 1985.

56. Kiel EA, Van Devanter SH, Readinger RI, et al. Aortic balloon valvuloplasty with transluminal venous balloon inflow occlusion. *Pediatr Cardiol* 7:103–105, 1986.

57. Meier B, Friedli B, Oberhänsli I. Trefoil balloon for aortic valvuloplasty. *Br Heart J* 56:292–293, 1986.

58. Mullins CE. Transseptal left heart catheterization: experience with a new technique in 520 pediatric and adult patients. *Pediatr Cardiol* 4:239–245, 1983.

59. Rao PS. Balloon aortic valvuloplasty in children. *Clin Cardiol* 13:458–466, 1990.

60. Rao PS, Thapar MK, Wilson AD, et al. Intermediate-term follow-up results of balloon

aortic valvuloplasty in infants and children with special reference to causes of restenosis. *Am J Cardiol* 64:1356–1360, 1989.

61. Roberts WC. Good-Bye to thoracotomy for cardiac valvulotomy. *Am J Cardiol* 59:198–202, 1987.

62. Walls JT, Lababidi Z, Curtis JJ, et al. Assessment of percutaneous balloon pulmonary and aortic valvuloplasty. *J Thorac Cardiovasc Surg* 88:352–356, 1984.

63. Waller BF, McKay CR, Erny R, et al. Catheter balloon valvuloplasty of necropsy stenotic aortic valves: etiology of aortic stenosis is a major factor in early "restenosis". *J Am Coll Cardiol* 13:16A, 1989.

64. Choy M, Beekman RH, Rocchini AP, et al. Percutaneous balloon valvuloplasty for valvar aortic stenosis in infants and children. *Am J Cardiol* 59:1010–1013, 1987.

65. Sholler GF, Keane JF, Perry SB, et al. Balloon dilation (BD) of aortic stenosis (AS): influences of valve morphology and technique on outcome. *Circulation* 76 (suppl IV): IV-554, 1987.

66. Wessel DL, Keane JK, Fellows KE, et al. Fibrinolytic therapy for femoral arterial thrombosis after cardiac catheterization in infants and children. *Am J Cardiol* 58:347–351, 1986.

67. Waller BF, Girod DA, Dillon JC. Transverse aortic wall tears in infants after balloon angioplasty for aortic valve stenosis. Relation of aortic wall damage to diameter of inflated angioplasty balloon and aortic lumen in seven necropsy cases. *J Am Coll Cardiol* 4:1235–1241, 1984.

68. Newfeld EA, Muster AJ, Paul MH, et al: Discrete subvalvular aortic stenosis in childhood Study of 51 patients. *Am J Cardiol* 38:53–61, 1976.

69. Van Praagh R, Corwin RD, Dahlquist EH Jr, et al. Tetralogy of Fallot with severe left ventricular outflow tract obstruction due to anomalous attachment of the mitral valve to the ventricular septum. *Am J Cardiol* 26:93–101, 1970.

70. Van Mierop LHS. Pathology and pathogenesis of the common cardiac malformations. *Cardiovasc Clin* 2(1):27–59, 1970.

71. Roberts WC. Pathologic aspects of valvular and subvalvular (discrete and diffuse) aortic stenosis. In: Kidd BSL, Keith JD (eds). *The Natural History and Progress in Treatment of Congenital Heart Defects*, Springfield, Illinois, Charles C Thomas, Publisher 1971. pp. 221–244.

72. Pyle RL, Patterson DF, Chacko S. The genetics and pathology of discrete subaortic stenosis in the Newfoundland dog. *Am Heart J* 92:324–334, 1976.

73. Somerville J, Stone S, Ross D. Fate of patients with fixed subaortic stenosis after surgical removal. *Br Heart J* 43:629–647, 1980.

74. Freedom RM, Pelech A, Brand A, et al. The progressive nature of subaortic stenosis in congenital heart disease. *Int J Cardiol* 8:137–143, 1985.

75. Leichter DA, Sullivan I, Gersony WM. "Acquired" discrete subvalvular aortic stenosis: natural history and hemodyamics. *J Am Coll Cardiol* 14:1539–1544, 1989.

76. Ferrans VJ, Muna WFT, Jones M, et al. Ultrastructure of the fibrous ring in patients with discrete subaortic stenosis. *Lab Invest* 39:30–40, 1978.

77. Kelly DT, Wulfsberg E, Rowe RD. Discrete subaortic stenosis. *Circulation* 46:309–322, 1972.

78. Champsaur G, Trusler GA, Mustard WT. Congenital discrete subvalvar aortic stenosis. Surgical experience and long-term follow-up in 20 paediatric patients. *Br Heart J* 35:443–446, 1973.

79. Sung C-S, Price EC, Cooley DA. Discrete subaortic stenosis in adults. *Am J Cardiol* 42:283–290, 1978.

80. Chaikhouni A, Crawford FA, Sade RM, et al. Discrete subaortic stenosis. *Clin Cardiol* 7:289–293, 1984.

81. Reis RL, Peterson LM, Mason DT, et al. Congenital fixed subvalvular aortic stenosis. An anatomical classification and correlations with operative results. *Circulation* 43 (Suppl I):I-11–I-18, 1971.

82. Lemole GM, Tesler UF, Colombi M, et al. Subaortic stenosis caused by two discrete membranes. *Chest* 69:104–106, 1976.

83. Khan MM, Varma MPS, Cleland J, et al. Discrete subaortic stenosis. *Br Heart J* 46:421–431, 1981.

84. Fontana RS, Edwards JE. *Congenital Cardiac Disease: A Review of 357 Cases Studied Pathologically.* Philadelphia, WB Saunders, 1962. p. 219.

85. Wilcox WD, Seward JB, Hagler DJ, et al. Discrete subaortic stenosis. Two-dimensional echocardiographic features with angiographic and surgical correlation. *Mayo Clin Proc* 55:425–433, 1980.

86. Suarez de Lezo J, Pan M, Sancho M, et al. Percutaneous transluminal balloon dilatation for discrete subaortic stenosis. *Am J Cardiol* 58:619–621, 1986.

87. Arora R, Goel PK, Lochan R, et al: Percutaneous transluminal balloon dilatation in discrete subaortic stenosis. *Am Heart J* 116:1091–1092, 1988.

88. Alyousef S, Khan A, Lababidi Z, Mullins C: Percutaneous transluminal balloon dilatation of discrete membranous subvalvular aortic stenosis. *Herz* 13:32–35, 1988.

89. Biancaniello TM: Balloon dilation in discrete subaortic stenosis. *Am Heart J* 117:1397, 1989.

90. Hellenbrand WE: Balloon dilatation of six patients with discrete subaortic stenosis. Symposium on Advances in Interventional Catheterization. Presented at the 39th Annual Scientific Session of the American College of Cardiology, New Orleans, Louisiana, Mar. 18–22, 1990.

91. Chevers N. Observations on the diseases of the orifice and valves of the aorta. *Guy Hosp Rep* 7:387–442, 1842.

92. Denie JJ, Verheugt AP. Supravalvular aortic stenosis. *Circulation* 18:902–908, 1958.

93. Kreel I, Reiss R, Strauss L, et al. Supra-valvular stenosis of the aorta. *Ann Surg* 149:519–524, 1959.

94. Perou ML. Congenital supravalvular aortic stenosis. A morphological study with attempt at classification. *Arch Pathol* 71:453–466, 1961.

95. Roberts WC. Valvular, subvalvular and supravalvular aortic stenosis: morphologic features. *Cardiovasc Clin* 5(1):97–126, 1973.

96. Williams JCP, Barratt-Boyes BG, Lowe JB. Supravalvular aortic stenosis. *Circulation* 24:1311–1318, 1961.

97. Kahler RL, Braunwald E, Plauth WH Jr, et al. Familial congenital heart disease. Familial occurrence of atrial septal defect with A-V conduction abnormalities; supravalvular aortic and pulmonic stenosis; and ventricular septal defect. *Am J Med* 40:384–399, 1966.

98. Ino T, Nishimoto K, Iwahara M, et al. Progressive vascular lesions in Williams-Beuren syndrome. *Pediatr Cardiol* 9:55–58, 1988.

99. Peterson TA, Todd DB, Edwards JE. Supravalvular aortic stenosis. *J Thorac Cardiovasc Surg* 50:734–741, 1965.

100. Do Valle PV, Barcia A, Bargeron LM Jr, et al. Angiographic study of supravalvular aortic stenosis and associated lesions. Report of five cases and review of literature. *Ann Radiol* 12:779–796, 1969.

101. Martin EC, Moseley IF. Supravalvar aortic stenosis. *Br Heart J* 35:758–765, 1973.

102. Rastelli GC, McGoon DC, Ongley PA, et al. Surgical treatment of supravalvular aortic

stenosis. Report of 16 cases and review of literature. *J Thorac Cardiovasc Surg* 51:873–882, 1966.

103. Keane JF, Fellows KE, LaFarge CG, et al. The surgical management of discrete and diffuse supravalvar aortic stenosis. *Circulation* 54:112–117, 1976.

104. Doty DB, Polansky DB, Jenson CB. Supravalvular aortic stenosis. Repair by extended aortoplasty. *J Thorac Cardiovasc Surg* 74:362–371, 1977.

105. Tyagi S, Arora R, Kaul UA, et al. Percutaneous transluminal balloon dilatation in supravalvular aortic stenosis. *Am Heart J* 118:1041–1044, 1989.

CHAPTER **14**

ACQUIRED AORTIC STENOSIS

ALAIN CRIBIER
BRICE LETAC

The 1980s and early 1990s have brought an increasing development and application of balloon catheters and more recently other devices to provide nonsurgical treatment of vascular and valvular stenosis. We became interested in percutaneous balloon aortic valvuloplasty as an alternative to surgical valve replacement 6 years ago. We began to investigate the procedure in elderly patients with severe degenerative aortic stenosis who, because of their age and associated co-morbidities, were considered to be at a too high risk for surgical valve replacement.[1] Our initial experience showed that the procedure was feasible at an acceptably low risk with immediate benefit in most patients, and this experience has been confirmed at other centers.[2-6]

As we have refined the technique and begun using specifically designed catheters and guidewires, the spectrum of patients included in our protocol was widened. We included younger patients who had contraindications to surgery or were at high surgical risk. We also subsequently included patients who were good candidates for surgery, either to defer the surgical valve replacement or because the patients refused to have surgery unless the valvuloplasty failed.[7,8] With continued experience and the analysis of a large series of patients, we[8] and others[9] began to recognize the limitations of the procedure. The high rates of residual aortic stenosis and restenosis, have led us again to restrict our selection of patients.

The findings of the Mansfield Multicenter Registry, in which we participated, were reported in the literature in 1991.[10-17] These data had been reviewed by the U.S. Food and Drug Administration (FDA) and in 1990 the procedure was approved for U.S. patients who are not considered to be surgical candidates.

Currently in our institution, the majority of patients selected for balloon aortic valvuloplasty are either very old (usually 80 years or older) or have severe left ventricular dysfunction (balloon aortic valvuloplasty being used as a bridge to surgery). Other indications include patients with significant noncardiac illness, patients who need an urgent noncardiac operation under general anesthesia, and patients who refuse surgery.

In this chapter, we provide a review of the technique and an update of the role of balloon aortic valvuloplasty in our experience, emphasizing the two major indications for the procedure: age of 80 years or more and critical illness.

TECHNIQUE

At our center, balloon aortic valvuloplasty is performed by passing the balloon catheter through the femoral artery and then retrograde across the aortic valve over a guidewire. We use a series of balloons of increasing diameter to obtain the largest possible valve area. Usually our goal is to increase the valve area by at least 100% and to achieve a valve area of at least 1 cm^2.

Initially, we used 9-Fr. Mansfield balloon catheters designed for dilatation of peripheral arterial stenosis or pulmonary valve stenosis. We used very small balloon diameters of 8, 10, and 12 mm only in the very first patients.[1] We then began to use balloons with diameters of 15, 18, and 20 mm, and subsequently 23 mm and even 25 mm.[7,8] These balloons were 3 or 4 cm long. Since September 1987 we have used a balloon catheter specifically designed for aortic valvuloplasty (Boston Scientific). The balloon is configured with a proximal segment 3.5 cm long which abruptly tapers to a more narrow distal segment 2 cm long. It is available in two sizes. The most frequently used balloon has a 20-mm proximal diameter and a 15-mm distal diameter (Fig. 14.1). A larger balloon has a 23-mm proximal diameter and 18-mm distal diameter. The catheter has a lumen proximal and distal to the balloon, allowing us to monitor central aortic pressure, measure transaortic valvular gradient, and perform contrast injections with the same device. Similar catheters with a single-size balloon of 15, 18, 20, or 23 mm are also available. A pigtail tip adds stability and safety to this device. At the time of this writing, however, these triple-lumen pigtail-tip catheters are not yet approved in the United States. We will therefore describe our earlier method in addition to the technique using the newer device.

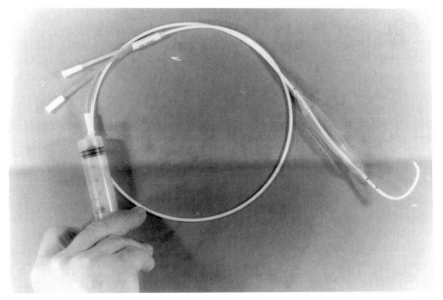

Figure 14.1 9-Fr. triple lumen, double-size (15- and 20-mm), pigtail-tip balloon catheter for percutaneous balloon aortic valvuloplasty.

Earlier Technique

The method first used in our laboratory is still currently used in many catheterization laboratories in the United States. The single-size straight-tipped Mansfield balloon catheter, previously approved only for pulmonary valvuloplasty procedures, has now been approved by the U.S. FDA also for aortic valvuloplasty.

Baseline hemodynamic measurements are obtained by performing a right heart catheterization with a thermodilution balloon flotation catheter from the femoral vein approach. Then, a 7-Fr. pigtail catheter is positioned in the ascending aorta through an 8-Fr. sheath in a femoral artery. Through this catheter, central aortic pressure is measured and aortograms are performed before the aortic valve is crossed and after the aortic valve has been dilated. An 8-Fr. sheath is introduced into the contralateral femoral artery. We prefer to use a 7-Fr. Sones catheter over 0.035-inch straight-tipped guidewire to cross the aortic valve, although several preformed catheter shapes are now available to facilitate crossing the valve. The transvalvular aortic pressure gradient is measured, cardiac output is obtained by means of the thermodilution technique, and the valve area is calculated by the computer using Gorlin's formula.[18] After the baseline hemodynamic measurements have been obtained, a left ventricular angiogram is performed in the right anterior oblique projection. This can be accomplished using the Sones catheter or a pigtail catheter by exchanging it over a long wire. Whenever we exchange catheter in the left ventricle over a wire, we first form an exaggerated curve in the distal extremity to protect the endocardium from perforation. This is particularly important with the use of straight-tipped balloons and stiffer wires.

The diagnostic catheter is removed over a 0.038-inch wire and the 8-Fr. sheath is removed at the same time. Additional lidocaine is infiltrated into the insertion site and 0.5 mg atropine is given intravenously to avert vagal reaction, which might otherwise occur during manipulation of the catheters and sheaths at the femoral entry site. A large introducer sheath, 12 or 14 Fr. (Schneider, UMI) is placed into the femoral artery with careful attention to the position of the wire near the left ventricular apex. The first balloon catheter, usually with a 15-mm diameter, is advanced over the wire and positioned across the aortic valve. Exerting traction on the wire by holding it fixed while the balloon is being advanced is helpful in negotiating tortuous iliac arteries and crossing severely stenosed valves. Careful attention to the position of the wire near the left ventricle apex, and to potential blood loss from the sheath is necessary during manipulation of the catheter.

The balloon is purged of air and the lumen is flushed with heparinized saline before the procedure. We use a 50:50 mixture of contrast medium and saline at the start, but often dilute the contrast further during the procedure if necessary to facilitate balloon deflation.

The balloon is inflated two or three times, and each balloon inflation is maintained for about 30 seconds or until the aortic pressure falls below 60 mmHg. The balloon is then simultaneously deflated and withdrawn into the ascending aorta, care being taken not to pull the guidewire into the aorta. It is also necessary to deflate the balloon promptly if the patient develops symptoms of near syncope, hypotension, bradycardia, arrhythmias, or significant ST-segment depression.

We judge the adequacy of the inflation pressure to the balloon by observing its shape as seen on the fluoroscope, trying to achieve a cylindrical or slightly bulging appearance. After this first series of inflations, the balloon catheter is removed over an exchange guidewire and replaced with a pigtail catheter. The aortic valve area is estimated from repeat measurement of the transaortic gradient and the thermodilution cardiac output. If the result is not satisfactory, the procedure is repeated with an 18-mm, a 20-mm, and then a 23-mm balloon catheter when necessary. Finally, the transaortic gradient and cardiac output for the final valve area are determined.

When a satisfactory result is obtained, or a decision is reached to terminate the procedure, the right heart pressures are remeasured, ventriculography is often performed, and a pullback gradient measurement is obtained. Aortography is repeated to look for postprocedure appearance or aggravation of aortic regurgitation. Coronary angiograms are usually done prior to the procedure. At this point, we generally remove all the catheters and sheaths before the patient leaves the laboratory. Hemostasis is obtained with manual pressure at the puncture site. We no longer use therapeutic doses of heparin, unless the patient has severely depressed myocardial function, severe coronary artery disease, or both. In such cases, the usual dose of 5,000 IU of heparin is reversed with protamine sulfate prior to catheter removal..

Updated Technique

The procedure has been remarkably simplified subsequent to the availability of the triple-lumen double-size balloon catheter.[19] Fewer catheter exchanges are required because pressure measurements, contrast injections, and serially sized balloon inflations can all be carried out using the same device. Also, the low profile of this balloon catheter, which fits through a 14-Fr. sheath, has further decreased trauma to the femoral arteral entry site, significantly reducing the incidence of local complications.

Using the new devices, the technique is currently performed as follows: With the distal end of the Sones catheter inside the left ventricle, the straight 0.035-inch guidewire is replaced with a .038-inch "extra stiff" guidewire (Schneider-Medintag). This is a 270-mm long exchange wire with a very stiff core. The distal 3 cm are flexible and shaped with a dull instrument into an exaggerated pigtail curve. The point in the wire where the stiff core and the distal flexible end join should be curved slightly by hand to avoid a sharp bend capable of injuring the left ventricle. With constant fluoroscopic visualization of the guidewire in the left ventricle, the Sones catheter is removed. Careful fluoroscopic monitoring of all catheter and sheath exchanges is very important, both to avoid the chance of the guidewire being pulled out from the left ventricle and to prevent injury to the myocardium.

An extra dose of local anesthetic is administered at the arterial entry site to diminish discomfort and vagal reaction during sheath exchange. The 8-Fr. arterial sheath is removed while hemostasis is obtained with hand compression. The femoral artery is catheterized with a 14-Fr. sheath (Schneider-Medintag). This special sheath has a proximal diaphragm that allows minimal blood leakage around the guidewire when the balloon catheter is not in place. Except for the 25-mm balloon catheters, all valvuloplasty catheters, when deflated, can be introduced and removed through this sheath. This diminishes trauma and discomfort with fewer vascular complications and less vagal reaction. The occlusive effect of the sheath in the femoral artery prevents bleeding without the need for constant groin compression throughout the procedure.

The chosen balloon is purged of air and kept completely deflated by applying strong negative pressure with an empty 20-mL syringe. It is introduced through the 14-Fr. sheath with a counterclockwise rotation which by design will keep the balloon profile at its minimum.

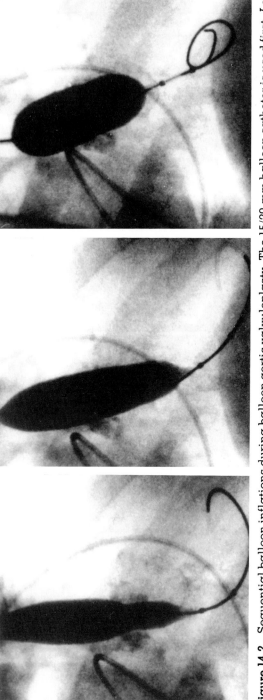

Figure 14.2 Sequential balloon inflations during balloon aortic valvuloplasty. The 15/20-mm balloon catheter is used first. *Left* and *center,* the balloon is first inflated on the 15-mm distal segment and then on the proximal 20-mm segment. *Right,* A single 23-mm balloon size catheter is then used. The transvalvular gradient is measured between series of balloon inflations and at the end of the procedure with the same catheter by positioning the 2 markers across the valve distal to the balloon, after removal of the guidewire.

Under fluoroscopic visualization of the tip of the guidewire the balloon catheter is rapidly advanced until the pigtail end reaches the left ventricle. Two distal markers are placed over the aortic valve calcifications to indicate the optimal position for accurate recording of the transvalvular gradient (Fig. 14.2). Once the catheter is well positioned the guidewire is removed and the aortic transvalvular gradient recorded. At this time the cardiac output is measured by thermodilution and the aortic valve area is calculated by Gorlin's formula on the computer.

The extra-stiff guidewire is readvanced up to the tip of the catheter but not protruding beyond it. This guidewire allows the balloon catheter to track better across the aortic valve and also supports the balloon in a stable position during inflation. The distal, smaller-diameter segment of the balloon is advanced and positioned across the aortic valve. Balloon inflations are performed with a hand-held syringe filled with a 50:50 mixture of contrast medium and saline. When using balloons larger than 20 mm we dilute this mixture further to allow faster deflation times. We begin balloon inflation slowly with a 20-mL syringe while the primary operator fixes the balloon in a stable position. Once fixation is obtained the balloon is rapidly inflated to its premaximal diameter with a 10-mL syringe.

During balloon inflation we constantly monitor three surface electrocardiographic leads and the aortic blood pressure via the proximal catheter lumen. If inflation is well tolerated and if no contraindications exist for long inflation, the balloon is kept inflated for a total 20 to 40 seconds. The balloon is deflated immediately if significant hypotension occurs or if marked ST-segment shifts or arrhythmias are noted on the electrocardiographic monitor. Before the next inflation, time should be allowed for blood pressure and electrocardiographic changes to return to baseline. After two or three inflations with the smaller segment of the balloon, the guidewire is removed and a transvalvular gradient obtained. Sometimes no further dilatations are required because the gradient is abolished, but this is rare. In most cases, the transvalvular gradient has been reduced but further dilatations with a larger size balloon are necessary.

With the extra-stiff guidewire in place the proximal, larger segment of the balloon is positioned across the aortic valve. With the technique already described, this segment of the balloon is inflated. One must remember that with larger-diameter balloons the hemodynamic and electrocardiographic changes occur sooner and are more pronounced. It is important to reach the maximal balloon diameter with each inflation. This can be judged grossly under fluoroscopy as the balloon shape changes during inflation. At maximal diameter, the balloon will appear perfectly cylindrical and even overdistended.

After each inflation the balloon is carefully but rapidly pulled back into the aorta, leaving the pigtail end in the left ventricle. This maneuver allows for a faster return of systemic blood pressure and cardiac performance to normal. After two or three inflations, a transvalvular gradient and a valve area are obtained. If the result is still not satisfactory, the balloon is ruptured during the next inflation. At the time of rupture, the balloon reaches a maximal compliance diameter, which is 21 mm for a 20-mm balloon and 24 mm for a 23-mm balloon. The transaortic valve gradient and the aortic valve area are again measured. If the measurements are considered suboptimal, a still larger balloon is used (Fig. 14.3). The same balloon catheter used for aortic valvuloplasty serves for final gradient measurements including a transvalvular pullback recording and also adequate contrast studies, more particularly an aortography for detection and quantitation of aortic insufficiency. These studies can be obtained without need of additional catheters.

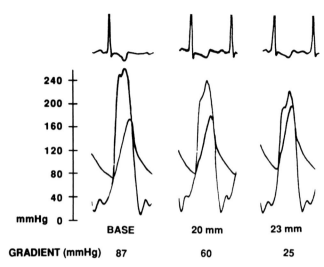

Figure 14.3 Effect of an increase in balloon size from 20-mm to 23-mm diameter on the transvalvular gradient reduction. The peak-to-peak gradient decreased from 87 to 60 mmHg after the 20-mm balloon inflation and further decreased to 25 mmHg with the use of the 23-mm balloon. Subsequently, the aortic valve area increased from 0.55 to 0.71 cm² and to 1.09 cm² after the 23-mm balloon inflation, a 100% increase.

Immediately after the procedure is completed, the catheters and arterial sheath are removed. The balloon profile allows the catheter to be removed through the sheath. Manual pressure is applied to the entry site until complete hemostasis is obtained. Patients remain supine in bed for 24 hours. The majority are discharged from the hospital 48 hours following balloon valvuloplasty.

We have now used the new devices in more than 300 patients. A 15- to 20-mm double-size balloon was used first in the majority of the patients. We then used a 23-mm single-size balloon if the results after the first dilatation were not satisfactory. The larger 18- to 23-mm balloon was used first only if the aortic annulus was found to be very large (>25 mm) on two-dimensional echocardiography. Nevertheless, considering the long inflation–deflation time with this balloon we now prefer using the 15- to 20-mm size followed by the 23-mm single size even in the case of a large annulus (Fig. 14.2). If the patient has a very small left ventricle, it may be dangerous to push the proximal segment across the aortic valve if there is not enough room for the distal segment and pigtail end of the balloon catheter. We prefer the single-size balloons in these cases.

Later in this review, we compare the results obtained when using the newer technique to those of our earlier experience. Briefly, we obtained improved results with a procedure that is completed faster, with less discomfort and risk to the patient..

Other Methods for Balloon Aortic Valvuloplasty

Several other methods for performing balloon aortic valvuloplasty have been proposed, using antegrade as well as retrograde techniques. The dual-balloon technique has been suggested as a method to obtain improved results.[20] In this method, two balloons are passed side by side across the aortic valve and then inflated simultaneously. The two catheters can be introduced through both femoral arteries, through a femoral artery and a brachial artery via cutdown, or even through the same femoral artery using cutdowns. Our experience with this particular technique is limited to a few patients, less than 5% of our series, when tortuous or stenotic iliac arteries would not allow passage of a 20-mm balloon and the brachial route has to be used, or when we were not satisfied with the results obtained with a 20-mm balloon and the 23-mm balloon was not available. In our experience the technique did not appear advantageous, except in the case of limited arterial access. The transseptal antegrade technique[21] would also be used if severe peripheral vascular disease limits access. Because of the added risk and longer duration of the procedure, however, we would consider it only for patients in whom neither the femoral nor the brachial arteries could be used.

RESULTS

Immediate Hemodynamic Results

Since 1985 the procedure has been performed in more than 600 patients in our institution. Because we had investigated a broad spectrum of indications, our first series of 406 patients was younger than all of the other published series of balloon aortic valvuloplasty for aortic stenosis in adults (mean age 73 yr; range 25–98 yr). The clinical and functional status of this population are shown in Table 14.1. Table 14.2 reports the technique used for balloon aortic valvuloplasty in this series.

Our hemodynamic results are presented in Figure 14.4. The transvalvular peak-to-peak gradient decreased by 60% and the aortic valve area improved by 100%. The mean absolute increase in valve area was 0.4 cm² (Fig. 14.5). Our results have been confirmed by other investigators (Table 14.3).[13,22-26] We have found the best results

Table 14.1 CLINICAL AND FUNCTIONAL STATUS OF THE FIRST 406 PATIENTS TREATED WITH BALLOON AORTIC VALVULOPLASTY IN THE ROVEN SERIES

Sex distribution:	199 M				
	207 F				
Mean age: 73 ± 11 (25–98)					
≤70:128	(32%)				
>70–80: 152	(37%)				
≥80:126	(31%)				
Etiology:					
unknown origin	363	(89%)			
rheumatic	36	(9%)			
congenital	7	(2%)			
Dyspnea (NYHA class III or IV)				256	(63%)
Syncopal attacks				85	(21%)
Angina pectoris				208	(51%)
Can HA class III or IV:		82	(20%)		
Asymptomatic				14	(3%)
Critical clinical condition (impending death)				61	(15%)

Table 14.2 TECHNICAL ASPECTS OF BALLOON AORTIC VALVULOPLASTY IN THE ROVEN SERIES OF 406 PATIENTS

Catheter insertion		
Femoral *(percutaneous)*	374	(92%)
Brachial *(cutdown)*	32	(8%)
Balloon catheter type		
Old	259	(64%)
New	147	(36%)
Largest balloon size used		
15 mm	18	
18 mm	57	(14%)
20 mm	219	(54%)
23 mm	90	(22%)
25 mm	7	(2%)
2 balloons	15	(4%)

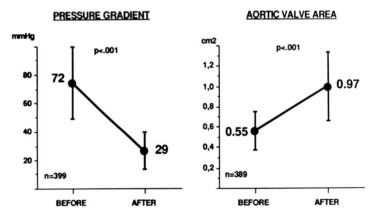

Figure 14.4 Decrease in peak-to-peak transvalvular gradient and increase in aortic valve area obtained after balloon aortic valvuloplasty in the Rouen series.

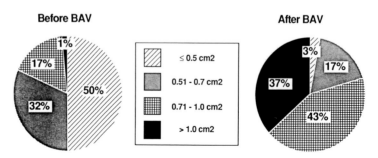

Figure 14.5 Aortic valve area distribution before (*left*) and after balloon aortic valvuloplasty (*right*) in the Rouen series.

Table 14.3 IMMEDIATE HEMODYNAMIC RESULTS OF BALLOON AORTIC VALVULOPLASTY (BAV) IN THE LARGEST REPORTED SERIES

Study	No. Pts.	AVA (cm²)		Gradient (mmHg)		
		Pre-BAV	Post-BAV	Pre-BAV	Post-BAV	
Safian et al[9] 1988	170	0.6 ± 0.2	0.9 ± 0.3	71 ± 20	36 ± 14	(p)
Block et al[35] 1988	162	0.5 ± 0.1	0.9 ± 0.2	61 ± 2	27 ± 1	(m)
McKay et al[24] 1988[a]	285	0.5	0.8	61	30	(m)
Powers et al[25] 1988[a]	155	0.5 ± 0.2	0.8 ± 0.4	58 ± 28	29 ± 16	(m)
Lancelin et al[26] 1989	92	0.47 ± 0.2	0.77 ± 0.2	62 ± 21	33 ± 14	(m)
Rouen 1989[b]	405	0.51 ± 0.2	0.98 ± 0.4	71 ± 20	28 ± 16	(p)
MSAVR[13] 1991[a]	492	0.50 ± 0.2	0.82 ± 0.3	60 ± 23	30 ± 13	(m)

AVA — aortic valve area. (p) — peak-to-peak transvalvular gradient. (m) — mean transvalvular gradient.

MSAVR — results of the Mansfield Scientific Aortic Valvuloplasty Registry.

[a] Results of a cooperative study.

[b] Results of the Rouen series (September 1985–December 1989).

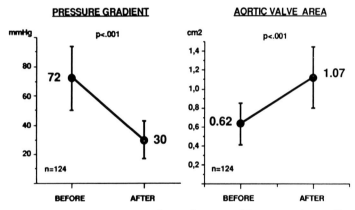

Figure 14.6 Changes in peak-to-peak gradient and increase in aortic valve area after balloon aortic valvuloplasty in a population of 124 patients below 70 years of age.

in younger patients whose valves were less calcified and who had slightly larger prevalvuloplasty valve areas (Fig. 14.6). There were more women in the older age group, and when corrected by body size, there was no difference in the results.

There is definitely a learning curve, and our results have improved with experience and better equipment (Fig. 14.7). In our first patients we were able to obtain a final valve area of 1.0 cm² or more in only 34% of the cases, whereas now we achieve that result in 47% of our cases. Also, in our first series, 22% of the patients were left with severe aortic stenosis (aortic valve area ≤ 0.7 cm²) after the procedure, but this has improved to only 12%.

To obtain the best results, the balloon must be maximally inflated while across the aortic valve, so that it generates the greatest dilating force. The force exerted by the expanded balloon ruptures calcific nodules, splits fused commissures, and stretches

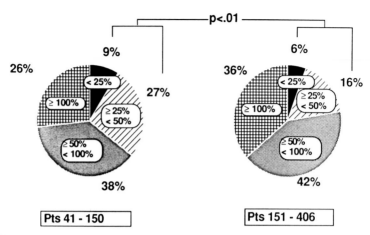

Figure 14.7 Improvement in percentage of increase in aortic valve area obtained after balloon aortic valvuloplasty with greater experience and better equipment in the Rouen series.

the valve structure. These mechanisms of improving the valve leaflet mobility and increasing the aortic valve orifice size have been previously described.[27,28] The maximal balloon diameter and dilating force are actually achieved just before the balloon ruptures. We routinely apply this amount of force in our procedures, and since the balloon is designed to split in a longitudinal tear, there have been no complications associated with bursting of the balloon.

Complications

Major Complications
When the first patients were done we had to overcome our fear of possible complications. Potentially lethal complications included embolic stroke, perforation of the heart, severe aortic regurgitation, disruption of the aortic annulus, myocardial infarction, malignant ventricular arrhythmias, or electromechanical dissociation.[8] Fortunately, in our series of patients, many of whom were very old and debilitated, the frequency of major complications was very low. Death occurred in 1%, pericardial tamponade (most likely due to myocardial perforation) in 1%, stroke in 0.7%, and complete heart block in 0.5%. The first 347 consecutive patients of our series had an aortic root angiogram routinely performed before and immediately after balloon aortic valvuloplasty. Severe or moderate aortic insufficiency was observed after the procedure in only 6 patients. No change or a slight increase or decrease of aortic regurgitation was seen in other patients. (Fig. 14.8). Although fatal aortic rupture has been reported in the literature,[29] it has not occurred in our series. We are aware, however, of a few cases of nonfatal aortic annulus disruptions which were discovered on subsequent evaluation at the time of valve replacement or necropsy in patients who had died of noncardiac causes.[27]

Minor Complications
Early in our experience, the femoral artery entry site was the most frequent source of complications. Since we have been using the 14-Fr. sheath, this complication rate has

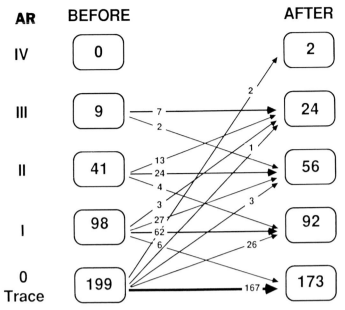

Figure 14.8 Angiographic changes in aortic regurgitation (*AR*) after balloon aortic valvuloplasty in our first 347 consecutive patients.

been reduced, and only 4% of patients with hematoma or femoral thrombosis need local surgery.

In-hospital Complications and Deaths

There were three additional major nonfatal complications prior to hospital discharge: two strokes and one myocardial infarction. Eleven additional patients died prior to discharge, increasing the total procedural and in-hospital mortality to 4%. These additional deaths were primarily due to end-stage heart failure but also included sepsis, stroke, renal failure, internal hemmorhage, cardiac arrest during general anesthesia for femoral repair.

Immediate Results in Our Most Recent Series

The results obtained in the last 100 patients of our previous series of 510 patients have been analyzed. The mean age of the population, 79 years (45–92 yr), was definitely higher than during our first experience and more comparable to other series of the literature. Sixty percent of this population was female. All procedures could be performed via the femoral route.

The maximal balloon size used for balloon aortic valvuloplasty was 20 mm in 62% of the cases and 23 mm in 38%. The transvalvular gradient decreased from 67 to 29 mmHg and the aortic valve area increased from 0.54 to 0.90 cm², an 81% increase.

Two patients died during the procedure and two additional deaths occurred during postprocedure hospitalization (a peri- and postprocedure mortality of 4%). One patient with severe cerebrovascular disease and previous neurologic events had a stroke during the balloon valvuloplasty. There were no other major complications. Minor complications were limited to hematomas at the femoral puncture site in 4 patients, requiring surgical femoral repair in 2. Thus, the total complication rate includng local complications was only 9%, 91% of the patients thus having an uneventful course. Taking into account the poor clinical condition of these elderly patients, we consider this relatively low complication rate acceptable. Nevertheless, it shows that despite considerable operator's experience and improved equipment, the risk of a major cardiac complication is always present in balloon aortic valvuloplasty.

Symptomatic Improvement and Survival

The remarkable and often dramatic symptomatic improvement after balloon aortic valvuloplasty is shown in Figure 14.9, which reports on improvement of dyspnea and angina in the first of 156 patients of our series, followed over a period of 16 ± 7 months, who had no repeat valvuloplasty or valve replacement. Similar results have been confirmed by other investigators.[6,12,30-33] Patients who were not critically ill at admission and who experienced no major complications had an average hospital stay of 5 days. Symptomatic improvement is certainly one of the most important issues in a population of very disabled elderly patients with aortic stenosis. After balloon aortic valvuloplasty, most of the patients are able to resume normal activities for their age within a few days and remain so for at least several months.

Survival of patients after balloon aortic valvuloplasty is related to their clinical status prior to the procedure. Figure 14.10 shows survival curves for the first 244 patients in our series. Patients who were less than 80 years old and who were considered to be good candidates for surgery had a 1-year mortality of 11%. Patients who were 80 years and older or who had associated diseases and were considered to be at increased surgical risk, had a 1-year mortality of 21%. Patients who had contraindications to surgical valve replacement had a 1-year mortality of 46%. Patients who died were older, had more severe clinical and hemodynamic deterioration, more severe aortic stenosis, and a very low ejection fraction. From our series, 185 patients were followed over a mean duration of 16 ± 7 months. Of these, 29 patients were candidates for surgery and had a subsequent valve replacement and 50 had a repeat balloon valvuloplasty. The remaining patients had sustained clinical improvement.

Restenosis

The recurrence of symptoms is often associated with restenosis, which had occurred in approximately half of our patients by 7 months.[8,34] In our early series of 300 patients, 96 had a repeat catheterization either for clinical restenosis (group 1, 31 patients; time elapsed postprocedure 6 ± 3 mo) or on the basis of a systematic control (group 2, 65 patients; time elapsed postprocedure 10 ± 7 mo). Restenosis (defined as a 50% loss of the gain in valve area) was 71% in group 1 and 37% in group 2. Restenosis rate was 52% for the entire series of 96 patients. Restenosis increases with time following the procedure, and in our series, it appeared to increase particularly after the ninth month.[8] However, we[8] and others[6,30] have observed that symptomatic improvement often persists despite the occurrence of restenosis. The occurrence and rate of restenosis are not predictable in a particular patient, but several factors may be related, including age >75 years, female gender, and the adequacy of the dilatation procedure.[34] In a series of 133 patients, Block[35] demonstrated a clinical restenosis rate of 59% at 7 months' followup in patients with a postvalvuloplasty valve area >0.7 cm^2 whereas the rate was 75% when the final valve area remained below 0.7 cm^2. In

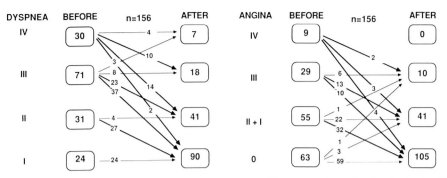

Figure 14.9 Symptomatic improvement after balloon aortic valvuloplasty in 156 patients followed over a period of 16 ± 7 months: dyspnea, New York Heart Association class I to IV *(left)*; angina: Canadian Heart Association class 0 to IV *(right panel).*

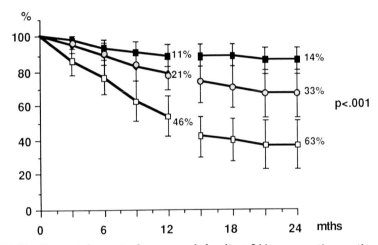

Figure 14.10 Actuarial survival curves of the first 244 consecutive patients of the Rouen series. *Black squares,* potentially good surgical candidates (up to 80 years of age), 92 patients. *Circles,* "High surgical risk patients" (above 80 years of age, depressed left ventricular function, associated diseases), 82 patients. *White squares,* Contraindications to surgery, 70 patients.

another series of 40 patients with clearly inadequate results (increase in valve area from 0.61 to 0.74 cm²), the restenosis rate was 100% at 12 months.[36]

Repeat Balloon Valvuloplasty

Balloon aortic valvuloplasty may have to be repeated in case of restenosis if surgery cannot be performed. Our series showed that the result of a repeat balloon aortic valvuloplasty are similar to those obtained during the first procedure. Of the patients in our early series, 67 of 363 had a repeat valvuloplasty 10 ± 6 months after the first procedure. The aortic valve area increased from 0.53 ± 0.18 cm² to 0.91 ± 0.32 cm² after the first procedure and from 0.60 ± 0.18 to 0.86 ± 0.18 cm² after the repeat procedure. These postprocedure results are comparable but they were obtained with the use of a larger balloon for repeat procedure in 38 patients. Other series have reported poorer results after repeat balloon aortic valvuloplasty despite the use of larger balloons.[37] The risk of the procedure appeared similar at the first and repeat balloon aortic valvuloplasty. Two patients with severe left ventricular dysfunction (ejection fraction of 15% and 26%) died in hospital from heart failure. One patient had pericardial effusion and three patients had femoral arterial complications. In uncomplicated cases, the mean in-hospital stay was 5 days after repeat balloon aortic valvuloplasty. Thus, in patients with a persistent contraindication to surgery, a second balloon aortic valvuloplasty may be considered as the best answer for optimal patient care.

THE MANSFIELD SCIENTIFIC AORTIC VALVULOPLASTY REGISTRY

The Mansfield Scientific Aortic Valvuloplasty Registry was established in 1986 to provide the U.S. FDA with data on safety and efficacy of balloon aortic valvuloplasty for "premarket approval." The registry consisted of 26 clinical centers in the United States and our center in Europe, with 492 patients enrolled as participants between December 1986 and October 1987. The results of this registry should thus be considered the early experience of this new technique.

The report summarizes the acute hemodynamic results of balloon aortic valvuloplasty,[13] the results according to patient's ages,[14] the procedural complications and predictors of long-term survival,[11,12,17] the results of followup recatheterization,[15] and the efficacy of repeated procedures.[16]

The mean age of this population was 79 ± 8.4 years, including 273 women (55%) and 219 men (45%). All patients were symptomatic with dyspnea associated with congestive heart failure (91.8%), angina (54.0%), or a history of syncope (22.4%); 45% of patients were in class III and 37% in class IV of the New York Heart Association classification; and 19% of patients were in severe congestive heart failure with pulmonary edema or pleural effusion, or both. All patients were at high risk for surgery because of advanced age (88% of the patients), severe coronary artery disease (23%), depressed ventricular function (30%), or associated medical conditions (23%).

Immediate Hemodynamic Changes

The procedures were performed from a femoral (92%), brachial (6%), or transseptal (2%) approach and employed either the single-balloon technique that we had described previously (72%) or a double-balloon technique (28%). The procedural factors that had affected the acute efficacy of balloon aortic valvuloplasty were also examined.

Overall, balloon aortic valvuloplasty increased the aortic valve area, reduced the mean aortic valve pressure gradient, increased the cardiac output, reduced the left ventricular systolic and end diastolic pressures, pulmonary capillary wedge pressure and mean pulmonary artery pressure, and increased the mean aortic pressure (Table 14.4). Serial aortography in 234 patients showed a moderate or severe increase in aortic regurgitation in only 2.1% of patients.

To study the effect of technique on the immediate results, six procedure-related variables were examined: use of single versus double balloons, the largest balloon diameter, the number of balloon inflations, the number of balloon exchanges, the

Table 14.4 IMMEDIATE HEMODYNAMIC RESULTS OF BALLOON AORTIC VALVULOPLASTY IN THE MANSFIELD SCIENTIFIC REGISTRY (492 PATIENTS)

	AVA (cm²)	Gr (mmHg)	CI (L/min/m²)	LVSP (mmHg)	LVEDP (mmHg)	CWP (mmHg)	PA (mmHg)	Ao (mmHg)
Pre Valvuloplasty	.50	60	3.86	201	19	23	30	88
	±.18	±23	±1.26	±42	±12	±12	±13	±18
Post Valvuloplasty	.82	30	4.05	173	17	16	28	91
	±.30	±13	±0.50	±32	±10	±18	±12	±20
p value	<.001	<.001	<.001	<.001	<.001	<.001	<.001	<.001

AVA: aortic valve area; Gr: mean transvalvular gradient; CI: cardiac index; LVSP: left ventricular systolic pressure; LVEDP: left ventricular end diastolic pressure; CWP: capillary wedge pressure; PA: mean pulmonary artery pressure; Ao: mean aortic blood pressure.

number of balloon inflations with the largest balloon used, and the mean inflation time. The results were analysed in relation to postvalvuloplasty aortic valve area and mean aortic valve gradient. The statistical analysis revealed that use of the double-balloon technique, more balloon inflations, and more frequent balloon exchanges improved hemodynamic outcome with respect to gradient reduction. However, the study cautions that patient-related variables are more important than techniques in determining the immediate hemodynamic results.

Procedural Complications and In-hospital Mortality

The overall rate of major and minor complications was 20.5%, with 101 patients experiencing a procedural complication.

Embolic events in the form of focal neurologic deficit occurred in 11 patients (2.2%), ventricular perforation with cardiac tamponade in 9 (1.8%), and severe aortic regurgitation in 5 (1%). The latter required emergent aortic valve replacement in 4 patients. Benign arrhythmias occurred in only 5 patients (1%). Local femoral arterial complications occurred in 52 (11%), requiring surgical intervention in 27. In the last series of 231 patients, a marked reduction in complication rate has been shown, from 25% in patients treated before July 1987 to 10% in those created thereafter (p <0.05). This difference may be attributed primarily to an improvement in low profile second-generation valvuloplasty balloon catheters that led to a large decrease in local vascular problems.

Catastrophic complications have been reported in 6.3% of patients in this latest series, being observed more frequently in females and with the use of double-balloon techniques. Fatal cardiac arrest occurred in 13 patients (2.6%), including 7 with cardiogenic shock and 4 with refractory ventricular tachyarrythmias during the procedure. Occlusion of the aortic valve orifice by the inflated balloon, myocardial stunning of the left ventricle during balloon inflation, or occlusion of the left or right coronary ostia during balloon inflation are the most likely mechanisms for fatal cardiac arrest during balloon aortic valvuloplasty.

The multivariate analysis studied by the registry identified important factors associated with increased in-hospital mortality related to the procedure. These included periprocedural complications, very depressed left ventricular function, low ventricular systolic pressure, low baseline cardiac output, and a smaller final aortic valve area. The more serious the complication, the higher the mortality, with myocardial perforation and ventricular fibrillation being the most lethal. Thus, improved patient selection alone can improve the risk benefit ratio in favor of better patient care.

Predictors of Long-Term Postprocedure Survival

The registry analyzed and reported the overall survival data and determinants of improved survival rates after balloon valvuloplasty in this severely symptomatic, elderly group of patients. The clinical status was determined in 488 of the 492 patients (99%) followed for a mean period of 7 months (range 0–19 mo). During this period, 117 patients died and 81 had repeat balloon valvuloplasty or valve replacement. The survival rate at 1 year was 64%. The functional status obtained in 304 of the 334 patients who survived >6 months revealed symptomatic improvement in 66%, and 26% were asymptomatic. Thus, even short-term clinical benefits justify balloon valvuloplasty as a therapeutic option for elderly patients who cannot be treated any other way. Eight variables were shown as predictors of improved probability of survival after balloon valvuloplasty: younger age, higher baseline cardiac output, better functional class, higher initial left ventricular systolic pressures, absence of coronary artery disease, greater final valve area, fewer balloon inflations, and lower left ventricular end-diastolic pressure. Those surviving longest after valvuloplasty would be the patients who had had no previous myocardial infarction and who had a less severe ventricular dysfunction, a lower systolic and mean pulmonary arterial pressure, and the largest initial aortic valve area. The sicker patients with heart failure and a smaller valve area are more likely to die.

From this report, subgroups of patients with lower and higher mortality could be identified. A patient survival probability at 1 year between 20% and 80% could be established. The findings revealed that only the final severity of aortic stenosis was prognostic and implied that successful balloon valvuloplasty indeed imparts an advantage to the survival of this subgroup of patients.

CURRENT INDICATIONS AND RESULTS

Balloon aortic valvuloplasty has two limiting factors that prevent its becoming a true alternative to surgical valve replacement. After a successful balloon aortic valvuloplasty procedure, some aortic stenosis remains and there is a high rate of restenosis in less than 1 year. Because of this, we began to employ more restrictive indications for the procedure. During the past 2 years we have been selecting patients who are very old (for example 80 years and older) and patients who are critically ill, particularly those requiring a bridge to surgery.

Current Indications: Age 80 or Older

Advances in surgical techniques, myocardial protection, and postoperative care have reduced the risk of aortic valve replacement, although the improved results reported in the literature are also related to patient selection. Given that balloon aortic valvuloplasty is a potential alternative to surgical valve replacement, interest in the application of surgical valve replacement in the elderly has been rekindled. Although the risks of surgery in older patients have been reduced, many physicians remain reluctant to refer their oldest patients to the cardiac surgeon. One reason has been a lack of published data to help the clinician reach a decision. Patient age above 70 has been recognized as a risk factor in cardiac surgery. Mortality rates published in the literature[38,39] for patients in their seventies range from 3 to 18%. Data for patients over 80 has been particularly limited. In a series of 100 patients 75 years and older[40] operative mortality was 3%; however, only 19 of the patients were aged 80 or older. More recently, there have been two reports of aortic valve replacement in very old patients.[41,42] In their series of open heart surgery in 100 patients over the age of 80 Edmunds and coworkers[41] reported a 90-day peri- and postoperative mortality of 29%. The mortality associated with an isolated aortic valve replacement was 30%; when aortic valve replacement was combined with coronary artery bypass graft surgery, the mortality was 24%. Early perioperative death was associated with a history of previous myocardial infarction, surgery performed as an emergency, cachexia, and severe heart failure. Actuarial mortality at 1, 2, and 5 years was 35%, 38%, and 50%, respectively.

Levinson and coworkers[42] reported a series of 64 patients with a mean age of 82 who had aortic valve replacement. These patients were selected because of their good preoperative clinical status. There were 6 surgery-related deaths (9.5%). Complications included permanent debilitating neurologic events in 9.5% and transient encephalopathy in 23% of the patients. Only 44% had an uncomplicated late outcome. The actuarial mortality was 17% and 35% at 1 and 5 years, respectively.

A review of these series of surgical patients confirms the observation of our larger series of very old patients that octogenarians are not a uniform group and that the preoperative status is a determinant of outcome. Some of these patients remain active and otherwise healthy despite their age, while others are frail with additional significant associated illnesses that substantially increase their predicted risk for surgery and often contraindicate major surgery of any kind. It is from this latter group of very old and frail patients, often with severely depressed left ventricular function requiring repeated hospitalizations because of refractory congestive heart failure, angina, and syncope that we select patients for balloon aortic valvuloplasty. Our goal in this group of patients is to palliate their symptoms so as to improve their quality of life.

We have reviewed the results of balloon aortic valvuloplasty obtained in our last series of 200 consecutive patients over the age of 80 years (mean 85 ± 4). The oldest patient was 98 years old. There was no selection bias, as the procedure was attempted in every patient referred regardless of the severity of the patient's clinical status.[43] In 20% of these patients there was a serious co-morbidity such as previous myocardial infarction, cancer, pulmonary insufficiency, or renal failure. Signs of severe heart failure (NYHA class III or IV) were present in 80%, syncope was present in 25%, and angina in 20%. The mean transvalvular aortic gradient decreased from 73 mmHg to 26 mmHg and the aortic valve area increased from 0.46 cm^2 to 0.98 cm^2. The procedure was a failure (less than 25% increase in valve area) in only 6%. Most patients were discharged 3 to 4 days after the procedure with evidence of clinical improvement.

Because the procedure has been simplified with the new devices, it has become shorter and safer during the past 3 years. We have compared the results of the current technique with our previous experience. The in-hospital complication rates are presented in Table 14.5. In the most recent series the in-hospital mortality had decreased from 6% to 1%. The total complication rate has decreased from 23% to 9%. Stroke occurred in 2% of the patients (who had previous neurologic events and cerebrovascular disease), myocardial infarction in 1%, and pericardial tamponade in 1%. No cases of aortic rupture or severe aortic regurgitation were observed. The rate of local complications at the femoral artery entry site improved, from 15% to 4%. The actuarial mortality in these elderly and severely ill patients at 3 months, 1 year, and 2

Table 14.5 INFLUENCE OF TECHNICAL IMPROVEMENT ON COMPLICATION RATE IN 200 CONSECUTIVE OCTOGENARIANS

	Group 1[a] (n = 98)	Group 2[b] (n = 102)
Death	6 (6%)	1 (1%)
Stroke	1 (1%)	2 (2%)
Myocardial infarction	0 (0%)	1 (1%)
Severe arrhythmias	1 (1%)	1 (1%)
Complications at site of femoral artery entry	15 (15%)	4 (4%)
Surgery required	6 (6%)	1 (1%)
Totals	*23%*	*9%*

[a] Patients in whom the initial technique was applied
[b] Patients in whom the updated technique was performed

years is 7%, 25%, and 50%, respectively. This compares favorably with a population of younger patients 10 year younger who were not operated on.[44,45]

Followup evaluation at a mean of 12 months revealed that 60% of the surviving patients had sustained marked clinical improvement, having returned to normal activities for their age. If symptoms recurred, restenosis was suspected and could be confirmed with echocardiographic techniques. Of 76 consecutives patients who had balloon aortic valvuloplasty in the recent series using the new equipment only 2 have required repeat valvuloplasty for restenosis. Three other patients subsequently showed sufficient clinical improvement to be accepted for surgical valve replacement 1, 2, and 6 months after the balloon aortic valvuloplasty. One of these patient died postoperatively.

Because of patient selection bias in other reported surgical series, it is not possible to compare our series of elderly patients treated with balloon aortic valvuloplasty directly with these findings. It seems apparent to us that octogenarians selected for balloon aortic valvuloplasty are not similarly ill to patients selected for surgical valve replacement. Most of the patients referred for valve replacement are otherwise healthy. Patients referred for balloon aortic valvuloplasty have symptoms of heart failure and usually other associated illnesses or debilitation which makes the risk of surgery too high. Balloon aortic valvuloplasty can provide a moderate increase in valve area sufficient to alleviate the symptoms of these patients. Sustained improvement at 1 year is seen in many of these patients. The palliation of symptoms is achieved at low risk and low cost. The procedure can be repeated if restenosis causes a recurrence of symptoms, and in some patients the subsequent clinical hemodynamic improvement may allow for a lower risk surgical valve replacement.

Although our data suggest that elderly patients have a lower risk with balloon aortic valvuloplasty than surgery and are likely to benefit from the procedure, we do not consider the patient's age alone. Despite our extensive experience with balloon aortic valvuloplasty, we recommend surgical valve replacement for octogenarians who are otherwise healthy. Balloon aortic valvuloplasty is indicated in the octogenarian patient with severe aortic stenosis associated with congestive heart failure, severe coronary disease, chronic debilitation, or other noncardiac disease that potentially could increase the risk of surgery or shorten the patient's life expectancy.

Current Indications: Critical Illness

It is well documented that left ventricular dysfunction and advanced New York Heart Association functional class are important predictors of operative mortality in patients who undergo aortic valve replacement. Patients who require emergent surgery and who present with clinical signs of cardiogenic shock are at particularly high risk.[46-48] Some of these patients may be considered unsuitable for surgery despite their predictably lethal spontaneous course.

Balloon aortic valvuloplasty has been shown to markedly improve left ventricular performance in patients with critical aortic stenosis associated with severe left ventricular dysfunction.[49-52] We reported a series of 55 patients with poor left ventricular function (ejection fraction <40%) who were treated with balloon aortic valvuloplasty.[49] Repeat catheterization was performed 6 months later in 20 patients. The ejection fraction had increased from $39 \pm 10\%$ to $52 \pm 10\%$ in the 11 patients who had no restenosis. Recently we reported a series of 34 patients (mean age 76 yr) with "end-stage" heart failure who had balloon aortic valvuloplasty performed as a last resort treatment.[53] Aortic valve replacement was considered to be high-risk in these patients. Balloon aortic valvuloplasty was successfully performed in each case. The transaortic gradient decreased from 59 to 21 mmHg, the cardiac index increased from 1.77 to 2.1 L/min/m^2, and the aortic valve area increased from 0.42 to 0.85 cm^2. The left ventricular ejection fraction also showed immediate improvement from 28% to 35%. No deaths or strokes occurred during the procedure. Two patients had no improvement after the procedure and died while in the hospital. Another 2 patients who showed some clinical improvement but had continued heart failure were subjected to surgical valve replacement. One patient died and the other had a good surgical outcome. Thirty patients were discharged after an average stay of 10 days, significantly improved. The patients were followed for 15 ± 7 months. During this time there were 15 deaths at an average 6 ± 5 months following the procedure. None of these patients were surgical candidates. The 15 remaining survivors had sustained functional improvement. Three of the younger patients (50, 59, and 53 years old) subsequently had elective aortic valve replacement at an average of 9 months following balloon aortic valvuloplasty, but at a much lower surgical risk than that which would have been predicted had they presented with profound heart failure.

Cardiogenic shock due to cardiac failure in patients with severe aortic stenosis is associated with a lethal outcome or a very short predicted survival. Balloon aortic valvuloplasty has been carried out in 10 patients of our series who were moribund when they were transferred to our laboratory. Each patient was reviewed by the cardiac surgeon, who declined to operate because of the very high surgical risk. The balloon aortic valvuloplasty was performed without any procedural deaths. The valve area increased from 0.47 ± 0.1 cm^2 to 0.95 ± 0.3 cm^2, comparable to the results achieved in the total series. Dyspnea improved immediately, and signs of cardiogenic shock diminished within hours. In one patient, early restenosis led to a recurrence of cardiogenic shock, causing death 2 days later. Another patient who had a partial remission of cardiac failure had a successful aortic valve replacement 8 days later. The other 8 patients continued to show clinical improvement after balloon aortic valvuloplasty and were discharged after an average length of stay of 10 days. An example of such a dramatic improvement in shown in Figure 14.11. Followup catheterization showed an improved left ventricular ejection fraction. Aortic valve replacement was recommended and successfully carried out in 6 of the patients at an average of 9 months after the balloon aortic valvuloplasty procedure. They all had an excellent

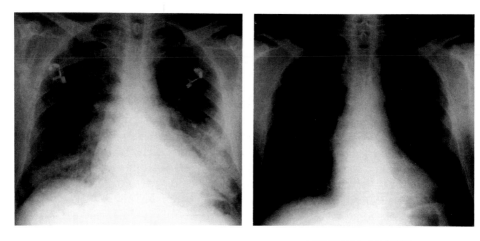

PRE-BAV   POST-BAV : 21 DAYS

Figure 14.11   Resolution of pulmonary edema seen on chest x-rays 21 days after balloon aortic valvuloplasty (BAV) in a 54-year-old man who had the procedure done in the emergency department while he was in cardiogenic shock refractory to vasopressive drugs. With the use of a 23-mm balloon catheter, the mean gradient decreased from 53 to 26 mmHg and the valve area increased from 0.38 to 1.35 cm². BAV was followed by a dramatic clinical improvement. The ejection fraction was 19% before BAV; it was 50% before valve replacement which was performed 8 months later. The patient remained asymptomatic until surgery was performed.

surgical outcome. Two of the patients refused to have the recommended surgery and were still surviving with sustained clinical improvement 24 and 48 months after balloon aortic valvuloplasty. Similar results have been reported in patients with cardiogenic shock by Desnoyers.[52]

It is possible to perform balloon aortic valvuloplasty safely in critically ill patients with aortic stenosis; balloon aortic valvuloplasty is particularly indicated in patients who present in cardiogenic shock. The indications should be flexible in the consideration of young patients with an advanced degree of heart failure or unstable hemodynamic situations. The technique could be lifesaving in these patients, and may serve as a useful "bridge to surgery."

Once the patient has obtained clinical improvement and the risk of surgery is acceptably low, aortic valve replacement should be recommended.

Other Indications: Young Patients With Congenital or Rheumatic Aortic Stenosis

In November 1982, balloon aortic valvuloplasty emerged as a potential alternative to surgical treatment of severe congenital aortic valvular stenosis in children.[54] Since then, several authors[55-58] have also reported their experiences with this procedure in congenital and rheumatic aortic stenosis in children and young adults. In these cases, the mechanism of balloon aortic valvuloplasty has been shown to be a splitting of both noncalcified and calcified fused aortic commissures, similar to the results reported in rheumatic mitral valve stenosis. Ribeiro for example,[58] in an in vitro study, have

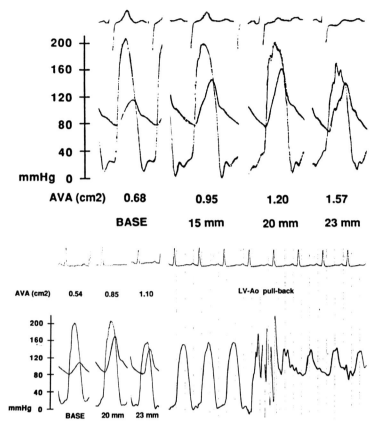

Figure 14.12   Representative example of the improvement in aortic valve area (*AVA*) obtained after balloon aortic valvuloplasty in a 38-year-old man with rheumatic aortic stenosis (*upper panel*) and in a 49-year-old man with congenital aortic stenosis (*lower panel*).

demonstrated an optimal commissural splitting in the aortic valve with an increase of 57% in mean aortic valve area after double-balloon aortic valvuloplasty, showing that the technique have palliative effects similar to those of surgical valvotomy.

We have attempted balloon aortic valvuloplasty in 19 young patients, 12 to 49 years old, as an alternative to surgical valvotomy or valve replacement. Ten of these patients had congenital and 9 had rheumatic aortic valve stenosis (Figs. 14.12 and 14.13). Two had membranous discrete subvalvular stenosis and one had a restenosis following surgical valvotomy performed 10 years before. All patients had moderate to severe dyspnea at exertion and one had had several episodes of syncope.

We used the double-balloon technique in the first 4 patients of this series and thereafter the single-balloon technique. The immediate results obtained after balloon aortic valvuloplasty are shown in Figure 14.14. The peak transvalvular gradient was decreased from 82 ± 22 mmHg to 48 ± 22 mmHg and the aortic valve area increased from 0.71 ± 0.25 cm^2 to 1.23 ± 0.34 cm^2.

Aortic insufficiency was the only complication of the procedure and was observed after balloon aortic valvuloplasty in all patients, grade 1 or 2 in 15 and grade 3 in 4. In

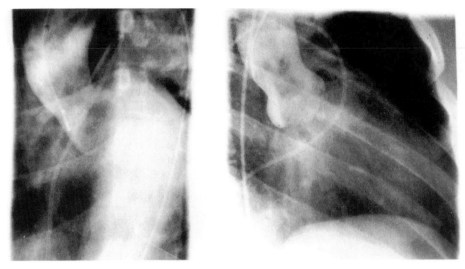

Figure 14.13 Representative example of the improvement in aortic valve opening observed in a 16-year-old patient with congenital aortic valve stenosis. Typical doming of the aortic valve with a central "jet" as seen on the supravalvular aortogram before balloon aortic valvuloplasty during systole (*left panel*). After balloon aortic valvuloplasty, no doming could be seen and the aortic valve orifice appeared clearly enlarged. In this patient, the gradient was decreased from 80 to 25 mmHg and aortic valve area was increased from 0.7 to 1.4 cm². No restenosis was demonstrated on Doppler echocardiography 1 year post-balloon aortic valvuloplasty.

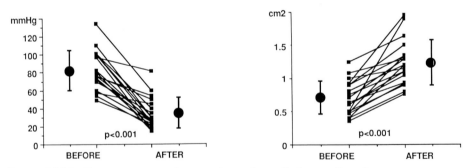

Figure 14.14 Decrease in peak-to-peak gradient (*left panel*) and increase in aortic valve area (*right panel*) observed in a series of 19 young patients (below 50 years of age) with congenital or rheumatic aortic valve stenosis.

one patient, a 39-year-old man with rheumatic aortic valve stenosis, a valve replacement was done 3 months after balloon aortic valvuloplasty because of the severity of aortic insufficiency. Another patient, a 30-year old woman who had a very severe congenital aortic stenosis and who presented with syncope at the time of balloon aortic valvuloplasty, had an uneventful pregnancy and delivery in the year following the procedure. However, she had a valve replacement 3 years later because of progressive left ventricular enlargement resulting from a grade 3 aortic regurgitation. Valve replacement was performed on two additional patients because balloon aortic valvuloplasty failed to reduce the gradient below 60 mmHg. The remaining patients have been followed 38 ± 11 months (1 to 70 months) clinically and by Doppler echocardiography. One of these patients, who was 36 years old at the time of balloon aortic valvuloplasty, had clinical and echocardiographic signs of restenosis 5 years after the procedure and is now scheduled for valve replacement.

In young adults with aortic valve stenosis of congenital or rheumatic origin, balloon aortic valvuloplasty may be attempted in selected cases as a palliative procedure aimed at postponing surgery for some years. More particularly, balloon aortic valvuloplasty should be considered in women who wish to become pregnant in the near future and in still-growing adolescents.

Severe aortic insufficiency does represent a major potential complication in these patients. For this reason, we recommend that aortic root angiography be performed after each series of balloon inflations and before increasing the size of the balloon to prevent induction of significant aortic regurgitation. In this subset of patients, a suboptimal result with a gradient of 40 mmHg should be acceptable in most situations.

FUTURE DIRECTIONS

The technique and technology of balloon aortic valvuloplasty are still under investigation, and its clinical application is therefore still in evolution. Percutaneous cardiopulmonary support has been proposed as a means to assist balloon aortic valvuloplasty in high-risk patients,[59] but we have not found this to be very necessary in our series. Other investigators have proposed novel approaches to valvuloplasty with new devices such as lithotripsy[60] or laser balloon.[61] Restenosis remains the major challenge, and as the morphologic and histologic basis of restenosis becomes better understood[62] perhaps a more direct attack on the pathophysiologic mechanism of restenosis will become feasible in the future.

CONCLUSION

In adult aortic stenosis, we consider balloon aortic valvuloplasty to be a palliative procedure which should be restricted to patients who are considered to be poor candidates for surgical aortic valve replacement, mainly because of very advanced age. It may also be the only therapeutic option for critically ill patients with severe aortic stenosis.

The therapeutic goal in these patients is to improve the quality of life and possibly to improve survival. On patients with severe left ventricular dysfunction, the technique can be used as a "bridge to surgery," allowing valve replacement to be performed at a lower risk after cardiac function has improved.

Balloon aortic valvuloplasty has a limited role in patients who are good surgical candidates; it should be considered only when general anesthesia is required for an emergent noncardiac intervention or when surgical valve replacement is absolutely refused by the patient.

REFERENCES

1. Cribier A, Savin T, Saoudi N, et al: Percutaneous transluminal valvuloplasty of acquired aortic stenosis in elderly patients: an alternative to valve replacement? *Lancet.* 1:63–67, 1986.

2. McKay RG, Safian RD, Lock JE, et al: Balloon dilatation of calcific aortic stenosis in elderly patients: postmortem, intraoperative, and percutaneous valvuloplasty studies. *Circulation.* 74:119–125, 1986.

3. Isner JM, Salem DN, Desnoyers MR, et al: Treatment of calcific aortic stenosis by balloon valvuloplasty. *Am J Cardiol.* 59:313–317, 1987.

4. Drobinski G, Lechat P, Metzger JP, et al: Results of percutaneous catheter valvuloplasty for calcified aortic stenosis in the elderly. *Eur Heart J.* 8:322–328, 1987.

5. Jackson G, Thomas S, Monaghan M, et al: Inoperable aortic stenosis in the elderly: benefit from percutaneous transluminal valvuloplasty. *Br Med J.* 294:83–86, 1987.

6. Schneider JF, Wilson M, Gallant TE: Percutaneous balloon aortic valvuloplasty for aortic stenosis in elderly patients at high risk for surgery. *Ann Intern Med.* 106:696–699, 1987.

7. Cribier A, Savin T, Berland J, et al: Percutaneous transluminal balloon valvuloplasty of adult aortic stenosis: report of 92 cases. *J Am Coll Cardiol.* 9:381–386, 1987.

8. Letac B, Cribier A, Koning R, et al: Results of percutaneous transluminal valvuloplasty in 218 adults with valvular aortic stenosis. *Am J Cardiol.* 62:598–605, 1988.

9. Safian RD, Berman AD, Diver DJ, et al: Balloon aortic valvuloplasty in 170 consecutive patients. *N Engl J Med.* 319:125–130, 1988.

10. O'Neill WW: Seminar on balloon aortic valvuloplasty, I:introduction. *J Am Coll Cardiol.* 17:187–188, 1991.

11. Holmes DR Jr, Nishimura RA, Reeder GS: In-hospital mortality after balloon aortic valvuloplasty: frequency and associated factors. *J Am Coll Cardiol.* 17:189–192, 1991.

12. O'Neill WW for the Mansfield Scientific Aortic Valvuloplasty Registry Investigators: Predictors of long-term survival after percutaneous aortic valvuloplasty: report of the Mansfield Scientific Balloon Aortic Valvuloplasty Registry. *J Am Coll Cardiol.* 17:193–198, 1991.

13. McKay RG for the Mansfield Scientific Aortic Valvuloplasty Registry Investigators: The Mansfield Scientific Aortic Valvuloplasty Registry: overview of acute hemodynamic results and procedural complication. *J Am Coll Cardiol.* 17:485–491, 1991

14. Reeder GS, Nishimura RA, Holmes DR Jr, et al: Patient age and results of balloon aortic valvuloplasty: the Mansfield Scientific Registry experience. *J Am Coll Cardiol.* 17:909–913, 1991.

15. Bashore TM, Davidson CJ and the Mansfield Scientific Aortic Valvuloplasty Registry Investigators: Follow-up recatheterization after balloon aortic valvuloplasty. *J Am Coll Cardiol.* 17:1188–1195, 1991.

16. Ferguson JJ, Garza RA, and the Mansfield Scientific Aortic Valvuloplasty Registry Investigators: Efficacy of multiple balloon aortic valvuloplasty procedures. *J Am Coll Cardiol.* 17:1430–1435, 1991.

17. Isner, JM and the Mansfield Scientific Aortic Valvuloplasty Registry Investigators: Acute catastrophic complications of balloon aortic valvuloplasty. *J Am Coll Cardiol.* 17:1436–1444, 1991.

18. Gorlin R, Gorlin SG: Hydraulic formula for calculation of the area of the stenotic mitral valve, other cardiac valves, and central circulatory shunts. I. *Am Heart J.* 41:1–29, 1951.

19. Cribier A, Gerber L, Berland J, et al: Percutaneous balloon aortic valvuloplasty: the state of the art. a review of two years' experience in Rouen. *J Intervent Cardiol.* 1:237–250, 1988.

20. Dorros G, Lewin RF, King JF, et al: Percutaneous transluminal valvuloplasty in calcific aortic stenosis: the double balloon technique. *Cathet Cardiovasc Diagn*. 13:151–156, 1987.

21. Block PC, Palacios IF: Comparison of hemodynamic results of anterograde versus retrograde percutaneous balloon aortic valvuloplasty. *Am J Cardiol*. 60:659–662, 1987.

22. Bashore TM, Davidson CJ: Acute hemodynamic effects of percutaneous balloon aortic valvuloplasty. In: Bashore TM, Davidson CJ. *Percutaneous Balloon Valvuloplasty and Related Techniques*. Baltimore: Williams & Wilkins, 1991, p 103.

23. Orme EC, Wray RB, Barry WH, et al: Comparison of three techniques for percutaneous balloon aortic valvuloplasty of aortic stenosis in adults. *Am Heart J*. 117:11–17, 1989.

24. McKay RG for the Mansfield Scientific Aortic Valvuloplasty Registry: Balloon aortic valvuloplasty in 285 patients: initial results and complications. *Circulation*. 78(suppl II):II-594, 1988.

25. Powers ER for the NHLBI Balloon Valvuloplasty Registry: Early Results of aortic valvuloplasty from the NHLBI Balloon Valvuloplasty Registry. *Circulation*. 78(suppl II):II-594, 1988.

26. Lancelin B, Chevalier B, Bourdin T, et al: Suivi à moyen terme après valvuloplastie aortique percutanèe du sujet âgè: ètude clinique à propos de 102 procèdures. *Arch Mal Coeur*. 82:1397–1404, 1989.

27. Letac B, Gerber LI, Koning R: Insights on the mechanism of balloon valvuloplasty of aortic stenosis. *Am J Cardiol*. 62:1241–1247, 1988.

28. Safian RD, Mandell VS, Thurer RE, et al: Postmortem and intraoperative balloon valvuloplasty of calcific aortic stenosis in elderly patients: mechanisms of successful dilation. *J Am Coll Cardiol*. 9:655–660, 1987.

29. Lembo NJ, King SB III, Roubin GS, et al: Fatal aortic rupture during percutaneous balloon valvuloplasty for valvular aortic stenosis. *Am J Cardiol*. 60:733–736, 1987.

30. Block PC, Palacios IF: Clinical and hemodynamic follow-up after percutaneous aortic valvuloplasty in the elderly. *Am J Cardiol*. 62:760–763, 1988.

31. Serruys PW, Luijten HE, Beatt KJ, et al: Percutaneous balloon valvuloplasty for calcific aortic stenosis. A treatment 'sine cure'? *Eur Heart J*. 9:782–794, 1988.

32. Lewin RF, Dorros G, King JF, et al: Percutaneous transluminal aortic valvuloplasty: acute outcome and follow-up of 125 patients. *J Am Coll Cardiol*. 14:1210–1217, 1989.

33. Holmes DR Jr, Nishimura RA, Reeder GS, et al: Clinical follow-up after percutaneous aortic balloon valvuloplasty. *Arch Intern Med*. 149:1405–1409, 1989.

34. Cribier A, Gerber LI, Letac B: Percutaneous balloon aortic valvuloplasty: the French experience. In: Topol EJ. *Textbook of Interventional Cardiology*. Philadelphia: WB Saunders, 1990, pp 849–867.

35. Block PC, Palacios IF: Percutaneous aortic balloon valvuloplasty (PAV) in the elderly: update of immediate results and follow-up. *Circulation*. 78(suppl II:II-593, 1988.

36. Meany BT, Sprigings D, Chambers J, et al: Aortic valvuloplasty in the elderly: is re-stenosis inevitable? *Circulation*. 78(suppl II):II-531, 1988.

37. Ross TC, Banks AK, Collins TJ, et al: Repeat balloon aortic valvuloplasty for aortic valve restenosis. *Cathet Cardiovasc Diagn*. 18:96–98, 1989

38. Bergdahl L, Bjork VO, Jonasson R. Aortic valve replacement in patients over 70 years. *Scand J Thorac Cardiovasc Surg*. 15:123–128, 1981.

39. Santinga JT, Flora J, Kirsh M, et al: Aortic valve replacement in the elderly. *J Am Geriatr Soc*. 31:211–212, 1983.

40. Blakeman BM, Pifarrè R, Sullivan HJ, et al: Aortic valve replacement in patients 75 years old and older. *Ann Thorac Surg*. 44:637–639, 1987.

41. Edmunds LH Jr, Stephenson LW, Edie RN, et al: Open-heart surgery in octogenarians. *N Engl J Med*. 319:131–136, 1988.

42. Levinson JR, Akins CW, Buckley MJ, et al: Octogenarians with aortic stenosis: outcome. after aortic valve replacement. *Circulation.* (Suppl I):I-49–I-56, 1989.

43. Letac B, Cribier A, Koning R, et al: Aortic stenosis in elderly patients aged 80 or older: treatment by percutaneous balloon valvuloplasty in a series of 92 cases. *Circulation.* 80:1514–1520, 1989.

44. O'Keefe JH, Vlietstra RE, Bailey KR, et al: Natural history of candidates for balloon aortic valvuloplasty. *Mayo Clin Proc.* 62:986–991, 1987.

45. Turina J, Hess O, Sepulcri F, et al: Spontaneous course of aortic valve disease. *Eur Heart J.* 8:471–483, 1987.

46. Scott WC, Miller DC, Haverich A, et al: Determinants of operative mortality for patients undergoing aortic valve replacement. Discriminant analysis of 1479 operations. *J Thorac Cardiovasc Surg.* 89:400–413, 1985.

47. Carabello BA, Green LH, Grossman W, et al: Hemodynamic determinants of prognosis of aortic valve replacement in critical aortic stenosis and advanced congestive heart failure. *Circulation.* 62:42–48, 1980.

48. Smith N, McAnulty JH, Rahimtoola SH: Severe aortic stenosis with impaired left ventricular function and clinical heart failure: results of valve replacement. *Circulation.* 58:255–264, 1978.

49. Berland J, Cribier A, Savin T, et al: Percutaneous balloon valvuloplasty in patients with severe aortic stenosis and low ejection fraction. Immediate results and 1-year follow-up. *Circulation.* 79:1189–1196, 1989.

50. McKay RG, Safian RD, Lock JE, et al: Assessment of left ventricular and aortic valve function after aortic balloon valvuloplasty in adult patients with critical aortic stenosis. *Circulation.* 75:192–203, 1987.

51. Safian RD, Warren SE, Berman AD, et al: Improvement in symptoms and left ventricular performance after balloon aortic valvuloplasty in patients with aortic stenosis and depressed left ventricular ejection fraction. *Circulation.* 78:1181–1191, 1988.

52. Desnoyers MR, Salem DN, Rosenfield K, et al: Treatment of cardiogenic shock by emergency aortic balloon valvuloplasty. *Ann Intern Med.* 108:833–835, 1988.

53. Cribier A, Lafont A, Eltchaninoff H, et al: La valvuloplastie aortique percutanée réalisée en dernier recours chez les patients atteints de rétrécissement aortique en état critique. *Arch Mal Coeur.* 83:1783–1790, 1990.

54. Lababidi Z: Aortic balloon valvuloplasty. *Am Heart J.* 106:751–752, 1983.

55. Choy M, Beekman RH, Rocchini AP, et al: Percutaneous balloon valvuloplasty for valvar aortic stenosis in infants and children. *Am J Cardiol.* 59:1010–1013, 1987.

56. Scholler GF, Keane JF, Perry SB, et al: Balloon dilation of congenital aortic valve stenosis. Results and influence of technical and morphological features on outcome. *Circulation.* 78:351–360, 1988.

57. Ribeiro PA, Al Zaibag M, Halim M, et al: Percutaneous single- and double-balloon aortic valvotomy in adolescents and young adults with congenital aortic stenosis. *Eur Heart J.* 9:866–873, 1988.

58. Ribeiro PA, Al Zaibag M, Rajendran V: Double balloon aortic valvotomy for rheumatic aortic stenosis: in vitro studies. *Eur Heart J.* 10:417–422, 1989.

59. Vogel RA: The Maryland experience: angioplasty and valvuloplasty using percutaneous cardiopulmonary support. *Am J Cardiol.* 62:11K–14K, 1988.

60. Erny RE, Waller BF: Potential use of lithotripsy in balloon aortic valvuloplasty. *Circulation.* (suppl II):II-529, 1988.

61. McMath L, Rezkalla S, Spears JR: Laser balloon valvuloplasty: in vitro feasibility in canine aortic valves. *Circulation.* 80(suppl II):II-359, 1989.

62. Essed C, Van den Brand M, Plante S, et al: Histologic findings in aortic valves previously subjected to percutaneous balloon aortic valvuloplasty. *Eur Heart J.* 11(abstract suppl):228, 1990.

CHAPTER **15**

Pulmonic Stenosis

P. SYAMASUNDAR RAO

Stenosis of the pulmonary valve constitutes 7.5 to 9.0% of all congenital heart defects.[1,2] Children with pulmonic stenosis usually present with asymptomatic murmurs, but they may also present with signs of congestive heart failure due to severe right ventricular dysfunction or cyanosis because of right-to-left shunting across the atrial septum. Clinical findings of ejection systolic click and ejection systolic murmur at the left upper sternal border, right ventricular hypertrophy on an electrocardiogram, a prominent main pulmonary artery segment on a chest roentgenogram, and increased Doppler flow velocity in the main pulmonary artery are characteristic for this anomaly. When the pulmonary valvar obstruction is moderate to severe, relief of the obstruction is recommended to treat symptoms, if present, or to prevent right ventricular fibrosis and dysfunction. Until recently, surgical valvotomy was the only treatment available, but pulmonary valve obstruction can now be relieved by percutaneous balloon valvuloplasty.

Rubio and Limon Lason[3] in 1954 described a technique by which pulmonic valve stenosis could be relieved via a catheter; they used a ureteral catheter with a wire. Twenty-five years later, Semb and his associates[4] used a Berman balloon angiographic catheter to rupture the pulmonary valve (commissures); they withdrew an inflated balloon from the main pulmonary artery to the right ventricle and reduced the pulmonary valve gradient. More recently, Kan and her associates[5] used a static dilatation technique (similar to that used by Dotter and Judkins[6] and Grüntzig and his associates[7,8]) in which they introduced a deflated balloon across the pulmonic valve and inflated the balloon; the radial forces of balloon inflation produced relief of pulmonary valve obstruction. This static dilatation technique is what is currently used. This chapter presents the current state of the art of percutaneous balloon pulmonary valvuloplasty; personal experience with this procedure, including that reported previously,[9-26] and the experiences reported in the literature are used as supportive material. Although the majority of the presentation focuses on the isolated pulmonic valvular stenosis, the use of transcatheter methods in the treatment of pulmonic stenosis associated with complex heart defects and valvular pulmonary atresia are included at the conclusion of the chapter.

INDICATIONS

By and large, the indications for percutaneous balloon dilatation of pulmonic stenosis are essentially the same as those used for surgical intervention. The indications for surgical pulmonary valvotomy are reasonably clear; patients with stenosis of moderate to severe degree irrespective of the symptoms are candidates for surgical relief of the obstruction.[27,28] The indications for balloon valvuloplasty appear less clear and are rarely defined.[29] Careful examination in 1988[18] of all the available studies[5,29-38] revealed that many patients with what may be considered mild pulmonic stenosis (natural history study definition[28]: gradient <25 mmHg = trivial; 25–49 mmHg = mild, 50–79 mmHg = moderate; and ≥ 80 mmHg = severe) underwent balloon valvuloplasty. A review of the results of balloon valvuloplasty in patients with mild stenosis revealed that residual right ventricular peak systolic pressures at followup were $75 \pm 18\%$ of prevalvuloplasty values.[18] Furthermore, natural history studies of pulmonic stenosis[28,39,40] indicated that mild pulmonary stenosis remains mild on followup. Therefore, the advisability of balloon valvuloplasty for mild obstruction can be questioned. My recommendations are to consider the indications for balloon valvuloplasty to be the same as those used for surgical valvuloplasty and that balloon dialatation should not be performed in patients with gradients of less than 50 mmHg. Because noninvasive echo-Doppler estimates of pulmonary valve gradients are reasonably accurate,[41-43] patients with mild stenosis can be kept under observation; once the Doppler estimate of the gradient is in excess of 50 mmHg, they can undergo balloon valvuloplasty. Although there is some wisdom in using valve areas for setting criteria for intervention, gradients are adequate for estimating stenosis of the pulmonary valve provided cardiac indices are measured during prevalvuloplasty catheterization and are shown to be within normal range.

Some investigators consider dysplastic pulmonary valves as a relative contraindication for balloon valvuloplasty.[44,45] On the basis of the results of others[36,46] and our own data,[17] balloon valvuloplasty is the initial treatment of choice; perhaps large balloons to produce a balloon:annulus ratio of 1.4 to 1.5 should be used.[17] Our experience indicates that the procedure is also successful in patients with Noonan's syndrome. Patients whose pulmonary valves have restenosed after a previous surgical pulmonary valvotomy also respond favorably to balloon pulmonary valvuloplasty. In conclusion, moderate to severe pulmonic valvular stenosis (gradient ≥ 50 mmHg) irrespective of previous surgical intervention and pulmonary valve dysplasia is an indication for percutaneous balloon pulmonary valvuloplasty.

TECHNIQUE

The diagnosis and assessment of the pulmonary valve obstruction are made by the usual clinical, roentgenographic, electrocardiographic, and echo-Doppler data. Once a moderate to severe obstruction has been diagnosed, cardiac catheterization and cineangiography are performed percutaneously to confirm the clinical impression and to evaluate the feasibility of balloon dilatation of the pulmonic valve. The indications for catheter intervention (described above) are usually those prescribed for surgical intervention. Once balloon dilatation is decided upon:

1. A 5-Fr. to 7-Fr. multi-A-2 (Cordis) catheter is introduced percutaneously into

the femoral vein and advanced across the pulmonic valve and then into the left pulmonary artery.

2. A 0.014- to 0.035-inch J-shaped guidewire is passed through the catheter into the distal left pulmonary artery.

3. A 4-Fr. to 9-Fr. balloon dilatation catheter is advanced over the guidewire and the balloon is positioned across the pulmonic valve.

4. The balloon is inflated with diluted contrast material to approximately three to five atmospheres of pressure (Figure 15.1) (The recommended duration of inflation is 5 seconds. Usually a total of three to four balloon inflations are performed, 5 minutes apart. We use a double-balloon technique — two balloons simultaneously inflated across the stenotic region — when the valve annulus is too large to dilate with a commercially available single balloon).

5. Measurement of pressure gradients across the pulmonic valve and angiographic demonstration of the relief of obstruction are performed.

Heart rate, systemic pressure, and cardiac index are recorded prior to and after balloon dilatation to ensure that the change in pressure gradient is not related to a change in cardiac index but is indeed related to procedure.

We generally perform this procedure with the patient sedated (usually with a mixture of meperidine, promethazine, and chlorpromazine, given intramuscularly), although others use ketamine[37] or general anesthesia.[29,47]

Other aspects of importance for successfully accomplishing balloon valvuloplasty are as follows:

Difficult femoral venous access: Sometimes it may be difficult to cannulate the femoral vein percutaneously either because of technical problems or because of

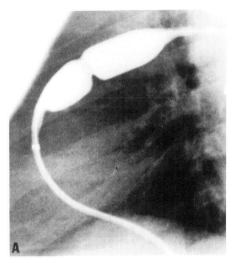 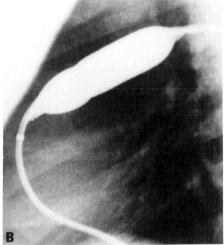

Figure 15.1 Selected cineradiographic frames of a balloon dilatation catheter placed across the pulmonic valve. Note "waisting" of the balloon during the initial phases of balloon inflation (*A*) which is almost completely abolished during the later phases of balloon inflation (*B*).

femoral venous thrombosis secondary to previous catheterization or surgery. Cutdown and isolation of the saphenous vein–femoral vein junction may be performed and catheterization and balloon valvuloplasty can be accomplished via saphenous venous bulb. When femoral venous access is not possible, balloon pulmonary valvuloplasty may be performed via an axillary venous[34,48] or internal jugular venous[49] approach. The latter two approaches are also useful in the presence of infrahepatic interruption of the inferior vena cave with azygos or hemiazygos continuation.

Passing an end-hold catheter across the pulmonic valve: This may be difficult in some patients, particularly in young children and neonates. In such occasions, we employ several maneuvers: (1) An end-hole catheter (usually a multi-A-2), may be positioned just underneath the pulmonary valve and the floppy end of a straight guidewire advanced through the tip of the catheter into the main pulmonary artery. (2) A balloon-wedge catheter is positioned just beneath the pulmonic valve, the balloon is quickly deflated, and the catheter is advanced into the main pulmonary artery. Failing this, we use a guidewire, as described earlier. (3) A flexible, steerable coronary guidewire is passed through an end-hole catheter. (4) We have encountered one child in whom we could not advance any catheter across the right ventricular infundibulum because of severe infundibular constriction. In this child, administration of propranolol (0.1 mg/kg IV slowly) made it possible to pass a catheter across the pulmonary valve and eventually to carry out balloon pulmonary valvuloplasty.[25]

Choice of size of balloon dilatation catheter: The current recommendations are to use a balloon that is 1.2 to 1.4 times the size of the pulmonary valve annulus. These recommendations are formulated on the basis of immediate[35] and followup[12,15,20] results. For further discussion of reasoning behind such recommendations, the reader is referred to these publications.[12,15,20,22] Balloons larger than 1.5 times the size of the pulmonary valve annulus are not recommended because of potential damage to the right ventricular outflow tract caused by use of large balloons.[50] However, it may be advisable to use large balloon to produce a balloon:annulus ratio of 1.5:1 when pulmonary valve dysplasia is present.[17]

When the pulmonary valve annulus is too large to dilate with a single balloon, valvuloplasty with simultaneous inflation of two balloons across the pulmonary valve annulus should be performed. When two balloons are used, the following formula is used to calculate the effective balloon size[12]:

$$\frac{D_1 + D_2 + \pi\left(\dfrac{D_1}{2} + \dfrac{D_2}{2}\right)}{\pi}$$

where D_1 and D_2 are diameters of the balloons used.

Although we do not believe that double-balloon technique is superior to single-balloon technique,[15,21,51] it does reduce injury to the femoral veins because smaller catheters can be used.

Some workers[52-54] have advocated trefoil balloons with the idea that there will be forward flow around the balloon during balloon inflation. Such attempts to allow forward flow during balloon inflation are laudable, but I do not believe that there will be any significant forward flow since the balloons used for pulmonary valve dilatation are larger than the valve annulus.

Difficulty in advancing the balloon valvuloplasty catheter across the pulmonic valve: It is important to avoid kinking or looping of the guidewire to prevent such a problem. Replacement of the guidewire with an extra-stiff Amplatz guide may circumvent the difficulty.

Sometimes it may not be feasible to advance an appropriate-sized balloon dilatation catheter across the pulmonic valve even after having a guidewire across it. In such situations, we use a smaller 4- to 6-mm balloon on a 4- or 5-Fr. catheter initially to predilate and then use larger, more appropriate-sized balloons.

IMMEDIATE RESULTS

Several groups of investigators,[29-36,54-65] including our group,[9,10,14,20,22,51] have reported excellent immediate relief of pulmonic valve obstruction following balloon valvuloplasty. From our group, 71 infants and children, aged 2 days to 20 years (median 5 years), underwent balloon dilatation of pulmonic valvular stenosis during a 7.5-year period ending March 1991. Following valvuloplasty, the peak systolic pressure in the right ventricle decreased from 108 ± 41 (mean $\pm$ SD) to 53 ± 22 mmHg ($p < 0.001$), as did the peak systolic gradient across the pulmonic valve, from 91 ± 41 to 26 ± 19 mmHg ($p < 0.001$) (Figure 15.2). The cardiac index did not change ($p > 0.1$). Width of the jet of the contrast material through the pulmonary valve as

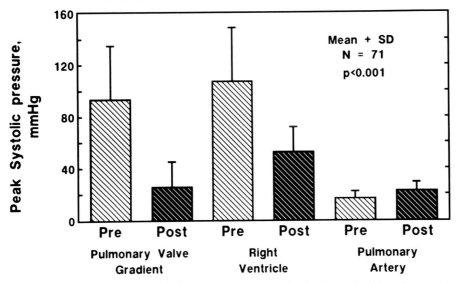

Figure 15.2 Acute results of balloon pulmonary valvuloplasty in 71 patients showing a significant ($p < 0.001$) decrease in the peak-to-peak systolic pressure gradient across the pulmonic valve and peak systolic pressures in the right ventricle. Also, note a significant ($p<0.001$) increase in the peak systolic pressure in the pulmonary artery.

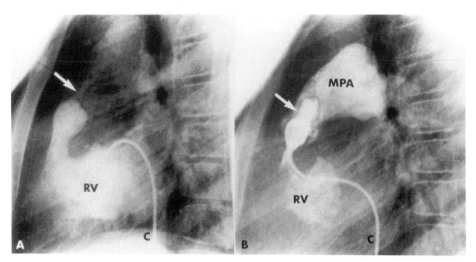

Figure 15.3 Selected frames from lateral views of right ventricular (*RV*) cine-angiogram prior to (*A*) and after (*B*) balloon pulmonary valvuloplasty. Note extremely thin jet (*arrow*) prior to balloon dilatation (*A*) which increased to a much wider jet (*arrow*) after valvuloplasty (*B*), opacifying the main pulmonary artery (*MPA*). C—catheter. (From: Rao PS: Balloon angioplasty and valvuloplasty in infants, children, and adolescents. *Curr Probl Cardiol.* 14:417–497, 1989. With permission.)

Table 15.1 INTERMEDIATE-TERM FOLLOWUP CATHETERIZATION RESULTS OF BALLOON PULMONARY VALVULOPLASTY (BPV) FROM THE LITERATURE

Study	No. Patients Undergoing BPV	No. Patients With Followup	Duration of Followup, Mean (Range), Months	
Kan et al,[31] 1984	20	11	7	(2–12)
Tynan et at,[29] 1985	27	6	no data	(2–6)
Kveselis et al,[32] 1985	19	7	12	(9–13)
Miller,[33] 1985	16	7	4	(3–6)
Sullivan et al,[34] 1985	23	12	5.5	(0.25–6)
Ali Khan et al,[57] 1986	32	14	10	(6–14)
Shrivastava et al,[55] 1987	32	21	no data	(3–18)
Rey et al,[36] 1988	51	23	no data	(1–17)
Fontes et al,[58] 1988	100	44	12	(3–14)
Schmaltz et al,[63] 1989	273	53	11	(−)
Rao, 1991	71	45	11	(6–34)

[a] Poor result is defined as pulmonary valve gradient in excess of 30 mmHg at followup.

[b] The pulmonary valve gradient ranged between 31 and 52 mmHg with a mean of 38 mmHg.

[c] Poor result is defined as gradient ≥ 40 mmHg.

visualized in the lateral view of the cineangiogram (Figure 15.3) increased. Less doming and much more "free" movement of the pulmonary valve leaflets occurred after the valvuloplasty in each case. Surgical intervention was avoided in all cases. Most patients were discharged home within 24 to 48 hours following the procedure. Though not studied by us, an improvement in the function of both the right and left ventricles[66] is expected.

FOLLOWUP RESULTS

Several authors[29,31-34,36,55,57,58,63] have conducted studies in which recatherization was performed on 6 to 53 patients, 1 week to 18 (mean) months following balloon valvuloplasty. They reported significant residual gradients (> 30 mm) in 14 to 100% of patients (Table 15.1). We recatheterized 45 children 6 to 34 months (mean, 11.0 months) following balloon valvuloplasty. For the group of children for whom followup catheterization data were available, the peak systolic pressure gradient across the pulmonic valve (92 ± 43 vs 29 ± 23 mmHg, $p < 0.001$) and the peak systolic pressure in the right ventricle (109 ± 41 vs. 56 ± 22 mmHg, $p < 0.001$) decreased after balloon dilatation. The cardiac index (3.3 ± 0.9 vs 3.2 ± 0.7 L/min/m^2, $p > 0.1$) remained unchanged. Upon followup approximately 11 months later, systolic pressure gradient across the pulmonic valve (29 ± 23 mmHg, $p < 0.001$) remains improved when compared to predilatation value (Figure 15.4). The cardiac index (3.5 ± 0.8 L/min/m^2) did not change significantly ($p > 0.1$). Despite improvement as a group, several children had significant residual gradients (Fig. 15.5) across the pul-

Poor Result[a] on Followup, No. (%)	Comments
2 (18)	The failure was in patients with dysplastic valve or after previous Brock procedure.
2 (33)	Both patients underwent surgery.
7 (100)[b]	Repeat BPV in 1 patients with 52 mmHg gradient with reduction to 34 mmHg.
1 (14)	2 patients with gradients of 24 and 22 mmHg at followup underwent repeat BPV with excellent results.
6 (50)	Repeat valvuloplasty in 4 patients with good results.
2 (14)	None
9 (43)	None
5 (22)	Repeat BPV in 5 patients with satisfactory results.
10 (23)	
14 (26)[c]	Repeat BPV in 14 patients; successful in 10, remaining 4 with dysplastic valves required surgery.
9 (20)	Repeat BPV in 6 patients with good results.

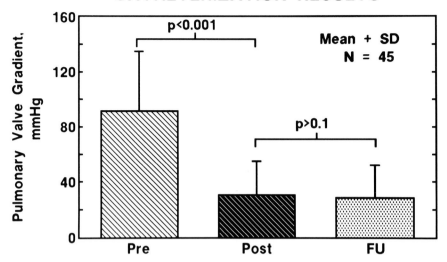

Figure 15.4 Acute and follow-up results of the 45 unselected patients (from among 71 patients undergoing balloon valvuloplasty—Figure 15.2) who underwent cardiac catheterization 11 months (mean) following balloon pulmonary valvuloplasty. Note significant (p < 0.001) fall in the peak systolic pressure gradient across the pulmonary valve immediately after the procedure which remained unchanged (p > 0.1) at follow-up (FU); the latter continues to be significantly (p < 0.001) lower than the prevalvuloplasty gradient. The gradients represented are valvular gradients without any regard to infundibular gradients.

monic valve, hereafter referred to as restenosis. Nine out of 45 children who were restudied had pulmonary valve gradients in excess of 30 mmHg. Six of these children underwent repeat balloon valvuloplasty with larger balloons (Fig. 15.5), and the pulmonary valve gradients were reduced from 96 ± 40 to 40 ± 22 mmHg (p < 0.01). The other three children with residual gradients of 45, 50, and 60 mmHg are being followed clinically. Repeat followup catheterization (in 4) or echo-Doppler studies (in 4) were available in 8 children (24 months after first balloon valvuloplasty) and the residual pulmonary valve gradients were 28 ± 12 mmHg.

The restenosis rate (9 of 45, 20%) in our group, though high, is comparable to the 14 to 100% reported by other workers (Table 15.1). It should be noted however, that we initially recommended that recatheterization be performed routinely 6 to 12 months after balloon valvuloplasty. More recently we have not employed routine postoperative catheterization, ordering it only when the echo-Doppler estimate of the residual gradient is high. On this basis we conclude that restenosis occurred in 9 of the 70 patients for whom followup catheterization data, echo-Doppler data, or both are available, i.e., a 12.9% recurrence rate. Electrocardiographic and echo-Doppler followup studies, which are also reflective of the pressure gradient relief,[11,16] are discussed later in this chapter.

BALLOON PULMONARY VALVULOPLASTY
POOR RESULTS GROUP

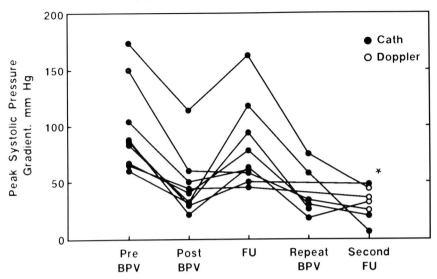

Figure 15.5 Sequential pulmonary valvular gradients are shown for each of the 9 patients who had gradients in excess of 30 mmHg at followup catheterization. Repeat balloon dilatation at the time of followup (*FU*) catheterization in 6 of these children produced a fall in the gradient in each patient. At a second followup study (catheterization or Doppler), the gradients remained low. *Solid circles,* Gradients measured at cardiac catheterization. *Open circles,* Doppler-estimated peak instantaneous gradients. 43. *BPV*—balloon pulmonary valvuloplasty.

Apart from the pressure gradient relief, there are other benefits. Right-to-left interatrial shunting that was present prior to balloon valvuloplasty has completely disappeared in most patients. Right ventricular dysfunction and tricuspid insufficiency are alleviated. Figures 15.6 and 15.7 illustrate improvement in the cardiac size and tricuspid insufficiency following balloon valvuloplasty.

These intermediate-term followup results appear encouraging and lead me to recommend balloon valvuloplasty as a procedure of choice for treatment of isolated valvular pulmonic stenosis. Further refinement of the catheter technology and a better understanding of the use of balloon catheters with appropriate choices for specific situations may decrease or abolish the recurrence rate. Despite these good results, much longer-term (10 years) followup data are necessary to further confirm long-term effectiveness of balloon pulmonary valvuloplasty for relief of valvular pulmonic stenosis.

APPLICABILITY TO ALL AGE GROUPS

Although balloon pulmonary valvuloplasty is used most frequently in children, it has also been used in neonates[13,36,64,67-74] and in adults.[75-81]

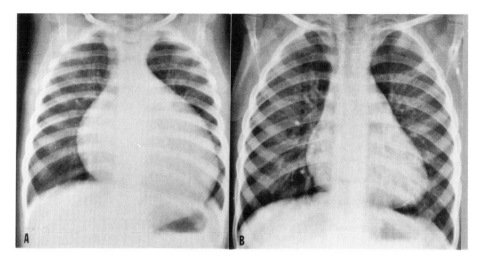

Figure 15.6 Chest roentgenogram, posteroanterior view, showing cardiomegaly (*A*) prior to balloon pulmonary valvuloplasty. The cardiomegaly has improved on a chest x-ray taken 1 year following balloon valvuloplasty (*B*).

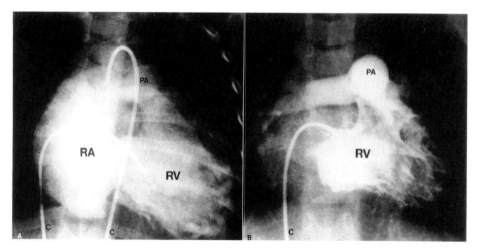

Figure 15.7 Right ventricular (*RV*) cineangiogram posteroanterior views prior to (*A*) and 1 year following (*B*) balloon pulmonary valvuloplasty. Note difference of tricuspid insufficiency at followup (*B*). The right ventricular cineangiograms correspond to *A* and *B* of Fig. 15.6. *C*—catheter. *PA*—pulmonary artery. *RA*—right atrium.

Neonates

Experience with balloon pulmonary valvuloplasty in the neonate with critical pulmonary stenosis is limited. The series with largest numbers contain 6,[69] 8,[36] and 20[73] patients. The procedure is more technically difficult but can be accomplished by the use of end-hold balloon-wedge catheters, small-sized, high-torque guidewires, low profile balloon catheters, and progressive dilatation with small balloons.

Occlusion of pulmonary outflow tract during balloon valvuloplasty is made tolerable by continuous administration of prostaglandins to maintain ductal patency. Once the ductus is closed, progressive dilatation of the stenotic pulmonary valve[70] may be of benefit. The overall result is perhaps not as favorable as in children. Right ventricular hypoplasia, severe infundibular obstruction, pulmonary valve ring hypoplasia, or pulmonary valve dysplasia may tend to adversely affect the results of balloon valvuloplasty in the neonate with critical pulmonary stenosis.

Adults

Relief of pulmonary stenosis in adult patients has been accomplished by balloon valvuloplasty.[75-81] Because of the physical size of the pulmonary valve ring, many adult patients may require balloon valvuloplasty using two balloons.[78,79] However, as pointed out elsewhere[15,21] double-balloon technique is comparable but not superior to single-balloon technique when equivalent balloon:annulus ratios are compared.

Immediate results of balloon valvuloplasty[75-81] are similar to those reported in children. A successful result has even been documented in the seventh decade of life.[81] Our own experience with teenagers[14,23] and that of others with adult patients[75,78,80] suggests that infundibular obstruction following balloon valvuloplasty is more common in older patients than in young patients — probably because of longstanding right ventricular hypertension and consequent right ventricular hypertrophy in older patients. Followup results, though documented in few studies,[79,80] do indicate persistent relief after a mean followup of 1 to 2 years.

In summary, it appears that successful balloon valvuloplasty is feasible in all age groups.

APPLICABILITY IN RESTENOSIS AFTER PREVIOUS SURGICAL PULMONARY VALVOTOMY

Some authors[29,33] observed poor results in balloon valvuloplasty in patients with previous surgical pulmonary valvotomy; in some of these,[29] pulmonary valve dysplasia is associated with a lack of success. Poor results of balloon valvuloplasty have also been reported in patients with previous surgical pulmonary valvotomy for pulmonary atresia with an intact ventricular system.[31,34,65] Others[36,37,80] did not specifically comment on the results of balloon valvuloplasty in patients with previous surgery.

In our patient population, only two children, aged 3 and 14 years, had had previous surgical pulmonary valvotomy, 1 and 4 years prior to balloon valvuloplasty, respectively. The pulmonary valvular gradients of 120 and 146 mmHg were reduced respectively to 48 and 34 mmHg immediately after valvuloplasty. In the 3-year-old patient, the pulmonary valve gradient fell further to 25 mmHg at a 10-month followup catheterization.

The available data indicate that successful balloon valvuloplasty can be expected even after recurrence following previous surgical valvotomy. Therefore, I believe balloon valvuloplasty is the treatment of choice for this application.

COMPARISON WITH SURGICAL RESULTS

Over the years, the risk associated with surgical correction of cardiac defects has diminished markedly. Even so, the surgical repair of cardiac defects has many disadvantages, including prolonged hospitalization, frightening postoperative appearance (especially to the parents), residual scars, possible psychological trauma to the child or parents, and expense. For these reasons, it is better to correct these defects by catheter techniques, provided morbidity and mortality figures and recurrence rates are better than, or at least comparable to, those for surgical therapy. However, comparison of immediate and followup results of surgical versus balloon therapy is fraught with problems because of (1) the small number of balloon valvuloplasty patients available for followup, (2) the shorter duration currently available for followup studies in balloon valvuloplasty patients, and (3) possible inaccuracy of comparing older surgical studies with those employing current balloon dilatation techniques.

Surgical treatment for valvular pulmonic stenosis has been available for 40 years since the first description by Brock.[82] Eight representative reports of surgical pulmonary valvuloplasty[28,83-89] were chosen for comparison with balloon valvuloplasty. These authors followed 46 to 234 patients for months to 30 years after surgical relief of pulmonary valve obstruction. Operative mortality ranged from 3% to 14%; the cooperative study involving several institutions had only a 3% mortality in 304 patients presented.[28] Poor results at followup were noted in 0 to 8%.[28,83-89] Again, the cooperative study had the lowest rate: 4% poor results at followup. A poor result at followup is defined as a pulmonary valvar gradient in excess of 50 mmHg. Pulmonary valve insufficiency was reported in all studies. Followup catheterization studies after balloon valvuloplasty[29,31-34,36,55,57,58,63], including the current study, involved recatheterization in 6 to 53 patients 1 week to 34 months after valvuloplasty (Table 15.1) and reported varying degrees of recurrence.

No significant mortality has been reported following balloon valvuloplasty.[64] The mortality figures and morbidity appear higher following surgery, but the recurrence rate appears higher following the balloon procedure. With refinement of balloon techniques, as indicated elsewhere,[15,19,20] recurrence rate can be brought down to extremely low levels: Of the 32 dilatations with balloons larger than 1.2 times the size of the pulmonary valve annulus,[20] none required repeat valvuloplasty and none had pressure gradients in excess of 30 mmHg at followup. On the basis of the available information, it is likely that both immediate and followup results are better with balloon than with surgical pulmonary valvuloplasty. Such a sweeping statement can be substantiated when 5- and 10-year followup studies of balloon valvuloplasty confirm the current intermediate findings.

MECHANISM OF VALVULOPLASTY

Inflation of a balloon placed across an obstructive lesion exerts radial forces upon the stenotic lesion without any axial component.[90] Several physical principles of the "dilating force" are important in the mechanism of action and should be understood for successful application of the balloon dilatation technique.[90]

1. At the same pressure, a larger diameter balloon exerts a greater dilating force than does a smaller diameter balloon.

2. For the same pressure, longer balloons exert greater dilating force than shorter balloons.

3. For the same size balloon, the higher the inflation pressure, the greater is the dilating force; these are related in a linear fashion.

4. For the same pressure, a tighter stenotic area will receive a greater dilating force than a less tight stenosis.

5. For the same pressure, a large stenotic area will receive a higher dilating force than a small stenotic area.

6. High inflation pressures will not significantly increase the diameter of the balloon: The balloon material (specially treated polyethylene in most pediatric dilatation balloons) does not expand because the yield strength (the force at which permanent deformation of the material occurs) and the ultimate tensile strength (the force necessary to break the material) of the balloon material are nearly equal.

On the basis of these principles and our experience with balloon dilatations in children, we now routinely perform sequential balloon inflation with 3, 4, and 5 atmospheres of pressure of five-second duration, five minutes apart. If "waisting" of balloon can not be abolished, we sequentially increase pressure of inflation to 6, 7, and 8 atmospheres; this was required on only two occasions (both native coarctations) of a total experience in excess of 250 balloon dilatations in children.

Walls and associates[91] investigated the mechanism of balloon valvuloplasty by inspecting the valve mechanism by direct vision at surgery. They found tearing of the valve raphae, tearing of the valve leaflets; and avulsion of the valve leaflets; all are conceivably the mechanisms by which pulmonary or aortic valve obstruction can be relieved. Direct visual observations by others,[13,29-31] though limited in numbers, as well as echocardiographic observations,[37] indicate similar mechanisms. The circumferential dilating force exerted by balloon inflation is likely to rupture (tear) the weakest part of the valve structure. It is likely that the fused commissures are the weakest links that can be broken with balloon dilatation. However, in a given patient, when the fused commissures are strong and cannot be torn, tears in the valve leaflets[92] or avulsion of the valve leaflets[91] can occur. The latter events may worsen semilunar valve insufficiency. Morphologic studies[93,94] of postmortem specimens with valvular pulmonic stenosis suggests that commissural splitting is feasible. However, abnormality of the valve annulus and dysplastic pulmonary valve leaflets have been identified in these studies.[93,94] If severe, these conditions may preclude successful balloon pulmonary valvuloplasty.

COMPLICATIONS

Acute Complications

The complications seen during and immediately after balloon pulmonary valvuloplasty have been remarkably minimal. Transient bradycardia, premature beats, and a fall in systemic pressure during balloon inflation have been uniformly noted by all workers, particularly with valvular dilatations. These signs return rapidly back to normal following balloon deflation (Figure 15.8). Minimal systemic hypotension may occur during balloon inflation in the presence of a patent foramen ovale because of

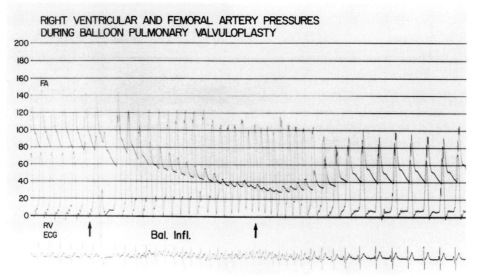

Figure 15.8 Simultaneous recording of the right ventricular (*RV*) and femoral artery (*FA*) pressure during balloon dilatation of stenotic pulmonary valve. Note a marked increase in the RV pressure, presumably related to complete obstruction of the right ventricle. There is a simultaneous fall in the FA pressure, again related to complete obstruction to flow during balloon valvuloplasty. Following deflation of the balloon, the FA pressure returns toward normal. The 10-second period of balloon inflation (*Bal. Infl.*) is marked with *arrows.* Now we use only 5 seconds of balloon inflation with which we observe less fall in FA pressure with more prompt return toward normal than when we were using 10-second balloon inflation. (From: Rao PS, Mardini MK: Pulmonary valvotomy without thoracotomy: the experience with percutaneous balloon pulmonary valvuloplasty. *Ann Saudi Med.* 5:149–155, 1985. With permission.)

the right-to-left shunting across it, filling the left ventricle.[95] To allow egress of blood from the ventricle during balloon inflation, some authors advocate the use of double balloons[76] and a trefoil or a bifoil balloon.[52-54] Others[15,21] suggest shorter periods (5 sec) of inflation to minimize systemic hypotension. Having had experience with each of these techniques, the author believes that short periods of balloon inflation (5 s or less) are most effective without compromising immediate or followup results.

Blood loss necessitating transfusion has been reported in many studies. Complete right bundle branch block,[68] transient or permanent complete heart block,[29,96] cerebrovascular accident,[36] loss of consciousness,[29] cardiac arrest,[97] convulsions,[29] balloon rupture at high inflation pressures,[30,36,57] tricuspid valve papillary muscle rupture,[98] and severe infundibular obstruction necessitating propranolol administration[14,23,25,36,57] or surgical intervention,[57,99] though rare, have been reported. Some of these complications may be unavoidable. However, meticulous attention to the details of the technique, use of an appropriate length of the balloon, avoiding extremely high inflation pressures, and short inflation/deflation cycles may prevent or reduce the complications.

Holter monitoring for 24 hours following balloon valvuloplasty[32] revealed premature ventricular contractions (grade 1, Lown criteria) in one third of the 12 patients so studied. It is not clear from this study[32] whether the premature beats were present prior to balloon valvuloplasty and for how long after valvuloplasty the premature beats persisted.

Transient prolongation of the QT_c interval following balloon angioplasty and valvuloplasty[100] may be a potential hazard for the development of R-on-T phenomenon in children with ventricular ectopy. Holter findings[32] of premature beats following valvuloplasty may have a significance in the light of prolongation of the QT_c interval.[100] No patients from our series or many other studies have been known to develop ventricular arrhythmias, although two cases of sudden death from ventricular fibrillation shortly after balloon angioplasty in aortic coarctation have been reported.[101,102] Whether these arrhythmias are related to QT_c prolongation is not known, However, patient monitoring following balloon valvuloplasty or angioplasty is warranted.[100]

Although multiple complications were listed, the Valvuloplasty and Angioplasty of Congenital Anomalies Registry reported only a 0.24% death rate and a 0.35% major complication rate from the 822 balloon pulmonary valvuloplasty procedures from 26 member institutions.[64] These figures attest to the safety of the procedure.

Complications at Followup

At the intermediate-term followup, femoral venous occlusion, pulmonary valve insufficiency, and pulmonary valve restenosis have been noted. Restenosis is discussed in the next section. Anywhere between 10 and 29%[14,32,36] of femoral veins through which balloon valvuloplasty has been performed were found to be occluded at followup. In the present series, 3 out of 45 patients (7%) whom we restudied following pulmonary valvuloplasty had blocked femoral vein. It is the consensus that femoral venous occlusion is more common in small infants.[32,36,97]

Auscultatory evidence for pulmonary valve insufficiency has not been thoroughly scrutinized. Doppler evidence for pulmonary insufficiency appears sensitive but has been studied by only a few investigators.[14,32,37,103] Rocchini and Beekman[103] reported pulmonary insufficiency in 31 of 37 (84%) patients, whereas Robertson and associates[37] found mild pulmonary insufficiency in all 29 patients studied. When we last reviewed this finding from our group,[22] 34 of 43 patients (79%) had Doppler-demonstrable pulmonary insufficiency. However, the pulmonary insufficiency is minimal as evidenced by an absence of right ventricular overloading (normal-sized right ventricle and no paradoxical septal motion) in this group of patients as well as by equilibrium-gated radionuclide angiograms reported by Tynan.[29] Although the long-term followup studies should be scrutinized for progressive right ventricular volume overloading, the current data suggest that the pulmonary insufficiency produced by balloon valvuloplasty is unlikely to be problematic.

CAUSES OF RESTENOSIS

Recurrence of valvular stenosis following balloon pulmonary valvuloplasty has been reported,[29,31-34,36,55,57,58,63,65] but the reasons for the restenosis at intermediate-term followup have been studied only to a limited degree.[29,31-34] We have systemically investigated the cause of recurrence of pulmonic stenosis following balloon valvuloplasty.[19,24] On the basis of results from followup catheterizations conducted from 6 to 34 months after valvuloplasty, 40 children were divided into group 1 with good results (pulmonary valve gradient 30 mmHg or less), 33 patients; and group 2 with poor results (gradient greater than 30 mmHg), 7 patients (Table 15.2). Fourteen biographical, anatomic, physiological, and technical factors (Table 15.3) were examined by multivariate logistic regression analysis to identify factors associated with restenosis. The identified risk factors were:

1. Residual pulmonary valve gradient in excess of 30 mmHg immediately following balloon valvuloplasty.
2. Balloon:pulmonary valve annulus ratio less than 1.2:1.

Dysplastic pulmonary valves did not seem to influence recurrence possibly because large balloons were used with dysplastic valves. The data suggested that a balloon:annulus ratio of less than 1.2 is the cause for pulmonary valve restenosis at intermediate-term followup and that such recurrences can be predicted in patients with immediate postvalvuloplasty pulmonary valve gradients in excess of 30 mmHg. We suggested the use of progressively larger balloons to reduce the valve gradient to less than 30 mmHg.[19,24,51]

Pulmonary valve dysplasia and pulmonary valve annular hypoplasia may well be significant factors in the recurrence of pulmonary valve obstruction. These conditions did not seem to have an adverse effect in our study group, however, perhaps because of the narrow ranges of such abnormalities in our study group.

INFLUENCE OF TECHNICAL FACTORS

Balloon Size

Radtke[35] and we[12] evaluated the influence of balloon size on the results of pulmonary valvuloplasty and recommended a balloon:pulmonary valve annulus ratio of 1.2:1 to 1.4:1. Such recommendations are arbitrary and were based on (1) small number of patients with immediate results,[12,35] (2) no followup results,[35] or (3) followup results on a few patients.[12] Our experience with 64 consecutive balloon dilatation procedures performed in 56 patients with isolated valvular pulmonic stenosis and 39 followup catheterizations in 36 patients was reviewed to examine this issue.[15,20,22] Five repeat valvuloplasty procedures were performed at followup catheterization and three patients had valvuloplasty sequentially with balloons resulting in increasingly larger balloon:annulus ratios. Thus, there were 64 valvuloplasty procedures in 56 patients. These were divided into two groups: group 3, those in which the balloon:annulus ratio was 1.0:1.0 or less, 12 dilatations; and group 4, those in which the ratio was more than 1.0:1.0, 52 dilatations (see Table 15.2). Table 15.3 lists the variables examined.

The two groups had similar prevalvuloplasty valvular gradients (Table 15.4). Immediately after valvuloplasty, there was a significant reduction in pulmonary valve gradient in both group 3 and group 4 although the fall in the gradient was greater in group 4 with larger balloons. On intermediate-term followup (which ranged between 6 and 34 months), residual pulmonary valvular gradients were significantly lower in group 4 than in group 3, suggesting restenosis in group 3 with small balloons (Table 15.4). At followup, repeat balloon valvuloplasty was required in 4 group 3 patients and only 1 from group 4. Similarly, a higher number of patients with residual pulmonary

Table 15.2 GROUPINGS USED IN THE TEXT

Group 1	Good results group (at followup) with catheterization pulmonary valve gradients ≤ 30 mmHg, 33 children
Group 2	Poor results group (at followup) with catheterization pulmonary valve gradients > 30 mmHg, 7 patients
Group 3	Balloon dilatations in which balloon:annulus ratio was 1.0:1 or less (0.89 ± 0.08; range 0.76 to 1.0), 12 dilatations
Group 4	Balloon dilatations in which balloon:annulus ratio was more than 1.0:1 (1.31 ± 0.19; range, 1.01 to 1.8), 44 dilatations
Group 5	Balloon dilatations in which balloon:annulus ratio was 1.2:1 or less (1.03 ± 0.13; range, 0.76 to 1.2), 32 dilatations
Group 6	Balloon dilatations in which balloon:annulus ratio was more than 1.2:1 (1.43 ± 0.13; range, 1.21 to 1.8), 32 dilatations
Group 7	Balloon valvuloplasties in which balloon:annulus ratio was between 1.21 and 1.5:1 (1.36 ± 0.08), 23 dilatations
Group 8	Balloon valvuloplasties in which balloon:annulus ratio was between 1.51 and 1.8:1 (1.6 ± 0.09), 9 dilatations
Group 9	Double-balloon valvuloplasty (balloon:annulus ratio, 1.19 ± 0.14:1, range, 1.01 to 1.53), 12 patients
Group 10	Single-balloon valvuloplasty, matched with group 9 for balloon:annulus ratio (1.19 ± 0.15:1, range 1.0 to 1.53), 12 patients
Groups 11	Dysplastic pulmonary valves, 13 patients
Groups 12	Nondysplastic pulmonary valves, 43 patients

Modified from: Rao PS: Balloon pulmonary valvuloplasty: a review. *Clin Cardiol.* 12:55–74, 1989. Copyrighted and reprinted with the permission of Clinical Cardiology Publishing Co. Inc., and/or the Foundation for Advances in Medicine and Science (FAMS), Box 832, Mahwah, New Jersey 07430, USA.

Table 15.3 VARIABLES EXAMINED BY MULTIVARIATE LOGISTIC REGRESSION ANALYSIS TO IDENTIFY FACTORS RESPONSIBLE FOR PULMONARY VALVE RESTENOSIS FOLLOWING BALLOON VALVULOPLASTY

Age at valvuloplasty

Duration of followup

Pulmonary valve dysplasia, severe or mild

Pulmonary valve ring hypoplasia

Right ventricular hypoplasia

Angiographic infundibular stenosis

Right ventricular peak systolic pressure prior to balloon valvuloplasty

Pulmonary valve peak systolic pressure gradient prior to balloon valvuloplasty

Right ventricular infundibular pressure gradient prior to balloon valvuloplasty

Pulmonary valve peak systolic pressure gradient immediately after balloon valvuloplasty

Balloon:pulmonary valve annulus ratio

Maximum pressure achieved in the balloon

Number of balloon dilatations

Total duration of balloon inflation

Modified from: Rao PS: Balloon pulmonary valvuloplasty: a review. *Clin Cardiol.* 12:55–74, 1989.

Table 15.4   COMPARISON OF GROUP 3 WITH BALLOON:ANNULUS RATIO OF 1.0:1 OR LESS WITH GROUP 4 WITH BALLOON: ANNULUS RATIO > 1.0:1

	Group 3, mean ± SD	Group 4, mean ± SD	p-value
Pulmonary valve gradient prevalvuloplasty, mmHg	84.3 ± 39.2	92.8 ± 41.2	> 0.1
Pulmonary valve gradient immediately after valvuloplasty, mmHg	43.6 ± 26.8[a]	22.4 ± 13.6[b]	< 0.01
Pulmonary valve gradient at followup, mmHg	75.0 ± 49.4[c]	20.8 ± 18.5[b]	< 0.001

[a] p < 0.02 when compared with prevalvuloplasty gradients

[b] p < 0.001 when compared with prevalvuloplasty gradients

[c] p > 0.1 when compared with prevalvuloplasty gradients

SD – standard deviation.

Modified from: Rao PS: How big a balloon and how many balloons for pulmonary valvuloplasty? *Am Heart J.* 116:577–580, 1988. With permission.

Table 15.5   PREVALANCE OF REPEAT VALVULOPLASTY AND SIGNIFICANT RESIDUAL GRADIENTS IN SELECTED GROUPS

Groups	No. Patients Needing Repeat Valvuloplasty	p-value[a]	No. Patients With Pulmonary Valve Gradient > 30 mmHg	p-value[a]
Group 3 N = 7	4		5	
		0.002		0.001
Group 4 N = 32	1		2	
Group 5 N = 21	5		7	
		0.005		0.002
Group 6 N = 18	0		0	

N – Number of patients with intermediate-term followup catheterization

[a] Fisher's exact test

Modified from: Rao PS: How big a balloon and how many balloons for pulmonary valvuloplasty. *Am Heart J.* 116:577–580, 1988. With permission.

valvular gradients in excess of 30 mmHg were present in group 3 than in group 4 (Table 15.5). These data suggest that although good immediate results are seen with either small or large balloons, balloons larger than the pulmonary valve annulus produce a more sustained relief of pulmonary stenosis.

Second, the balloon:annulus ratio cutoff point was increased to 1.2:1.0 and balloon valvuloplasties were divided into another two groups (see Table 15.2): Group 5, those in whom the ratio was 1.2:1 or less and group 6, those in whom the ratio was more than 1.2:1. In group 5, consisting of 32 dilatations, the mean ratio was 1.03 ± 0.13, whereas in group 6, which also consisted of 32 balloon dilatations, the ratio was 1.43 ± 0.13. Both these groups had similar prevalvuloplasty gradients, and both groups had a significant (p < 0.001) reduction in pulmonary valvular gradients both immediately after valvuloplasty and at followup (Table 15.6). However, the followup gradients in group 6 with larger balloons were lower than those in group 5 with small balloons. Five patients from group 5 required repeat balloon dilatation at followup

Table 15.6 COMPARISON OF GROUP 5 WITH BALLOON:ANNULUS RATIO OF 1.2:1 OR LESS WITH GROUP 6 WITH BALLOON: ANNULUS RATIO > 1.2:1

	Group 5, mean ± SD	Group 6, mean ± SD	p-value
Pulmonary valve gradient prevalvuloplasty, mmHg	93.4 ± 40.5	89.1 ± 42.8	> 0.1
Pulmonary valve gradient immediately after valvuloplasty, mmHg	34.3 ± 23.5[a]	27.0 ± 18.5[a]	> 0.1
Pulmonary valve Gradient at followup, mmHg	42.3 ± 41.6[a]	16.7 ± 7.9[a]	< 0.01

[a] p < 0.001 when compared with prevalvuloplasty gradient

SD – standard deviation.

Modified from: Rao PS: How big a balloon and how many balloons for pulmonary valvuloplasty? *Am Heart J.* 116:577–580, 1988. With permission.

Table 15.7 COMPARISON OF GROUP 6 WITH BALLOON:ANNULUS RATIO OF 1.21 TO 1.5:1 WITH GROUP 7 WITH BALLOON: ANNULUS RATIO 1.51 TO 1.8:1

	Group 7, mean ± SD	Group 8, mean ± SD	p-value
Pulmonary valve gradient prevalvuloplasty, mmHg	91.8 ± 45.2	82.1 ± 37.4	> 0.1
Pulmonary valve gradient immediately after valvuloplasty, mmHg	26.7 ± 20.4[a]	27.8 ± 13.3[a]	> 0.1
Pulmonary valve gradient at followup, mmHg	17.2 ± 8.4[a]	14.0 ± 5.6[a]	> 0.1

[a] p < 0.001 when compared with prevalvuloplasty gradient

SD – standard deviation.

Modified from: Rao PS: How big a balloon and how many balloons for pulmonary valvuloplasty? *Am Heart J.* 116:577–580, 1988. With permission.

whereas none from group 6 required repeat valvuloplasty (see Table 15.5). Also, 7 patients from group 5 had gradients in excess of 30 mmHg whereas none in group 6 had that high a gradient at followup (Table 15.5). On the basis of these data, the use of balloons smaller than 1.2 times the pulmonary valve annulus is associated with a significant chance of residual pulmonary stenosis at followup, and as such, is not recommended.

Finally, the results of balloon valvuloplasty with a balloon:annulus ratio of 1.21 to 1.5:1 (group 7) were compared with those in which the ratio was in excess of 1.5:1 (group 8), because balloons larger than 1.5 times the size of the valve annulus are reported to damage the right ventricular outflow tract.[50] Group 7, with a mean balloon:annulus ratio of 1.36 ± 0.08, consisted of 23 patients while group 8, with a mean balloon:annulus ratio of 1.6 ± 0.09, consisted of 9 patients (see Table 15.2). Table 15.7 summarizes the data from these groups. The pulmonary valve gradients were similar prior to valvuloplasty in both groups. A significant (p < 0.01) reduction of gradient occurred in both groups immediately after valvuloplasty as well as at followup catheterization. Residual pulmonary valvular gradients immediately after balloon dilatation and on followup were similar. No patient in either group required repeat balloon dilatation nor did any patient have a residual pulmonary valvular gradient in excess of 30 mmHg. These data signify that balloons larger than 1.5 times the size of the pulmonary valve annulus do not offer any advantage over balloons with a ratio of 1.21 to 1.5:1.

To summarize: The data presented in this section indicate that balloons larger than 1.2 times the diameter of the pulmonary valve annulus should be used for pulmonary valvuloplasty if restenosis is to be prevented and that there is no advantage in the use of balloons larger than 1.5 times the size of the pulmonary valve annulus.

Balloon Length

The majority of workers use balloons 30 mm long for pulmonary valvuloplasty. There are no data either from our own series or from the literature to assess whether shorter (20 mm) or longer (40 mm or longer) balloons have any advantages or disadvantages over the conventional 30-mm length balloons. Balloons 20 mm long are too short to maintain the balloon center over the pulmonary valve annulus during balloon inflation. Therefore, they are not advisable in children and adolescents, though they are appropriate for neonates and infants. Balloons 40 mm and longer may impinge upon the tricuspid valve mechanism and may injure it. Two experiences, one causing avulsion of the papillary muscle[98] and another causing complete heart block[96] when balloons 60 and 40 mm long, respectively, were used, suggest that these long balloons should not be used for balloon pulmonary valvuloplasty. Based on this discussion, it may be concluded that balloons 30 mm long should be used in children for valvuloplasty until data to the contrary become available.

Number of Balloons

Although single balloons are used in the majority of cases, several groups have reported valvuloplasty with simultaneous inflation of two balloons placed across the stenotic pulmonary valve when the pulmonary valve annulus is too large to dilate with a single balloon.[10,12,14,21,35,38,57,78] Indeed, some authors[78] advocate use of double-balloon valvuloplasty as a procedure of choice, especially in adults. To evaluate this issue, 12 patients from our series who underwent double-balloon valvuloplasty (group 9) were compared with 12 patients with single-balloon valvuloplasty who were matched for the balloon:annulus ratio (group 10) (see Table 15.2). Effective balloon diameter with double balloons was calculated by a formula that we previously proposed[12]; this formula was given in the section on technique.

Table 15.2 and Figure 15.9 summarize the findings. The balloon:annulus ratio in group 9 with double balloons was similar to that in group 10 with a single balloon. The two groups had similar prevalvuloplasty pulmonary valvular gradients and peak right ventricular systolic pressures. Immediately following valvuloplasty, there was a significant reduction (p < 0.001) in pulmonary valvular gradients in both groups. The improvement was maintained at 6- to 14-month followup catheterization (Figure 15.10). Residual pulmonary valvular gradients immediately after valvuloplasty and at followup catheterization were similar in both groups (Figure 15.11). These data indicate that results of double-balloon valvuloplasty, though excellent, are comparable but not superior to those observed with single-balloon valvuloplasty. The bal-

DATA PRIOR TO BALLOON DILATION

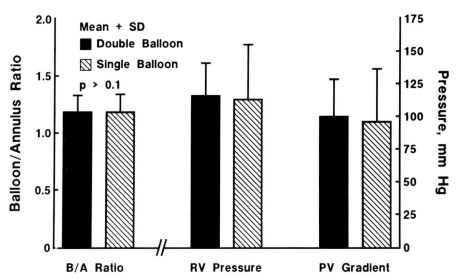

Figure 15.9 Prevalvuloplasty comparison of double- and single-balloon groups. Balloon to pulmonary valve annulus (B/A) ratios of double-balloon group are similar (p > 0.1) to those of the single-balloon group. The right ventricular (RV) peak systolic pressure and pulmonary valve (PV) peak systolic pressure gradients in both groups were similar prior to balloon valvuloplasty; these data suggest that severity of pulmonary valve stenosis is similar in both groups. (From: Rao PS, Fawzy ME: Double balloon technique for percutaneous balloon pulmonary valvuloplasty: comparison with single balloon technique. *J Intervent Cardiol.* 1:257–262, 1988. With permission.)

loon:pulmonary valve annulus ratio as presented in the earlier part of the discussion is perhaps a better determinant of relief of pulmonary valve stenosis than whether a single- or double-balloon technique is used. The specific formula that we used to calculate balloon size and balloon:annulus ratio may be criticized, but this formula was concurrently and independently advocated by us[12] and others,[35,104,105] and it fits the best available geometric model. Therefore, I believe that the comparison of double-balloon data with single-balloon data is justified.

The suggestion by Al Kasab and his associates[78] that a double-balloon technique is preferable is based on immediate- and short-term (6-week followup only) results (but without single-balloon controls) and less systemic hypotension and bradycardia during balloon inflation. Initially, we inflated the balloon(s) for 10 seconds[9] for valvuloplasty. We also noticed hypotension[9] during balloon inflation, but the blood pressure promptly returned to normal after balloon deflation. More recently,[14,22] we have used 5-second inflation, which induced a lesser degree of hypotension not too different from that reported with the double-balloon technique[38,78] and without a sacrifice in result. Although we and others[38] did not find a significantly higher complication rate with double-balloon technique, it does indeed prolong the procedure and involves the use of an additional femoral venous site with the attendant

IMMEDIATE AND FOLLOW-UP RESULTS
OF BALLOON PULMONARY VALVULOPLASTY

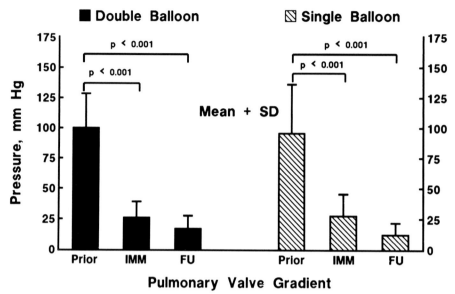

Figure 15.10 The pulmonary valve peak systolic pressure gradient fell (p < 0.001) immediately (*IMM*) following balloon valvuloplasty with two balloons as well as with one balloon. On intermediate-term follow-up (*FU*), the gradient remains low (p < 0.001) when compared to prevalvuloplasty values in both groups. These data suggest excellent immediate and intermediate-term results of pulmonary valvuloplasty both with double- and single-balloon techniques. (From: Rao PS, Fawzy ME: Double balloon technique for percutaneous balloon pulmonary valvuloplasty: comparison with single balloon technique. *J Intervent Cardiol.* 1:257–262, 1988. With permission.)

potential complications. Therefore, we would recommend that the double-balloon technique be used when the pulmonary valve annulus is too large to dilate with a commercially available single balloon or when a single balloon cannot be safely passed across the femoral vein,[38] not because the double-balloon technique gives a better result. Bifoil- and trefoil-balloon catheters[52-54] may help resolve the problem, but our limited personal experience suggests that these catheters are too bulky and the advantage of less hypotension during valvuloplasty is minimal.

In conclusion, the immediate and followup results of balloon pulmonary valvuloplasty with two balloons are excellent, but these results are similar to those seen with equivalent-size single-balloon valvuloplasty. Double balloons offer no additional advantage over single balloons. There are no data to support the contention that a double-balloon technique is superior to single-balloon pulmonary valvuloplasty. I suggest that a double-balloon technique be used when the pulmonary valve annulus is to too large to dilate with a commercially available single balloon.

DATA FOLLOWING BALLOON VALVULOPLASTY

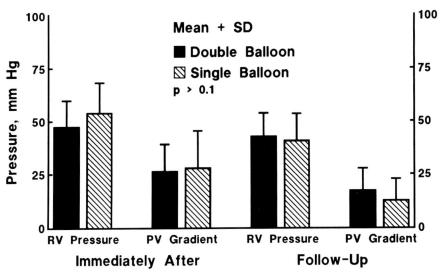

Figure 15.11 Residual right ventricular (*RV*) pressures and pulmonary valvular (*PV*) peak systolic pressure gradients immediately after balloon pulmonary valvuloplasty and at intermediate-term followup were similar ($p > 0.1$) in both double-balloon and single-balloon groups. The data suggest good results whether a double- or single-balloon technique was used for pulmonary valvuloplasty provided that balloon: annulus ratios are similar. (From: Rao PS, Fawzy ME: Double balloon technique for percutaneous balloon pulmonary valvuloplasty: comparison with single balloon technique. *J Intervent Cardiol.* 1:257–262, 1988. With permission.)

Pressure, Number, and Duration of Balloon Inflation(s)

Recommendations for pressure of inflation of the balloon range between 2 to 8.5 atm.[5,9,14,30,31,34-36,38,69] Suggested duration of each inflation ranges 5 to 20 seconds. Anywhere from one to four, balloon inflations, 2 to 5 minutes apart, have been suggested. Clearly, no data are available for deciding on which is the best method of inflation. We compared the inflation characteristics in the group 1 with good results (see Table 15.2) with those of group 2 with poor results (Table 15.8). As can be seen, there were no significant differences between the groups, suggesting that the outcome of valvuloplasty is not related to these balloon inflation characteristics. We have also looked at the data with arbitrary division of maximum pressure, number of balloon inflations, and total duration of balloon inflation (Tables 15.9 through 15.11). We found that higher pressure, larger number, and longer duration of balloon inflation did not favorably influence residual gradients at followup, especially when the influence of balloon:annulus ratio was removed.

Table 15.8 BALLOON INFLATION CHARACTERISTICS IN GROUP 11 WITH GOOD RESULTS AND GROUP 12 WITH POOR RESULTS

Inflation Characteristic	Group 11, mean ± SD	Group 12, mean ± SD	p-value
Maximum pressure in the balloon, atm	4.6 ± 0.2	4.0 ± 1.4	> 0.1
Number of balloon inflations	4.4 ± 1.1	4.0 ± 1.0	> 0.1
Total duration of balloon inflation, sec	36.2 + 13.5	37.9 + 13.5	> 0.1

SD – Standard deviation.

From: Rao PS: Balloon pulmonary valvuloplasty: a review. *Clin Cardiol.* 12:55–74, 1989. Copyrighted and reprinted with the permission of Clinical Cardiology Publishing Co. Inc., and/or the Foundation for Advances in Medicine and Science (FAMS), Box 832, Mahwah, New Jersey 07430, USA.

Table 15.9 INFLUENCE OF MAXIMAL PRESSURE OF BALLOON INFLATION ON THE IMMEDIATE AND FOLLOWUP RESIDUAL PULMONARY VALVE GRADIENTS

	Maximum Pressure of Balloon Inflation, atm			
	≤ 3	4–5	> 5	p-value[a]
Pre-BPV gradient, mmHg, mean ± SD	94.8 ± 51.8	90.1 ± 29.5	97.6 ± 45.6	> 0.1
Post-BPV gradient, mmHg, mean ± SD	29.9 ± 19.8	26.8 ± 15.6	33.3 ± 26.2	> 0.1
FU gradient, mmHg, mean ± SD	43.0 ± 46.5	18.1 ± 15.5	30.1 ± 36.4	> 0.1
FU gradient, mmHg (BA ratio > 1.0:1), mean ± SD	26.4 ± 35.4	18.3 ± 16.1	20.6 ± 13.4	> 0.1

[a] The p-value was derived by comparing ≤ 3 with 4–5, 4–5 with > 5.0, and > 5 with ≤ 3 atm groups.

BA – balloon:annulus ratio. BPV – balloon pulmonary valvuloplasty. FU – followup. SD–standard deviation.

From: Rao PS: Balloon pulmonary valvuloplasty: a review. *Clin Cardiol.* 12:55–74, 1989. Copyrighted and reprinted with the permission of Clinical Cardiology Publishing Co. Inc., and/or the Foundation for Advances in Medicine and Science (FAMS), Box 832, Mahwah, New Jersey 07430, USA.

Table 15.10 INFLUENCE OF NUMBER OF BALLOON DILATATIONS ON THE IMMEDIATE AND FOLLOWUP RESIDUAL PULMONARY VALVE GRADIENTS

	Number of Balloon Dilatations			
	3	4	5–7	p-value[a]
Pre-BPV gradient, mmHg, mean ± SD	77.9 ± 20.1	101.0 ± 52.4	97.0 ± 36.0	> 0.05
Post-BPV gradient, mmHg, mean ± SD	22.0 ± 9.0	33.2 ± 25.6	29.6 ± 19.7	> 0.05
FU gradient, mmHg, mean ± SD	42.3 ± 50.3	32.9 ± 37.1	19.1 ± 15.3	> 0.1
FU gradient, mmHg, (BA Ratio > 1.0:1), mean ± SD	27.2 ± 38.0	20.7 ± 13.5	19.1 ± 15.3	> 0.1

[a] The p-value was derived by comparing 3 with 4, 4 with 5–7, and 5–7 with 3 dilatation groups.

BA – balloon:annulus ratio. BPV – balloon pulmonary valvuloplasty. FU – followup. SD–standard deviation.

From: Rao PS: Balloon pulmonary valvuloplasty: a review. *Clin Cardiol.* 12:55–74, 1989. Copyrighted and reprinted with the permission of Clinical Cardiology Publishing Co. Inc., and/or the Foundation for Advances in Medicine and Science (FAMS), Box 832, Mahwah, New Jersey 07430, USA.

Table 15.11 **INFLUENCE OF TOTAL DURATION OF BALLOON INFLATION ON THE IMMEDIATE AND FOLLOW-UP RESIDUAL PULMONARY VALVE GRADIENT**

	Total Duration of Balloon Inflation, sec			
	≤ 25	26–40	> 40	p-value[a]
Pre-BPV gradient, mmHg, mean $\pm$ SD	87.3 ± 47.6	99.4 ± 40.5	96.2 ± 35.2	> 0.1
Post-BPV gradient, mmHg, mean $\pm$ SD	25.7 ± 18.0	29.5 ± 23.9	36.0 ± 20.2	> 0.1
FU gradient, mmHg, mean $\pm$ SD	25.5 ± 25.3	34.4 ± 42.2	22.7 ± 16.7	> 0.1
FU gradient, mmHg, (BA Ratio $> 1.0{:}1$), mean $\pm$ SD	25.4 ± 25.3	16.9 ± 15.0	22.7 ± 16.7	> 0.1

[a] The p-value was derived by comparing ≤ 25 with 26–40, 26–40 with > 40, and > 40 with ≤ 25 s groups.

BA – balloon:annulus ratio. BPV – balloon pulmonary valvuloplasty. FU – followup. SD – standard deviation.

From: Rao PS: Balloon pulmonary valvuloplasty: a review. *Clin Cardiol.* 12:55–74, 1989. Copyrighted and reprinted with the permission of Clinical Cardiology Publishing Co. Inc., and/or the Foundation for Advances in Medicine and Science (FAMS), Box 832, Mahwah, New Jersey 07430, USA.

Some investigators[30] recommend pressures of 7 to 8.5 atm which, in our opinion, has a good chance for balloon rupture and potential problems associated with rupture. In our own experience, the "waisting" of the balloon was noted to disappear even at 2 atm with a resultant good valvuloplasty.[9] We now routinely perform valvuloplasty sequentially at 3, 4, and 5 atm of pressure inflation. The "waisting" usually disappears at 3 or 4 atm. With this protocol, we have had no balloon ruptures. Initially, we used a 10-second inflation and now we use a 5-second inflation. With the shorter interval, there is less hypotension, which returns to normal a few seconds after deflation.

After a successful valvuloplasty, we usually repeat the procedure twice. We agree with Yeager's observation[106] that pressures much higher than those required to abolish "waisting" of the balloon offer no advantage, especially because the polyethylene balloons are designed to maintain a relatively uniform diameter even at high pressures. Furthermore, high pressures tend to lead to balloon rupture. Shorter inflation–deflation cycles produce minimal hemodynamic disturbances during balloon valvuloplasty.

On the basis of the data presented and on our own experience, we would recommend sequential balloon inflation with 3, 4 and 5 atm of pressure of 5-second duration, 5 minutes apart.

NONINVASIVE FOLLOWUP EVALUATION

Electrocardiographic Studies

Kveselis,[32] Fontes,[58] Lloyd,[107] and we[16] have previously reported electrocardiographic changes following balloon pulmonary valvuloplasty. Kveselis[32] observed significant decrease in R-wave voltage in lead V_1 and a leftward shift of frontal plane mean QRS vector in 13 patients, 16 ± 9 months following balloon pulmonary valvuloplasty. Fontes and associates[58] reported a shift of frontal plane mean vector (axis) from $118 \pm 31°$ to $86 \pm 31°$ in 56 patients during a followup from 6 to 52 months following balloon pulmonary valvuloplasty. They also found regression of right ventricular hypertrophy in 16 cases (29%) while mild to moderate hypertrophy persisted in 29 cases (52%). Lloyd and Donnerstein[107] noted reversion to normal (inversion) of T waves in lead V_1 in 17 of 19 (89%) patients under 12 years of age, in whom the T wave had been upright prior to balloon valvuloplasty. They attributed this change in T-wave polarity to favorable alteration of the relationship between myocardial oxygen consumption and coronary blood flow following pressure gradient relief produced by balloon valvuloplasty.

In a detailed study[16] of 35 patients with electrocardiographic followup 3 to 34 (mean 11) months following valvuloplasty, we made the following observations. When electrocardiograms obtained immediately before and after balloon valvuloplasty were compared, there was practically no change in mean vectors, QRS voltages, and T waves in any patient. The absence of T-wave changes in our study is in contradistinction to findings of Lloyd and Donnerstein[107]; however, most of our ECGs were obtained within a few hours of balloon valvuloplasty and probably did not allow sufficient time for regression of T waves. In 30 children with excellent relief of pulmonic stenosis at followup, the frontal plane means QRS vector moved toward the left, as did the horizontal plane means QRS vector (Table 15.12). The amplitude of the R wave in V_1 and V_2, decreased, as did S-wave amplitudes in V_5 and V_6. The improvement in the electrocardiogram is associated with a decrease in pulmonary valve gradient from 95 ± 50 to 29 ± 23 mmHg. In 5 children with a significant residual gradient, the electrocardiogram did not show any significant change.

Evaluation of the time course of the electrocardiographic changes in the group with good results revealed minimal improvement or none in electrocardiographic parameters at the 3-month followup visit ($p > 0.05$ to 0.2), whereas at 6-, 12-, and 18-month followup visits, there was a significant improvement ($p < 0.05$ to 0.001) (Figure 15.12).

Having concluded that the electrocardiogram improves after successful balloon pulmonary valvuloplasty, I was attempted to see if individual postvalvuloplasty electrocardiograms reflected a significant residual valve gradient at followup. Thirty sets of paired electrocardiographic and pulmonary valve pressure gradient data obtained

Table 15.12 ELECTROCARDIOGRAPHIC CHANGES AFTER BALLOON PULMONARY VALVULOPLASTY

	Pre-Valvuloplasty mean ± SD	Follow-Up mean ± SD	p value
Frontal plane mean QRS vector (°)	127 ± 25	81 ± 47	< 0.001
Horizontal plane mean QRS vector (°)	88 ± 36	27 ± 51	< 0.001
Amplitude of R wave in V_1 (mm)	19.0 ± 11.6	9.5 ± 5.9	< 0.001
Amplitude of R wave in V_2 (mm)	19.7 ± 12.2	11.3 ± 6.1	< 0.001
Amplitude of S wave in V_5 (mm)	10.5 ± 6.5	5.9 ± 3.9	< 0.01
Amplitude of S wave in V_6 (mm)	6.7 ± 4.7	2.9 ± 2.6	< 0.01

SD — standard deviation

Time course of Right precordial Voltage changes following Balloon Pulmonary Valvuloplasty

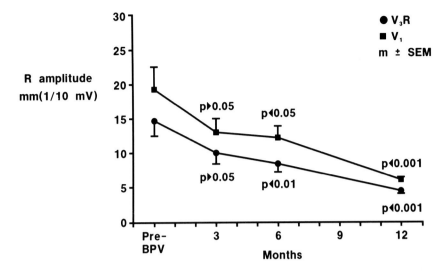

Time course of Left Precordial Voltage changes following Balloon Pulmonary Valvuloplasty

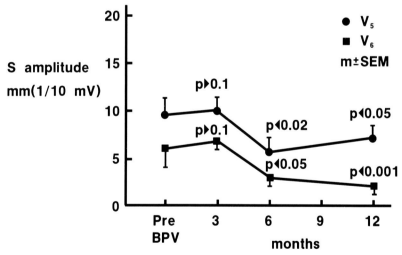

Figure 15.12 Precordial voltages, $R_{V_3}R$ and R_{V_1} (A) and S_{V_5} and S_{V_6} (B) prior to and 3, 6, and 12 months following balloon pulmonary valvuloplasty (BPV) in Group 1 with good results. Note that precordial voltages did not significantly change ($p > 0.05$ to $p > 0.1$) at 3-month followup, whereas at 6 and 12 months following BPV, there was a significant decrease ($p < 0.05$ to $p < 0.001$) in the right ventricular voltages. Electrocardiograms were available in all 30 group 1 patients prior to valvuloplasty. The followup data are based on electrocardiograms in 20, 24, and 22 patients, respectively, at 3-,6-, and 12-month followup. *SEM*—Standard error of mean. (From: Rao PS, Solymar L: Electrocardiographic changes following balloon dilatation of valvar pulmonic stenosis. *J Intervent Cardiol.* 1:189–197, 1988. With permission.)

within 24 hours of each other were available for analysis. Fifteen electrocardiograms were interpreted to be normal, and the corresponding pulmonary valve gradients were low: $18.3 + 8.2$ mmHg (range 4–30 mmHg) (Figure 15.13). These electrocardiograms and catheterization-measured gradients were recorded seven to 28 months (12.0 ± 5.5 mo) following balloon valvuloplasty. Ten electrocardiograms showed right ventricular hypertrophy and were not significantly different from prevalvuloplasty tracings. Right ventricular outflow gradients (valvular plus infundibular) obtained 6 to 23 months (10 ± 5 mo) following valvuloplasty ranged between 32 and 118 mmHg (55.8 ± 26.4 mmHg) and were higher than those seen in normal electrocardiographic group ($p < 0.01$) (Fig. 15.13). The remaining five electrocardiograms, obtained

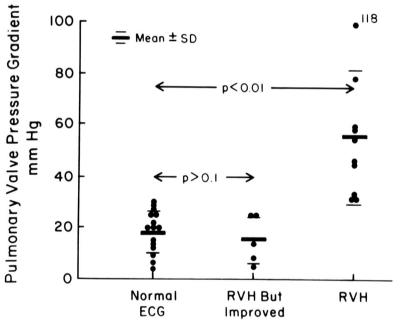

Figure 15.13 Relationship of postvalvuloplasty electrocardiograms with the residual pulmonary outflow tract (valvular plus infundibular) gradients. Note that in the presence of normal electrocardiogram (ECG), the pulmonary valve gradients were low, less than 30 mmHg (left-hand column.) The ECGs shown in the right-hand column, marked "RVH" (right ventricular hypertrophy), were obtained 6 months or more after balloon valvuloplasty and all had right ventricular outflow tract gradients in excess of 30 mmHg. The ECGs shown in the central column marked "RVH but improved" were obtained less than 6 months after balloon valvuloplasty and had right ventricular outflow gradients less than 30 mmHg. These data would suggest that a normal ECG would indicate right ventricular outflow gradient $\leq$ 30 mmHg whereas RVH would indicate significant (> 30 mmHg) right ventricular outflow gradients unless the ECG was obtained less than 6 months after valvuloplasty. (From: Rao PS, Solymar L: Electrocardiographic changes following balloon dilatation of valvar pulmonic stenosis. *J Intervent Cardiol.* 1:189–197, 1988. With permission.)

within 6 months following balloon valvuloplasty, showed right ventricular hypertrophy but were markedly improved when compared with prevalvuloplasty electrocardiograms. The pulmonary valve gradients at catheterization were 5 to 25 mmHg (15.2 ± 9.4 mmHg) and were not significantly different ($p > 0.1$) from the normal electrocardiogram group (Fig. 15.13). Three of these patients had repeat electrocardiograms 6 months later (1 year after valvuloplasty) and were found to be normal. Thus, pulmonary gradients less than 30 mmHg are likely to be present in patients who have normal electrocardiograms. If right ventricular hypertrophy is present and the electrocardiogram is obtained later than 6 months following valvuloplasty, a significant residual gradient could be expected. Right ventricular hypertrophy in an electrocardiogram obtained at or before 6 months following valvuloplasty does not accurately predict the pulmonary valve gradient.

In conclusion, electrocardiographic findings improve after successful pulmonary valvuloplasty, and the electrocardiogram is a useful adjunct in the evaluation of intermediate-term results of balloon pulmonary valvuloplasty. However, electrocardiographic evidence for hemodynamic improvement does not become apparent until after 6 months following balloon valvuloplasty.

Doppler & Echocardiographic Evaluation

Rocchini and associates,[32,103] Robertson and associates,[37] Mullins and associates,[59] and we[10,11,14,22] have previously reported Doppler and echocardiographic followup studies after balloon pulmonary valvuloplasty. Kveselis[32] reported results of Doppler examination in 11 patients 15 ± 19 months following balloon valvuloplasty: The calculated right ventricular outflow gradient was reduced from 86 ± 29 to 38 ± 9 mmHg immediately after balloon valvuloplasty. The gradients diminished, though to an insignificant degree, to 33 ± 7 mmHg, at followup. Doppler evidence for pulmonary insufficiency was present in 8 out of 11 patients. Similar improvement was noted in a subsequent publication[103] involving 28 patients with successful balloon valvuloplasty. Robertson and associates,[37] while analyzing the morphology of the right ventricular outflow tract following balloon valvuloplasty, reported followup (10.2 ± 5.6 mo) Doppler studies in 18 patients. The calculated pulmonary valvular gradient, having been reduced to 37 ± 23 from 72 ± 31 mmHg immediately following balloon valvuloplasty, decreased further to 31 ± 21 mmHg at followup.

Mullins and associates[59] obtained continuous-wave Doppler flow measurements in 30 of 63 children who underwent balloon pulmonary valvuloplasty at a mean of 13 months following valvuloplasty; the estimated residual gradient was 20 ± 8 mmHg.

We have echo-Doppler followup studies obtained in 43 children at 3 to 36 months (15 ± 6 mo) following balloon valvuloplasty. Two-dimensionally derived M-mode tracings of the right ventricle and left ventricle and pulsed- and continuous-wave Doppler flow velocity recordings from the right ventricular outflow tract and the main pulmonary artery were recorded, as previously reported,[11,14,42] initially, at 3- to 6-month intervals, and subsequently at 12-month intervals. The pulmonary valvular gradient was calculated by a modified Bernoulli equation (gradient $= 4V_2^2$, where V_2 is peak Doppler flow velocity in the main pulmonary artery). When the right ventricular outflow tract Doppler flow velocity (V_1) was in excess of 1.0 M/s, V_1 was incorporated into the Bernoulli equation (gradient $= 4\,(V_2^2 - V_1^2)$.

The echo-Doppler results were analyzed separately for group 1 (good-results group) and group 2 (poor-results group). Table 15.13 summarizes these findings.

Table 15.13   ECHO-DOPPLER RESULTS FOLLOWING BALLOON PULMONARY VALVULOPLASTY

	Pre mean ± SD	Post Mean ± SD	p value*	Follow-up mean ± SD	p value*
Group 1 (Good Results)					
RVEDD (mm)	19.3 ± 5.4	17.1 ± 5.2	> 0.05	15.7 ± 5.0	< 0.01
LVEDD (mm)	31.8 ± 7.6	31.2 ± 7.0	> 0.1	35.5 ± 7.7	< 0.01
Peak Doppler flow velocity in MPA (m/s)	4.16 ± 0.8	2.86 ± 0.64	< 0.001	2.38 ± 0.64	< 0.001
Group 2 (Poor results)					
RVEDD (mm)	22.1 ± 10.1	20.3 ± 8.3	> 0.1	23.2 ± 13.8	> 0.1
LVEDD (mm)	27.9 ± 5.9	30.3 ± 7.7	> 0.1	26.2 ± 5.7	> 0.1
Peak Doppler flow velocity in MPA (m/s)	3.74 ± 0.5	3.6 ± 0.54	> 0.1	3.5 ± 0.83	> 0.1

* Compares with pre-valvuloplasty values; Pre — prior to valvuloplasty; Post — immediately after valvuloplasty; SD — standard deviation

RVEDD — right ventricular end-diastolic dimension

LVEDD — left ventricular end-diastolic dimension

In group 1 patients the right ventricular end-diastolic dimension decreased, but not significantly immediately after balloon valvuloplasty, decreasing further at the last available followup. The left ventricular end-diastolic dimension did not change immediately after valvuloplasty, but at followup there was a significant increase. The Doppler flow velocity in the main pulmonary artery decreased immediately following valvuloplasty. On followup, this parameter was further improved, as was the pressure gradient. Doppler evidence for mild pulmonary insufficiency was present in 34 out of 43 patients for whom data were available. Longitudinal followup, Doppler flow velocities in the pulmonary artery are shown in Figure 15.14. These data show a rapid reduction of flow velocities immediately following valvuloplasty with further reduction at 3-month followup. Subsequently, there was minimal fall, if any.

By contrast, in group 2, the right ventricular end-diastolic dimension did not change either immediately after balloon valvuloplasty or at followup. Similarly, the left ventricular end-diastolic dimension did not change immediately following or several months after valvuloplasty. Peak Doppler flow velocity in the pulmonary artery prior to valvuloplasty remained essentially unchanged after valvuloplasty and on followup. (Table 15.13). Doppler evidence for pulmonary insufficiency was present in 2 of the 7 patients on followup. Of the 7 group 2 patients, 5 underwent repeat balloon valvuloplasty; 7 to 12 months following repeat valvuloplasty the Doppler flow velocity decreased to 2.5 ± 0.4 M/s ($p < 0.001$).

The ability of Doppler studies to predict pulmonary valvular gradients after balloon valvuloplasty was then evaluated. We had 37 paired sets of Doppler and catheterization data obtained within 24 hours of each other immediately following balloon pulmonary valvuloplasty. We then had 30 paired sets of Doppler and catheterization data obtained within 24 hours of each other at 6- to 36-month followup. Correlation between Doppler-calculated and catheterization-measured pulmonary valvular gradients at followup was excellent ($r = 0.9$), whereas correlation of data obtained immediately after valvuloplasty was less good ($r = 0.6$). These results are similar to those we reported in a smaller number of subjects.[42] No technical or

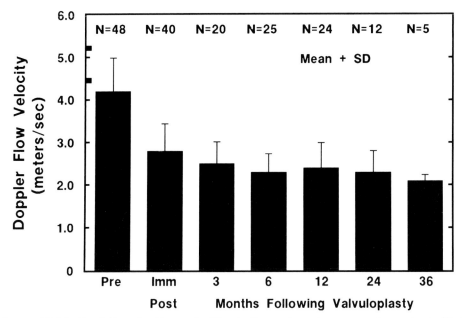

Figure 15.14 Peak Doppler flow velocities in the main pulmonary artery prior to (*Pre*) and immediately after (*Imm*) balloon pulmonary valvuloplasty and at followup are shown. *N* indicates the number of patients in whom the data were available at that particular interval. Note that a fall in the flow velocity occurred immediately after valvuloplasty with further reduction at 3-month followup. There was minimal, if any, change subsequent to 3-month followup. (From: Rao PS: Balloon pulmonary valvuloplasty: a review. *Clin Cardiol.* 12:55–74, 1989. With permission.)

clear anatomic reason was found.[42] Apparently, the right ventricular outflow is hyperreactive immediately after balloon valvuloplasty; this was shown in immediate postprocedure right ventricular angiography but without a demonstrable pressure gradient on pressure pullback tracings.

No significant changes in the ventricular sizes were observed immediately following balloon valvuloplasty, regardless of the quality of the results. Doppler flow velocity recording often overestimated the residual gradient, probably because of infundibular hyperreactivity. Therefore, echo-Doppler studies immediately following balloon valvuloplasty are not reflective of the favorable hemodynamic changes occurring at that time.

At followup, the echocardiographic size of the right ventricle, the Doppler flow velocity in the main pulmonary artery, and the calculated pulmonary valve gradient improved in patients with successful balloon valvuloplasty, whereas no such changes were observed in the group of patients with significant residual pulmonary stenosis. The data indicate that intermediate-term followup echo-Doppler studies are reflective of the hemodynamic improvement. These studies suggest that repeat cardiac catheterization to evaluate intermediate-term and long-term results of balloon pulmonary valvuloplasty may not be necessary.

Although our initial impression was the incidence of pulmonary valve insufficiency following balloon valvuloplasty was low,[10,11] the results of this larger study showed that 34 of 43 (79%) patients with successful balloon valvuloplasty developed pulmonary insufficiency on intermediate-term followup. This is understandable, because the balloon valvuloplasty produces commissural splitting and tearing or avulsion of valve leaflets.[91] However, the pulmonary insufficiency is minimal and unlikely to be problematic; there was no evidence for right ventricular volume overloading (near-normal right ventricle size and no paradoxical septal motion) in our echocardiographic studies and by equilibrium-gated radionuclide angiograms reported by Tynan and associates.[29] Although the long-term followup studies should be scrutinized for progressive right ventricular volume overload, the current data suggest that pulmonary insufficiency produced by balloon dilatation is unlikely to be problematic.

OTHER ISSUES

Dysplastic Pulmonary Valve

Several studies have implicated dysplastic pulmonary valves as a cause of failure following balloon pulmonary valvuloplasty.[29,31-34,36,65,103] More recently, detailed reports of balloon valvuloplasty in patients with dysplastic pulmonary valves[44,45] suggested that poor results may be expected if dysplasia is present. A summary of experience reported in the literature is tabulated in Table 15.14. Our experience with dysplastic pulmonary valves is contrary to that reported in these papers. Therefore, we previously reviewed[17] the results of balloon valvuloplasty in 13 patients with dysplastic pulmonary valves (group 11, Table 15.2) from our total experience with 56 patients to assess the outcome of balloon valvuloplasty in dysplastic valves. These results were compared with valvuloplasty results in 43 patients with nondysplastic pulmonary valves (group 12). Assessment of dysplasia of the pulmonary valve was based on the criteria outlined by Jeffery and Koretzky and their associates[108,109]:

Table 15.14 SUMMARY OF RESULTS OF BALLOON VALVULOPLASTY IN PATIENTS WITH PULMONARY VALVE DYSPLASIA FROM THE LITERATURE

Study	No. of patients with DPV	Immediate Success (%)		Follow-up Success (%)	
Kan et al,[31] 1984	1	0	(0)	0	(0)
Tynan et at,[29] 1985	3	0	(0)	0	(0)
Miller,[33] 1985	1	0	(0)	—	
Sullivan et al,[34] 1985	2	1	(50)	0	(0)
Rocchini & Beekman,[103] 1986	7	0	(0)	3	(43)
Musewe et al,[44] 1987	5	1	(20)	1	(20)
DiSessa et al,[45] 1987	3	0	(0)	—	
Rey et al,[36] 1988	4	3	(75)	3	(75)
Marantz et al,[46] 1988	4	3	(75)	2	(50)
Rao et al,[17] 1988	13	9	(69)	10	(77)
Ballerini et al,[65] 1990	9	2	(22)	3	(33)
Total	52	19	(37)	22	(47)[a]

[a] Patients without followup were excluded for the purpose of calculation of percentage of success.

DPV — dysplastic pulmonary valves.

1. Angiographic appearance of nodular and uneven thickening and poor doming of the valve leaflets (Fig. 15.15)
2. Valve ring hypoplasia (less than mean value for the given body surface area as defined by Rowlatt et al.[110])
3. No poststenotic dilatation

When all three criteria were present, the pulmonary valve was considered dysplastic. If the valve leaflets fulfilled criteria 1 without the presence of one or both of the other criteria, the valve was considered mildly dysplastic. A total of 13 dysplastic pulmonary valves were identified; 7 were severely dysplastic and 6 were mildly dysplastic.

Table 15.15 summarizes these data. Balloon valvuloplasty in 13 patients, aged 6 days to 12 years (median 1 yr), with dysplastic pulmonary valves (group 11) led to an improvement in the pulmonary valve gradient that was maintained at 6- to 19-month (mean, 10 mo) followup. Valvuloplasty in 43 patients with nondysplastic pulmonary valves (group 12) also led to a sustained improvement in the valvular gradient at 6- to 34-month followup in 23 patients. Immediate and long-term findings in the two groups were similar. A slightly higher mean balloon:annulus ratio was used in the patients with dysplastic pulmonary valves, this difference did not attain statistical significance ($p > 0.1$). Two of the 13 patients with dysplasia and 3 of the 23 patients without dysplasia required repeat valvuloplasty at followup catheterization. Residual

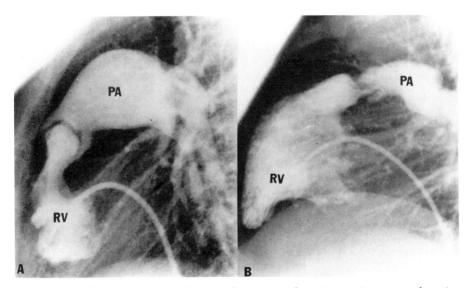

Figure 15.15 Selected frames from right ventricular cineangiograms of patients without (*A*) and with (*B*) dysplastic pulmonary valves. *A*, Thickened and domed pulmonary valve leaflets are seen. Note poststenotic dilatation of the pulmonary artery. *B*, Pulmonary valve leaflets are markedly and unevenly thickened without doming. There was no jet formation and no poststenotic dilatation of the pulmonary artery. The pulmonary valve ring is small when compared to norms described by Rowlatt and associates.[110] (From: Rao PS: Indications for balloon pulmonary valvuloplasty. Am Heart J. 116:1168–1173, 1988. With permission.)

Table 15.15 COMPARISON OF GROUP 11 WITH DYSPLASTIC PULMONARY VALVES WITH GROUP 12 WITH NO PULMONARY VALVE DYSPLASIA

	Group 11, mean ± SD	Group 12, mean ± SD	p-value
Pulmonary valve gradient prevalvuloplasty, mmHg	77.2 ± 44.2	94.3 ± 41.0	> 0.1
Pulmonary valve gradient immediately after valvuloplasty, mmHg	26.8 ± 17.0[a]	31.1 ± 22.4[a]	> 0.1
Pulmonary valve gradient at followup, mmHg	34.9 ± 34.6[b]	29.2 ± 33.5[a]	> 0.1

[a] p < 0.001 when compared to prevalvuloplasty gradient

[b] p < 0.02 when compared to prevalvuloplasty gradient

SD — standard deviation.

From: Rao PS: Balloon dilatation in infants and children with dysplastic pulmonary valves: short-term and intermediate-term results. *Am Heart J.* 116:1168–1173, 1988. With permission.

pulmonary valvular gradients in excess of 30 mmHg at follow-up were present, respectively, in 3 of 13 and 4 of the 23 patients with and without dysplastic valves.

As shown in Table 15.2 all balloon pulmonary valvuloplasties were divided into those with good results (gradient ≤ 30 mmHg at followup), 29 patients (group 1) and poor results (gradient > 30 mmHg at followup), 7 patients (group 2). The prevalence of dysplastic pulmonary valves was 10 in group 1 and 3 in group 2. This prevalence was similar (p > 0.1). In the 10 patients with dysplastic pulmonary valves with good results, the balloon:annulus ratio (1.37 ± 0.22) used for balloon valvuloplasty was larger than that (10.4 ± 0.17) used in the 3 patients with poor results (p < 0.01). These data suggest that (1) the results of balloon valvuloplasty in patients with dysplastic valves are comparable to those in patients with nondysplastic valves; (2) the dysplastic valves were not responsible for recurrence of valve stenosis; and (3) the use of large balloons in patients with dysplastic valves may have reduced the chance for recurrence.

Marantz and associates[46] compared immediate and followup results of balloon valvuloplasty in 4 patients with dysplastic pulmonary valves with those of 32 patients with nondysplastic valves and concluded that significant palliation or relief of gradient occurred following valvuloplasty. These investigators suggested that patients with dysplastic pulmonary valves should not be excluded from an attempt at balloon valvuloplasty.

The reason for the discrepancy between different studies in the results of balloon valvuloplasty in patients with dysplastic pulmonary valves is not clear. It may be related to interpretation of clinical and angiographic data in labeling a given patient as having dysplastic pulmonary valves, or it may be related to variations in degrees of pulmonary valve dysplasia[44,111,112] or to the presence of commissural fusion mixed with dysplasia.[44,45,111] It is generally considered that splitting of commissural fusion[91] is one of the major mechanisms by which balloon dilatation relieves valvular stenosis. Therefore, it is somewhat surprising that some patients with dysplastic valves would have good results. However, variations in the extent of dysplasia and dysplasia mixed with commissural fusion[44,45,109,111,112] can to some extent explain these results. Musewe and associates[44] suggested that if echocardiographic features of commissural fusion are present, catheterization and angiography should be performed to confirm commissural fusion, and, if it is present, balloon valvuloplasty should be performed.

We agree with this approach. However, these results[17] and those observed by Marantz and associates[46] lead us to recommend balloon valvuloplasty for relief of pulmonary valve obstruction even with angiographic features of pulmonary valve dysplasia. Also, it seems reasonable to use larger balloons than are recommended for non-dysplastic pulmonary valves; we personally tend to use balloons large enough to produce a balloon:annulus ratios of 1.4 to 1.5:1 and tend to avoid ratios in excess of 1.5 for fear of damage to the right ventricular outflow tract.[50]

Infundibular Obstruction

Many reports identify infundibular obstruction as a complicating feature immediately following balloon valvuloplasty.[9,10,14,34-37,57-59,75,80,95,99,113] We studied this problem further to define the prevalence and significance of infundibular obstruction in patients undergoing balloon valvuloplasty for valvular pulmonic stenosis[23]; we used the data of 62 children who had undergone balloon valvuloplasty during a 55-month period ending May 1988.

Of the 62 children, 13 (21%) had infundibular pressure gradients prior to balloon valvuloplasty; these ranged between 10 and 137 mmHg (49 ± 42 mmHg). Following valvuloplasty, infundibular gradients disappeared in 5 patients (Fig. 15.16). The

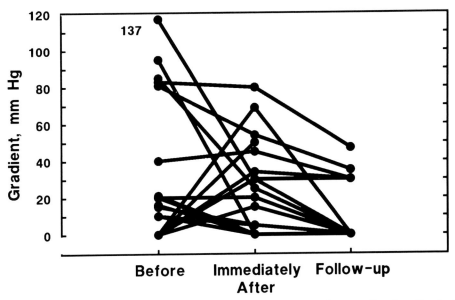

Figure 15.16 Sequential infundibular gradients before and immediately after balloon pulmonary valvuloplasty and at followup are shown. Thirteen children had initial gradients, five of which disappeared following valvuloplasty. New gradients appeared in five other patients. The gradients either disappeared or improved at followup. (From: Thapar MK, Rao PS: Significance of infundibular obstruction following balloon valvuloplasty for valvar pulmonic stenosis. *Am Heart J.* 118:99–103, 1989. With permission.)

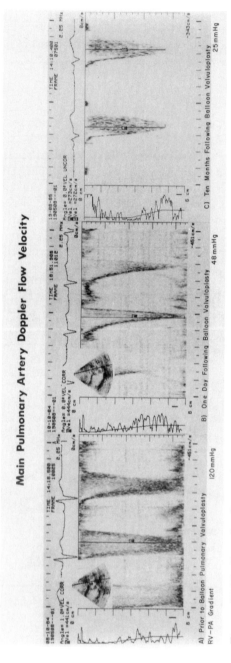

Figure 15.17 Doppler flow velocity recordings from the main pulmonary artery prior to (*left*), and 1 day (*center*) and 10 months (*right*) following balloon pulmonary valvuloplasty are shown. Note that there is no significant fall in the peak flow velocity immediately after valvuloplasty, but there is a characteristic triangular pattern, indicative of infundibular obstruction. At 10-month followup, the flow velocity markedly diminished, suggesting resolution of infundibular obstruction. (From: Thapar MK, Rao PS: Significance of infundibular obstruction following balloon valvuloplasty for valvar pulmonic stenosis. *Am Heart J* 118:99–103, 1989. With permission.)

infundibular gradient in the remaining 8 patients was 33 ± 26 mmHg with a range of 5 to 80 mmHg. In 6 of these 8 patients, the infundibular gradients diminished as compared with prevalvuloplasty gradients. In one child, the gradient remained unchanged at 20 mmHg, and in the final patient the infundibular gradient increased from 40 to 45 mmHg. In 5 additional patients without infundibular gradients but with angiographic infundibular narrowing, an infundibular gradient appeared after valvuloplasty; new infundibular gradients were 15, 30, 34, 50, and 69 mmHg (40 ± 21 mmHg) (Fig. 15.16). Thus, 18 of 62 (29%) patients had infundibular gradients prior to or immediately after valvuloplasty. Examples of severe infundibular reaction demonstrated by Doppler echocardiography and cineangiography are shown in Figures 15.17 and 15.18.

One child received propranolol prior to balloon pulmonary valvuloplasty. Two other children, with what was thought to be successful balloon valvuloplasty, developed systemic-level pressures in the right ventricle because of severe infundibular reaction. Propranolol at a dosage of 0.1 mg/kg, was slowly administered intravenously with a decrease in the right ventricular pressures and infundibular gradients. These 3 patients and three others with infundibular stenosis were given oral propranolol, 2 to 3 milligrams per kilogram per day in three or four divided doses, for approximately 3 months. None of our patients required surgical infundibular resection.

The gradients disappeared at followup in 7 of the 13 patients with infundibular gradients at the end of ballon valvuloplasty. No followup data were available in one

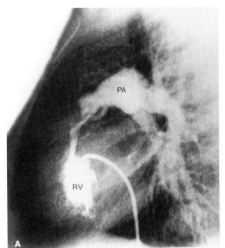
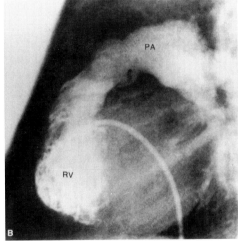

Figure 15.18 Selected frames from lateral view of the right ventricular (*RV*) cineangiogram showing severe infundibular reaction (*A*) immediately following balloon valvuloplasty (corresponding to Fig. 15.17. *center*). Note wide-open right ventricular outflow tract (*B*) at 10-month postvalvuloplasty catheterization (corresponds to Fig. 15.17, *right*). The peak-to-peak pulmonary valvular pressure gradient at followup catheterization was 20 mmHg; there was no infundibular gradient. *PA*—pulmonary artery. (From: Thapar MK, Rao PS: Significance of infundibular obstruction following balloon valvuloplasty for valvar pulmonic stenosis. *Am Heart J.* 118:99–103, 1989. With permission.)

child. In the remaining 5 patients with persistent infundibular gradients at followup, the gradients were low, range 10 to 47 mmHg (mean 29 mmHg); in each patient the gradient at followup was lower than the immediate postvalvuloplasty gradient (Fig. 15.16).

We also investigated the influence of severity of pulmonary valve obstruction and the age of the patient on the development of infundibular obstruction. The patients with infundibular obstruction (n = 18) had higher pulmonary valve gradient. (119 ± 51 mmHg) than those (n = 44) without infundibular gradient (83 ± 35 mmHg) (p < 0.01). When the prevalence of infundibular obstruction was scrutinized (Table 15.16), patients with a higher degree of obstruction had a greater prevalence of infundibular stenosis. The age distribution of patients with and without infundibular gradients (9.8 ± 7.1 vs 8.2 ± 6.4 yr) was similar (p > 0.01). However, the prevalence of infundibular gradient was higher in older patients than in younger patients (p < 0.01) (Table 15.16).

Several authors have reported either persistence of right ventricular infundibular gradients or appearance of such gradients following balloon pulmonary valvuloplasty.[9,14,34-37,57,65,75,95,99,113] When such infundibular obstruction was severe, propranolol was administered by several groups of workers[14,36,57,80,113] with variable result. Infundibular resection by surgery was required in two patients.[57,99] In a few studies with followup catheterization, the infundibular obstruction improved.[14,34-36,75,113]

The absence of a pressure gradient across angiographically narrow right ventricular infundibula in the presence of a more severe distal obstruction (valvular stenosis) is well known.[114-116] This atypical behavior of multiple obstructions may be due to "forced vibration" with greater energy transfer into the cardiovascular segment upstream of the proximal obstruction than into the segment upstream to the distal obstruction.[115,116] The elastic and pulsatile characteristics of the cardiovascular system are important for expressing this property.[115,116] Once the valvular (distal) gradient was relieved, an infundibular (proximal) gradient appeared.

Infundibular gradients immediately following valvuloplasty appear to be related to infundibular hyperreactivity. If severe (producing near-systemic pressure in the right ventricle), treatment with propranolol may be necessary. We did indeed observe significant improvement in the gradient following intravenous administration of propranolol. This response is similar to that observed in patients with surgical

Table 15.16 RELATIONSHIP BETWEEN SEVERITY OF PULMONARY VALVULAR STENOSIS AND AGE WITH THE PREVALENCE OF INFUNDIBULAR GRADIENTS

	No. of Patients in the Specified Group	No. With Infundibular Gradients	p-value[a]
Pulmonary valve gradient $\geq$ 100 mmHg	21	9	< 0.01
Pulmonary valve gradient < 100 mmHg	41	9	
Pulmonary valve gradient $\geq$ 80 mmHg	32	12	< 0.01
Pulmonary valve gradient < 80 mmHg	30	6	
Age $\geq$ 5 Years	40	14	< 0.01
Age < 5 Years	22	4	

[a] Chi-square

From: Thapar MK, Rao PS: Significance of infundibular obstruction following balloon valvuloplasty for valvar pulmonic stenosis. *Am Heart J.* 118:99–103, 1989. With permission.

pulmonary valvotomy.[117] Although we were able to manage all our patients without surgical resection of the infundibular obstruction, an occasional patient may require infundibular resection.[57,99] Oral propranolol therapy may be required in some patients with significant infundibular obstruction; patients with an infundibular gradient in excess of 50 mmHg, as suggested by Fontes and associates,[113] may be candidates for such therapy. The infundibular obstruction is expected to regress with time as has been observed following surgical pulmonary valvotomy[118,119] and balloon valvuloplasty.[10,14,34,75] Whether propranolol has any effect in enhancing regression of infundibular obstruction cannot be answered by this study.

Al Kasab and associates [80] observed that 5 patients receiving propranolol prior to balloon dilatation developed insignificant infundibular gradients (12 ± 4 mmHg) following valvuloplasty, whereas 6 other patients not receiving propranolol developed more severe infundibular gradients (45 ± 27 mmHg.) In the latter group, gradients diminished (9 ± 4 mmHg) following propranolol. Although these authors did not recommend routine use of propranolol therapy prior to valvuloplasty, they implied the potential use of beta blockade. At this time, there is not, in my opinion, sufficient evidence to advocate routine use of beta-blocking agents prior to valvuloplasty.

In summary, infundibular gradients in association with balloon pulmonary valvuloplasty were documented in 29% (18 out of 62) of patients. The prevalence of such gradients appears to be more frequent with increasing age and severity of valvular stenosis. Some of these children may develop systemic or suprasystemic pressures in the right ventricle because of hyperreactivity of the right ventricular infundibulum and may need beta blockade. The infundibular stenosis does regress to a great degree at follow-up. The potential for development of infundibular gradient after balloon valvuloplasty should not deter physicians from use of this technique in the treatment of valvular pulmonic stenosis.

CYANOTIC CONGENITAL HEART DEFECTS

Cyanotic heart defects, as a group, contribute up to from one fifth to one fourth of all congenital heart defects.[2] In many of these patients, pulmonic stenosis is an integral part of the cardiac malformation causing right-to-left shunting. These patients usually present with symptoms in the neonatal period or early infancy. The degree of cyanosis and the level of hypoxemia determine the symptomatology. Physical findings and laboratory data depend upon the defect complex and are reasonably characteristic for each defect complex. Total surgical correction or, if that is not feasible, palliation by some type of systemic–pulmonary artery anastomosis to augment pulmonary blood flow and to improve oxygenation is usually recommended. With the availability of transluminal balloon dilatation, we and others have used this technique to augment pulmonary flow instead of the initial or repeat systemic–pulmonary shunts. This was accomplished by balloon pulmonary valvuloplasty or by dilating previously created but narrowed Blalock-Taussig shunts.[120] Issues relating to dilating these shunts are not discussed in this chapter.

Indications

The indications for balloon pulmonary valvuloplasty that we have used[13] were cardiac defects not amenable to surgical correction at the age and size at the time of presentation but at the same time requiring palliation for pulmonary oligemia.

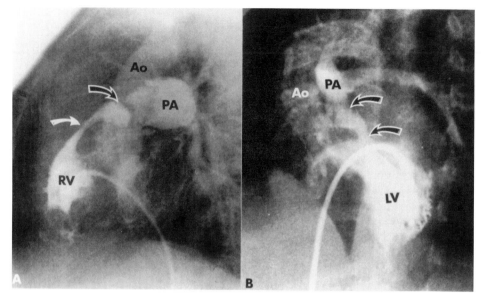

Figure 15.19 Selected cineangiographic frames from patients with tetralogy of Fallot (*A*) and transposition of the great arteries (*B*) demonstrating two sites of pulmonary outflow obstruction (*two arrows*). When the pulmonary obstruction is relieved by balloon valvuloplasty, the subvalvular obstruction remains and prevents flooding of lungs. *Ao*—aorta. *LV*—left ventricle. *PA*—pulmonary artery. *RV*—right ventricle.

Symptoms related to hypoxemia and progressive polycythemia are indications for intervention. The presence of two or more sites of obstruction to pulmonary blood flow (Fig. 15.19) was considered a prerequisite when employing balloon pulmonary valvuloplasty because if valvular stenosis is the sole obstruction, relief of such an obstruction may cause a marked increase in pulmonary blood flow and elevation of pulmonary artery pressure.

Technique

The technique of balloon valvuloplasty in patients with complex cyanotic heart defects is similar (Fig. 15.20) to that described in the beginning of the chapter and in the section dealing with isolated pulmonary stenosis, although at times, it may be more difficult to accomplish balloon valvuloplasty in this group than in simple pulmonary stenosis group. We use a balloon that is 1.2 to 1.4 times the pulmonary valve annulus.

Immediate Results

We[13] and others[56,121-124] have used balloon pulmonary valvuloplasty to augment pulmonary blood flow in infants with cyanotic heart defects and pulmonary oligemia. Boucek and associates[121] performed balloon pulmonary valvuloplasty in 7 children and increased their oxygen saturation from $72 \pm 5\%$ to $83 \pm 5\%$ (p < 0.005). Both pulmonary arterial pressure and pulmonary blood flow increased. Qureshi and associ-

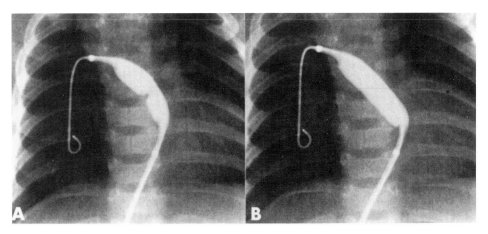

Figure 15.20 Selected cineradiographic frames demonstrating the position of balloon dilatation catheter across the pulmonic valve in a patient with tetralogy of Fallot. Note the indentation (waist) of the balloon (*A*) which disappeared (*B*) following full inflation. Although we prefer to place the guidewire in the left pulmonary artery, balloon valvuloplasty can also be successfully performed with the guidewire positioned in the right pulmonary artery, as in the illustrated case.

ates[122] reported their observations after balloon dilatation of the pulmonary valve in 15 patients with tetralogy of Fallot; the systemic arterial saturation increased in the majority of patients. In 4 of these children, either no significant change or a deterioration of oxygen saturation occurred. Six children required no further intervention, and 4 children received a systemic-to-pulmonary artery shunt 1.6 months (0–3 mo) after the procedure. Qureshi's group concluded that balloon dilatation may be useful in the management of infants with severe tetralogy of Fallot and that it should be considered for the initial palliative treatment. Mehta and Perlman[123] reported a single patient with tetralogy of Fallot in whom pulmonary balloon valvuloplasty increased oxygen saturation from 80% to 90%.

Our experience with this procedure, including that reported previously,[13,124] was in 12 infants with congenital cyanotic heart defects, aged 3 days to 24 months, weighing 2.9 to 12.0 kg, who underwent percutaneous balloon pulmonary valvuloplasty as a palliative procedure to alleviate pulmonary oligemia. The diagnoses in these cases were tetralogy of Fallot in 5; transposition of the great arteries (S, D, D) with ventricular septal defect and valvular and subvalvular pulmonic stenosis in 3; critical pulmonary stenosis with intact ventricular septum and hypoplastic right ventricle in 3; and ventricular inversion, ventricular septal defect, and valvular and subvalvular pulmonic stenosis in one. Following balloon valvuloplasty, increases were as follows:

Arterial oxygen saturation ($65.9 \pm 9.7\%$ vs 78.4 ± 13.6, $p < 0.05$)
Pulmonary blood flow index (1.83 ± 0.55 to 3.14 ± 0.6 L/min/m^2, $p < 0.05$)
Pulmonary:systemic flow ratio (0.62 ± 0.35 to 1.2 ± 0.6, $p < 0.05$)
Pulmonary artery pressure (16.8 ± 7.2 to 29.2 ± 11.1 mmHg, $p < 0.02$)

Immediate surgical intervention was avoided in all 12 patients.

Followup Results

Followup data are limited. Boucek and associates[121] reported 0.5- to 2.8-year followup results; 4 tetralogy patients underwent surgical correction, 1 patient underwent a systemic-to-pulmonary shunt procedure, and the other 2 did not require surgical intervention. Qureshi[122] reported followup observations after balloon valvuloplasty of 15 tetralogy of Fallot patients; 7 children required no further palliation during a mean followup period of 12.9 months (3.5–26 mo). Four children required a systemic-to-pulmonary artery shunt operation 1 day to 3 months (mean 1.6 months) after valvuloplasty. The final 4 patients had a corrective operation 6 to 10 months (mean 8 mo) after balloon dilatation.

Of our group of patients on followup 4 to 26 months after balloon valvuloplasty, all infants were thriving well with decreased hypoxemia and polycythemia. Followup catheterization data are available for all 12 patients, 3 to 15 months following valvuloplasty, and in all, the immediate improvement after balloon valvuloplasty persisted or further improvement was noted. None of the patients had significant elevation of pulmonary arterial systolic pressure (23.1 ± 5.8 mmHg; range 12–28 mmHg). Four infants with tetralogy of Fallot underwent successful total surgical correction 6 and 24 months following balloon valvuloplasty. Two infants with transposition of the great arteries showed evidence for increase in the size of the pulmonary arteries (Fig. 15.21), but because persistent hypoxemia, a Blalock-Taussig shunt was performed 6 months following initial balloon valvuloplasty. The other 4 infants were doing well clinically with continued palliation of pulmonary oligemia. In 4 of these children, we noted a significant improvement in the size of the pulmonary artery (Fig. 15.22), making safer surgical correction feasible. Parsons and associates[125] also reported enlargement of the pulmonary artery in tetralogy of Fallot patients after balloon valvuloplasty. These data suggest that pulmonary valvuloplasty offers an excellent palliation of pulmonary oligemia in cyanotic heart defects, thereby avoiding the risks of immediate surgical palliation and preparing for a better result of eventual total surgical correction.

Battistessa and associates[126] reported their observations at surgery of tetralogy of Fallot patients who had previously undergone balloon pulmonary valvuloplasty. Results in 27 patients (which included 15 patients previously reported by Qureshi[122]) were scrutinized. Anatomic alterations in the right ventricular outflow tracts were observed in 20 patients (74%) while no change was found in 7 (26%). They also noted that there was no evidence for significant growth of the pulmonary valve annulus and that the need for a transannular patch at the time of intracardiac repair is not abolished. However, the surgery was performed 15.6 (3 to 39) months after balloon valvuloplasty, indicating that these infants achieved palliation for a significant period. These are important observations, although the authors did not report the total number of patients who underwent balloon valvuloplasty from whom the 27 patients presented were derived. In addition, significant complications such as a pulmonary arterial tear[127] and right ventricular outflow tract disruption[126] were reported.

Comments

In view of the available data, it would seem that balloon pulmonary valvuloplasty in tetralogy of Fallot (or any other cyanotic heart defect) should be performed in only selected patients and not in all. General criteria that we propose are the following:

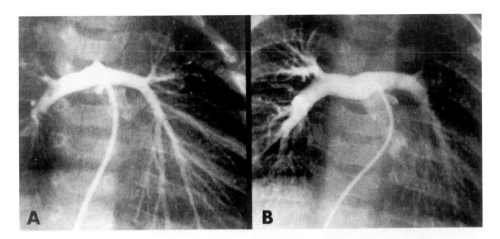

RPA — 5.0 mm   RPA — 9.4 mm
LPA — 3.3 mm   LPA — 7.8 mm

Figure 15.21 Pulmonary arteriogram immediately before (*A*) and 6 months after (*B*) balloon pulmonary valvuloplasty in an infant with transposition of the great arteries, ventricular septal defect, and valvular and subvalvular pulmonic stenosis. Note increase in the size of the pulmonary arteries after pulmonary valvuloplasty. There were differences in the magnification between the two cineangiographic frames; catheters in both frames were 5-Fr. After correcting for magnification, the right pulmonary artery size increased from 5.0 mm to 9.4 mm whereas the left pulmonary artery increased from 3.3 mm to 7.8 mm. Part of the enlargement was attributed to an increase in forward flow following balloon valvuloplasty. *RPA*—right pulmonary artery. *LPA*—left pulmonary artery. (From: Rao PS, Brais M.: Balloon pulmonary valvuloplasty for congenital cyanotic heart defects. *Am Heart J.* 115:1105–1110, 1988. With permission.)

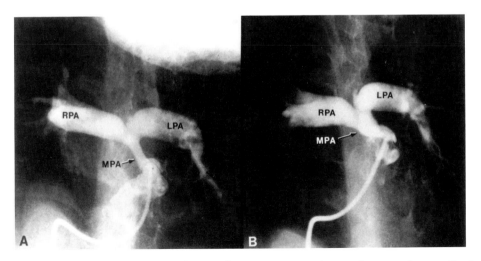

Figure 15.22 Selected frames from pulmonary artery cineangiograms in a patient with tetralogy of Fallot prior to (*A*) and 12 months following (*B*) balloon pulmonary valvuloplasty. Note significant improvement in the size of pulmonary valve annulus and main and branch pulmonary arteries following valvuloplasty.

1. The child requires palliation of pulmonary oligemia but is not a candidate for total surgical correction either because of the type of defect or because of anatomic variations.
2. Valvular obstruction is a significant component of the right ventricular outflow obstruction.
3. Multiple obstructions in series (see Fig. 15.19) are present so that there is residual obstruction after relief of pulmonary valvular obstruction and flooding of the lungs is prevented.
4. The balloon:annulus ratio should be approximately 1.2:1 to 1.4:1

New Developments

Obstruction to the pulmonary outflow tract is usually at several levels in tetralogy of Fallot; the sites of obstruction are the hypoplastic pulmonary arteries, pulmonary valve leaflets, pulmonary valve ring, and infundibulum. Relief of valvular obstruction can in some patients increase forward flow and encourage growth of the pulmonary valve ring and pulmonary arteries (see Fig. 15.22). If severe infundibular stenosis is present, relief of pulmonary valve stenosis alone may not accomplish the objectives of relieving systemic hypoxemia and encouraging growth of the pulmonary arteries.

Qureshi and associates[128] used a Simpson coronary atherectomy catheter[129] to perform infundibular myectomy in a 14-month-old child with tetralogy of Fallot. The systemic arterial saturation improved from 78% prior to the procedure to 85% a month later, and the right ventricular outflow tract became wider. They suggested that this type of transcatheter resection of the infundibulum may be important in the palliation of tetralogy of Fallot. Further clinical trials in selected patients seem to be indicated.

PULMONARY ATRESIA

Pulmonary atresia may be present with or without a ventricular septal defect. Sequential palliative surgical procedures are usually necessary prior to any corrective surgery.[130,131] Some of the surgical procedures can be avoided if transcatheter methods can open the atretic pulmonary valve to allow forward flow. Perforation of the atretic pulmonary valve with blunt wire, though feasible, is not generally used (Wexler L, personal communication 1989). Lee[132] and Riemenschneider[133] and their associates applied laser irradiation to relieve obstructed valves and create atrial septal defects in animal models and human postmortem specimens. Arapov and associates[134] used a laser intraoperatively for pulmonary valvotomy. Qureshi and associates[135] used a laser via a catheter to perforate an atretic pulmonary valve and followed this with balloon enlargement of the pulmonary valve. They were successful in perforating the pulmonary valve with an Nd:YAG laser wire in four of the five patients in whom they tried this procedure. Perforation of the right ventricle with immediate cardiac tamponade occurred in the remaining patient. An increase in the pulmonary artery pressure and a decrease in right ventricular pressure occurred in all four patients. At 2- to 6-month followup, forward flow across the laser-opened pulmonary valve was demonstrated; there was a residual gradient of from 50 to 70 mmHg across the pulmonic valve. The oxygen saturations ranged from 70% to 87%.

These preliminary observations are of interest. With further refinement of the technique and additional clinical trials, the laser techniques are likely to be useful in the management of these complex pulmonary atresia patients.

PORCINE HETEROGRAFT STENOSIS

Calcification and development of stenosis of bioprosthetic valves, particularly in children, is well documented. Such calcification and valve dysfunction may require replacement of the heterograft. However, balloon dilatation of the stenotic porcine valve may avoid or postpone reoperation. Several authors have reported dilatation of the bioprosthetic valves in the pulmonary, aortic, mitral, and tricuspid positions.

Waldman and associates[136] reported four children who developed stenosis of the porcine valves in pulmonary position 10 to 24 months after their insertion and who underwent balloon dilatation. The average valve gradient was reduced from 48 to 25 mmHg, and there was only mild pulmonary insufficiency after balloon valvuloplasty. Lloyd and associates[137] presented results of balloon dilatation in six children who developed stenosis of the bioprosthetic valves inserted 4 to 14 years previously. In three children, systolic gradients were reduced significantly and no surgical intervention was required. In the other three patients the balloon dilatation did not significantly reduce the gradients. Two of these patients required conduit replacement; the remaining patient has only a modest amount of stenosis and is being followed clinically. Similar results have been supported by Ensing,[138] Zeevi,[139] Unwala,[140] and their associates. We had experience with dilating four porcine heterografts in pulmonary position which had been placed 4, 6, 12, and 13 years prior to dilatation. In three children, gradients of 73, 68, and 40 mmHg were respectively reduced to 40, 11, and 10 mmHg; these patients are being followed clinically. In the fourth child, who had a gradient of 79 mmHg, there were no significant reduction in the gradient. This patient, who also appeared to have diffuse narrowing of the conduit presumably related to peel formation, subsequently underwent replacement of the conduit with an aortic homograft, with good results. No complications were encountered in these patients.

The mechanism for relief of porcine valve stenosis appears to be related to separating valve fusion that is seen in some of these patients.[136,141] Peel formation, causing conduit stenosis, is not amenable to balloon valvuloplasty.

On the basis of our experience and that reported, it seems prudent to try to balloon-dilate stenotic porcine valves in the pulmonary position in an attempt to prevent or postpone second replacement of a calcified, stenotic valve. If this is not feasible, valve replacement may be required.

SUPRAVALVULAR PULMONIC STENOSIS

Stenosis of the main pulmonary artery may occur as an isolated anomaly or may be a component of other right ventricular outflow obstructive lesions such as valvular pulmonic stenosis and tetralogy of Fallot. It may also occur secondary to rubella syndrome. Supravalvular pulmonic stenosis may also develop at the site of anastomosis in the neopulmonary artery following arterial switch procedure for transposition of the great arteries, or it may be a residual after removal of a previously placed pulmonary artery band. There is only a limited experience in the balloon dilatation of supravalvular pulmonary artery stenotic lesions.[51,139,142,143]

The indications for balloon angioplasty of these lesions should, in my opinion, be similar to those recommended for valvular pulmonic stenosis[18]: a moderate to severe peak-to-peak systolic pressure gradient ($\geq$ 50 mmHg) across the narrowed area in the face of a normal cardiac index. Although there are no definitive guidelines, the size of the balloon should be at least two times the diameter of the narrowest site of obstruction.

To the best of my knowledge, there are no reports of dilatation of native supravalvular pulmonary artery stenosis other than that utilized for cyanotic heart defects, discussed earlier in this chapter (for example, Fig. 15.22).

We have attempted balloon dilatation in three patients, aged 4, 6, and 19 years and have reduced the gradients across the supravalvular stenosis (Fig. 15.23); in two, the result was excellent and in the third the gradient reduction was minimal. Two of these children manifested supravalvular pulmonary stenosis 4 and 15 years following surgical pulmonary valvotomy, and it is not clear whether the supravalvular stenosis was native or developed secondary to surgery. The third child exhibited pulmonary artery narrowing 1 year following arterial switch procedure for transposition of the great arteries. There was angiographic (Fig. 15.24) and pressure gradient (Fig. 15.25) relief in this child.[51] No followup data are available for these children.

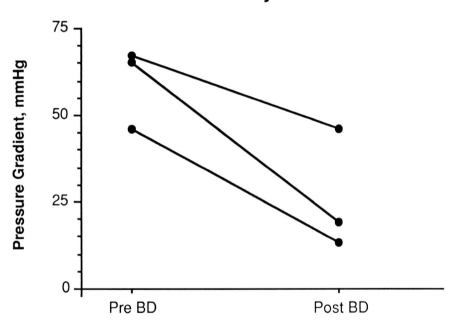

Figure 15.23 The effect of balloon angioplasty on pressure gradients in three patients with supravalvular pulmonary stenosis. In two patients, the residual gradients were minimal while in the third there was significant residual gradient. *BD—balloon dilatation.*

Schranz and associates[142] successfully balloon-dilated supravalvular pulmonary stenosis in a single patient who developed it following arterial switch procedure. Zeevi and associates[139] attempted balloon angioplasty of postarterial switch supravalvular stenosis in five children and produced a gradient reduction of 1 to 75%. Their assessment was that only one patient had a successful result with reduction of the peak-to-peak systolic pressure gradient from 79 mmHg to 20 mmHg. Of the four patients with a poor result, three underwent surgical relief 1 day to 6 months after angioplasty. Saxena and associates[143] attempted eight balloon dilatations in five children who developed supravalvular pulmonary stenosis following arterial switch procedure for transposition of the great arteries. In none of these dilatations was there

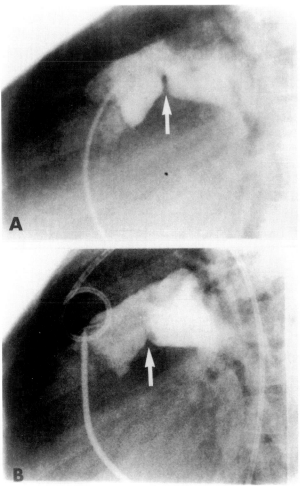

Figure 15.24 Cine frames from pulmonary artery cineangiograms, lateral view, showing supravalvular pulmonary stenosis (*arrow*) following arterial switch procedure (*A*) which improved markedly following balloon angioplasty (*B*). (From: Rao PS: Balloon angioplasty and valvuloplasty in infants, children, and adolescents. *Curr Probl Cardiol.* 14:417–497, 1989. With permission.)

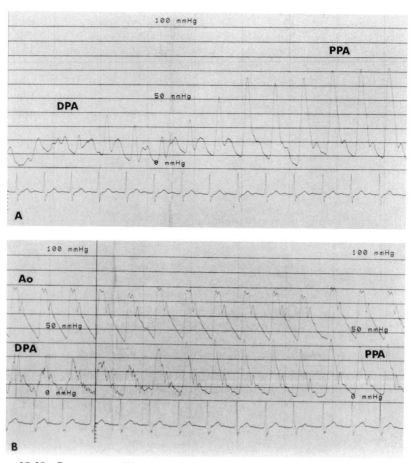

Figure 15.25 Pressure pullback tracings across supravalvular pulmonary stenosis (shown in Fig. 15.24) showing significant pressure gradient (*A*) which diminished markedly following balloon angioplasty (*B*). Aortic pressure is also shown in (*B*). Ao—aorta. DPA—distal pulmonary artery. PPA—proximal pulmonary artery. (From: Rao PS: Balloon angioplasty and valvuloplasty in infants, children, and adolescents. *Curr Probl Cardiol.* 14: 417–497, 1989. With permission.)

any improvement in the pressure gradient across the area of obstruction, nor was there any significant angiographic change.[143]

The limited experience thus far documented[51,139,142-144] suggests that discrete narrowing at the suture lines in the neopulmonary artery is likely to be relieved by balloon dilatation, whereas diffuse narrowings secondary to anteroposterior flattening[139] or shrinkage and retraction of the pericardial patch[143] used in the enlargement of a neopulmonary artery are unlikely to respond to balloon angioplasty.

Balloon dilatation was attempted in two patients with residual supravalvular pulmonary stenosis following removal of a previously placed pulmonary artery band.[139] The peak-to-peak systolic pressure gradient was reduced from 60 to 38 mmHg in one and from 65 to 35 mmHg in the other. These data were interpreted as indicating partially successful balloon dilatation.[139]

In summary, supravalvular pulmonary stenosis that develops following previous surgery can be relieved by balloon dilatation if it is a discrete narrowing. Balloon angioplasty should probably not be attempted if the obstruction is diffuse.[144] There are no similar data for native supravalvular pulmonic stenosis.

SUMMARY AND CONCLUSIONS

The technique of balloon dilatation of stenotic pulmonary valves has been available since 1982. Balloon pulmonary valvuloplasty has been used successfully over the last few years for the relief of moderate to severe pulmonic valvular stenosis in neonates, infants, children, and adults. Both immediate and intermediate-term followup results have been well documented by cardiac catheterization and Doppler studies. Electrocardiographic and echo-Doppler evaluation at followup is reflective of the results and may avoid the need for recatheterization. The results of balloon valvuloplasty are either comparable to or better than those reported with surgical valvuloplasty.

Complications of the procedure have been minimal. The causes of restenosis have been identified and appropriate modifications in the technique, particularly use of a balloon:annulus ratio of 1.2 to 1.5:1 should provide better results than previously documented. Further refinement of the catheters and technique may further reduce the complication rate and prevalence of restenosis.

The major mechanism by which relief of pulmonary obstruction is relieved by balloon valvuloplasty appears to be commissural splitting although occasional tearing or avulsion of valve leaflets may occur.

The indications for balloon valvuloplasty have not been clearly defined but should probably be similar to those used for surgical valvotomy; only patients with moderate to severe pulmonic valvular stenosis are candidates for balloon valvuloplasty. Previous surgery, pulmonary valve dysplasia, and Noonan syndrome are not contraindications for balloon valvuloplasty. The procedure is also applicable to pulmonary stenosis associated with other complex cardiac defects and stenosis of bioprosthetic valves in the pulmonary position.

Infundibular reaction may be present in older patients and in patients with severe obstruction and can most often be managed with adequate valvuloplasty and beta-blocking drugs with rare need for surgery.

Use of atherectomy catheter devices to relieve infundibular pulmonic stenosis and laser-assisted balloon dilatation of atretic pulmonary valve are new and exciting developments in this arena.

Miniaturization of the balloon/catheter systems, further refinement of the procedure, and meticulous attention to details of the technique may further reduce the complication rate and increase the safety. Documentation of the favorable results at 5- to 10-year followup is necessary. Transcatheter techniques are excellent alternatives to open or closed heart surgery in most, if not all, patients with pulmonary stenosis.

Acknowledgments: The author wishes to acknowledge with thanks the contributions to this material by the past and present colleagues in pediatric cardiology and cardiovascular surgery, including Drs. M. Brais, P.S. Chopra, M.E. Fawzy, F. Kutayli, J. Levy, M.K. Mardini, L. Solymar, M.K. Thapar, and A.D. Wilson. Thanks are also due to Nanette Kelsey for her assistance in the preparation of the manuscript.

This work was supported in part by a grant from Oscar Rennebohm Foundation, Inc., Madison, WI.

REFERENCES

1. Nadas AS, Fyler DC: *Pediatric Cardiology*. 3rd ed. Philadelphia: WB Saunders Co, 1972, p 683.

2. Keith JD, Rowe RD, Vlad P: *Heart Disease in Infancy and Childhood*. 3rd ed. New York: Macmillan, 1978, pp 4–6.

3. Rubio V, Limon Lason R: Treatment of pulmonary valvular stenosis and of tricuspid stenosis using a modified catheter. Second World Congress of Cardiology, Washington DC, 1954, Program abstracts II, p 205.

4. Semb BKH, Tjönneland S, Stake G, et al: "Balloon valvulotomy" of congenital pulmonary valve stenosis with tricuspid valve insufficiency. *Cardiovasc Radiol*. 2:239–241, 1979.

5. Kan JS, White RI Jr, Mitchell SE, et al: Percutaneous balloon valvuloplasty: a new method for treating congenital pulmonary valve stenosis. *N Engl J Med*. 307:540–542, 1982.

6. Dotter CT, Judkins MP: Transluminal treatment of arteriosclerotic obstruction. Description of a new technic and a preliminary report of its application. *Circulation*. 30:654–670, 1964.

7. Zeitler E, Grüntzig A, Schoop W: *Percutaneous Vascular Recanalization: Technique, Application, Clinical Results*. Berlin: Springer-Verlag, 1978.

8. Grüntzig AR, Senning A, Siegenthaler WE: Nonoperative dilatation of coronary-artery stenosis. Percutaneous transluminal coronary angioplasty. *N Engl J Med*. 301:61–68, 1979.

9. Rao PS, Mardini MK: Pulmonary valvotomy without thoracotomy: the experience with percutaneous balloon pulmonary valvuloplasty. *Ann Saudi Med*. 5:149–155, 1985.

10. Rao PS: Transcatheter treatment of pulmonary stenosis and coarctation of the aorta: experience with percutaneous balloon dilatation. *Br Heart J*. 56:250–258, 1986.

11. Rao PS: Value of echo-Doppler studies in the evaluation of the results of balloon pulmonary valvuloplasty. *J Cardiovasc Ultrasonography*. 5:309–312, 1986.

12. Rao PS: Influence of balloon size on short-term and long-term results of balloon pulmonary valvuloplasty. *Tex Heart Inst J*. 14:57–61, 1987.

13. Rao PS, Brais M: Balloon pulmonary valvuloplasty for congenital cyanotic heart defects. *Am Heart J*. 115:1105–1110, 1988.

14. Rao PS, Fawzy ME, Solymar L, et al: Long-term results of balloon pulmonary valvuloplasty of valvar pulmonic stenosis. *Am Heart J*. 115:1291–1296, 1988.

15. Rao PS: How big a balloon and how many balloons for pulmonary valvuloplasty? *Am Heart J*. 116:577–580, 1988.

16. Rao PS, Solymar L: Electrocardiographic changes following balloon dilatation of valvar pulmonic stenosis. *J Intervent Cardiol*. 1:189–197, 1988.

17. Rao PS: Balloon dilatation in infants and children with dysplastic pulmonary valves: short-term and intermediate-term results. *Am Heart J*. 116:1168–1173, 1988.

18. Rao PS: Indications for balloon pulmonary valvuloplasty. *Am Heart J*. 116:1661–1662, 1988.

19. Rao PS, Thapar MK, Kutayli F: Causes of restenosis after balloon valvuloplasty for valvular pulmonary stenosis. *Am J Cardiol*. 62:979–982, 1988.

20. Rao PS: Further observations on the effect of balloon size on the short term and

intermediate term results of balloon dilatation of the pulmonary valve. *Br Heart J*. 60:507–511, 1988.

21. Rao PS, Fawzy ME: Double balloon technique for percutaneous balloon pulmonary valvuloplasty: comparison with single balloon technique. *J Intervent Cardiol*. 1:257–262, 1988.

22. Rao PS: Balloon pulmonary valvuloplasty: a review. *Clin Cardiol*. 12:55–74, 1989.

23. Thapar MK, Rao PS: Significance of infundibular obstruction following balloon valvuloplasty for valvar pulmonic stenosis. *Am Heart J*. 118:99–103, 1989.

24. Rao PS: Causes of restenosis following balloon angioplasty/valvuloplasty: a review. *Pediatr Rev Commun*. 4:157–172, 1990.

25. Thapar MK, Rao PS: Use of propranolol for severe dynamic infundibular obstruction prior to balloon pulmonary valvuloplasty (a brief communication). *Cathet Cardiovasc Diagn*. 19:240–241, 1990.

26. Rao PS, Thapar MK: Balloon pulmonary valvuloplasty. – Reply *Am Heart J*. 121:1839–1840, 1991.

27. Nadas AS: Pulmonic stenosis – indications for surgery in children and adults. *N Engl J Med*. 287:1196–1197, 1972.

28. Nugent EW, Freedom RM, Nora JJ, et al: Clinical course in pulmonary stenosis. *Circulation*. 56(suppl I):I-38–I-47, 1977.

29. Tynan M, Baker EJ, Rohmer J, et al: Percutaneous balloon pulmonary valvuloplasty. *Br Heart J*. 53:520–524, 1985.

30. Lababidi Z, Wu JR: Percutaneous balloon pulmonary valvuloplasty. *Am J Cardiol*. 52:560–562, 1983.

31. Kan JS, White RI Jr, Mitchell SE, et al: Percutaneous transluminal balloon valvuloplasty for pulmonary valve stenosis. *Circulation*. 69:554–560, 1984.

32. Kveselis DA, Rocchini AP, Snider AR, et al: Results of balloon valvuloplasty in the treatment of congenital valvar pulmonary stenosis in children. *Am J Cardiol*. 56:527–532, 1985.

33. Miller GAH: Balloon valvuloplasty and angioplasty in congenital heart disease. *Br Heart J*. 54:285–289, 1985.

34. Sullivan ID, Robinson PJ, Macartney FJ, et al: Percutaneous balloon valvuloplasty for pulmonary valve stenosis in infants and children. *Br Heart J*. 54:435–441, 1985.

35. Radtke W, Keane JF, Fellows KE, et al: Percutaneous balloon valvotomy of congenital pulmonary stenosis using oversized ballons. *J Am Coll Cardiol*. 8:909–915, 1986.

36. Rey C, Marache P, Francart C, et al: Percutaneous transluminal balloon valvuloplasty of congenital pulmonary valve stenosis, with a special report on infants and neonates. *J Am Coll Cardiol*. 11:815–820, 1988.

37. Robertson M, Benson LN, Smallhorn JS, et al: The morphology of the right ventricular outflow tract after percutaneous pulmonary valvotomy: long term followup. *Br Heart J*. 58:239–244, 1987.

38. Mullins CE, Nihill MR, Vick GW II, et al: Double balloon technique for dilation of valvular or vessel stenosis in congenital and acquired heart disease. *J Am Coll Cardiol*. 10:107–114, 1987.

39. Tinker J, Howitt G, Markman P, et al: The natural history of isolated pulmonary stenosis. *Br Heart J*. 27:151–160, 1965.

40. Mody MR: The natural history of uncomplicated valvular pulmonic stenosis. *Am Heart J*. 90:317–321, 1975.

41. Stevenson JG, Kawabori I: Noninvasive determination of pressure gradients in children: two methods employing pulsed Doppler echocardiography. *J Am Coll Cardiol*. 3:179–192, 1984.

42. Rao PS: Doppler ultrasound in the prediction of transvalvar pressure gradients in patients with valvar pulmonary stenosis. *Int J Cardiol.* 15:195–203, 1987.

43. Kosturakis D, Allen HD, Goldberg SJ, et al: Noninvasive quantification of stenotic semilunar valve areas by Doppler echocardiography. *J Am Coll Cardiol.* 3:1256–1262, 1984.

44. Musewe NN, Robertson MA, Benson LN, et al: The dysplastic pulmonary valve: echo-cardiographic features and results of balloon dilatation. *Br Heart J.* 57:364–370, 1987.

45. DiSessa TG, Alpert BS, Chase NA, et al: Balloon valvuloplasty in children with dysplastic pulmonary valves. *Am J Cardiol.* 60:405–407, 1987.

46. Marantz PM, Huhta JC, Mullins CE, et al: Results of balloon valvuloplasty in typical and dysplastic pulmonary valve stenosis: Doppler echocardiographic follow-up. *J Am Coll Cardiol.* 12:476–479, 1988.

47. Chaffe A, Fairbrass MJ, Chatrath RR: Anaesthesia for valvuloplasty. *Anaesthesia.* 43:359–361, 1988.

48. Sideris EB, Baay JE, Bradshaw RL, et al: Axillary vein approach for pulmonic val-vuloplasty in infants with iliac vein obstruction. *Cathet Cardiovasc Diagn.* 15:61–63, 1988.

49. Chaara A, Zniber L, Haitem NE, et al: Percutaneous balloon valvuloplasty via the right internal jugular vein for valvular pulmonic stenosis with severe right ventricular failure. *Am Heart J.* 117:684–685, 1989.

50. Ring JC, Kulik TJ, Burke BA: Morphologic changes induced by dilation of the pulmonary valve anulus with overlarge balloons in normal newborn lambs. *Am J Cardiol.* 55:210–214, 1985.

51. Rao PS: Balloon angioplasty and valvuloplasty in infants, children, and adolescents. *Curr Probl Cardiol.* 14:417–497, 1989.

52. Van den Berg EJM, Niemeyer MG, Plokker TWM, et al: New triple-lumen balloon catheter for percutaneous (pulmonary) valvuloplasty. *Cathet Cardiovasc Diagn.* 12:352–356, 1986.

53. Meier B, Friedli B, Oberhaensli I, et al: Trefoil balloon for percutaneous valvuloplasty. *Cathet Cardiovasc Diagn.* 12:277–281, 1986.

54. Thanopoulos BD, Margetakis A, Papadopoulos G, et al: Valvuloplasty with large trefoil balloons for the treatment of congenital pulmonary stenosis. *Acta Paediatr Scand.* 78:742–746, 1989.

55. Shrivastava S, Sundar AS, Mukhopadhyaya S, et al: Percutaneous transluminal balloon pulmonary valvoplasty—long-term results. *Int J Cardiol.* 17:303–314, 1987.

56. McCredie RM, Lee CL, Swinburn MJ, et al: Balloon dilatation pulmonary valvuloplasty in pulmonary stenosis. *Aust N Z J Med.* 16:20–23, 1986.

57. Ali Khan MA, Al Yousef S, Mullins CE: Percutaneous transluminal balloon pulmonary valvuloplasty for the relief of pulmonary valve stenosis with special reference to double-balloon technique. *Am Heart J.* 112:158–166, 1986.

58. Fontes VF, Sousa JEMR, Esteves CA, et al: Pulmonary valvoplasty—experience of 100 cases. *Int J Cardiol.* 21:335–342, 1988.

59. Mullins CE, Ludomirsky A, O'Laughlin MP, et al: Balloon valvuloplasty for pulmonic valve stenosis—two-year follow-up: hemodynamic and Doppler evaluation. *Cathet Cardiovasc Diagn.* 14:76–81, 1988.

60. Yeager SB, Neal WA, Balian AA, et al: Percutaneous balloon pulmonary valvuloplasty. *W V Med J.* 82:169–171, 1986.

61. Hsieh KS, Ou TY, Hwang B, et al: Percutaneous balloon pulmonary valvuloplasty in children. *Chung Hua I Hsueh Tsa Chih.* 39:247–254, 1987.

62. Mashru MR, Loya YS, Sharma S: Percutaneous balloon valvuloplasty for pulmonary valve stenosis using single or double balloon technique. *J Assoc Physicians India.* 36:546–550, 1988.

63. Schmaltz AA, Bein G, Grävinghoff L, et al: Balloon valvuloplasty of pulmonary stenosis in infants and children — co-operative study of the German Society of Pediatric Cardiology. *Eur Heart J.* 10:967–971, 1989.

64. Stanger P, Cassidy SC, Girod DA, et al: Balloon pulmonary valvuloplasty: results of the Valvuloplasty and Angioplasty of Congenital Anomalies Registry. *Am J Cardiol.* 65:775–783, 1990.

65. Ballerini L, Mullins CE, Cifarelli A, et al: Percutaneous balloon valvuloplasty of pulmonary valve stenosis, dysplasia, and residual stenosis after surgical valvotomy for pulmonary atresia with intact ventricular septum: long-term results. *Cathet Cardiovasc Diagn.* 19:165–169, 1990.

66. Stenberg RG, Fixler DE, Taylor AL, et al: Left ventricular dysfunction due to chronic right ventricular pressure overload. Resolution following percutaneous balloon valvuloplasty for pulmonic stenosis. *Am J Med.* 84:157–161, 1988.

67. Tynan M, Jones O, Joseph MC, et al: Relief of pulmonary valve stenosis in first week of life by percutaneous balloon valvuloplasty. *Lancet.* 1:273, 1984.

68. Zeevi B, Keane JF, Fellows KE, et al: Balloon dilation of critical pulmonary stenosis in the first week of life. *J Am Coll Cardiol.* 11:821–824, 1988.

69. Ali Khan MA, Al-Yousef S, Huhta JC, et al: Critical pulmonary valve stenosis in patients less than 1 year of age: treatment with percutaneous gradational balloon pulmonary valvuloplasty. *Am Heart J.* 117:1008–1114, 1989.

70. Qureshi SA, Ladusans EJ, Martin RP: Dilatation with progressively larger balloons for severe stenosis of the pulmonary valve presenting in the late neonatal period and early infancy. *Br Heart J.* 62:311–314, 1989.

71. Robida A, Pavcnik D: Perforation of the heart in a newborn with critical valvar pulmonary stenosis during balloon valvoplasty. *Int J Cardiol.* 26:111–112, 1990.

72. Gordon LS: Neonatal Cardiology Casebook: emergency pulmonary balloon valvuloplasty of congenital pulmonary valve stenosis. *J Perinatol.* 10:86–89, 1990.

73. Caspi J, Coles JG, Benson LN, et al: Management of neonatal critical pulmonic stenosis in the balloon valvotomy era. *Ann Thorac Surg.* 49:273–278, 1990.

74. Latson L, Cheatham J, Kugler J, et al: Balloon valvuloplasty in pulmonary valve atresia and critical pulmonary stenosis. *J Am Coll Cardiol.* 15:241A, 1990.

75. Pepine CJ, Gessner IH, Feldman RL: Percutaneous balloon valvuloplasty for pulmonic valve stenosis in the adult. *Am J Cardiol.* 50:1442–1445, 1982.

76. Khalilullah M, Bahl VK, Choudhary A, et al: Pulmonary balloon valvuloplasty for the non-surgical management of valvular pulmonary stenosis. *Indian Heart J.* 37:150–153, 1985.

77. Gibbs JL, Stanley CP, Dickinson DF: Pulmonary balloon valvuloplasty in late adult life. *Int J Cardiol.* 11:237–239, 1986.

78. Al Kasab S, Ribeiro P, Al Zaibag M: Use of a double balloon technique for percutaneous balloon pulmonary valvotomy in adults. *Br Heart J.* 58:136–141, 1987.

79. Fawzy ME, Mercer EN, Dunn B: Late results of pulmonary balloon valvuloplasty in adults using double balloon technique. *J Intervent Cardiol.* 1:35–42, 1988.

80. Al Kasab S, Ribeiro PA, Al Zaibag M, et al: Percutaneous double balloon pulmonary valvotomy in adults: one- to two-year follow-up. *Am J Cardiol.* 62:822–824, 1988.

81. Flugelman MY, Halon DA, Lewis BS: Pulmonary balloon valvuloplasty in the seventh decade of life. *Isr J Med Sci.* 24:112–113, 1988.

82. Brock RC: Pulmonary valvulotomy for the relief of congenital pulmonary stenosis: report of three cases. *Br Med J.* 1:1121–1126, 1948.

83. Campbell M, Brock R: The results of valvotomy for simple pulmonary stenosis. *Br Heart J.* 17:229–246, 1954.

84. Mirowski M, Shah KD, Neill CA, et al: Long-term (10 to 13 years) follow-up study after transventricular pulmonary valvulotomy for pulmonary stenosis with intact ventricular septum. *Circulation.* 28:906–914, 1963.

85. Engle MA, Ito T, Goldberg HP: The fate of the patient with pulmonic stenosis. *Circulation.* 30:554–561, 1964.

86. Reid JM, Coleman EN, Stevenson JG, et al: Long-term results of surgical treatment for pulmonary valve stenosis. *Arch Dis Child.* 51:79–81, 1976.

87. McNamara DG, Latson LA: Long-term follow-up of patients with malformations for which definitive surgical repair has been available for 25 years or more. *Am J Cardiol.* 50:560–568, 1982.

88. Kopecky SL, Gersh BJ, McGoon MD, et al: Long-term outcome of patients undergoing surgical repair of isolated pulmonary valve stenosis. Follow-up at 20–30 years. *Circulation.* 78:1150–1156, 1988.

89. Vogel M, Eger R, Klinner W, et al: Brock transventricular pulmonary valvotomy in patients with pulmonary stenosis: long-term results. *Pediatr Cardiol.* 11:191–194, 1990.

90. Abele JE: Balloon catheters and transluminal dilatation: technical considerations. *AJR.* 135:901–906, 1980.

91. Walls JT, Lababidi Z, Curtis JJ, et al: Assessment of percutaneous balloon pulmonary and aortic valvuloplasty. *J Thorac Cardiovasc Surg.* 88:352–356, 1984.

92. Lucas RV Jr, Burke BA, Edwards JE: Anatomic sequelae of balloon angioplasty in congenital heart disease. *Semin Intervent Radiol.* 1:225–236, 1984.

93. Becker AE, Hoedemaker G: Balloon valvuloplasty in congenital and acquired heart disease: morphologic considerations. *Z Kardiol.* 76(Suppl 6):73–79, 1987.

94. Gikonyo BM, Lucas RV, Edwards JE: Anatomic features of congenital pulmonary valvar stenosis. *Pediatr Cardiol.* 8:109–116, 1987.

95. Shuck JW, McCormick DJ, Cohen IS, et al: Percutaneous balloon valvuloplasty of the pulmonary valve: role of right to left shunting through a patent foramen ovale. *J Am Coll Cardiol.* 4:132–135, 1984.

96. Lo RNS, Lau KC, Leung MP: Complete heart block after balloon dilatation for congenital pulmonary stenosis. *Br Heart J.* 59:384–386, 1988.

97. Fellows KE, Radtke W, Keane JF, et al: Acute complications of catheter therapy for congenital heart disease. *Am J Cardiol.* 60:679–683, 1987.

98. Attia I, Weinhaus L, Walls JT, et al: Rupture of tricuspid valve papillary muscle during balloon pulmonary valvuloplasty. *Am Heart J.* 114:1233–1235, 1987.

99. Ben-Shachar G, Cohen MH, Sivakoff MC, et al: Development of infundibular obstruction after percutaneous pulmonary balloon valvuloplasty. *J Am Coll Cardiol.* 5:754–756, 1985.

100. Martin GR, Stanger P: Transient prolongation of the QT_c interval after balloon valvuloplasty and angioplasty in children. *Am J Cardiol.* 58:1233–1235, 1986.

101. Kan JS, White RI Jr, Mitchell SE, et al: Treatment of restenosis of coarctation by percutaneous transluminal angioplasty. *Circulation.* 68:1087–1094, 1983.

102. Suarez de Lezo J, Fernandez R, Sancho M, et al: Percutaneous transluminal angioplasty for aortic isthmic coarctation in infancy. *Am J Cardiol.* 54:1147–1149, 1984.

103. Rocchini AP, Beekman RH: Balloon angioplasty in the treatment of pulmonary valve stenosis and coarctation of the aorta. *Tex Heart Inst J.* 13:377–382, 1986.

104. Yeager SB: Balloon selection for double balloon valvotomy. *J Am Coll Cardiol.* 9:467–468, 1987.

105. Butto F, Amplatz K, Bass JL: Geometry of the proximal pulmonary trunk during dilation with two balloons. *Am J Cardiol.* 58:380–381, 1986.

106. Yeager SB: Occlusion time and inflation pressure in pulmonary valvuloplasty. *Am J Cardiol.* 55:619–620, 1985.

107. Lloyd TR, Donnerstein RL: Rapid T-wave normalization after balloon pulmonary valvuloplasty in children. *Am J Cardiol.* 64:399–400, 1989.

108. Koretzky ED, Moller JH, Korns ME, et al: Congenital pulmonary stenosis resulting from dysplasia of valve. *Circulation.* 40:43–53, 1969.

109. Jeffery RF, Moller JH, Amplatz K: The dysplastic pulmonary valve: a new roentgenographic entity. With a discussion of the anatomy and radiology of other types of valvular pulmonary stenosis. *Am J Roentgenol Ther Radium Nucl Med.* 114:322–339, 1972.

110. Rowlatt UF, Rimoldi HJA, Lev M: The quantitative anatomy of the normal child's heart. *Pediatr Clin North Am.* 10:499–588, 1963.

111. Linde LM, Turner SW, Sparkes RS: Pulmonary valvular dysplasia. A cardiofacial syndrome. *Br Heart J.* 35:301–304, 1973.

112. Schneeweiss A, Blieden LC, Shem-Tov A, et al: Diagnostic angiocardiographic criteria in dysplastic stenotic pulmonic valve. *Am Heart J.* 106:761–762, 1983.

113. Fontes VF, Esteves CA, Sousa JEMR, et al: Regression of infundibular hypertrophy after pulmonary valvuloplasty for pulmonic stenosis. *Am J Cardiol.* 62:977–979, 1988.

114. Brock R: Control mechanisms in the outflow tract of the right ventricle in health and disease. *Guy's Hosp Rep.* 104:356–379, 1955.

115. Silove ED, Vogel JHK, Grover RF: The pressure gradient in ventricular outflow obstruction: influence of peripheral resistance. *Cardiovasc Res.* 2:234–242, 1968.

116. Rao PS, Linde LM: Pressure and energy in the cardiovascular chambers. *Chest.* 66:176–178, 1974.

117. Moulaert AJ, Buis-Liem TN, Geldof WC, et al: The postvalvulotomy propranolol test to determine reversibility of the residual gradient in pulmonary stenosis. *J Thorac Cardiovasc Surg.* 71:865–868, 1976.

118. Danielson GK, Exarhos ND, Weidman WH, et al: Pulmonic stenosis with intact ventricular septum. Surgical considerations and results of operations. *J Thorac Cardiovasc Surg.* 61:228–234, 1971.

119. Griffith BP, Hardesty RL, Siewers RD, et al: Pulmonary valvulotomy alone for pulmonary stenosis: results in children with and without muscular infundibular hypertrophy. *J Thorac Cardiovasc Surg.* 83:577–583, 1982.

120. Rao PS, Levy JM, Chopra PS: Balloon angioplasty of stenosed Blalock-Taussig anastomosis: role of balloon-on-a-wire in dilating occluded shunts. *Am Heart J.* 120:1173–1178, 1990.

121. Boucek MM, Webster HE, Orsmond GS, et al: Balloon pulmonary valvotomy: palliation for cyanotic heat disease. *Am Heart J.* 115:318–322, 1988.

122. Qureshi SA, Kirk CR, Lamb RK, et al: Balloon dilatation of the pulmonary valve in the first year of life in patients with tetralogy of Fallot: a preliminary study. *Br Heart J.* 60:232–235, 1988.

123. Mehta AV, Perlman PE: Palliative percutaneous balloon valvuloplasty in a cyanotic child with tetralogy of Fallot. *South Med J.* 83:360–361, 1990.

124. Rao PS: Percutaneous balloon valvotomy/angioplasty in congenital heart disease. In: Bashore TM, Davidson CJ. *Percutaneous Balloon Valvuloplasty and Related Techniques.* Baltimore: Williams & Wilkins, 1991, pp 251–277.

125. Parsons JM, Ladusans EJ, Qureshi SA: Growth of the pulmonary artery after neonatal balloon dilatation of the right ventricular outflow tract in an infant with the tetralogy of Fallot and atrioventricular septal defect. *Br Heart J.* 62:65–68, 1989.

126. Battistessa SA, Robles A, Jackson M, et al: Operative findings after percutaneous pulmo-

nary balloon dilatation of the right ventricular outflow tract in tetralogy of Fallot. *Br Heart J.* 64:321–324, 1990.

127. Lamb RK, Qureshi SA, Arnold R: Pulmonary artery tear following balloon valvoplasty in Fallot's tetralogy. *Int J Cardiol.* 15:347–349, 1987.

128. Qureshi SA, Parsons JM, Tynan M: Percutaneous transcatheter myectomy of subvalvar pulmonary stenosis in tetralogy of Fallot: a new palliative technique with an atherectomy catheter. *Br. Heart J.* 64:163–165, 1990.

129. Simpson JB, Selmon MR, Robertson GC, et al: Transluminal atherectomy for occlusive peripheral vascular disease. *Am J Cardiol.* 61:96G–101G, 1988.

130. Rao PS: Comprehensive management of pulmonary atresia with intact ventricular septum. *Ann Thorac Surg.* 40:409–413, 1985.

131. Puga FJ, Leoni FE, Julsrud PR, et al: Complete repair of pulmonary atresia, ventricular septal defect, and severe peripheral arborization abnormalities of the central pulmonary arteries. Experience with preliminary unifocalization procedures in 38 patients. *J Thorac Cardiovasc Surg.* 98:1018–1029, 1989.

132. Lee G, Ikeda RM, Kozina J, et al: Laser-dissolution of coronary atherosclerotic obstruction. *Am Heart J.* 102:1074–1075, 1981.

133. Riemenschneider TA, Lee G, Ikeda RM, et al: Laser irradiation of congenital heart disease: potential for palliation and correction of intracardiac and intravascular defects. *Am Heart J.* 106:1389–1393, 1983.

134. Arapov AD, Vishnevskii AA Jr, Abdullaev FZ, et al: A preliminary report on laser application in cardiosurgery. *Eksp Khir Anesteziol* 4:10–12, 1974.

135. Qureshi SA, Rosenthal E, Tynan M, et al: Transcatheter laser–assisted balloon pulmonary valve dilation in pulmonic valve atresia. *Am J Cardiol.* 67:428–431, 1991.

136. Waldman JD, Waldman J, Jones MC: Failure of balloon dilatation in mid-cavity obstruction of the systemic venous atrium after the Mustard operation. *Pediatr Cardiol.* 4:151–154, 1983.

137. Lloyd TR, Marvin WJ Jr, Mahoney LT, et al: Balloon dilation valvuloplasty of bioprosthetic valves in extracardiac conduits. *Am Heart J.* 114:268–274, 1987.

138. Ensing GJ, Hagler DJ, Seward JB, et al: Caveats of balloon dilation of conduits and conduit valves. *J Am Coll Cardiol.* 14:397–400, 1989.

139. Zeevi B, Keane JF, Perry SB, et al: Balloon dilation of postoperative right ventricular outflow obstructions. *J Am Coll Cardiol.* 14:401–408, 1989.

140. Unwala AA, Mintz GS, Kimbiris D: Balloon valvuloplasty of a stenotic bioprosthesis in the pulmonic position. *J Invasive Cardiol.* 2:73–76, 1990.

141. McKay CR, Waller BF, Hong R, et al: Problems encountered with catheter balloon valvuloplasty of bioprosthetic aortic valves. *Am Heart J.* 115:463–465, 1988.

142. Schranz D, Jüngst BK, Huth R, et al: Supravalvular pulmonary stenosis after arterial switch operation for complete transposition of the great arteries: report of a successful balloon-dilatation. *Z Kardiol.* 77:743–745, 1988.

143. Saxena A, Fong LV, Ogilvie BC, et al: Use of balloon dilation to treat supravalvar pulmonary stenosis developing after anatomical correction for complete transposition. *Br Heart J.* 64:151–155, 1990.

144. Rao PS: Balloon angioplasty of supravalvar pulmonic stenosis following arterial switch procedure for complete transposition. *Br Heart J.* in press.

CHAPTER **16**

Tricuspid Stenosis

FRANCIS Y. K. LAU
DAVID JOSEPH
FRANK GAVINI
CARLOS E. RUIZ

Successful percutaneous balloon valvuloplasty for pulmonic stenosis was first reported by Kan and associates[1] in 1982, for mitral stenosis by Inoue and associates[2] in 1984, for aortic stenosis in children by Labadidi[3] in 1983, and in adults by Cribier and associates[4] in 1986. Percutaneous balloon valvuloplasty for tricuspid stenosis was first attempted in a patient with a porcine bioprosthesis and reported by Feit and associates[5] in 1986. Zaibag and associates[6] reported the first successful balloon valvuloplasty for native tricuspid stenosis in 1987.

Tricuspid stenosis is usually of rheumatic etiology. Autopsy studies indicate that it occurs much more frequently than it is suspected or diagnosed, although the incidence in postmortem studies of patients with rheumatic heart disease varies widely. In seven combined series, 240 of a total of 806 patients with rheumatic heart disease (30%) were found to have tricuspid stenosis.[7-11] In 340 cases of rheumatic valvular disease, Smith and Levine[10] noted a 9.4% incidence of tricuspid stenosis. In a clinical series Coombs[7] noted an incidence of 14%. Kitchin and Turner[12] noted an incidence of 3.1% of severe tricuspid stenosis in patients who had undergone mitral valvotomy. Guyer and associates[13] noted a prevalence of 9.5% tricuspid stenosis in a group of 147 patients with rheumatic heart disease who had echocardiograms.

Although tricuspid stenosis is most frequently associated with rheumatic multivalvulitis,[14] it can occur as a single-valve lesion[15] in rare instances. Other etiologic considerations are degenerated biological artificial valves, carcinoid disease,[16] tumors (cardiac or metastatic),[17-19] echinococcal cysts,[20] congenital defects,[21] endocardial fibroelastosis,[22] endomyocardial fibrosis,[23] infective endocarditis,[24] systemic lupus erythematosus,[25] Ebstein's anomaly,[26] constrictive pericarditis,[27] and even pericardial tamponade[28] involving the right atrium.

DIAGNOSIS

Ever since the surgical relief of mitral stenosis became available in the 1950s, the index of suspicion for concommitant tricuspid stenosis has been entertained if there were signs of right-sided failure (distended neck veins, liver enlargement, ascites, peripheral edema) out of proportion to the degree usually associated with mitral stenosis. The diastolic rumbling murmur and opening snap associated with tricuspid stenosis are usually most intense between the fourth and fifth interspaces at the left sternal border. The echocardiographic findings[13] are distinct and may be more diagnostic than the hemodynamic findings unless provocative fluid challenges[29] are used. If the use of transthoracic echo-transducer sampling sites is impeded by anatomic problems, transesophageal echocardiographic recordings may be of more diagnostic significance.

A reasonable approach to diagnostic testing for suspected tricuspid stenosis is to appreciate the physical findings of right-sided heart failure and overload that are out of proportion to the degree of pulmonary hypertension. The heart murmur may be indistinguishable from that of mitral stenosis. The right atrial enlargement seen on electrocardiograms and chest x-rays is usually out of proportion to that seen with isolated mitral stenosis, the usual cause of secondary tricuspid regurgitation.

At cardiac catheterization, meticulous care should be taken to calibrate the right atrial and right ventricular catheters, strain gauges, and connecting lines. Simultaneous recordings of the right atrial and right ventricular pressures are essential,

Table 16.1 NATIVE TRICUSPID VALVULOPLASTIES

Study	No. Patients	Age	Sex	Etiology	Mean Gradient Across TV, mmHg		Cardiac Index, L/min/M²	
					Pre	Post	Pre	Post
Zaibag et al,[6] 1987	1	45	M	Rheumatic	6.3	2.1	2.1	2.3
Khalilullah et al,[31] 1987	1	36	F	Rheumatic	7	1.5	2.1	2.6
Ribero et al,[32] 1988	1	—	—	Rheumatic	5	2	unavailable	
	2	—	—	Rheumatic	5	2	unavailable	
	3	—	—	Rheumatic	8	1	unavailable	
Rico Blazquez et al,[33] 1988	1	54	F	Rheumatic	6	0	unavailable	
Goldenberg et al,[34] 1989	1	40	F	Rheumatic	7	2	2.97[a]	3.05[a]
Bourdillon et al,[35] 1989	1	35	F	Rheumatic	14	9.5	4.4[a]	4.5[a]
Mullins et al,[16] 1990	1	77	F	Carcinoid	10.5	7.6	unavailable	

[a] Cardiac output
TV — tricuspid valve.
AVB — atrioventricular block

since even mild errors in recordings could lead to a false diagnosis. The normal tricuspid valve area is about 7 cm², and the mean gradient across the tricuspid valve is usually <2 mmHg. Significant tricuspid stenosis occurs when the valve area is less than 2 cm². A valve area less than 1.5 cm² is defined as moderately severe tricuspid stenosis. Patients with echocardiographic features of tricuspid stenosis without a significant gradient across the tricuspid valve should undergo provocative fluid challenge to identify hemodynamically significant tricuspid stenosis.[29] Right atrial angiography may show a thickened, domed tricuspid valve with a narrow jet diagnostic of tricuspid stenosis.[30]

The classic treatment for severe tricuspid stenosis involves surgery. Sodium restriction and diuretic therapy, which alleviates symptoms and improves hepatic function, constitute the main medical management. The surgical options are commissurotomy or tricuspid valve replacement if commissurotomy is not successful. A bioprosthesis is preferred to a mechanical prosthesis because of the higher risk of thrombosis in the tricuspid position, although the bioprosthesis may need to be replaced in 5 to 10 years.

Balloon valvuloplasty for tricuspid stenosis has been used in both bioprosthetic and native valves. Table 16.1 lists reviews of the literature on reported cases of native tricuspid valvuloplasty Table 16.2 lists reviews of bioprosthetic tricuspid val-

Tricuspid Valve Area, cm²		Balloon(s), Used, mm	Tricuspid Regurgitation		Comments
Pre	Post		Pre	Post	
0.9	2.0	15 + 20	Trivial	No change	5-mo followup improvement persists.
1.2	2.6	20 + 20	None	None	Transient 3° AVB which resolved in 12 h.
0.6	1.4	18 + 18	Moderate	Moderate	Cardiac output increased from 2.5 ± 0.6 to 3.6 ± 1 L/min
0.7	1.4	18 + 20	Moderate	Moderate	A short-term followup improvement persists.
0.8	2.5	20 + 20	Trivial	Trivial	
—	—	21 + 21 + 15	Moderate	—	Postvalvuloplasty ventriculography was not performed.
0.82	1.64	20 + 20	Moderate	Moderate	At 3-mo followup clinical improvement persists.
0.78	0.95	20 + 20	Mild to moderate	Increased	Recurrence of symptoms at 6 mo. and underwent tricuspid and mitral valve replacement.
0.9	1.4	18 + 15	Moderate	—	Followup echocardiogram at 1 mo showed no increase in gradient or severity of tricuspid regurgitation.

Table 16.2   PROSTHETIC TRICUSPID VALVULOPLASTIES

Study	No. Patients	Age	Sex	Mean Gradient Across TV, mmHg		Cardiac Index, L/min/M²		Tricuspid Valve Area, cm²	
				Pre	Post	Pre	Post	Pre	Post
Feit et al,[5] 1986	1	46	M	22	15	2.33	3.55	0.69	1.22
Wren et al,[36] 1989	1	19	F	8–12	4–6	3.4	3.2	0.52	0.65
Same pt. 3 mo later				9–11	4–8	2.8	2.8	0.43	0.58
Attubato et al,[37] 1990	1	35	F	11	6	1.4	3.6	0.6	1.5
	2	29	F	8	4	3.1	2.7	1.0	1.6
Chow et al,[36] 1990	1	67	F	6	2.5	2.76[a]	2.86[a]	0.93	4.42
Benedick et al,[24] 1990	1	37	F	21	7	2.7[a]	4.6[a]	0.3	1.2

[a] Cardiac output (L/min)
TV – tricuspid valve.
TEE – transesophageal echocardiography.
TVR – tricuspid valve replacement.

vuloplasties. Table 16.3 summarizes reports of cases in which balloon valvuloplasty was employed in more than one valve. In a total of 25 cases of balloon tricuspid valvuloplasty published in the literature, including our own (Table 16.4), no directly procedure-related deaths have occurred. One patient[24] was in moribund condition owing to fungal endocarditis of the bioprosthetic valve. Balloon valvuloplasty was offered as a last resort. The patient developed a cerebral hemorrhage 5 days after the procedure and died 20 days later. Another patient[31] developed a third-degree atrioventricular block that resolved in 12 hours. A minimal to mild increase in tricuspid regurgitation was seen in 20 to 25% of patients who underwent balloon valvuloplasty.

TECHNIQUE

The patient is premedicated with meperidine and diphenhydramine hydrochloride. The right and left groins are surgically prepared and draped. Using 1% lidocaine as

Type of Prosthetic Valve	Balloon(s) Used, mm	Tricuspid Regurgitation		Comments
		Pre	Post	
#31 Hancock porcine	20	Mild	Mildly increased	At 1-mo followup patient showed markedly improved exercise tolerance.
#29 Ionescu-Shiley	20	Minimal	Minimal	Recurrence of symptoms 3 mo later.
#29 Ionescu-Shiley	23	Trace	Trace	Recurrence of symptoms 6 mo later and underwent TVR (St. Jude valve)
Carpentier-Edwards	20 + 15	Present	Not increased	Symptomatic improvement continues following discharge.
Carpentier-Edwards	20 + 15	Present	Not increased	
#29 Carpentier-Edwards	23	None	Minimal	At 6-mo followup marked improvement in exercise tolerance.
#27 Carpentier-Edwards	15 + 15	Minimal	Mild	Patient with acute fungal (*Candida*) endocarditis. TEE showed large vegetation on TV. Patient considered inoperable due to multisystem failure. Balloon valvuloplasty performed as bridge to surgery. After slow clinical improvement 5 days postvalvuloplasty patient developed intracerebral hemorrhage and died 20 days later.

local anesthesia, 8F hemaquet sheaths (USCI, Billerica, MA) are inserted in the right and left femoral veins using a modified Seldinger technique. A 6F sheath is inserted in the left femoral artery for monitoring of systemic pressure during the procedure. Right heart catheterization is performed using a 7F Swan-Ganz thermodilution catheter via the left femoral vein sheath. An 8F double-lumen pigtail catheter (Cordis, Miami, FL) is advanced via the sheath in the right femoral vein and the pigtail is positioned in the apex of the right ventricle. The transducers are calibrated and rechecked on both catheter lumens to assure accuracy and absence of an intrinsic catheter-induced gradient. Simultaneous right ventricular and right atrial pressures are recorded at 100 m/s paper speed and 40-mmHg range to assess the mean gradient across the tricuspid valve in diastole. If there is no significant gradient at rest, a fluid challenge of 500 to 1000 mL can be used to elicit an occult gradient. Cardiac output is determined by thermodilution technique unless there is moderate tricuspid regurgitation in which case a Fick cardiac output determination is necessary. Since most of the patients with tricuspid stenosis are of rheumatic etiology and have mild to moderate concurrent tricuspid regurgitation, calculation of the valve area by the Gorlin formula tends to underestimate the valve area. Underestimation occurs because the gradient

Table 16.3 NATIVE DOUBLE AND TRIPLE VALVULOPLASTIES

| | | | | | Mitral Valve | | | |
| | | | | | Mean Gradient, mmHg | | Valve Area, cm^2 | |
Study	No. Patients	Age	Sex	Etiology	Pre	Post	Pre	Post
DOUBLE VALVULOPLASTY								
Shrivastava et al,[39] 1988	1	21	F	Rheumatic	30	14	0.71*	1.2*
Romao et al,[40] 1989	1	21	F	Rheumatic	34	1	0.6	3.5
Berland et al,[41] 1990	1	22	F	Rheumatic	12	4	1.1	2.8
	2	13	M	Rheumatic	15	1	0.6	2.5
	3	18	M	Rheumatic	20	2	1.0	2.7
Bethencourt et al,[42] 1990	1	48	F	Rheumatic	14	5.2	1.0	1.8
Chen et al,[43] 1988	1	55	F	Congenital				

| | | | | Mitral Valve Area cm^2 | | Aortic Valve Area cm^2 | |
| **TRIPLE VALVULOPLASTY** | | | | | | | |
Author & Year	Age	Sex	Etiology	Pre	Post	Pre	Post
Konugres et al,[42] 1990	35	F	Rheumatic	0.8	2.9	0.5	3.2

* Valve area index
** Not reported in the article
TR — tricuspid regurgitation.
AS — aortic stenosis.
AVR — aortic valve replacement.
MVA — mitral valve area.
TVA — tricuspid valve area.

across tricuspid valve in diastole is based on total flow whereas the cardiac output as obtained by thermodilution technique gives only forward cardiac output.

The severity of tricuspid regurgitation should be analyzed both by echocardiography and cineangiography; if it is greater than 2 +, surgical replacement of the valve is recommended. Since the tricuspid valve has the largest valve area, the double-balloon technique usually gives better results than the single-balloon technique. The effective balloon dilating diameter when using two balloons is less than the sum of the two balloons and can be determined[45] by cineangiography and two-dimensional echocar-

| Tricuspid Valve | | | | Pulmonic Valve | | Valve Area, cm² | | Balloon(s) | Comments |
| Mean Gradient, mmHg | | Cardiac Output L/min | | Peak Gradient, mmHg | | | | Used, mm | |
Pre	Post	Pre	Post	Pre	Post	Pre	Post		
DOUBLE VALVULOPLASTY									
11.5	5.0	4.0	3.5			1.6*	2.4*	25	No increase in TR.
5	3	—**	—**			—**	—**	Trefoil 3 × 10 + 19	No increase in TR.
6	2	4.4	4.1			1.3	2.4	20 + 20	
6	1	3.0	5.5			1.1	2.7	Trefoil 3 × 10 + 18	
6	3	—**	—**			1.0	2.7	Trefoil 3 × 10 + 19	
13	4	3.05	4.5			0.81	2.0	Bifoil 2 × 19	Moderate TR which did not increase after valvuloplasty.
16	1	2.08	2.15	9	4	—**	—**	Inoue 27.5	TR increased from grade I/VI to grade II/VI by auscultation.

TRIPLE VALVULOPLASTY

| Tricuspid Valve Area cm² | | Cardiac Output L/min | | Balloons Used in Tricuspid Position mm | Comments: |
Pre	Post	Pre	Post		
1.0	4.0	2.63	3.03	25 + 23	Trace to 1 + TR. Symptomatic at 12 mo followup with recurrent AS; AVR with St. Jude valve was done. MVA = 2.2cm² TVA = 3.5cm²

diography. These modalities are also used to assess the valve ring size. The tricuspid annulus is usually oversized by 25%.

A double-lumen 8F wedge balloon catheter (Arrow International, Reading, PA) can be advanced via the right femoral vein through an 8F sideport sheath and placed in the apex of the right ventricle. Via this catheter two 0.038-inch Lau-Ruiz tapered core guidewires (Schneider, Minneapolis, MN) are placed in the right ventricular apex. By re-forming the tip of the guidewire into a pigtail with a $3\frac{1}{2}$ turns, this wire can be placed in the right ventricular apex to prevent the Mansfield percutaneous balloon catheters from perforating the right ventricular wall when inflated. Two Mansfield balloon catheters, 20- to 25-mm diameter, 4-cm length, are inserted by means of the guidewires to dilate the tricuspid valve until the "waists" on the balloons induced by narrow commissures are no longer noted and the gradient across the

Table 16.4   ILLUSTRATIVE NATIVE MULTIVALVE VALVULOPLASTIES

| | Cardiac Output, L/min | | Mitral Valve | | | |
| | | | Gradient, mmHg | | Valve Area, cm^2 | |
	Pre	Post	Pre	Post	Pre	Post
Case 1[a]	4.54	6.39	15	5	1.10	3.40
Case 2[a]					0.8	2.9
Case 3[a]	3.0	—	13	—	2.0	—

[a] See text.

tricuspid valve is less than 2 to 3 mmHg. The balloon is centered across the tricuspid valve by partially inflating one balloon and then centering both balloons so that they neither cross the pulmonic valve nor are caught in a chorda. Guidewires may be placed in the pulmonary artery to stabilize the balloon catheters, but care must be taken to ensure that the balloons are not caught in the chordae or across the pulmonary valve.

After dilatation the balloon catheters are replaced with monitoring pigtail catheters for simultaneous right atrial and right ventricular pressure measurements. Cardiac output measurements are repeated. To assess tricuspid regurgitation after balloon valvuloplasty, right ventricular cineangiography is repeated at the flow rate and views used prevalvuloplasty. The catheters and sheaths are then removed and manual pressure is applied to achieve hemostasis. The patient is transferred to the regular unit for observation. Usually, the patients are discharged the same or the following day.

CASE STUDIES

Percutaneous tricuspid valvuloplasty may be easily accomplished if the pathology is primarily commissural and is not accompanied by severe fibrotic and calcific changes in the valve and subvalvular structures. The following cases illustrate the variation in the pathology of the tricuspid valve disease that may be encountered necessitating different approaches to accomplish the balloon valvuloplasty.

Case 1

A 33-year-old Chinese woman with a history of rheumatic heart disease with New York Heart Association (NYHA) class III functional impairment was noted to have severe mitral and tricuspid stenosis on Doppler echocardiographic studies. She underwent successful percutaneous double-balloon valvuloplasty of both the mitral and the tricuspid valve during the same procedure. Mitral valve area improved from 1.10 cm^2 to 3.40 cm^2 after dilatation with two 20-mm Mansfield balloons, and tricuspid valve area improved from 1.70 cm^2 to 3.95 cm^2 after dilatation with two 25-mm Mansfield balloons. Because this patient was young and both the valves were free from signifi-

Cardiac Output, L/min		Tricuspid Valve				Balloons Used, mm	Comments
		Gradient, mmHg		Valve Area cm²			
Pre	Post	Pre	Post	Pre	Post		
4.54	5.61	6.0	0	1.7	3.95	25 + 25	1 + tricuspid regurgitation after tricuspid valvuloplasty.
2.63	3.03	—	—	1.0	4.0	25 + 23	
3.0	6.2	17	11	0.5	1.1	23 + 23	Mitral valvuloplasty was not performed.

cant calcification, the procedure was extremely rewarding in terms of hemodynamic and clinical improvement with a rapid uncomplicated recovery.

Case 2

This patient was reported by Konugres and associates.[44] A 35-year-old native-born white woman with rheumatic heart disease had progressive shortness of breath on exertion and extreme fatigue over 5 years. She had NYHA class III symptoms despite medical therapy. Clinical and noninvasive evaluation indicated severe mitral and aortic stenosis with 2 + calcification of the aortic valve. Invasive evaluation with fluid challenge confirmed severe tricuspid stenosis. Three valves were successively dilated with gratifying results with no complications and with clinical improvement maintained for 12 months. Figure 16.1 depicts the hemodynamic change in tricuspid valve gradient.

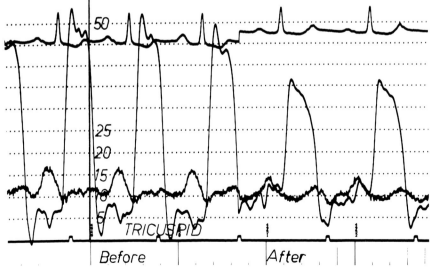

Figure 16.1 Case 2. Simultaneous pressure tracings of the right ventricle and right atrium showing the change in diastolic gradient before and after balloon valvuloplasty.

Mitral valve area 0.8 → 2.9 cm² (20-mm + 20-mm balloons)
Aortic valve area 0.5 → 3.2 cm² (18-mm + 18-mm balloons)
Tricuspid valve area 1.0 → 4.0 cm² (25-mm + 23-mm balloons)

After 12 months, her symptoms of shortness of breath returned and echocardiographic findings showed a return of her aortic stenosis requiring replacement with a St. Jude's valve. The mitral and tricuspid valve areas were 2.2 cm² and 3.5 cm², respectively. It has been our experience that calcification of the aortic valve usually predicts a shorter duration of improvement following balloon valvuloplasty. This patient is currently class II (NYHA) and is able to perform all her household duties as a mother of three young children.

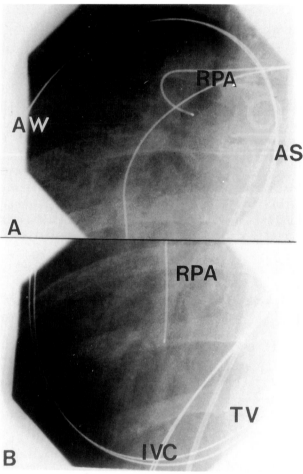

Figure 16.2 Case 3. Cine frames *A* and *B* depict the gigantic size of the right atrium. In the *lower frame*, the wires and the monitoring pigtail catheter enter from the intravenous catheter, encircle the right atrium, the septal wall, and the antero-lateral wall, pass through the tricuspid valve and the right ventricle, and are placed in the right pulmonary artery. The atrial septal wall could not be engaged by the transseptal equipment because of the marked septal displacement. *AS*—septal wall. *AW*—antero-lateral wall. *TV*—tricuspid valve. *RPA*—right pulmonary artery.

Case 3

A 62-year-old native-born female with progressive symptoms of shortness of breath and severe congestive heart failure refractory to medical therapy was admitted for evaluation. Two-dimensional echocardiography revealed severe tricuspid stenosis, moderate mitral stenosis, and a massively enlarged right atrium with 1+ to 2+ tricuspid regurgitation. The chest x-ray was significant for a massively enlarged right atrium filling most of right hemithorax (Fig. 16.2). Two cineframes (9-inch field) were required to cover the outlined area of the right atrium as noted by the guide wires. Doppler analysis of the tricuspid valve suggested mean gradient of 14 mmHg and an estimated tricuspid valve area of 0.5 cm^2.

Initially, crossing of the tricuspid valve was impeded by the massively enlarged right atrium and a 2+ tricuspid insufficiency. The use of a Mullins sheath and a balloon wedge catheter facilitated crossing of the tricuspid valve, and two guidewires were then placed in the pulmonary artery. The gradient was only partially relieved with two 20-mm Mansfield balloons. Two 23-mm Mansfield balloons were placed across the tricuspid valve with the guidewires placed at the apex of the right ventricle (Fig. 16.3 frames *A* and *B*). Percutaneous double-balloon dilatation was performed with an improvement in tricuspid valve area from 0.5 cm^2 to 1.1 cm^2. Tricuspid regurgitation increased from 1+ to 2+ (Fig. 16.3 frames *D* and *S*).

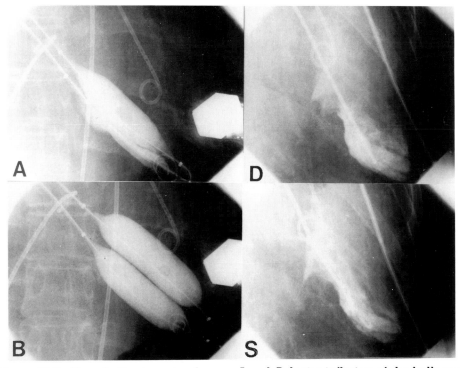

Figure 16.3 Case 3. The two cine frames *A* and *B* depict inflation of the balloons across the tricuspid valve with the guidewires at the apex of the right ventricle. The cine frames *D* and *S* show diastole and systole showing the 2+ tricuspid regurgitation at the close of the procedure.

Mitral valvuloplasty was not performed. The patient had a huge right atrium with bulging of the interatrial septum into left atrium. A transseptal catheterization procedure was attempted but the septum could not be engaged even with a marked C-curve in the transseptal needle.

The patient improved clinically over a period of 4 months and was then readmitted for surgical replacement of the mitral and tricuspid valves. The patient survived surgery but succumbed from respiratory complications.

The balloon valvuloplasty procedure for tricuspid stenosis can be accomplished most easily in patients with commissural disease. The older the patient is and the greater the involvement of the valve and subvalvular structures, the more difficult is the procedure and the less satisfactory the outcome. We have not had a long enough follow-up on our tricuspid valvuloplasties to give any estimate of the long-term results.

CURRENT STATUS

The decision to perform balloon valvuloplasty for tricuspid valve stenosis may be a difficult one. Usually these patients have multivalve disease, and surgery requires a coordinated team approach with a physician, nurse, and technician who are familiar with performing balloon valvuloplasties on the mitral, aortic, and pulmonic valves. Patient selection depends on (1) pathology that is found in the valve structures (commissures, leaflets, and subvalvular structures), (2) the presence or absence of calcification, (3) the degree of valvular regurgitation, and (4) the presence or absence of other disease to limit surgical intervention. The best candidate for immediate and long-term results of balloon valvuloplasty for tricuspid stenosis is the young patient with primarily commissural disease. Balloon valvuloplasty does provide a method for temporary relief of tricuspid stenosis that is reasonably efficacious, negligible in morbidity and mortality, and cost effective, and that requires neither general anesthesia nor thoracotomy.

REFERENCES

1. Kan JS, White RI, Mitchell SE, et al: Percutaneous balloon valvuloplasty: a new method for treating congenital pulmonary-valve stensis. *N Engl J Med.* 307:540–542, 1982.
2. Inoue K, Owaki T, Nakamura T, et al: Clinical application of transvenous mitral commissurotomy by a new balloon catheter. *J Thorac Cardiovasc Surg.* 87:394–402, 1984.
3. Labadidi Z: Aortic balloon valvuloplasty. *Am Heart J.* 106:751–752, 1983.
4. Cribier A, Savin T, Saoudi N, et al: Percutaneous transluminal valvuloplasty of acquired aortic stenosis in elderly patients: an alternative to valve replacement? *Lancet.* 1:63–67, 1986.
5. Feit F, Stecy PJ, Nachamie MS: Percutaneous balloon valvuloplasty for stenosis of a porcine bioprosthesis in the tricuspid valve position. *Am J Cardiol.* 58:363–364, 1986.
6. Zaibag MA, Ribeiro P, Kasab SA: Percutaneous balloon valvotomy in tricuspid stenosis. *Br Heart J.* 57:51–53, 1987.
7. Coombs CF: *Rheumatic Heart Disease.* New York: William Wood & Co, 1924, p 58.
8. Cabot RC: *Facts on the Heart.* Philadelphia: WB Saunders Co, 1926, pp 159–174.

9. Cooke WT, White PD: Tricuspid stenosis, with particular reference to diagnosis and prognosis. *Br Heart J.* 3:147–165, 1941.

10. Aceves S, Carral R: The diagnosis of tricuspid valve disease. *Am Heart J.* 34:114–130, 1947.

11. Smith JA, Levine SA: The clinical features of tricuspid stenosis. A study of trivalvular stenosis. *Am Heart J.* 23:739–760, 1942.

12. Kitchin A, Turner R: Diagnosis and treatment of tricuspid stenosis. *Br Heart J.* 26:354–379, 1964.

13. Guyer DE, Gillam LD, Foale RA, et al: Comparison of the echocardiographic and hemodynamic diagnosis of rheumatic tricuspid stenosis. *J Am Coll Cardiol.* 3:1135–1144, 1984.

14. Roberts WC, Sullivan MF: Combined mitral valve stenosis and tricuspid valve stenosis: morphologic observations after mitral and tricuspid valve replacements or mitral replacement and tricuspid valve commissurotomy. *Am J Cardiol.* 58:850–852, 1986.

15. Fujii S, Funaki K, Denzumi N: Isolated rheumatic tricuspid regurgitation and stenosis. *Clin Cardiol.* 9:353–355, 1986.

16. Mullins PA, Hall JA, Shapiro LM: Balloon dilatation of tricuspid stenosis caused by carcinoid heart disease. *Br Heart J.* 63:249–250, 1990.

17. Basso LV, Gradman M, Finkelstein S, et al: Tricuspid valve obstruction due to intravenous leiomyomatosis. *Clin Nucl Med.* 9:152–155, 1984.

18. Walters LL, Taxy JB: Malignant mesothelioma of the pleura with extensive cardiac invasion and tricuspid orifice occlusion. *Cancer.* 52:1736–1738, 1983.

19. Lyons HA, Kelly JJ Jr, Nusbaum N, et al: Right atrial myxoma. A clinical study of a patient in whom diagnosis was made by angiocardiography during life (surgically removed). *Am J Med.* 25:321–326, 1958.

20. Erol C, Candan I, Akalin H, et al: Cardiac hydatid cyst simulating tricuspid stenosis. *Am J Cardiol.* 56:833–834, 1985.

21. Gibbs KL, Reardon MJ, Strickman NE, et al: Hemodynamic compromise (tricuspid stenosis and insufficiency) caused by unruptured aneurysm of the sinus of Valsalva. *J Am Coll Cardiol.* 7:1177–1181, 1986.

22. Dennis JL, Hansen AE, Corpening TN: Endocardial fibroelastosis. *Pediatrics.* 12:130–139, 1953.

23. Davies JNP, Ball JD: The pathology of endomyocardial fibrosis in Uganda. *Br Heart J.* 17:337–359, 1955.

24. Benedick BA, Davis SF, Alderman E: Balloon valvuloplasty for fungal endocarditis induced stenosis of a bioprosthetic tricuspid valve. *Cathet Cardiovasc Diagn.* 21:248–251, 1990.

25. Gibson R, Wood P: The diagnosis of tricuspid stenosis. *Br Heart J.* 17:552–562, 1955.

26. Fasoli G, Scognamiglio R, Daliento L: Uncommon pattern of tricuspid stenosis in Ebstein's anomaly. *Int J Cardiol.* 9:488–492, 1985.

27. McGinn JS, Zipes DP: Constrictive pericarditis causing tricuspid stenosis. *Arch Intern Med.* 129:487–490, 1972.

28. Young SG, Gregoratos G, Swain JA, et al: Delayed postoperative cardiac tamponade mimicking severe tricuspid valve stenosis. *Chest.* 85:824–826, 1984.

29. Ribeiro PA, Zaibag MA, Kasab SA, et al: Provocation and amplification of the transvalvular pressure gradient in rheumatic tricuspid stenosis. *Am J Cardiol.* 61:1307–1311, 1988.

30. Yousof AM, Shafei MZ, Endrys G, et al: Tricuspid stenosis and regurgitation in rheumatic heart disease: a prospective cardiac catheterization study in 525 patients. *Am Heart J.* 110:60–64, 1985.

31. Khalilullah M, Tyagi S, Yadav BS, et al: Double-balloon valvuloplasty of tricuspid stenosis. *Am Heart J.* 114:1232–1233, 1987.

32. Ribeiro PA, Zaibag MA, Kasab SA, et al: Percutaneous double balloon valvotomy for rheumatic tricuspid stenosis. *Am J Cardiol.* 61:660–662, 1988.

33. Rico Blazquez J, Sobrino Daza N, Calvo Orbe L, et al: Percutaneous transluminal valvuloplasty in tricuspid valve stenosis. A case report. *Rev Esp Cardiol.* 41:636–638, 1988.

34. Goldenberg IF, Pedersen W, Olson J, et al: Percutaneous double balloon valvuloplasty for severe tricuspid stenosis. *Am Heart J.* 118:417–419, 1989.

35. Bourdillon PDV, Hookman LD, Morris SN, et al: Percutaneous balloon valvuloplasty for tricuspid stenosis: hemodynamic and pathologic findings. *Am Heart J.* 117:492–495, 1989.

36. Wren C, Hunter S: Balloon dilatation of a stenosed bioprosthesis in the tricuspid valve position. *Br Heart J.* 61:65–67, 1989.

37. Attubato MJ, Stroh JA, Bach RG, et al: Percutaneous double-balloon valvuloplasty of porcine bioprosthetic valves in the tricuspid position. *Cathet Cardiovasc Diagn.* 20:202–204, 1990.

38. Chow W-H, Cheung K-L, Tai Y-T, et al: Successful percutaneous balloon valvuloplasty of a stenotic tricuspid bioprosthesis. *Am Heart J.* 119:666–668, 1990.

39. Shrivastava S, Radhakrishnan S, Dev V: Concurrent balloon dilatation of tricuspid and calcific mitral valve in a patient of rheumatic heart disease. *Int J Cardiol.* 20:133–137, 1988.

40. Romao N, Prytzlik R, Salles Netto M, et al: Combined mitral and tricuspid valvuloplasty, case report. *Arq Bras Cardiol.* 53:333–338, 1989.

41. Berland J, Rocha P, Mechmeche R, et al: Percutaneous valvotomy in the combination of mitral and tricuspid valve stenosis. Report of 3 cases. *Arch Mal Coeur.* 83:1585–1589, 1990.

42. Bethencourt A, Medina A, Hernandez E, et al: Combined percutaneous balloon valvuloplasty of mitral and tricuspid valves. *Am Heart J.* 119:416–418, 1990.

43. Chen CR, Lo ZX, Huang ZD, et al: Concurrent percutaneous balloon valvuloplasty for combined tricuspid and pulmonic stenoses. *Cathet Cardiovasc Diagn.* 15:55–60, 1988.

44. Konugres GS, Lau FYK, Ruiz CE: Successive percutaneous double-balloon mitral, aortic, and tricuspid valvotomy in rheumatic trivalvular stenoses. *Am Heart J.* 119:663–666, 1990.

45. Rao PS: Influence of balloon size on short-term and long-term results of balloon pulmonary valvuloplasty. *Tex Heart Inst J.* 14:57–61, 1987.

CHAPTER **17**

Stenotic Porcine Bioprosthetic Valves

BRUCE F. WALLER
CHARLES MCKAY
JAMES VAN TASSEL
MARCUS ALLEN

During the last several years dilating balloons have been applied in the treatment of stenotic native cardiac valves. Initial morphologic studies [1-3] have indicated that "splitting" or "cracking" of fused commissures, stretching of surrounding structures (aortic walls, valve annuli), or both are mechanisms of action in dilating these native valves. Interest recently has been extended to bioprosthetic valves that have become stenotic. Application of balloon valvuloplasty to porcine prostheses could alleviate the need for repeat valve-replacement surgery. This chapter briefly reviews the underlying changes leading to stenosis of bioprosthetic valves and summarizes presently known morphologic studies concerning the application of catheter balloon valvuloplasty techniques to these prosthetic valves.

CAUSES OF VALVE FAILURE

The most widely used tissue-derived valve has been the flexible-stent-mounted porcine bioprosthesis which is derived from a glutaraldehyde-preserved pig aortic valve. Two popular porcine bioprosthetic valves include the Hancock and Carpentier-Edwards valves. Durability is similar in both prostheses. These two types of porcine bioprosthetic valves differ in the concentration of glutaraldehyde used in the tanning process, in stent composition, and in the manner of pig cusp modification.[4-6] In the pig, the right coronary cusp of the aortic valve is supported by a muscular shelf arising from the ventricular septum. A modified Hancock prosthesis substitutes a right cusp without a muscular ridge, whereas the Carpentier-Edwards type minimizes the amount of septal muscle incorporated in the prosthesis. Porcine aortic valve cusps contain three well-defined layers: the ventricularis, the central spongiosa, and the fibrosa. Collagen is an important element in each of these layers. Many of the changes occurring after implantation of the porcine prosthetic valve are related to a gradual breakdown in the collagen in these three layers.

Porcine bioprosthetic valves have no synthetic or renewal mechanism such as that provided by fibroblasts in native valves to replace the broken-down collagen. Eventual

Table 17.1   CAUSES OF DEGENERATION IN PORCINE BIOPROSTHETIC VALVES

Primary degeneration (intrinsic calcification, cusp tears and perforations) accounts for approximately 2 out of 3 failures. It may be divided into three subgroups:

- Calcification (accumulation of elemental calcium/phosphorus) is the most common cause of primary degeneration and appears related to cuspal collagen injury:
    Cuspal stiffness (stenosis) or disruption (regurgitation)
    Calcific deposits predominate at cuspal commissures and basal attachments (points of maximum flexion, stress)
- Cuspal tears from primary degeneration are found along the commissurial margins (secondary calcific deposits) or more centrally:
    Alteration and disruption of valvular collagen
    Calcification
- Cuspal thrombi (noninfected) are an uncommon form of primary degeneration (about 5% of porcine valves)
    Immobilizes cusp (stenosis)
    May calcify

effects of this gradual collagen breakdown can lead to cuspal loosening, cuspal delamination, cuspal tears, and perforation. Collagen also undergoes a time-dependent process of focal calcification.[3] These changes have been collectively termed *primary degeneration* (Table 17.1). Within a few days after implantation, the porcine valves become covered with a layer of fibrin, platelets, and erythrocytes, and microthrombi may develop. Reendotheliazation is a slow process, taking up to 5 or more years in some valves.

Indications for reoperation or causes of death in patients with porcine prosthetic valves have included: thromboemboli, cuspal thrombosis, infective endocarditis, and degenerative dysfunction. Thromboembolic complications for porcine prosthesis without anticoagulation range from 0.9 to 5.5 per 100 patient years.[4] Infective endocarditis is also an infrequent complication, occurring in 1 to 4% of patients.[4] In contrast to mechanical prosthetic valves, infective endocarditis of bioprosthetic valves destroys cuspal tissue.

Calcification (Figs. 17.1 through 17.6)

Calcification of cuspal tissue is the most common cause of primary degeneration. It has been recognized in up to 80% of prosthetic valves failing by primary degeneration.[4] Calcification, which becomes more prominent as the implantation time increases, represents an accumulation within porcine tissues of elemental calcium and phosphorus in various mineral phases. Calcific deposits are related to degeneration of cuspal collagen and connective tissue cells, to surface thrombi, or both.

Calcific deposits range in size from finely, friable granular material (Figs. 17.1, 17.3, and 17.4), to nodular yellow-white masses (Figs. 17.1, 17.5, and 17.6) with ulcerative surfaces. Intrinsic calcification may cause clinical failure by cuspal stiffening leading to stenosis, or by cuspal structural disruption resulting in regurgitation. Early calcific deposits frequently occur along the commissures and basal attachments (Figs. 17.1, 17.3, 17.4 and 17.5). As the process progresses, central cuspal tissue becomes involved. Factors predisposing to calcification of implanted porcine valves include

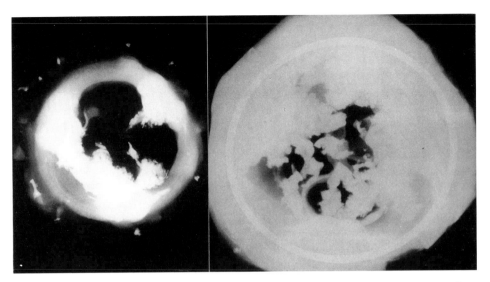

Figure 17.1 Primary degeneration: calcification. Radiographs of two porcine valves showing calcific deposits (*white areas*).

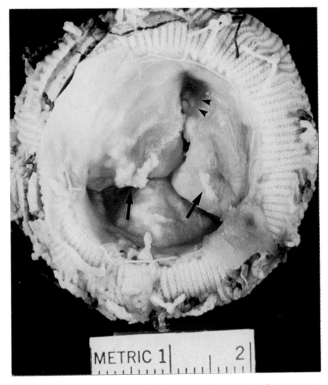

Figure 17.2 Primary degeneration: calcification. Bars of calcium extend along the cuspal surface (*arrows*) and within commissures (*arrowheads*). Figures 17.2 through 17.10 from Waller BF, et al: Catheter balloon valvuloplasty of stenotic porcine bioprosthetic valves. Part I: Anatomic considerations. *Clin Cardiol.* 14:686–691, 1991.

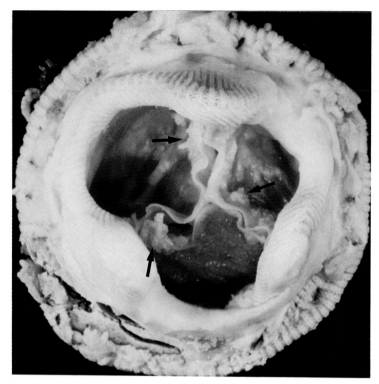

Figure 17.3 Primary degeneration: calcification. Focal areas of calcific deposits along commissures (*arrows*).

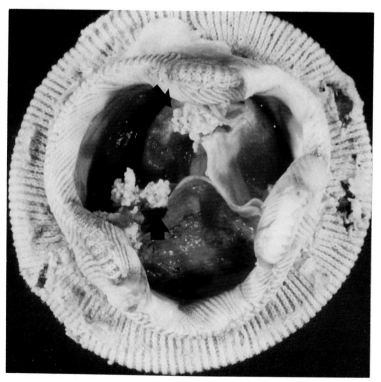

Figure 17.4 Primary degeneration: calcification. Nodular masses of calcium extend from commissural margins dangling freely within the valve cusp (*arrows*).

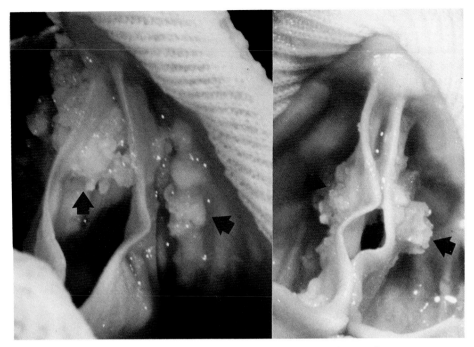

Figure 17.5 Primary degeneration: calcification. Closeup of cuspal margins at commissures showing calcific deposits (*arrows*).

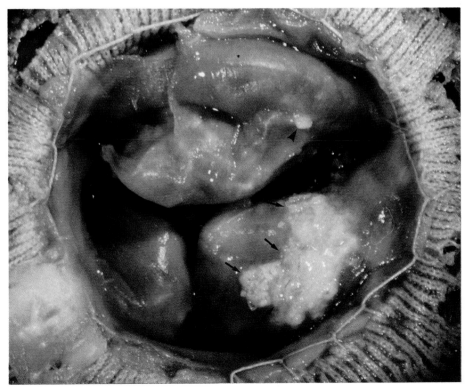

Figure 17.6 Primary degeneration: calcification. Sheet of calcium covers one of three porcine cusps (*arrows*). A small nodule of calcium is also present on adjacent cusp (*arrowhead*).

young age of patients (children), chronic renal disease, chronic hemodialysis, several etiologies of hyperparathyroidism, and infective endocarditis (so-called "extrinsic calcification")[4-6] The observation that calcification begins at areas of leaflet flexion (commissures) where deformations are maximal suggests that dynamic stress is also a factor in the calcification of bioprosthetic tissue.[4-6]

Tears and Perforations (Figs. 17.7 through 17.9)

Cuspal tears are a subtype of primary degeneration involving porcine prosthetic valves. Tears are frequently found along commissural margins (Fig. 17.7) or more centrally (Fig. 17.8). Some tears are adjacent to and probably secondary to calcific deposits. Other tears result from collagen disruption. Stress-induced collagen deterioration is seen by scanning electron microscopy as fraying and disruption of collagen fibers.[1-3] Cuspal tears are associated with clinical prosthetic valve regurgitation when the tears are large or if cuspal detachment has occurred (Fig. 17.9).

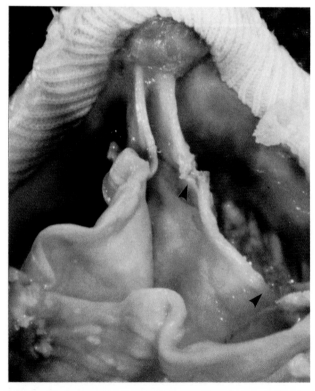

Figure 17.7 Primary degeneration: cuspal tears. Focal areas of cuspal tearing along the commissural margins (*arrows*) producing minimal if any regurgitation.

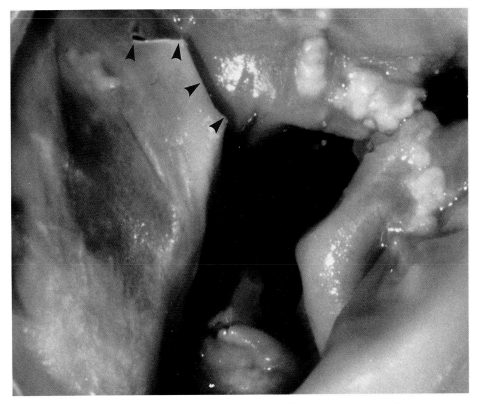

Figure 17.8 Primary degeneration: cuspal tears. Extensive tearing of porcine cusp (*arrows*) associated with regurgitation. The commissure is fused with calcific deposit.

Noninfective Cuspal Thrombus (Fig. 17.10)

Cuspal thrombus unassociated with infection is an uncommon form of primary degeneration accounting for less than 5% of failed porcine prosthetic valves.[4-6] Cuspal thrombus occurs on the concave surface of the valve, filling up 1 to 3 of the cusps. When present, the thrombus immobilizes one or more cusps and produces clinical stenosis. When disrupted, the thrombus may fragment and be the source of systemic or pulmonic emboli. Longstanding cuspal thrombi also may calcify.

PORCINE BIOPROSTHETIC VALVE VALVULOPLASTY

The use of nonsurgical balloon techniques in treating stenotic native cardiac valves[1-3] has shown that commissural cracking, leaflet or cuspal tears, and stretching are the mechanisms by which balloon valvuloplasty procedures act. Overstretching with

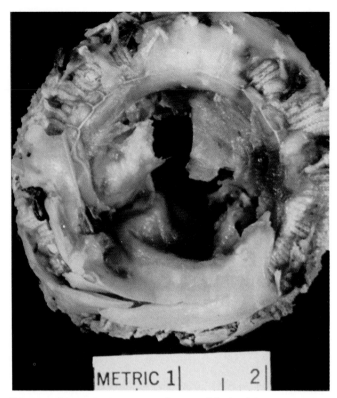

Figure 17.9 Primary degeneration: cuspal tears. Marked degenerative changes with extensive tearing and perforation of all three cusps producing severe regurgitation.

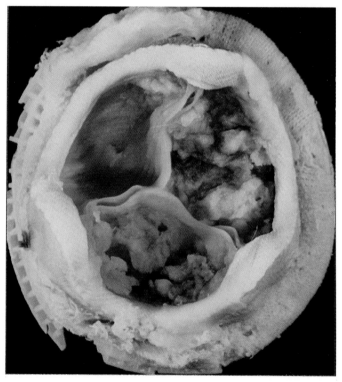

Figure 17.10 Primary degeneration: cuspal thrombus. Thrombi fill up two of three cusps producing prosthetic valve stenosis.

oversized or multiple balloons has occasionally led to aortic wall tearing (aortic dissection) or annular tearing (mitral annular separation).

Stenotic porcine prosthetic valves seemed initially to be ideally suited for balloon valvuloplasty techniques for 3 reasons:

1. The pathologic changes leading to primary degeneration of porcine bio-prosthetic valves, including cuspal stiffening and mild calcific deposits along with commissures occasionally producing commissural fusion, seemed suitable anatomy for balloon dilatation.
2. The rigid stent framework of the prosthetic valve would prevent annular tearing or rupture.
3. Annular stretching would seem remote and thus early "restenosis" from elastic recoil seems unlikely.

We therefore undertook a series of in vitro experiments to determine if the morphologic mechanisms of catheter balloon valvuloplasty of stenotic porcine bioprosthetic valves were similar to those applied to stenotic native cardiac valves.

Materials and Methods

Source of Porcine Bioprosthetic Valves

The Cardiovascular Pathology Registry at St. Vincent Hospital in Indianapolis represents a large collection of surgical and necropsy cardiovascular specimens. Twenty operatively excised degenerative stenotic porcine prosthetic valves were retrieved for analysis. Clinical information from each patient was also reviewed. All 20 operatively excised valves were radiographed and classified into types of degenerative changes.

Clinical Data (Table 17.2)

Of the 20 operatively excised porcine prosthetic valves, 14 (70%) were from mitral positions and 6 (30%) were from aortic positions. The patients were aged 26 to 68 years (mean 53) and 11 (55%) of the specimens were from men. Catheterization data obtained before surgery indicate that the mean end-diastolic gradient across mitral

Table 17.2 CLINICAL CHARACTERISTICS PERTAINING TO 20 OPERATIVELY EXCISED STENOTIC PORCINE BIOPROSTHETIC VALVES ON WHICH BALLOON VALVULOPLASTY WAS PERFORMED

Number dilated	
Mitral	14
Aortic	6
Patient age, yr	26–68 (mean 53)
Male: female ratio	11:9
Preexcision catheterization data	
Mitral prostheses: mean end-diastolic gradient, mmHg	12–17 (mean 14.2)
Aortic prostheses: peak systolic LV-Ao gradient, mmHg	58–112 (mean 85)
Implantation age of prosthesis, yr (insertion–excision interval)	1–10 (mean 6.6)
Internal diameter, mm	21–29 (mean 26)

LV — left ventricular Ao — aortic

prostheses ranged from 12 to 17 mmHg (mean 14.2). Peak systolic gradients (left ventricular–aortic) across prosthetic aortic valves ranged from 58 to 122 mmHg (mean 85). Internal diameters of porcine prostheses ranged from 21 to 29 mm (mean 26). The interval of implantation (age of prosthesis) ranged from 1 to 10 years (mean 6.6).

Morphologic Data (Table 17.3)
Of the 20 operatively excised stenotic porcine prostheses, two morphologic subgroups of degenerative changes were identified: primary degeneration (calcification, cuspal stiffness, and focal tears) in 18 (90%) and cuspal thrombus involving two or three of the cusps in 2 (10%) valves. Of the 18 valves with primary degeneration, 18 (100%) had commissural calcific deposits (friable, granular deposits or nodular deposits with or without ulcerative surfaces); 18 (100%) had severe cuspal stiffness with focal calcific deposits; and 3 (15%) had minor cuspal tears along the margin of closure insufficient to produce significant regurgitation. All 18 valves had variable amounts of commissural or cuspal calcific deposits, or both. Of the 2 valves with primary cuspal thrombi, neither had evidence of previous endocarditis (clinical or morphologic). One had two of three cusps filled with thrombus, and the other had all three cusps filled with thrombus. The thrombus was packed within the depths of the porcine aortic cusps. Neither valve had calcific deposits.

Methods of Valvuloplasty
Catheter balloon valvuloplasty was performed on the 20 stenotic prosthetic porcine valves using 20-mm dilating balloons inflated to a maximum of 3 atm (Fig. 17.11). Morphologic changes in prosthetic valve structures were recorded after *each* dilation. Following dilation, the prosthetic valves were reradiographed for comparison of previously located calcific deposits. Details of the dilation process were recorded using a split-image, (simultaneous front and back) closeup videorecording system.

Results of Valvuloplasty (Table 17.4, Figs. 17.11 through 17.25)
Table 17.4 shows dilation results in the 18 porcine prosthetic valves with primary degeneration as the cause for valve stenosis. All 18 valves had commissural "splitting"

Table 17.3 DEGENERATIVE CHANGES FOUND IN 20 OPERATIVELY EXCISED PORCINE BIOPROSTHETIC VALVES

	No. Valves
Type of degenerative change	
Primary degeneration	18
Commissural calcium	18
Cuspal stiffness	18
Minor tears	3
Cuspal thrombus producing valve stenosis (2 or 3/3 cusps)	2
Degree of radiographic calcification (0–4+)	
None	2
1–2+	4
3–4+	14

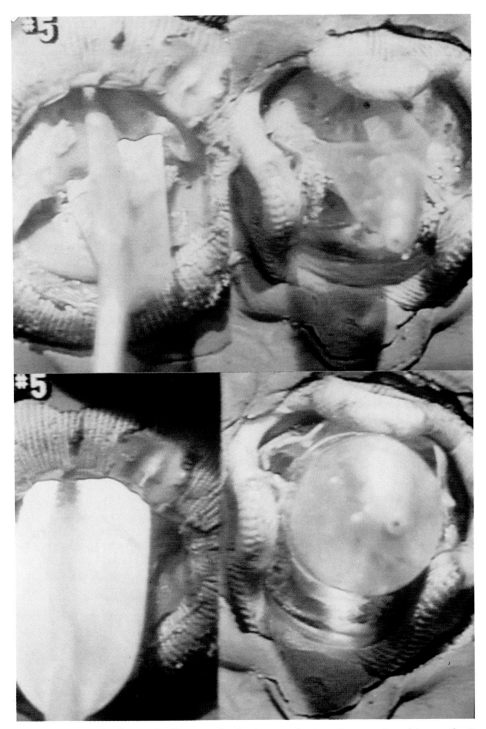

Figure 17.11 Catheter balloon valvuloplasty of stenotic porcine bioprosthetic valves. *Top* frames show insertion of balloon in simultaneous top and bottom views. Inflation of balloon (*lower* frames) shows splitting of fused calcified commissures (*lower right*). (Figures 17.11 through 17.23; 17.26 through 17.28 from Waller BF, et al: Catheter balloon valvuloplasty of stenotic porcine bioprosthetic valves. Part II. Mechanisms, complications and recommendations for clinical use. *Clin Cardiol.* 14:764–772, 1991.

Table 17.4 FINDINGS ON BALLOON DILATATION OF 20 OPERATIVELY EXCISED PORCINE BIOPROSTHETIC VALVES

	No. Valves
Primary degeneration producing valvular stenosis (N = 18)	
Commissural "splitting," "cracking"	18
Cuspal cracking/fracture	18
Cuspal cracking resulting in cusp tears (perforation)	
(major cusp fracture, = 3)	9
Dislodgement ("emboli") of calcific debris (commissures, cusps)	
with balloon inflation	10
Dislodgement ("emboli") of calcific nodules with insertion and	
removal of deflated balloon	6
Rupture of "annulus"	N/A
Cuspal thrombus producing valvular stenosis (N = 2)	
Thrombus crumbling	2
Thrombus dislodgement ("emboli") with balloon inflation	2
Cuspal tearing	1
Thrombus dislodgement ("emboli") with insertion or removal of	
delated balloon	0

or "cracking," and cuspal cracking or fracture was produced in 9 (50%) (Figs. 17.12 through 17.18). Extensive cuspal cracking resulting in major cuspal fractures and fragmentation (potential clinical emboli) occurred in 3 (33%) (Figs. 17.19 and 17.20). In 10 valves, balloon inflation also dislodged calcific debris. Six of these valves had a further dislodgement of calcific nodules or friable granular deposits with simple insertion or removal of the dilating balloon. "Annular" rupture was prevented by the rigid stent mounting structure.

Table 17.4 shows also the results of balloon valvuloplasty on two porcine prosthetic valves rendered stenotic by the presence of extensive intracuspal thrombus (Figs. 17.21 through 17.23). With inflation of the balloon (Fig. 17.21), "crumbling" of the thrombus occurred despite its well secured, well-impacted gross appearance (Figs. 17.22 and 17.23). Dislodgement of thrombi (potential clinical emboli) occurred in each of these two valves. None of the thrombi was dislodged during insertion or removal of the dilation balloon. Cuspal tearing occurred in one of these valves during balloon dilation.

Comments on In Vitro Experiments

Results of these in vitro balloon valvuloplasty experiments on human stenotic operatively excised porcine prosthetic valves indicate that dilation occurs by commissural splitting and cuspal cracking (Figs. 17.24 and 17.25). These mechanisms of action are similar to those of balloon valvuloplasty in stenotic native valves. Major differences in balloon dilation of porcine prosthetic valves, however, include:

- A high frequency of dislodgement of friable fragments of calcific deposits and thrombus during balloon inflation,

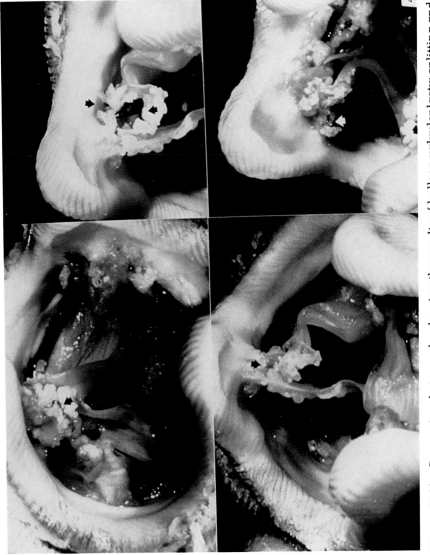

Figure 17.12 Composite photographs showing the results of balloon valvuloplasty: splitting and cracking of calcific nodules (*arrows*) and dislodgement of a calcific fragment (*upper right*).

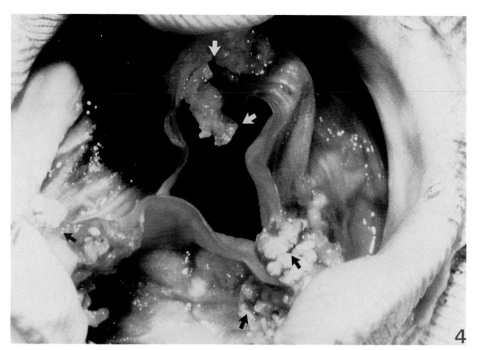

Figure 17.13 Closeup of fractured calcific nodules along the commissural margins (*arrows*).

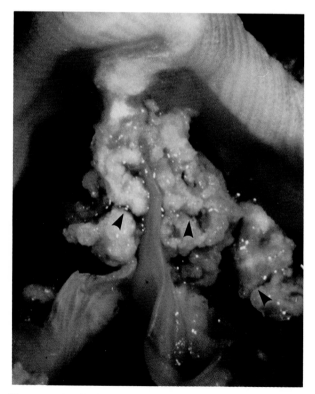

Figure 17.14 Closeup of calcified nodule following balloon valvuloplasty (*arrows*).

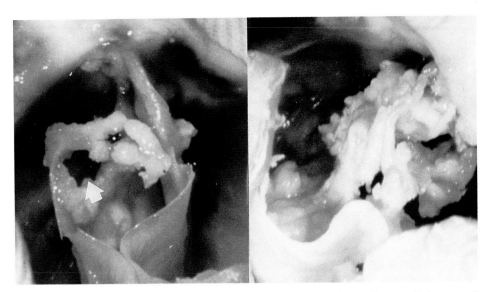

Figure 17.15 Closeup of split commissures showing perforated cusp (*left, arrow*) and fragmented calcific nodules (*right*). Reinsertion of wires or dilation balloons could pass through the cusp perforation and further injure the prosthetic cusp.

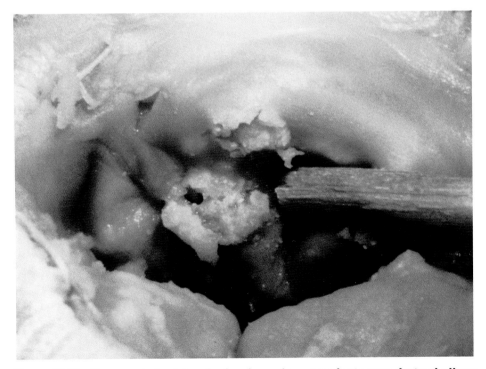

Figure 17.16 Fragment of calcium broken loose from prosthetic cusp during balloon dilation. These fragments may represent clinical emboli.

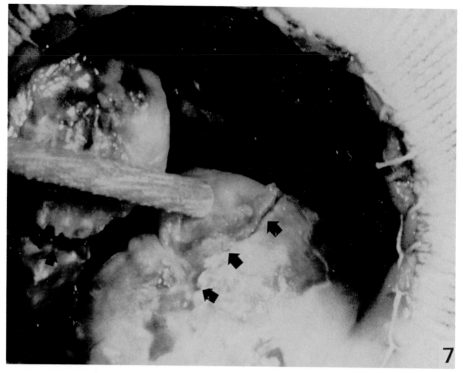

Figure 17.17 Stiff and calcified prosthetic cusp fractured (*arrows*) by balloon dilation.

- Dislodgement of calcific deposits simply during insertion and withdrawal of the deflated dilating balloon
- Fracture and dislodgement of portions of stiffened cusps.

The latter disadvantages far outweigh the single advantage of an absence of valve annular separation during dilation of bioprosthetic porcine valves. These findings suggest a limited and cautious role of catheter balloon valvuloplasty in the treatment of stenotic porcine prostheses.

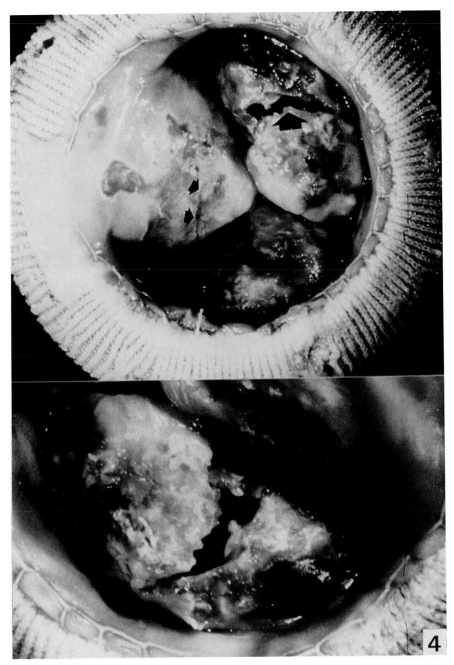

Figure 17.18 Stiff and calcified cusp severely cracked (*large arrows*) by balloon dilation. Smaller cuspal cracks (*small arrows*) also created by dilation.

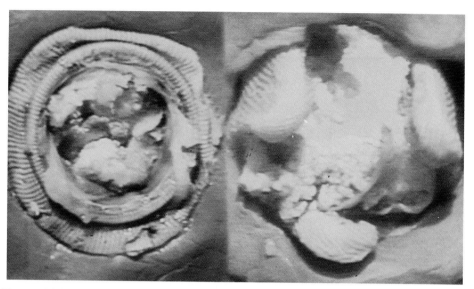

Figure 17.19 Large fragment of calcified cusp broken loose during balloon valvuloplasty. Clinically, this would have caused acute, severe valve regurgitation.

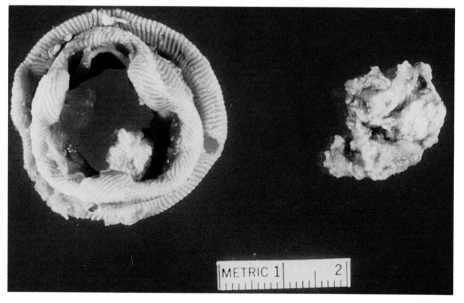

Figure 17.20 Dislodgement of two of three heavily calcified cusps during balloon dilation.

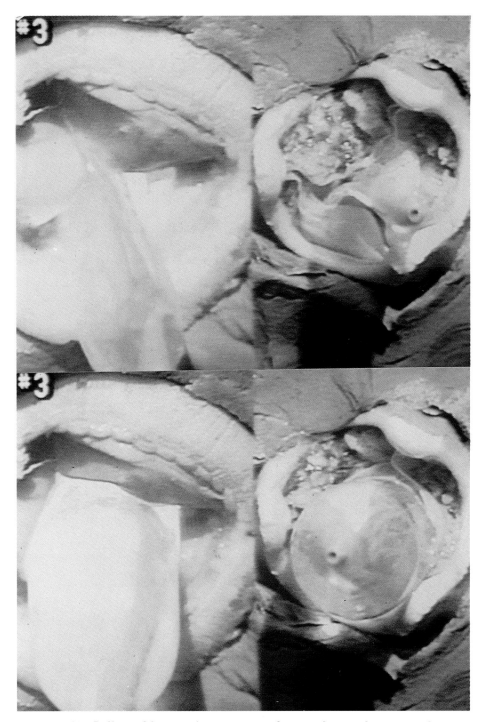

Figure 17.21 Balloon dilation of porcine prosthetic valve made stenotic by intra-cuspal thrombus. Inflation of balloon (*lower right*) crumbles cuspal thrombus.

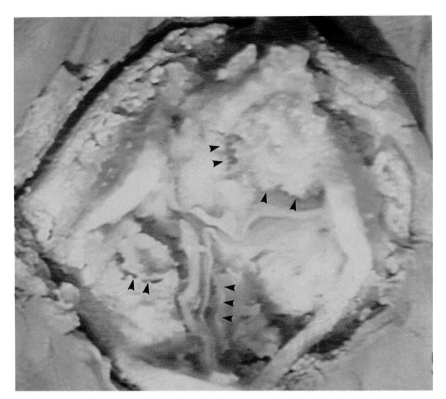

Figure 17.22 Results of balloon valvuloplasty of porcine bioprosthetic valve made stenotic by cuspal thrombus. The thrombus is broken (*arrowheads*) and crumbled and can easily be dislodged, potentially representing emboli.

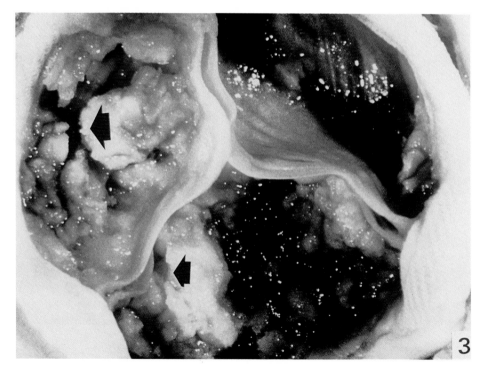

Figure 17.23 Large fractures (*arrows*) in intracuspal thrombus following balloon valvuloplasty.

Morphologic Effects of Balloon Valvuloplasty on Porcine
Bioprosthetic Valves Rendered Stenotic by Primary Degeneration

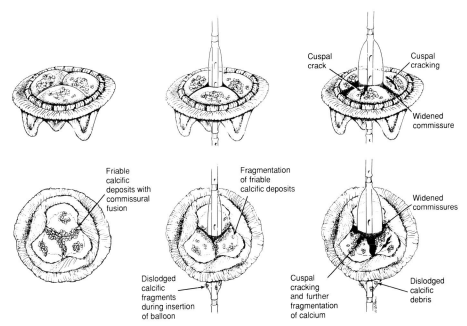

Figure 17.24 Mechanisms of balloon valvuloplasty in degenerative stenotic porcine bioprosthetic valves.

Morphologic Effects of Balloon Valvuloplasty on Porcine
Bioprosthetic Valves Rendered Stenotic by Cuspal Thrombus

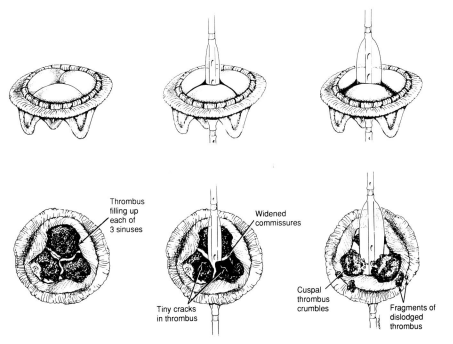

Figure 17.25 Mechanisms of balloon valvuloplasty in porcine bioprosthetic valves made stenotic by intracuspal thrombus.

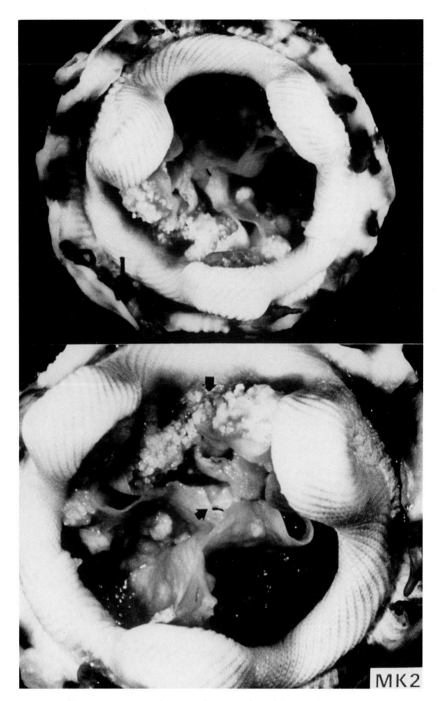

Figure 17.26 Stenotic porcine bioprosthetic valve dilated during life. Calcific nodule cracks (*arrows*), cuspal tears and perforation are identical to the in vitro studies.

Clinical Correlation

Clinical experience with balloon dilation of stenotic bioprosthetic valves has been limited. McKay and associates[7] reported the first two living patients undergoing dilation of stenotic aortic bioprosthesis (Figs. 17.26, 17.27, and 17.28). One patient required surgical replacement of the prosthetic valve shortly after dilation. Gross examination of the operatively excised Angell-Shiley porcine bioprosthesis showed that one of the three cusps had been immobilized by heavy calcific deposits. The free margin of the immobilized cusp had a 5-mm tear beneath the free margin, presumably from balloon dilation. The second patient died shortly after balloon dilation of the stenotic porcine aortic valve. Severe aortic regurgitation was noted immediately after dilation. At necropsy, the Hancock bioprosthetic valve showed perforations at all three cusps and broken, friable calcific deposits. The fractured calcific deposits and cuspal tears appeared to be the result of balloon valvuloplasty. One of the cusps was torn away from a previously fused commissure and accounted for the new, severe aortic regurgitation. These observations confirm the in vitro observations described earlier.

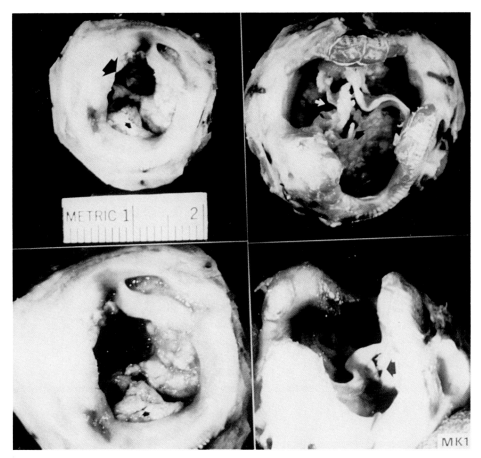

Figure 17.27 Stenotic porcine bioprosthetic valve dilated during life showing calcific nodule and cuspal cracks and tears (*arrows*).

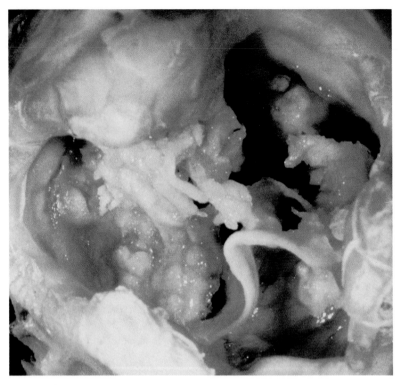

Figure 17.28 Closeup of prosthetic valve in Figure 17.27 showing severe cuspal tearing and perforation following balloon valvuloplasty resulting in new and severe clinical regurgitation.

Feit,[8] in contrast, dilated a stenotic Hancock porcine bioprosthesis in the tricuspid position. The procedure was clinically successful (clinical improvement, increased exercise tolerance, decreased peripheral edema), but no morphologic assessment was available to indicate the degree of injury.

CONCLUSIONS

Because of clinically unpredictable results, catheter balloon valvuloplasty of stenotic bioprosthetic valves should be restricted to highly selected patients who have no evidence of thrombosis and who have no regurgitation or subvalvular fibrous tissue ingrowth.[7,8]

Acknowledgement: The authors thank *Clinical Cardiology* for their permission to reproduce text and figures for this chapter.[9,10]

REFERENCES

1. Waller BF, Van Tassel JW, McKay C: Anatomic basis for and morphologic changes produced by catheter balloon valvuloplasty and valvotomy. In: Bashore TM, Davidson CJ,

eds. *Percutaneous Balloon Valvuloplasty and Related Techniques*. Baltimore: Williams & Wilkins. 1991 pp 10–36.

2. Waller BF, Van Tassel JW, McKay C: Anatomic basis for and morphologic results from catheter balloon valvuloplasty of stenotic mitral valves. *Clin Cardiol*. 13:655–661, 1990.

3. Reifart N, Nowak B, Baykut D, et al: Experimental mitral valvuloplasty of fibrotic and calcified valves with balloon catheters. *J Am Coll Cardiol*. 5:448, 1985.

4. Schoen FJ, Levy R: Bioprosthetic heart valve failure: pathology and pathogenesis. In: Waller BF, ed. Symposium on Cardiac Morphology. *Cardiol Clin*. 2(4):717–739, 1984.

5. Schoen FJ, Kujovich JL, Levy RJ, et al: Bioprosthetic valve failure. In: Waller BF, ed. Contemporary Issues in Cardiovascular Pathology. Cardiovascular Clinics Ser, Vol 18, No. 12. FA Davis, p 289–317, 1988.

6. Ferrans VJ, Tomita Y, Hilbert SL, et al: Evaluation of operatively excised prosthetic tissue valves: In: Waller BF, ed. Pathology of the Heart and Great Vessels. Contemporary Issues in Surgical Pathology Vol 12. Churchill Livingstone, p 311–329, 1988.

7. McKay CR, Waller BF, Hong R, et al: Problems encountered with catheter balloon valvuloplasty of bioprosthetic aortic valves. *Am Heart J*. 115:463–465, 1988.

8. Feit F, Stecy PJ, Nachamie MS: Percutaneous balloon valvuloplasty for stenosis of a porcine bioprosthesis in the tricuspid valve position. *Am J Cardiol*. 58:363–364, 1986.

9. Waller BF, McKay C, Van Tassel J, et al: Catheter balloon valvuloplasty of stenotic porcine bioprosthetic valves: Part I: anatomic considerations. *Clin Cardiol*. 14:686–691, 1991.

10. Waller BF, McKay C, Van Tassel J, et al: Catheter balloon valvuloplasty of stenotic porcine bioprosthetic valves: Part II: mechanisms, complications and recommendations for clinical use. *Clin Cardiol*. 14:764–772, 1991.

CHAPTER **18**

Conduits and Conduit Valves

DONALD J. HAGLER

The application of valved and nonvalved extracardiac conduits heralded the development of a new era in the management of complex forms of congenital heart disease. Its most important and persistent application has been in the treatment of patients who require an extracardiac communication between the right or pulmonary ventricle and the pulmonary artery. These pioneering efforts by Ross[1] and Rastelli[2] and their associates provided the mechanism for subsequent repair in many children with pulmonary atresia, ventricular septal defect or transposition of the great arteries with ventricular septal defect and pulmonary stenosis. Although truly gratifying results were obtained from these surgical interventions, the conduit itself remains an Achilles' heel because of recurring stenosis. Despite efforts to employ many different conduit materials, recurrent stenosis has been the eventual result.

Especially in children and adolescents, valved and nonvalved conduits often progressively calcify, or develop intimal peel, or both, leading to obstruction. Surgical replacement of conduits and grafts can be performed at relatively low mortality but is accompanied by morbidity associated with repeat thoracotomy and cardiotomy. If the conduit obstruction is predominantly at the valve, surgical exchange represents an easy solution; however, proximal and, to an even greater extent, distal conduit stenoses present more complex and challenging problems. Some efforts have been directed at graft replacement without associated valve replacement; however, many patients have variable degrees of pulmonary hypertension or limited pulmonary distribution in which a valved conduit is mandatory. To date, no valved conduit can guarantee reliable and persistent function with a long term that would allow freedom from recurrent stenosis and subsequent replacement. Thus, once a conduit valve has been replaced, one must anticipate that inevitably the countdown for eventual re-replacement has begun. Conduit stenosis may occur early when patient size may not allow replacement with an adult-sized conduit that would eventually be required. A method of interim palliation would be helpful to reduce the total number of cardiac operations required and to allow planning of such operations that would be more compatible with the patient's projected growth. In addition, delaying potential conduit replacements allows additional time before the projected life expectancy of the next conduit begins.

Balloon dilatation is now the therapy of choice for pulmonary valve stenosis and has been increasingly used to relieve stenoses in nearly every portion of the cardiovascular system. Since 1986, balloon dilatation of conduit valves has been used at the Mayo Clinic to provide an interim palliative method for relief of conduit valve stenosis.[3] Successful conduit valve balloon valvuloplasty requires significant attention to appropriate patient selection so that a relatively small number of patients have had balloon valvuloplasty. To date, 14 such patients have been included. Two additional patients with right atrium–right ventricle conduits have also undergone balloon valvuloplasty or angioplasty, so that a total of 10 male and 6 female patients with a mean age of 14.0 years have been included. Nine patients had had previous repair of pulmonary atresia with ventricular septal defect or complex tetralogy of Fallot. Three patients had a Rastelli repair of complete transposition of the great arteries with ventricular septal defect. One had a Damus-Stansel-Kaye repair of complete transposition with intact ventricular septum, one a Dacron graft enlargement of the pulmonary artery after a modified Fontan operation, and one a Hancock conduit from the right atrium to the right ventricle as a modified Fontan procedure. The mean time between conduit placement and balloon dilatation was approximately 6.5 years with a range of 3 to 9.8. The clinical data concerning these patients are summarized in Table 18.1.

Table 18.1 FEATURES OF 16 PATIENTS UNDERGOING BALLOON DILATION OF CONDUITS AND CONDUIT VALVES

Case	Age, yr	Gender	Diagnosis	Conduit
1	11	M	PA, VSD	18-mm Tascon[a]
2	19	F	PA, VSD	26-mm Ion-Shiley[b]
3	21	F	PA, VSD	22-mm Hancock
4	18	M	PA, VSD	22-mm Ion-Shiley
5	7	M	PA, VSD	18-mm Ion-Shiley
6	15	M	Tetralogy of Fallot	25-mm Hancock
7	14	M	Tetralogy of Fallot	25-mm Hancock
8	21	F	Rastelli – TGA, VSD	25-mm Hancock
9	12	F	Rastelli – TGA, VSD	22-mm Ion-Shiley
10	7	M	Kaye-Damus – TGA, IVS	18-mm C-Edwards[c]
11	14	M	Fontan – tricuspid atresia	Dacron graft
12	10	F	PA, VSD	18-mm Tascon
13	7	M	Rastelli – TGA, VSD	22-mm Tascon
14	18	F	PA, VSD	22-mm Hancock
15	15	M	Truncus	25-mm Hancock
16	20	M	Fontan – tricuspid atresia	23-mm Hancock

[a] Tascon (18-mm) conduit with porcine heterograft valve

[b] Ionescu-Shiley valve, Dacron conduit

[c] Dacron (18-mm) conduit with Carpentier-Edwards valve.

IVS – intact ventricular septum. PA – pulmonary atresia. TGA – transposition of great arteries.
VSD – ventricular septal defect.

PROCEDURE

Complete right heart catheterization data including cardiac output determination by indocyanine green dye curve or oximetry before dilatation has been obtained. Precise withdrawal recordings are obtained from the pulmonary artery through the conduit into the right ventricle to clearly delineate individual sites of conduit obstruction. Thus, pressure recordings should be obtained from the individual pulmonary arteries back to the main pulmonary artery, and subsequently into the distal conduit, proximal conduit, and finally the right ventricle. In this fashion, several sites of conduit obstruction should be delineated. Selective angiography also is critical to precise definition of sites of conduit obstruction. Multiple views may be necessary for clinical delineation of all aspects of the conduit and pulmonary artery anatomy. Patients who have severe proximal conduit obstruction secondary to sternal conduit compression or distortion of the conduit should be excluded from further consideration for conduit dilatation. In addition, those patients who have suggestive evidence of obstructive intraluminal peel are excluded.

Although distal conduit obstructions or branch pulmonary artery stenoses may be considered appropriate for balloon angioplasty procedures, this precise subject is not included in this discussion. Many of the patients included in this series did have conduit obstruction at more than one conduit site, and several had conduit obstruction at the distal anastomoses. In these patients attempts were made to dilate the distal conduit as well as the conduit valve itself. They were successful in 13 out of 14 patients with a reduction of the conduit gradient by an average of 59%.

Most patients had successful balloon dilatation using a single balloon catheter which was equal to or slightly larger than the predicted conduit diameter based on the manufacturer's classifications. Two balloons were used in two patients in an attempt to obtain easier access through the conduit valve. The computed combined catheter area equaled the predicted conduit valve area.

One or two 0.038-inch (0.097 cm) tight J-tipped exchange guidewires were advanced into the distal right or left pulmonary artery through an end-hole or balloon-wedge catheter. Although advancing the dilating balloon across the obstructed conduit was difficult in the 16 patients, it was accomplished in all but one. The most effective maneuver to facilitate balloon passage through the conduit valve was the use of an 0.038-inch extra-stiff exchange guidewire (Amplatz, Cook, Inc.) Additionally, silicone lubricant was applied directly to the balloon, Mullins transseptal sheath was placed in the right ventricular outflow tract to allow catheter advancement without catheter buckling, and a smaller balloon catheter was wedged in the valve commissure to facilitate the valve opening and subsequent advancement of a second, larger balloon across the central lumen.

Patients underwent two to eight inflations at 3.2 to 12 atm. Following the balloon dilatation, repeat measurements of pulmonary artery and right heart pressures and cardiac output determinations were obtained. Repeat right ventricular or selective conduit angiography should be obtained to assess the results of dilatation and to reaffirm the integrity of the proximal and distal conduit.

In 14 patients with a right ventricular–pulmonary artery conduit, the mean right ventricular peak systolic pressure before dilatation was 99 ± 21 mmHg. The mean right ventricle to pulmonary artery peak systolic gradient was 71 ± 20 mmHg, whereas the mean conduit valve peak systolic gradient was 51 ± 20 mmHg. The difference between the mean right ventricular to pulmonary artery and the mean conduit valve gradients thus represents the additional gradient either at the proximal or distal anastomotic sites or resulting from an intraluminal peel. Two of the patients had an additional peripheral pulmonary artery stenosis.

HEMODYNAMIC RESULTS OF BALLOON DILATATION (FIG. 18.1)

The mean conduit valve peak systolic gradient in 13 patients who underwent successful conduit valve dilatation decreased by 61% with a drop from 46 mmHg before to 18 mmHg after dilatation. The mean right ventricle to pulmonary artery gradient was reduced by only 42% from 65 to 38 mmHg, reflecting little change in the

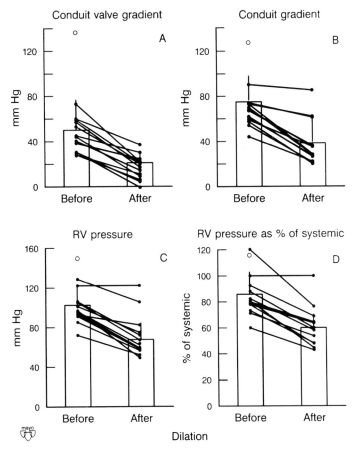

Figure 18.1 *A.* Conduit valve gradient before and after balloon dilatation in 13 patients. *B*, Right ventricle–pulmonary artery gradient before and after balloon dilatation. *C,* and *D,* Right ventricular (*RV*) pressure (*C*) and percentage of systemic pressure (*D*) before and after balloon dilatation. The *open circle* represents a 14th patient in whom the dilatation balloon could not be passed across the stenotic valve. The *vertical bar* represents standard deviation. (From: Ensing GJ et al: Caveats of balloon dilation of conduits and conduit valves. *J Am Coll Cardiol.* 14:397–400, 1989. With permission.)

associated proximal or distal conduit stenoses. The mean right ventricular pressure for these patients decreased by 28%, from 99 to 71 mmHg. Although all 14 patients had right ventricular systolic pressures greater than 70% of systemic pressure before dilatation, 9 patients had right ventricular systolic pressures less than 70% of systemic after dilatation.

In 12 of the 14 patients undergoing balloon conduit valve dilatation, surgery was either delayed or avoided. Two of these patients have subsequently returned for conduit replacement 1.5 and 4 years after balloon conduit valvuloplasty. In the latter patient, the initial valve gradient of 48 mmHg was reduced by the balloon valvuloplasty procedure to 21 mmHg. When the patient returned 4 years later, the conduit valve gradient had increased to approximately 30 mmHg. He underwent conduit replacement at that time because of increasing proximal and distal stenoses.

One patient with a known history of ventricular ectopy died suddenly, approximately 2 years following conduit valve balloon dilatation. Persistent distal conduit stenosis had been recognized at the time of his conduit valve dilatation. Two patients in this group underwent dilatation of a conduit placed from the right atrium to the right ventricle. One patient had a valveless Dacron graft. The conduit stenosis in this patient appeared to be at the distal conduit anastomosis; however, during dilatation, it was evident that the stenosis was secondary to an intraluminal peel and therefore not amenable to balloon dilatation. This patient had his graft replaced surgically. A second patient with a modified Fontan procedure had a 23-mm Hancock-valved conduit from the right atrium to the right ventricle. There was clear evidence of conduit valve stenosis with a peak end-diastolic gradient of 10 mmHg and a mean gradient of 7 to 9 mmHg. Following conduit valve balloon dilatation, the peak end-diastolic gradient was reduced to 5 mmHg with a mean diastolic gradient of 4 mmHg. Although the procedure was technically successful, this patient had persistently elevated right atrial and pulmonary artery pressures. He subsequently had surgical conduit replacement in association with left atrioventricular valve repair.

COMPLICATIONS

Significant complications of conduit dilatation can occur. Disruption of the intraconduit peel could lead to progressive conduit obstruction and acute hemodynamic deterioration. Disruption of the distal or proximal conduit anastomoses may cause formation of a false aneurysm. Dense periconduit fibrosis may have prevented this event in our patients. However, we avoided excessive balloon sizes (no greater than 1–2 cm larger than the conduit valve).

Balloon rupture occurs more commonly with conduit valve dilatation than with dilatation of native valves. We evaluated six balloon ruptures. Two types of balloon ruptures were of special concern (Fig. 18.2). In the patient with the stenotic right atrium–pulmonary artery graft after a Fontan operation, a portion (approximately 1.5 cm^2) of the ruptured dilation balloon was noted to be missing when the balloon was removed (Fig. 18.2A). The dilatation was unsuccessful, and the patient underwent reoperation several days later. Residual balloon fragments were not found. The patient was discharged after an uneventful postoperative course. Calcific spicules in the conduit may have lacerated the balloon.

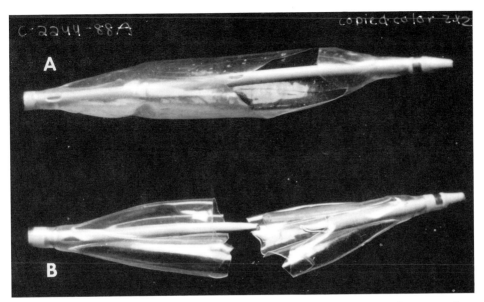

Figure 18.2 Atypical balloon ruptures. *A*, Absence of balloon fragment (*arrowheads*). *B*, Circumferential rupture with catheter separation. See text for details. (From: Ensing GJ et al: Caveats of balloon dilation of conduits and conduit valves. *J Am Coll Cardiol.* 14: 397–400, 1989. With permission.)

Another balloon rupture and complication occurred during successful dilatation of the stenotic Hancock conduit valve (Fig. 18.2*B*). A circumferential balloon rupture occurred at 3.8 atm, possibly in relation to high balloon wall tension located at the calcified conduit valve. On withdrawal, the distal balloon everted and lodged in the iliac vein, and further manipulation resulted in catheter breakage, with the distal part of the balloon and the catheter remaining in the femoral vein but on the wire that had been left in place. While direct pressure was held over the distal fragment and the supporting exchange wire to prevent embolic migration, a second wire loop was advanced over the fragment, through the same femoral vein but a different percutaneous site, and the distal wire and fragment were retrieved and brought to the second percutaneous site. The catheter fragment could be pulled into the femoral vein but had to be removed by surgical cutdown. The patient was discharged the following day, without problems secondary to this complication.

This experience is similar to that of Lloyd and associates,[5] who reported that balloon rupture occurred in more than half of their patients and that a transverse tear with evulsion of a balloon fragment requiring surgical removal from the iliac vein occurred in 1 of their 6 patients. The incidence of balloon rupture as well as atypical balloon rupture is increased with stenotic bioprosthetic conduits. As suggested by Lloyd and associates,[5] irregular calcification and calcific spicules likely cause asymmetrical balloon tension and increased balloon distortion in the region of the calcific deposits. This result predisposes to balloon rupture and to possible circumferential rupture or fragment loss. On the basis of this experience, our policy is never to overinflate the balloon catheter beyond recommended pressures during dilatation of prosthetic conduits and grafts.

DISCUSSION

Our results indicate that, although technically more challenging, balloon dilatation of stenotic heterograft valves and prosthetic conduits can be performed in most patients. The conduit valve gradient was reduced by 59%. This experience also was confirmed by Waldman and associates[4] and Lloyd and associates,[5] who used balloon dilatation successfully to reduce conduit valve gradient in 4 and 3 patients respectively.

Sources of Conduit Stenosis: Role of Balloon Dilatation

In an earlier pathologic study,[6,7] conduit valve stenosis alone was found to be the major obstruction in only 46% of patients, whereas 30% have a thick fibrous intimal peel and 24% have anastomotic stenoses. Dilatation of nonvalvular conduit stenosis due to either anastomotic stenosis or intraconduit peel may be unsuccessful. The noncompressibility of conduit peel was documented by Edwards and associates,[6] who described thick fibrous neointimal peel, sometimes with organized thrombi, in the area between the neointimal peel and the conduit wall. It seems unlikely that such fibrotic material and thrombi could be significantly compressed by direct lateral pressure. Additionally, the neointimal peel could be dislodged or dissected from the conduit wall during catheter manipulation or balloon dilatation. None of the patients in our series had this complication, but cautious catheter and wire manipulation would be advised. Conduit stenosis at distal anastomotic sites involves a circumferential suture line with associated fibrosis and scarring, and, especially when this suture line is attached to a fixed circumference of the prosthetic conduit, easy distention seems unlikely. Although suture lines have been successfully dilated in the descending aorta after repair of coarctation,[8,9] those stenoses typically do not have the circumferential fixed conduit at one end of the anastomosis.

Effect On Conduit Valve Regurgitation

The effect of balloon dilatation on conduit valve regurgitation was not assessed. Echocardiography has demonstrated that conduit valves may be nonfunctional, immobile, and regurgitant before dilatation. In the absence of substantial right ventricular dilatation or significantly elevated distal pulmonary artery pressures, this regurgitation should be well tolerated for the period of palliation that is being sought.

Technical Considerations

Crossing the obstructed conduit valve with balloon dilatation catheters is often challenging. In most recent cases, the extra-stiff exchange guidewire proved adequate to prevent catheter buckling. The use of one balloon "wedged" in the valve commissure to help direct the second dilating balloon to the central lumen, together with the use of silicone lubricant to allow less balloon distortion and easier passage (both through the skin and through the valve), allowed balloon passage and performance of dilatation in 13 of 14 patients with conduit valve obstruction.

CONCLUSIONS

Balloon dilatation of conduits and grafts can be performed safely and successfully to allow temporary reduction of right ventricular pressure and to delay conduit replacement, allow for more ideal surgical scheduling, and reduce the total number of thoracotomies. A substantial reduction in conduit valve gradient can be expected without a significant effect on proximal anastomotic stenoses or an intraconduit peel. Risk of balloon rupture as well as atypical balloon rupture with potential fragment loss seems to be increased in these patients, and inflation pressures should be limited to the level recommended by the manufacturer.

REFERENCES

1. Ross DN, Somerville J: Correction of pulmonary atresia with homograft aortic valve. *Lancet*. 2:1446–1447, 1966.
2. Rastelli GC, McGoon DC, Wallace RB: Anatomic correction of transposition of the great arteries with ventricular septal defect and subpulmonary stenosis. *J Thorac Cardiovasc Surg*. 58:545–551, 1969.
3. Ensing GJ, Hagler DJ, Seward JB, et al: Caveats of balloon dilation of conduits and conduit valves. *J Am Coll Cardiol*. 14:397–400, 1989.
4. Waldman JD, Schoen FJ, Kirkpatrick SE, et al: Balloon dilatation of porcine bioprosthetic valves in the pulmonary position. *Circulation*. 76:109–114, 1987.
5. Lloyd TR, Marvin WJ Jr, Mahoney LT, et al: Balloon dilation valvuloplasty of bioprosthetic valves in extracardiac conduits. *Am Heart J*. 114:268–274, 1987.
6. Edwards WD, Agarwal KC, Feldt RH, et al: Surgical pathology of obstructed, right-sided, porcine-valved extracardiac conduits. *Arch Pathol Lab Med*. 107:400–405, 1983.
7. Agarwal KC, Edwards WD, Feldt RH, et al: Clinicopathological correlates of obstructed right-sided porcine-valved extracardiac conduits. *J Thorac Cardiovasc Surg*. 81:591–601, 1981.
8. Lababidi ZA, Daskalopoulas DA, Stoeckle H Jr: Transluminal balloon coarctation angioplasty: experience with 27 patients. *Am J Cardiol*. 54:1288–1291, 1984.
9. Lock JE, Bass JL, Amplatz K, et al: Balloon dilation angioplasty of aortic coarctations in infants and children. *Circulation*. 68:109–116, 1983.

CHAPTER 19

Concurrent Multivalve Balloon Valvuloplasty

TSUNG O. CHENG

Begun as an isolated procedure for relief of stenosis of a single cardiac valve, percutaneous balloon valvuloplasty has recently been expanded to include patients with multivalve stenoses. As a matter of fact, Roberts[1] on January 1, 1987, predicted that balloon dilatation of more than one heart valve could be accomplished concurrently. One month later in February 1987, the first combined balloon valvuloplasty for aortic and pulmonic valves was reported from Brazil.[2] In August 1987 a group from the Massachusetts General Hospital, Boston, described combined valvuloplasty for mitral and aortic valves.[3] Concurrent valvuloplasty for combined mitral and tricuspid stenoses was reported from China in February 1988.[4] Concurrent tricuspid and pulmonic balloon valvuloplasty was also reported by the same group from China in July 1988.[5] The first successful triple-valve balloon dilatation in the same setting was reported from Brazil in 1987.[6] No case of concurrent balloon dilatation at same setting of all four heart valves has been reported as of this writing.

COMBINED AORTIC AND MITRAL VALVULOPLASTY

Rationale

Because of the frequent involvement of both mitral and aortic valves in rheumatic heart disease and the logistics of percutaneous balloon valvuloplasty, it is not difficult to understand why concurrent mitral and aortic valvuloplasty came to be the most frequently combined procedure performed to date. Patients with combined severe aortic and mitral stenoses require mechanical relief of their valvular obstructions. Until recently, the only option was surgery with either valve replacement or commissurotomy. Advanced age and other medical problems increase the morbidity and mortality of valvular surgery, especially when double valve replacements are considered. With the excellent results obtained by percutaneous balloon valvuloplasty on patients with either isolated mitral stenosis or isolated aortic stenosis, a combined procedure presents itself as a logical and attractive alternative for these patients.

Approaches

Both the aortic and mitral valves can be balloon-dilated by either the retrograde or antegrade approach. For percutaneous balloon aortic valvuloplasty, the retrograde technique is the usual approach. For simultaneous mitral valvuloplasty the technique described by Babic and associates,[7] in which the balloon catheter is inserted percutaneously from the left femoral artery over a long guidewire previously introduced into the right femoral vein, advanced transseptally to the left ventricle, and drawn out of the left ventricle by means of a retrieval device, has several obvious advantages. It avoids the creation of an iatrogenic interatrial septal defect, it allows easy placement of the balloon in the mitral valve orifice, and permits easy fixation of the balloon in place during inflation.

For percutaneous balloon mitral valvuloplasty the transseptal approach is an integral part of the procedure. Since balloon aortic valvuloplasty can also be performed by an antegrade approach,[8,9] both the mitral valve and aortic valve can be dilated transseptally, and the local arterial complications of the retrograde approach for balloon aortic valvuloplasty can thereby be avoided.

Sequence

The sequence of concurrent valve dilatation is usually the aortic first followed by the mitral valve. Many operators prefer this order for three reasons. First, if mitral valvuloplasty were performed before aortic dilatation, increased left ventricular diastolic filling might cause significant increases in both diastolic and systolic wall stress in a previously "protected" left ventricle. In the setting of unrelieved significant aortic stenosis, this increase in wall stress could lead to significant left ventricular subendocardial ischemia. Second, since mitral balloon valvuloplasty is commonly accompanied by a major and acute decline in systemic blood pressure during balloon inflation, it could be dangerous in the presence of critical aortic stenosis. Third, should significant mitral regurgitation occur following balloon mitral valvuloplasty, the hemodynamic consequences may be serious if unrelieved significant aortic stenosis is present. With this sequence, it is important to emphasize that the transseptal catheterization should be performed before the aortic valvuloplasty to obviate the need for and risks of systemic anticoagulation prior to attempted transseptal puncture.

On the other hand, others prefer to dilate the mitral valve before the aortic for four reasons. First, because transseptal puncture should be performed in a nonanticoagulated patient, the performance of the procedure is simpler if mitral valvuloplasty has been carried out first. Second, by enhancing the forward flow of blood with mitral valvuloplasty one can prevent the hypotension that may occur during balloon aortic valvuloplasty. Third, should significant aortic regurgitation result from balloon aortic valvuloplasty, any mitral regurgitation that might otherwise be inconsequential after balloon mitral valvuloplasty may be poorly tolerated. Fourth, in a patient with combined aortic and mitral stenoses it sometimes may be difficult to assess the relative hemodynamic severity of each lesion, especially in a patient with a reduced cardiac output in whom the gradient across the aortic valve may be either underestimated in the presence of concomitant mitral stenosis or overestimated in the presence of coexistent regurgitation.[10] By first performing percutaneous balloon mitral valvuloplasty one can then be in a better position to assess the severity of the coexistent aortic stenosis and the need for intervention by either balloon valvuloplasty or valve replacement.

The issue of a preferred sequence of valve dilatation in combined mitral and aortic stenoses is therefore not entirely settled and may be answered only by further clinical experience.

Results

Percutaneous balloon valvuloplasty for combined mitral and aortic stenoses has generally yielded very gratifying results.[3,11-13] Hemodynamic improvement is usually instantaneous (Fig. 19.1) It has several other advantages over combined valve replacement. First, it is a nonsurgical procedure. Second, it has a lower morbidity and mortality, a shorter hospital stay, and lower hospital costs than combined mitral and aortic valve replacement. Third, there is no need to make a therapeutic decision — a difficult one at times especially in young, pregnant patients and in women of child-bearing age — between the choice of a bioprosthesis and a mechanical prosthesis for a given valve. Fourth, in patients with a small mitral valve annulus and a narrow aortic root, valve replacement with a small prosthesis may be followed by a high residual gradient.[12] Fifth, with balloon valvuloplasty there is no need of long-term anti-coagulant therapy with its attendant complications. Sixth, if restenosis should occur, the percutaneous procedure of balloon valvuloplasty can be easily repeated for both valves. In this regard balloon valvuloplasty is ideally suited for treatment of mitral restenosis following either closed or open commissurotomy[14-16] (also see Chapter 12). With an operative mortality for repeat surgical commissurotomy as high as 10%,[16] percutaneous balloon valvuloplasty offers an attractive alternative. Seventh, in a critically ill patient with combined mitral and aortic stenoses, double valvuloplasty by the percutaneous balloon technique allows time for hemodynamic stabilization of the patient for later elective single or double valve replacement should it prove necessary.

COMBINED MITRAL AND TRICUSPID VALVULOPLASTY

Combined mitral and tricuspid stenosis is not uncommon in patients with rheumatic heart disease. Since successful balloon valvuloplasty is possible for pure mitral stenosis and isolated tricuspid stenosis, combined valvuloplasty for coexisting mitral and tricuspid stenosis has become an attractive alternative to surgical therapy[4,17-21] (Figs. 19.2 and 19.3).

The sequence of dilatation is first the mitral valve, then the triscuspid. This is because of the concern that concomitant mitral stenosis may lead to worsening pulmonary congestion once obstruction at the tricuspid valve is relieved by balloon valvuloplasty. On the other hand, in the presence of significant tricuspid stenosis with marked elevation of right atrial pressure, a prompt decrease of left atrial pressure following successful balloon mitral valvuloplasty may bring about an abrupt right-to-left shunting across the atrial septum, thereby inducing serious systemic hypoxemia.[21] Therefore it is recommended that two Cournand catheters be placed in the pulmonary artery to facilitate quick exchange and prompt dilatation of the stenotic tricuspid valve should such an emergency situation arise.[21]

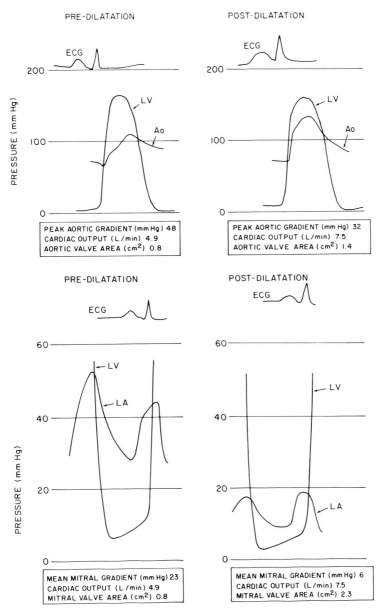

Figure 19.1 Patient with combined aortic and mitral stenoses. Aortic pressure gradients (*top*) and mitral pressure gradients (*bottom*) before and after concurrent aortic and mitral valvuloplasty. *Ao*—aortic pressure. *ECG*—electrocardiogram. *LA*—left atrial pressure. *LV*—left ventricular pressure. *POST*—after dilatation. *Pre*—before dilatation. Valve areas and cardiac outputs are listed below. (From: Berman AD et al: Combined aortic and mitral balloon valvuloplasty in patients with critical aortic and mitral stenosis: results in six cases. *J Am Coll Cardiol.* 11:1213–1218, 1988. With permission.)

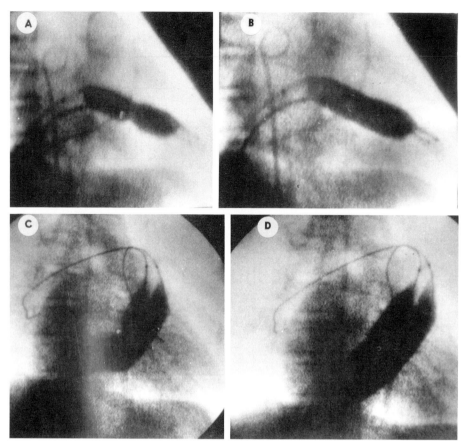

Figure 19.2 Patient with combined mitral and tricuspid stenoses undergoing concurrent percutaneous double balloon mitral (*top*: A—before, *B*—after) and tricuspid (*bottom: C*—before, *D*—after) valvuloplasty. (From: Sharma S et al: Concurrent double balloon valvotomy for combined rheumatic mitral and tricuspid stenosis. *Cathet Cardiovasc Diagn.* 23:42–46, 1991. Reprinted by permission of Wiley-Liss, a division of John Wiley & Sons, Inc. © 1991.)

Percutaneous balloon mitral valvuloplasty is a well-established technique and has been thoroughly covered in Chapters 9–12. The technique of balloon dilatation of a stenotic tricuspid valve (see also Chapter 16) merits some discussion. One of the problems likely to be encountered with balloon tricuspid valvuloplasty is determining the optimal balloon size to achieve the best results. Dilatation by a single balloon may not be adequate to relieve the obstruction; using two balloons may lead to significant tricuspid regurgitation. Therefore the tricuspid annulus should be measured either by echocardiography or angiocardiography[21] and the appropriate double-balloon combination selected as described by Dorros and associates.[22] Alternatively, the size of the balloon may be determined by repeatedly measuring gradients until optimal reduction is achieved.

The other problem during balloon tricuspid valvuloplasty is the precise position of the balloon across the tricuspid valve so that the waist of the stenotic valve is at the center of the balloon. Shrivastava and associates[17] determined the site of the tricuspid valve orifice by withdrawing the end-hole catheter from the right ventricle to the

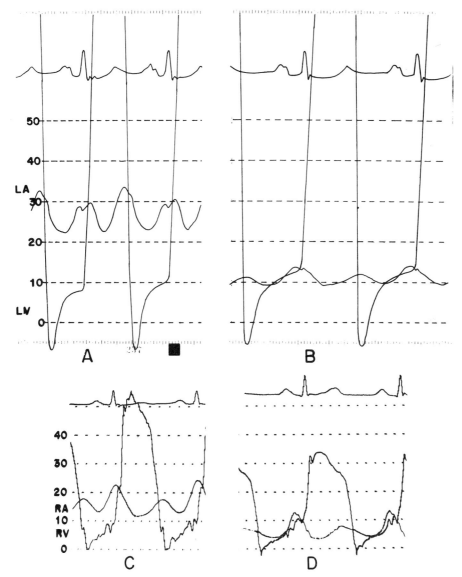

Figure 19.3 *A, B,* Transmitral and *C, D,* transtricuspid gradients before (left) and after (right) concurrent balloon mitral and tricuspid valvuloplasty. (From: Sharma S et al: Concurrent double balloon valvotomy for combined rheumatic mitral and tricuspid stenosis. *Cathet Cardiovasc Diagn.* 23:42–46, 1991. Reprinted by permission of Wiley-Liss, a division of John Wiley & Sons, Inc. © 1991.)

right atrium; this allowed positioning the center of the balloon catheter at the transition of the right ventricular pressure tracing to the right atrial tracing. Al Zaibag and associates[23] determined the site of the tricuspid orifice by injecting contrast medium into the right atrium. Sharma and associates[21] located the tricuspid valve annulus by freezing the right ventricular cineangiographic images on the video screen in 10° right anterior oblique projection.

The long-term results of combined mitral and tricuspid balloon valvuloplasty are not yet known. However, so far the accumulated experience indicates that the procedure appears to be an effective alternative to operation. Palliation with combined balloon valvuloplasty is particularly advantageous for women during their childbearing period.

COMBINED TRICUSPID AND PULMONIC VALVULOPLASTY

Combined right-sided valvular stenoses are not common. They represent either congenital heart disease[5] or carcinoid heart disease.[24]

Congenital Heart Disease

Chen and associates[5] reported in 1988 the first case of concurrent percutaneous balloon valvuloplasty for combined tricuspid and pulmonic stenoses $11\frac{1}{2}$ years following open valvotomies. Their patient was a 55-year-old Chinese woman who had undergone open valvotomies for congenital tricuspid and pulmonic stenoses $11\frac{1}{2}$ years earlier. She remained well for $6\frac{1}{2}$ years and then developed right-sided failure which was refractory to digoxin and diuretic therapy. Because the patient refused reoperation, percutaneous balloon valvuloplasty was offered as an alternative. Right heart catheterization confirmed the presence of combined tricuspid and pulmonic stenoses. Right heart angiograms (Fig. 19.4) revealed marked right atrial enlargement, moder-

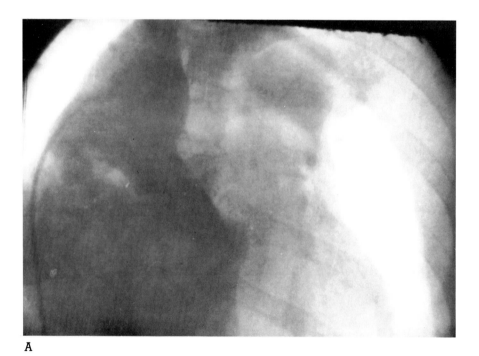

A

Figure 19.4 Cineangiograms of right atrium (A) and right ventricle (B) before and of right ventricle (C) after concurrent percutaneous balloon valvuloplasty for combined tricuspid and pulmonic stenoses. (From: Chen CR et al: Concurrent percutaneous

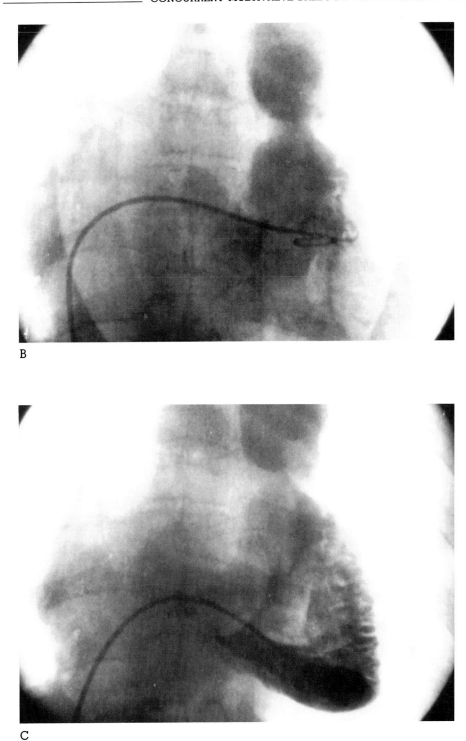

B

C

balloon valvuloplasty for combined tricuspid and pulmonic stenoses. *Cathet Cardiovasc Diagn.* 15:55–60, 1988. Reprinted by permission of Wiley-Liss, a division of John Wiley & Sons, Inc. © 1988.)

ately severe tricuspid stenosis with mild tricuspid regurgitation, and moderately severe pulmonic stenosis.

Following the same principle as in combined left-sided valvular stenosis the pulmonic valve was dilated first by means of the Inoue balloon catheter, followed by the tricuspid valve (Fig. 19.5). There is a technical reason for dilating the pulmonic valve first. As mentioned earlier, it may be difficult to align the balloon properly across the tricuspid valve, not only because the valve plane may be difficult to establish with certainty under fluoroscopy but also because the relatively small size of the right ventricle makes alignment of balloon toward the ventricular apex difficult. Therefore, passing the guidewire first out the pulmonic valve into the pulmonary artery as in balloon pulmonic valvuloplasty will give better stability to the balloon.[25]

At the end of the combined pulmonic and tricuspid valvuloplasty, pressure measurements showed a decrease of the pulmonic valve systolic gradient from 9 to 4 mmHg, of right atrial mean pressure from 18 to 5 mmHg, and of the tricuspid valve diastolic gradient from 16 to 1 mmHg. Right ventriculography showed the diameter of the pulmonic valve orifice to have increased from 6 to 14 mm and the diameter of the tricuspid valve orifice to have increased from 13 to 27 mm with a slight increase in tricuspid regurgitation (see Fig. 19.4–C). The patient's functional status improved from New York Heart Association class III to II, and her leg edema, ascites, and peripheral cyanosis all disappeared. On a two-dimensional echocardiogram taken 7 weeks following balloon valvuloplasty, the diameter of the right atrium decreased from 100 to 81 mm (Fig. 19.6). Her cardiac rhythm was subsequently converted by oral quinidine from atrial fibrillation to sinus rhythm (Fig. 19.7).

Carcinoid Heart Disease

The characteristic valvular lesions in carcinoid heart disease are pulmonic stenosis and tricuspid regurgitation.[24] However, tricuspid stenosis also may occur, either in association with tricuspid regurgitation[24] or as a predominent lesion, in which case it may be amenable to balloon valvuloplasty.[26] In the case reported by Rajan and associates,[27] the stenosis across either the pulmonic valve or the tricuspid valve was not considered severe enough to warrant balloon valvuloplasty.

Percutaneous balloon valvuloplasty of both pulmonic and tricuspid stenoses caused by carcinoid heart disease is a feasible and viable alternative to surgical treatment. The prognosis of the underlying disease for these patients is poor; if palliative cardiac surgery could be avoided, the patients' qualify of life could be much improved by this nonsurgical approach.[28]

COMBINED PULMONIC AND AORTIC VALVULOPLASTY

Congenital stenoses of both the pulmonic and aortic valves may coexist in the same patient. Fontes and associates[2] reported successful percutaneous balloon valvuloplasty in a 10-year-boy with stenoses of both the pulmonic and aortic valves during the same

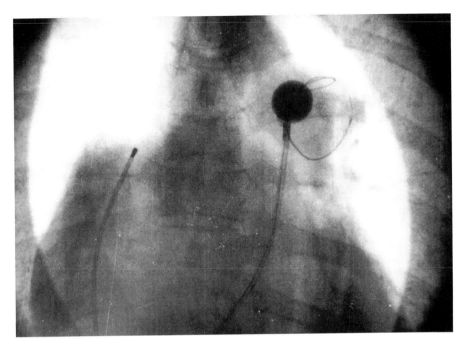

A

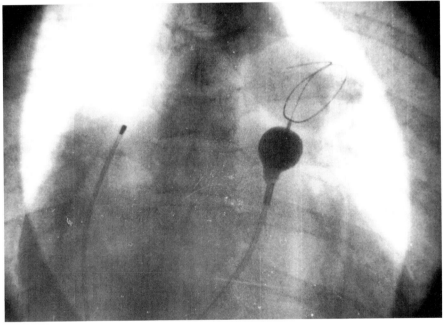

B

Figure 19.5 Concurrent balloon valvuloplasty of stenotic pulmonic (*A,B,C*) and tricuspid (*D,E,F*) valves. During pulmonic valvuloplasty, the distal portion of the balloon above the pulmonic valve on inflation expanded first (*A*), followed by the proximal portion (*B*) as inflation continued. Balloon indentation produced by the stenotic pulmonic valve nearly disappeared after the second inflation (*C*).

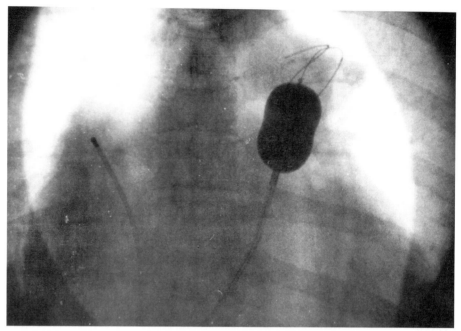

C

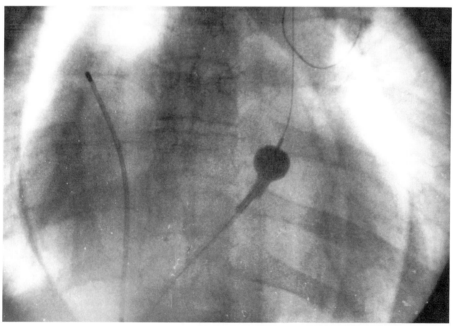

D

Figure 19.5 (continued)   For tricuspid valvuloplasty, the distal portion of the balloon was situated in the inflow portion of the right ventricle (*D*). Balloon indentation at the level of the stenotic tricuspid valve was nearly obliterated after the first inflation (*E*),

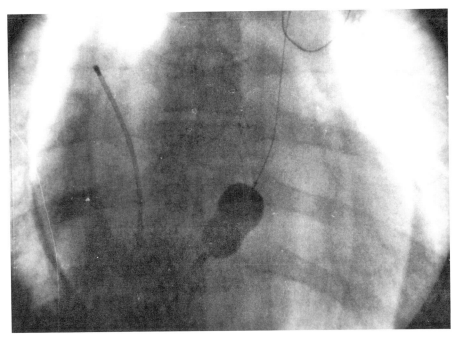

E

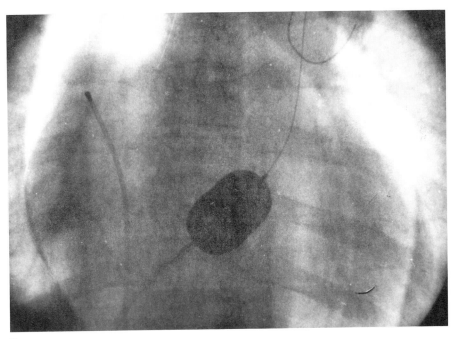

F

and completely obliterated after the second inflation. (*F*). (From: Chen CR et al: Concurrent percutaneous balloon valvuloplasty for combined tricuspid and pulmonic stenoses. *Cathet Cardiovasc Diagn.* 15:55–60, 1988. Reprinted by permission of Wiley-Liss, a division of John Wiley & Sons, Inc. © 1988.)

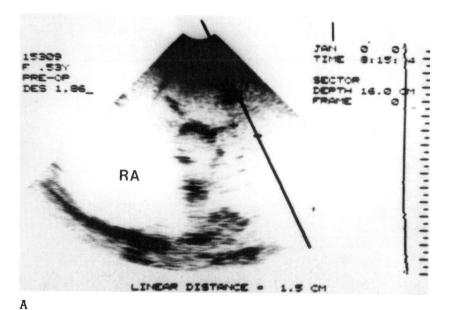

Figure 19.6 Two-dimensional echocardiograms before (*A*) and after (*B*) concurrent percutaneous balloon tricuspid and pulmonic valvuloplasty. *RA*—right atrium. *LA*—left atrium. *Ao*—aorta. (From: Chen CR et al: Concurrent percutaneous balloon valvuloplasty for combined tricuspid and pulmonic stenoses. *Cathet Cardiovasc Diagn.* 15:55–60, 1988. Reprinted by permission of Wiley-Liss, a division of John Wiley & Sons, Inc. © 1988.)

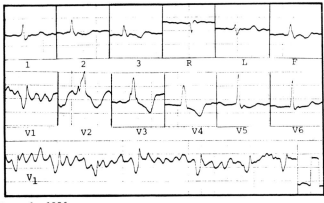

Dec. 1, 1986

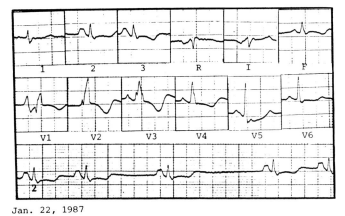

Jan. 22, 1987

Figure 19.7 Electrocardiograms before (*top*) and after (*bottom*) concurrent percutaneous balloon valvuloplasty for combined tricuspid and pulmonic stenosis. (From: Chen CR et al: Concurrent percutaneous balloon valvuloplasty for combined tricuspid and pulmonic stenoses. *Cathet Cardiovasc Diagn.* 15:55–60, 1988. Reprinted by permission of Wiley-Liss, a division of John Wiley & Sons, Inc. © 1988.)

session of a cardiac catheterization. They were able to reduce the systolic pressure gradient across the pulmonic valve from 78 to 15 mmHg (Fig. 19.8, *upper*), and across the aortic valve from 75 to 30 mmHg (Fig. 19.8, *lower*).

Although Fontes and associates chose to dilate the pulmonic valve first and then the aortic valve, the distal valve should preferably be dilated before the proximal one, ie, the aortic valve before the pulmonic valve. The reasons are the same as those for choosing the aortic valve as the site of initial balloon dilatation in combined aortic and mitral stenoses (see foregoing discussion). However, the interposition of the pulmonary capillary bed between the pulmonic and aortic valves makes such a choice less crucial.

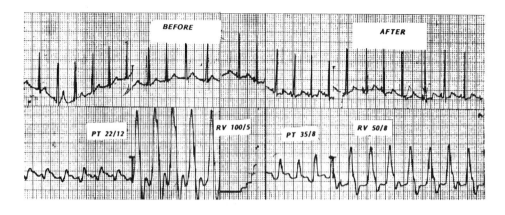

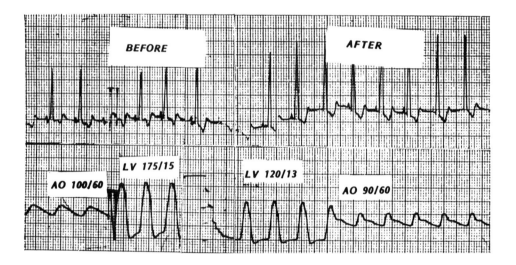

Figure 19.8 Transpulmonic systolic gradient was reduced from 78 to 15 mmHg (*top*) and transaortic systolic gradient from 75 to 30 mmHg (*bottom*) following concurrent percutaneous balloon pulmonic and aortic valvuloplasty. (From: Fontes VF et al: Double valvuloplasty with aortic and pulmonary balloon catheter. A case report. *Arq Bras Cardiol.* 48:105–107, 1987. With permission.)

COMBINED TRICUSPID AND AORTIC VALVULOPLASTY

Combined stenosis of the tricuspid and aortic valves is unusual. Buchler[29] in 1987 reported one such combination in a 20-year-old woman. Using a 20-mm balloon for both valves (Fig. 19.9), he reduced her tricuspid end-diastolic gradient from 4 to 0 mmHg and her aortic peak systolic gradient from 40 to 20 mmHg in the same procedure. This patient later underwent combined percutaneous balloon mitral and tricuspid valvuloplasty too. (Buchler JR, personal communication, April 23, 1991).

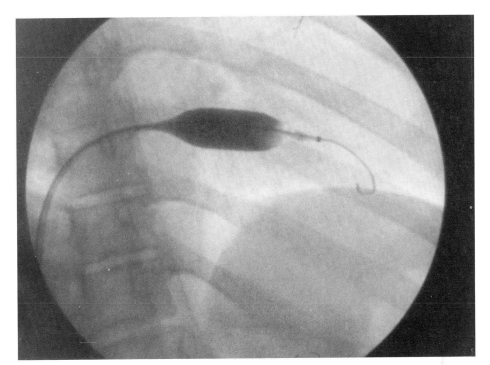

A

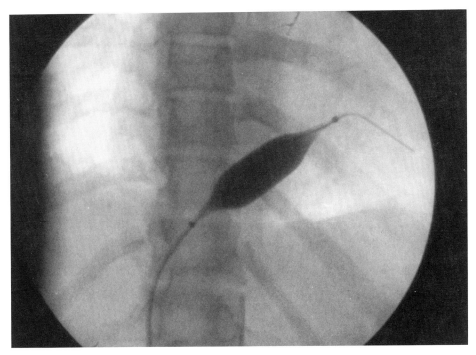

B

Figure 19.9 Concurrent percutaneous balloon valvuloplasty for combined stenosis of tricuspid (*A* and *B*) and aortic (*C* and *D*) valve. The "waist" produced by the stenosis at the beginning of balloon inflation is far less apparent with the tricuspid (*A*) than the aortic (*C*) valve owing to the comparatively larger orifice size of the former than the latter. (Courtesy of Jorge Roberto Buchler, M.D.)

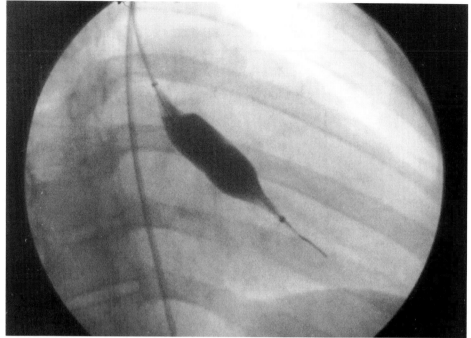

C

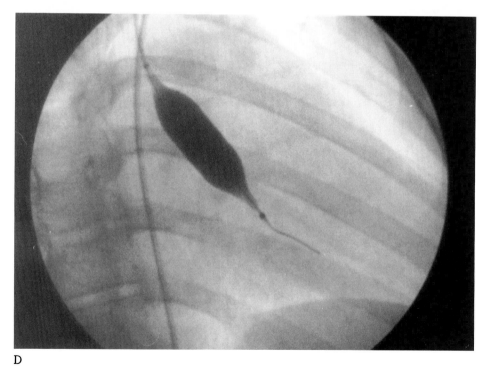

D

Figure 19.9 (Continued)

COMBINED AORTIC, MITRAL, AND TRICUSPID VALVULOPLASTY

Triple valve involvement of clinical significance is rare but exists in rheumatic heart disease. In 1989 Cheng[30] mentioned that his colleagues in China considered a 34-year-old Chinese woman for triple valvuloplasty by the percutaneous balloon technique for relief of aortic stenosis, mitral stenosis, and tricuspid stenosis resulting from rheumatic fever in childhood. However, the procedure was deferred because of coexistence of moderate tricuspid regurgitation.

In 1990 the group from Loma Linda University[31] described the successful sequential dilatation in the same procedure of mitral, aortic and tricuspid valves using the percutaneous double-balloon technique (Fig. 19.10, *upper*). In a 35-year-old native-born white woman with rheumatic mitral, aortic, and tricuspid stenoses, Konugres and associates[31] were able to increase the mitral valve area from 0.8 cm^2 to 2.9 cm^2, the aortic valve area from 0.5 cm^2 to 3.2 cm^2, and the tricuspid valve area from 1.0 cm^2 to more than 4.0 cm^2. Admittedly, with three stenotic valves in tandem, the measurement of cardiac output, pressure gradient, and valve area is rather difficult to assess: Not only are all dependent on the effective cardiac output, which may change significantly from beat to beat, but also the reduction of one valvular obstruction changes the entire hemodynamic effect of the other two valves. Nevertheless, the reduction in the pressure gradients across the three valves was impressive. (Fig. 19.10, *lower*).

The Loma Linda group chose to dilate the mitral valve first for two reasons: (1) to enhance the forward flow of blood with venous loading to prevent hypotension and (2) because transseptal puncture should be done in a nonanticoagulated patient. Of note was the fact that the peak baseline aortic systolic gradient rose from 64 to 74 mmHg following balloon mitral valvuloplasty, illustrating once again how the gradient across the aortic valve may be underestimated in the presence of concomitant mitral stenosis.[10]

One other patient has been reported in the literature to have undergone successful concurrent balloon valvuloplasty of mitral, aortic, and tricuspid valves.[6] In this case from Brazil a single balloon was used, and both the aortic and mitral dilatations were accomplished by the transarterial retrograde technique.

COMBINED PULMONIC, AORTIC, AND MITRAL VALVULOPLASTY

Al Zaibag[32] successfully performed a triple-valve balloon dilatation of pulmonic, aortic, and mitral valves in one patient (Fig. 19.11, *top*). Marked reduction of the transvalvular gradient across each of the three cardiac valves was achieved by concurrent percutaneous balloon valvuloplasty (Fig. 19.11, *bottom*).

COMPLICATIONS

Complications of multivalve percutaneous balloon valvuloplasty may or may not exceed those of a single valve procedure, depending on the circumstances. Mitral regurgitation, a most feared complication of percutaneous balloon mitral valvulo-

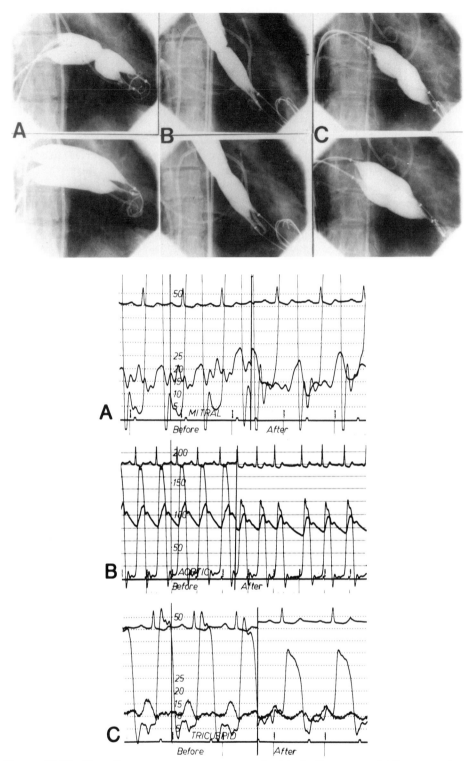

Figure 19.10 *Top,* Concurrent percutaneous double-balloon mitral (*A*), aortic (*B*), and tricuspid (*C*) valvuloplasty. *Bottom,* Simultaneous pressure tracings before and after concurrent percutaneous balloon mitral (*A*), aortic (*B*), and tricuspid (*C*) valvuloplasty, showing marked reduction of all the transvalvular gradients after successful balloon trivalvular dilatations. (From: Konugres GS et al: Successful percutaneous double-balloon mitral, aortic and tricuspid valvotomy in rheumatic trivalvular stenosis. *Am Heart J.* 119:663–666, 1990. With permission.)

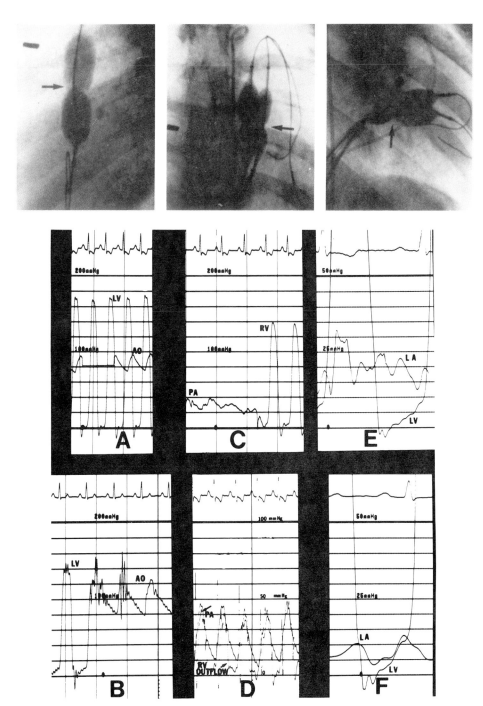

Figure 19.11 *Top,* Balloons across the stenotic aortic (*left*), pulmonary (*middle*), and mitral (*right*) valves in lateral, anteroposterior, and right anterior oblique views, respectively. Note the indentations around the balloons in early inflation (*arrows*). Bottom, Simultaneous pressure tracings before (*upper panel*) and after (*lower panel*) percutaneous balloon valvuloplasty of the aortic (*A* and *B*), pulmonary (*C* and *D*), and mitral (*E* and *F*) valves, showing the marked reduction of the transvalvular gradients across the three cardiac valves after successful balloon dilatations. *AO*—aorta. *LA*—left atrium. *LV*—left ventricle. *PA*—pulmonary artery. *RV*—right ventricle. (From: Topol EJ: *Textbook of Interventional Cardiology.* Philadelphia: WB Saunders Co, 1990. With permission.)

plasty, is usually not significant[33]; as a matter of fact, mitral regurgitation tends to improve either immediately following balloon valvuloplasty[34] or at followup.[33] However, massive mitral regurgitation has been reported to result from tearing of the anterior mitral leaflet during percutaneous balloon mitral valvuloplasty[35] or from rupture of mitral chordae during percutaneous balloon aortic valvuloplasty.[36] When this occurs, the hemodynamic consequences may be significant either in the presence of unrelieved aortic stenosis or with concomitant aortic regurgitation following concurrent balloon aortic valvuloplasty.

On the right side of the heart, rupture of tricuspid valve papillary muscle during balloon pulmonic valvuloplasty has been reported.[37] On a theoretical grounds there may be an increased risk of producing tricuspid regurgitation in combined pulmonic and tricuspid valvuloplasty in which the long balloon may straddle portions of both valves in the presence of a hypertrophied right ventricle with a small cavity. Whereas isolated pulmonic regurgitation following pulmonic balloon valvuloplasty or iatrogenic tricuspid regurgitation following tricuspid balloon valvuloplasty is usually well tolerated, combined pulmonic and tricuspid regurgitation may not be.

CONCLUSIONS

Percutaneous balloon valvuloplasty seems to be a very effective alternative for patients with multivalve stenoses, especially in young women of childbearing age in whom the anticoagulant therapy that is required following prosthetic valve replacement poses hazards to both the mother and the fetus. Furthermore, morbidity and mortality of multiple valve replacement are rather high. Then there is a big cost difference. Therefore percutaneous balloon valvuloplasty is an ideal form of therapy for multivalve stenoses, especially in developing countries where rheumatic heart disease is still common, open heart surgical facilities are either unavailable or inaccessible, and resources in health care delivery are generally limited.

The evolution of percutaneous multivalve balloon valvuloplasty parallels that of percutaneous multivessel balloon coronary angioplasty. When percutaneous transluminal coronary angioplasty was first introduced over a decade ago, its use was restricted to patients with single-vessel coronary artery disease. As experiences increased, percutaneous transluminal coronary angioplasty has subsequently become a routine procedure in multivessel coronary disease. So has percutaneous balloon valvuloplasty, which has now been expanded from treatment of stenosis of a single heart valve to combined valve stenoses. Another parallelism is the fact that whereas percutaneous balloon angioplasty has been successfully applied to coronary artery bypass grafts, percutaneous balloon valvuloplasty has also been employed with some degree of success in stenoses of bioprosthetic valves (see Chapter 17).

I predict that percutaneous balloon valvuloplasty of two or three cardiac valves will become a common practice in the near future. With increased operative expertise and technical improvements of the balloon catheters, the radiation time for multivalve balloon valvuloplasty as well as the risk should become acceptable.

The sequence in which concurrent balloon dilatation in multivalve stenoses should be carried out is always the most distal first. In other words:

1. In double valve stenoses affecting both aortic and mitral valves, the aortic valve should be dilated first.

2. In double valve stenoses affecting one left-sided and one right-sided valve, the left-sided stenosis should be dilated first.

3. In combined stenoses of the right-sided valves, the pulmonic valve should be dilated first.

4. In triple valve involvement, dilatation of the left-sided valve(s) should precede the right, and aortic (or pulmonic) valvuloplasty should precede mitral (or tricuspid) valvuloplasty.

REFERENCES

1. Roberts WC: Good-bye to thoracotomy for cardiac valvulotomy. *Am J Cardiol.* 59:198–202, 1987.

2. Fontes VF, Esteves CA, Silva MVD, et al: Double valvuloplasty with aortic and pulmonary balloon catheter. A case report. *Arq Bras Cardiol.* 48:105–107, 1987.

3. Kritzer GL, Block PC, Palacios I: Simultaneous percutaneous mitral and aortic valvotomies in an elderly patient. *Am Heart J.* 114:420–423, 1987.

4. Chen CR, Lo ZX, Huang ZD, et al: Percutaneous double balloon valvuloplasty for a patient with mitral and tricuspid stenoses. *Guangdong Med J.* 9(2):29–30, 1988.

5. Chen CR, Lo ZX, Huang ZD, et al: Concurrent percutaneous balloon valvuloplasty for combined tricuspid and pulmonic stenoses. *Cathet Cardiovasc Diagn.* 15:55–60, 1988.

6. Buchler JR: Percutaneous balloon dilation of rheumatic mitral stenosis by the transarterial approach. *J Am Coll Cardiol.* 10:1366–1367, 1987.

7. Babic UU, Pejcic P, Djurisic Z, et al: Percutaneous transarterial balloon valvuloplasty for mitral valve stenosis. *Am J Cardiol.* 57:1101–1104, 1986.

8. Block PC, Palacios IF: Comparison of hemodynamic results of anterograde versus retrograde percutaneous balloon aortic valvuloplasty. *Am J Cardiol.* 60:659–662, 1987.

9. Grollier G, Commeau Ph, Agostini D, et al: Anterograde percutaneous transseptal valvuloplasty in a case of severe aortic stensis. *Eur Heart J.* 8:190–193, 1987.

10. Cheng TO: *The International Textbook of Cardiology.* New York: Pergamon Press, 1987, pp 494–495.

11. Berman AD, Weinstein JS, Safian RD, et al: Combined aortic and mitral balloon valvuloplasty in patients with critical aortic and mitral valve stenosis: results in six cases. *J Am Coll Cardiol.* 11:1213–1218, 1988.

12. McKay CR, Kawanishi DT, Chatterjee S, et al: Stenotic aortic and mitral valves treated with catheter balloon valvuloplasty in a patient with small valve anuli. *Ann Intern Med.* 108:568–569, 1988.

13. Medina A, Bethencourt A, Coello I, et al: Combined percutaneous mitral and aortic balloon valvuloplasty. *Am J Cardiol.* 64:620–624, 1989.

14. Medina A, Suarez De Lezo J, Hernandez E, et al: Balloon valvuloplasty for mitral restenosis after previous surgery: a comparative study. *Am Heart J.* 120:568–571, 1990.

15. Rath PC, Berland J, Gamra H, et al: Balloon mitral valvotomy for mitral restenosis after surgical commissurotomy: immediate result and followup. *J Am Coll Cardiol.* 17:253A, 1991.

16. Rediker DE, Block PC, Abascal VM, et al: Mitral balloon valvuloplasty for mitral restenosis after surgical commissurotomy. *J Am Coll Cardiol.* 11:252–256, 1988.

17. Shrivastava B, Radhakrishnan S, Dav V: Concurrent balloon dilatation of tricuspid and calcified mitral valve in a patient of rheumatic heart disease. *Int J Cardiol.* 20:133–137, 1988.

18. Romao N, Prytzlik R, Salles Netto M, et al: Mitral and tricuspid valvuloplasty with balloon catheterization in the same procedure. A case report. *Arq Bras Cardiol.* 53:333–338, 1989.

19. Berland J, Rocha P, Mechmeche R, et al: Percutaneous valvulotomy for combined mitral and tricuspid stenosis. Results in 3 cases. *Arch Mal Coeur.* 83:1585–1589, 1990.

20. Bethencourt A, Medina A, Hernandez E, et al: Combined percutaneous balloon valvuloplasty of mitral and tricuspid valves. *Am Heart J.* 119:416–418, 1990.

21. Sharma S, Loya YS, Daxini BV, et al: Concurrent double balloon valvotomy for combined rheumatic mitral and tricuspid stenosis. *Cathet Cardiovasc Diagn.* 23:42–46, 1991.

22. Dorros G, Lewin RF, King JF, et al: Percutaneous transluminal valvuloplasty in calcific aortic stenosis: the double balloon technique. *Cathet Cardiovasc Diagn.* 13:151–156, 1987.

23. Al Zaibag M, Ribeiro P, Al Kasab S: Percutaneous balloon valvotomy in tricuspid stenosis. *Br Heart J.* 57:51–53, 1987.

24. Ross EM, Robert WC: The carcinoid syndrome: comparison of 21 necropsy subjects with carcinoid heart disease to 15 necropsy subjects without heart disease. *Am J Med.* 79:339–354, 1985.

25. Hurst JW: *The Heart.* New York:McGraw-Hill, 1990, p 2175.

26. Mullins PA, Hall JA, Shapiro LM: Balloon dilatation of tricuspid stenosis caused by carcinoid heart disease. *Br Heart J.* 63:249–250, 1990.

27. Rajan A, Titus T, Venkitachalam CG, et al: Tricuspid and pulmonary valve involvement in carcinoid syndrome. *Indian Heart J.* 40:67–71, 1988.

28. Cheng TO: Nonsurgical treatment of carcinoid heart disease. *Ann Thorac Surg.* 51:1046–1047, 1991.

29. Buchler JR: Percutaneous balloon dilation of rheumatic mitral stenosis by the transarterial approach. *J Am Coll Cardiol.* 10:1366–1367, 1987.

30. Cheng TO: Multivalve percutaneous balloon valvuloplasty. *Cathet Cardivasc Diagn.* 16:109–112, 1989.

31. Konugres GS, Lau FYK, Ruiz CE: Successive percutaneous double-balloon mitral, aortic, and tricuspid valvotomy in rheumatic trivalvular stenosis. *Am Heart J.* 119:663–666, 1990.

32. Al Zaibag M, Ribeiro PA: The future of balloon valvotomy. In: Topol EJ. *Textbook of Interventional Cardiology.* Philadelphia: WB Saunders Co, 1990, pp 923–924.

33. Abascal VM, Wilkins GT, Choong CY, et al: Echocardiographic evaluation of mitral valve structure and function in patients followed for at least 6 months after percutaneous balloon mitral valvuloplasty. *J Am Coll Cardiol.* 12:606–615, 1988.

34. Chen CR, Lo ZX, Huang ZD, et al: Percutaneous transseptal balloon mitral valvuloplasty: the Chinese experience in 30 patients. *Am Heart J.* 115:937–947, 1988.

35. Cequier A, Bonan R, Crepeau J, et al: Massive mitral regurgitation caused by tearing of the anterior leaflet during percutaneous mitral balloon valvuloplasty. *Am J Med.* 85:100–103, 1988.

36. Baudouy PY, Masquet C, Eiferman C, et al: An exceptional complication of percutaneous aortic valvuloplasty: rupture of an aberrant mitral chorda. *Arch Mal Coeur.* 81:227–230, 1988.

37. Attia I, Weinhaus L, Walls JT, et al: Rupture of tricuspid valve papillary muscle during balloon pulmonary valvuloplasty. *Am Heart J.* 114:1233–1235, 1987.

Concurrent Balloon Valvuloplasty and Coronary Angioplasty

RICHARD M. POMERANTZ
DANIEL J. DIVER
ROBERT D. SAFIAN

Valvular heart disease is frequently associated with coronary artery disease, particularly in elderly patients. Significant coronary artery disease occurs in 20 to 60% of patients with aortic stenosis, depending on the population studied.[1] Similarly, symptomatic coronary artery disease occurs in 10 to 20% of patients with mitral stenosis, although the incidence may approach 35 to 50% at necropsy in patients older than 30 years.[2] Therefore, treatment of concomitant coronary artery disease may be necessary in some patients considered for percutaneous balloon valvuloplasty.

RISKS OF SURGICAL AND NONSURGICAL INTERVENTIONS

Risks of Open Heart Surgery

There are no direct comparisons of open heart surgery and catheter-based techniques in patients with valvular heart disease and concomitant coronary artery disease. Available data suggest that aortic valve replacement is the procedure of choice for most adult patients with symptomatic aortic stenosis, in whom the perioperative mortality rate is less than 1 to 3%. Although the need for concomitant coronary artery bypass surgery increases the risks of open heart surgery, perioperative mortality is less than 5% in most patient populations. However, octogenarians with aortic stenosis have a perioperative mortality of 9 to 30%,[3,4] and the need for concomitant bypass surgery may result in a two- to fourfold increase in perioperative mortality in these elderly patients.[5]

Some patients with rheumatic mitral stenosis may be candidates for open commissurotomy, and recent studies suggest a perioperative mortality of less than 1%.[6] Patients who are not suitable candidates for open commissurotomy may require mitral valve replacement, which is usually associated with a perioperative mortality of 4 to 10%,[7] and the need for concomitant coronary artery bypass grafting may further increase the perioperative mortality to 3 to 20%.[7]

Risks of Balloon Valvuloplasty

Even though balloon aortic valvuloplasty is usually applied to elderly patients with advanced heart failure, the incidence of procedure-related complications is relatively low. The risk of death is 1 to 5%; of stroke, myocardial infarction, or damage to the aortic valve or annulus 1%; and of cardiac perforation 0.5%.[8] Although the immediate risks of balloon aortic valvuloplasty compare favorably to the perioperative risks of aortic valve replacement, the long-term results of balloon aortic valvuloplasty are limited by the high rate of restenosis, which approaches 80% at 2 years. Thus, patients with aortic stenosis should be considered for balloon aortic valvuloplasty (with or without concomitant coronary angioplasty) if they are not candidates for aortic valve replacement.

For patients with mitral stenosis, the immediate risks of balloon mitral valvuloplasty also compare favorably to those reported for open commissurotomy or mitral valve replacement: The risk of death is 2%; of stroke or damage to the mitral valve apparatus 1%; and of cardiac perforation 2%.[9] However, the best immediate and long-term results of balloon mitral valvuloplasty and open commissurotomy are achieved in patients with low echocardiographic scores ($\leq$ 8), based on leaflet mobility, leaflet thickening, calcification, and subvalvular disease.[9] In patients with high echocardiographic scores ($\geq$ 12), the long-term results of mitral valvuloplasty (and open commissurotomy) may be suboptimal, and mitral valve replacement may be the preferred treatment.

TECHNIQUE AND SEQUENCE OF COMBINED PROCEDURE

In general, patients should be considered for combined percutaneous balloon valvuloplasty and percutaneous transluminal coronary angioplasty if they meet the usual indications for each procedure. We do not recommend coronary angioplasty of asymptomatic coronary artery disease or of lesions of sufficient complexity to preclude coronary angioplasty under usual circumstances. There are two approaches to the technique of concomitant balloon valvuloplasty and coronary angioplasty. These procedures may be performed sequentially at the same sitting, or as staged procedures on separate days. In most cases it is possible to identify the most significant lesion on the basis of the patient's symptoms, hemodynamic data, and angiographic findings. We prefer to approach the most significant lesion first, followed by the second procedure, in a sequential or staged manner as clinically indicated. A staged approach is preferred in situations where the indications for the second procedure are not clear, or in situations where complications or technical problems arise during the first procedure.

Sequential Balloon Aortic Valvuloplasty and Coronary Angioplasty

Theoretically, it might be preferable to perform aortic valvuloplasty prior to coronary angioplasty to decrease wall stress and subendocardial ischemia. On the other hand, balloon valvuloplasty could lead to transient hypotension, and the transient decrease in coronary perfusion pressure could cause significant ischemia in the presence of a severe coronary stenosis. In fact, Rosseau and coworkers[11] demonstrated significant "low flow" ischemia in patients undergoing aortic valvuloplasty, manifested by decreases in coronary blood flow and myocardial oxygen uptake, and increases in myocardial lactate production. However, these parameters were not influenced by the presence or absence of coronary artery disease. Clinical experience in large numbers of patients suggests that significant ischemia is rare in patients with severe aortic stenosis and coronary artery disease undergoing balloon aortic valvuloplasty.

In elderly patients with syncope and congestive heart failure, we generally recommend balloon aortic valvuloplasty via the retrograde femoral approach, followed by coronary angioplasty as indicated. If symptoms are limited to angina alone, it may be difficult to determine whether aortic stenosis or coronary artery disease is most important. In this situation, we prefer to perform balloon aortic valvuloplasty first, since balloon aortic valvuloplasty is generally well tolerated in patients with severe coronary artery disease, and since abrupt closure following coronary angioplasty may be poorly tolerated in patients with critical aortic stenosis. However, factors that favor coronary angioplasty prior to balloon aortic valvuloplasty might include a history of unstable angina, angiographic demonstration of impaired flow (TIMI grade ≤ 2) or presence of intraluminal thrombus, and disease involving the ostium of the right coronary artery.

Sequential Balloon Mitral Valvuloplasty and Coronary Angioplasty

In most patients with severe mitral stenosis and coronary artery disease the transseptal puncture should be completed before the administration of heparin. Then, balloon mitral valvuloplasty can be performed safely via the antegrade approach, followed by coronary angioplasty via the retrograde approach, as indicated.

RESULTS

Hemodynamic and Angiographic Results

Although the data on balloon valvuloplasty and concomitant coronary angioplasty are limited, the immediate results and complications of the combined procedures are similar to those of the procedures performed individually. Hamad and associates[12] and Ports and associates[13] reported successful sequential coronary angioplasty and balloon aortic valvuloplasty with good results. Hamad and associates[14] and Vandormeael and associates[15] reported successful outcomes of staged balloon aortic valvuloplasty and coronary angioplasty. McKay and coworkers[16] reported the results of balloon aortic valvuloplasty and concomitant coronary angioplasty in 9 patients with symptomatic aortic stenosis and single-vessel coronary artery disease. Eight of nine patients had coronary angioplasty and balloon aortic valvuloplasty as a single procedure and one patient had aortic valvuloplasty followed by coronary angioplasty 10 days later. Coronary angioplasty was successful in all nine patients with a reduction in the diameter of stenosis from 91% to 29%. Balloon aortic valvuloplasty reduced the mean gradient from 60 to 39 mmHg, and increased the aortic valve area from 0.7 to 1.1 cm². In-hospital followup revealed no change in radionuclide left ventricular ejection fraction but eight of nine patients had significant symptomatic improvement.

One patient with persistent angina required aortic valve replacement and coronary artery bypass grafting.

Complications

Complications of the combined procedures are similar to those of the procedures performed individually. Although distal embolization is uncommon during both mitral and aortic valvuloplasty,[8,9] occasional episodes of systemic embolization to cerebral, hepatic, and coronary arterial circulations have been reported. Deligonul and coworkers[17] reported acute lateral wall myocardial infarction immediately after aortic valve dilatation; it was caused by embolic occlusion of an obtuse marginal branch of the left circumflex artery (Fig. 20.1). Romanello and coworkers[18] reported

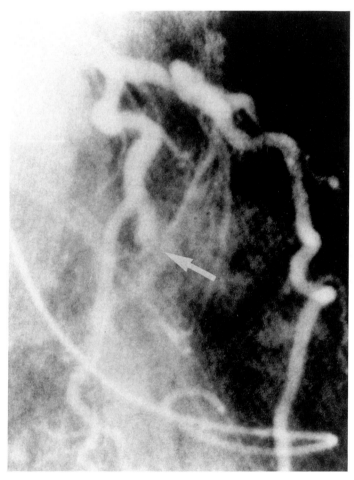

Figure 20.1 Coronary angiogram showing abrupt cutoff of the obtuse marginal branch of the left circumflex artery secondary to coronary embolus following percutaneous balloon aortic valvuloplasty. (From Deligonul U et al: Acute myocardial infarction during percutaneous aortic balloon valvuloplasty. *Cathet Cardiovasc Diagn.* 15:164–168, 1988. With permission.)

embolic occlusion of the proximal left anterior descending artery 10 minutes after balloon aortic valvuloplasty and emergent coronary angioplasty restored flow to the distal vessel with subsequent relief of ischemia (Fig. 20.2). Thus coronary angioplasty could be used as a "salvage" procedure in the rare event of coronary embolization or thrombosis following balloon valvuloplasty.

CONCLUSIONS

Valvular stenosis and concomitant coronary artery disease are often found within the population of patients referred for balloon valvuloplasty. Coronary angioplasty and percutaneous balloon valvuloplasty can be performed safely as a single or staged procedure with results and complications similar to those of the procedures done individually.

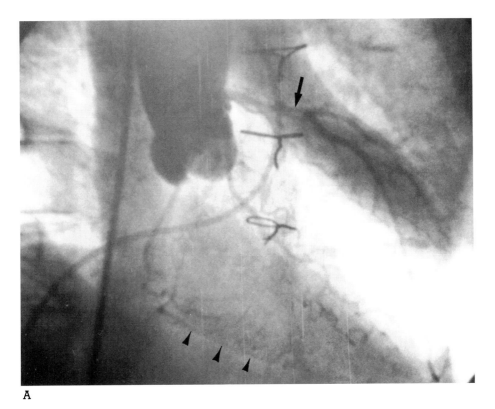

A

Figure 20.2 *A,* Aortogram prior to percutaneous balloon aortic valvuloplasty revealing good filling of the left anterior descending artery with a proximal severe stenosis (*arrow*). Collateral filling of a totally occluded right coronary artery is also noted (*arrowheads*). *B,* Aortogram following percutaneous balloon aortic valvuloplasty revealing an absence of dye beyond the proximal left anterior descending arterial obstruction (*arrow*). *C,* Post-dilatation angiogram with the angioplasty guidewire in the left anterior descending artery, revealing successful restoration of flow beyond the proximal stenosis. The diminution in distal flow (*arrows*) is due to either distal migration of the embolus or guidewire-induced spasm.

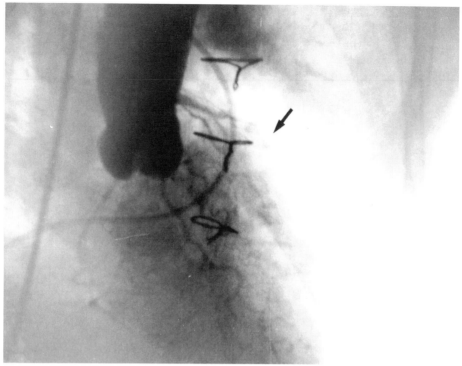

B

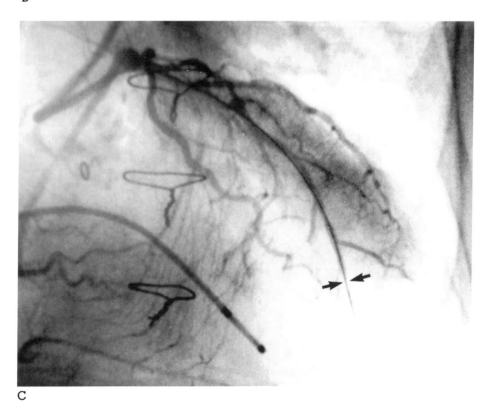

C

Figure 20.2 (Continued) (From: Romanello PP et al: Acute myocardial infarction complicating percutaneous aortic valvuloplasty successfully treated by percutaneous coronary angioplasty. *Am Heart J.* 119:953–955, 1990. With permission.)

REFERENCES

1. Exadactylos N, Sugrue DD, Oakley CM: Prevalence of coronary artery disease in patients with isolated aortic valve stenosis. *Br Heart J*. 51:121–124, 1984.

2. Reis RN, Roberts WC: Amounts of coronary arterial narrowing by atherosclerotic plaques in clinically isolated mitral valve stenosis: analysis of 76 necropsy patients older than 30 years. *Am J Cardiol*. 57:1117–1123, 1986.

3. Levinson JR, Akin CW, Buckley MJ, et al: Octogenarians with aortic stenosis: outcome after aortic valve replacement. *Circulation*. 80 (suppl I):I-49–I-56, 1989.

4. Edmunds LH Jr, Stephenson LW, Edie RN, et al: Open-heart surgery in octogenarians. *N Engl J Med*. 319:131–136, 1988.

5. Magovern JA, Pennock JL, Campbell DB, et al: Aortic valve replacement and combined aortic valve replacement and coronary artery bypass grafting: predicting high risk groups. *J Am Coll Cardiol*. 9:38–43, 1987.

6. Cohn LH, Allred EN, Cohn LA, et al: Long-term results of open mitral valve reconstruction for mitral stenosis. *Am J Cardiol*. 55:731–734, 1985.

7. Karp RB, Mills N, Edmunds LH Jr: Coronary artery bypass grafting in the presence of valvular disease. *Circulation*. 79 (suppl I): I-182–I-184, 1989.

8. Safian RD, Kuntz RE, Berman AD: Aortic valvuloplasty. *Cardiol Clin*. 9:289–299, 1991.

9. Block PC, Palacios IF: Aortic and mitral balloon valvuloplasty: the United States experience. In: Topol EJ. *Textbook of Interventional Cardiology*. Philadelphia: WB Saunders Co, 1990, p 861.

10. Mock MB, Holmes DR Jr, Vlietstra RE, et al: Percutaneous transluminal coronary angioplasty (PTCA) in the elderly patient: experience in the National Heart, Lung and Blood Institute PTCA Registry. *Am J Cardiol*. 53:89C–91C, 1984.

11. Rousseau MF, Wyns W, Hammer F, et al: Changes in coronary blood flow and myocardial metabolism during aortic balloon valvuloplasty. *Am J Cardiol*. 61:1080–1084, 1988.

12. Hamad N, Pichard A, Salomon J, et al: Combined percutaneous aortic valvuloplasty and coronary angioplasty. *Am Heart J*. 115:176–177, 1988.

13. Ports TA, Srebro JP, Manubens SM, et al: Simultaneous percutaneous aortic valvuloplasty and coronary artery angioplasty in an elderly patient. *Am Heart J*. 115:672–675, 1988.

14. Hamad N, Pichard A, Lindsay J: Combined coronary angioplasty and aortic valvuloplasty. *Am J Cardiol*. 60:1184–1186, 1987.

15. Vandormael M, Deligonul U, Gabliani, G, et al: Percutaneous balloon valvuloplasty and coronary angioplasty for the treatment of calcific aortic stenosis and obstructive coronary artery disease in an elderly patient. *Cathet Cardiovasc Diagn*. 14:49–52, 1988.

16. McKay RG, Safian RD, Berman AD, et al: Combined percutaneous aortic valvuloplasty and transluminal coronary angioplasty in adult patients with calcific aortic stenosis and coronary artery disease. *Circulation*. 76:1298–1306, 1987.

17. Deligonul U, Kern MJ, Bell ST, et al: Acute myocardial infarction during percutaneous aortic balloon valvuloplasty. *Cathet Cardiovasc Diagn*. 15:164–168, 1988.

18. Romanello PP, Moses JW, Wilentz JR, et al: Acute myocardial infarction complicating percutaneous aortic valvuloplasty successfully treated by percutaneous coronary angioplasty. *Am Heart J*. 119:953–955, 1990.

CHAPTER 21

Nonvalvular Lesions

CHARLES E. MULLINS

Attempts have been made to dilate almost all narrowed structures or orifices which occur in, or with, cardiac or vascular disease. Dilation of the four valves of the heart is discussed in other chapters. This chapter deals with the dilation of most other structures within the heart and great vessels. Many different areas have been attempted, some with reproducible success and others with only occasional success or even total failure. The information in this chapter is based on the experience at Texas Children's Hospital, from some personal communications, the data from the Valvuloplasty and Angioplasty of Congenital Anomalies (VACA) Registry,[1-7] and the literature.

COARCTATION OF THE AORTA

Experience with dilation of coarctation of the aorta — both recoarctation[8] and native lesions[9-13] — has been vast.

Recoarctation

Along with pulmonary valve stenosis, recoarctation of the aorta was one of the two earliest lesion to be dilated clinically.[8] The results in individual series and in the VACA data[5] were remarkably successful, with approximately 80% of 190 patients adequately reported having a reduction in the gradient across the coarctation to less than 20 mmHg and an 85% average increase in coarctation area diameter. In the VACA data there was no correlation between results and balloon/coarctation diameter, inflation pressure of the balloon, age at initial surgery, or the time interval between surgery and dilation. The type of previous surgery did not seem to affect results except that the coarctations repaired in conjunction with a Norwood-type procedure did seem to have a slightly better outcome from dilation.[5] Although interruption of the aortic arch is a different and usually more complex lesion, the types of repair in infancy and the mechanism of restenosis are the same, and the results of dilation seem to be the same. This lesion is therefore included in the discussion of dilation of recoarctation of the aorta.

The technique for dilating recoarctation of the aorta usually involves a single-balloon dilation using a balloon approximately the same size as the *smallest* adjacent "normal"-sized vessel. Because of the extensive guidewire manipulation and time within the left heart and ascending aorta plus the trauma to the femoral artery from the balloon introduction, these patients are systemically heparinized. At Texas Children's Hospital a prograde balloon catheter is advanced from the left ventricle into the ascending aorta and into the aortic arch proximal to the coarctation. A small monitoring cannula is placed in both femoral arteries at the beginning of the procedure. The diagnostic data and angiocardiograms are obtained, and the coarctation and the adjacent segments of the aorta are measured precisely using either a calibrated marker catheter or calibration grids. An end-hole catheter is passed from one femoral artery, retrograde across the coarctation, around the arch, and into the ascending aorta, with care being taken to stay out of the coronary arteries. An exchange wire is passed through this catheter and positioned securely in the ascending aorta. The appropriate balloon catheter is advanced to the area of coarctation and the balloon is inflated until its maximal pressure is reached or until the "waist" on the balloon disappears. The balloon is deflated in any case after 10 to 15 seconds. The balloon need merely be withdrawn out of the coarcted area to assess hemodynamic response. The catheter previously positioned in the aortic arch and the cannula in the opposite femoral artery allow immediate assessment of hemodynamic response with or without angiocardiography. The balloon need not be removed from the vessel, and catheters or wires need not be passed repeatedly through the recently dilated area. When the operator is satisfied with the results of the dilation, the wire is carefully withdrawn into the catheter and the balloon catheter is withdrawn out of the coarcted segment. Once the balloon tip is within the abdominal aorta the wire is readvanced several centimeters out of the balloon catheter and the balloon is withdrawn out of the vessel.

In the VACA series, there was a relatively high incidence of complications, including five deaths (2 vagal, 1 vessel rupture, 1 cerebrovascular accident and 1 shock of unknown cause) and 8.5% arterial injury. Changes in technique, added precautions, and improved balloon design have virtually eliminated these complications. The success of the procedure over the years, the reduction in complications, and the difficulties with repeat surgery[14] on these patients have made dilation of recoarctation the procedure of choice in most centers.[15,16]

Native Coarctation

Dilation of native coarctation, although acutely even more successful and having fewer acute complications than recoarctation dilation, remains more controversial. With native coarctation dilation the enlargement of the coarctation segment is better and the drop in gradient is greater than with recoarctation. The acute complications are significantly fewer and are mostly introductory-site vessel problems.[17] No long-term sequelae and only one death, in a sick infant, have been reported.[4] Even in the initial series, however, there were six reported "aneurysms" at the site of coarctation dilation.[18] Four of these patients went to surgery, not because of any acute problem, but because of the unknown and theoretical concern about these lesions. Pathologic examination of the removed aneurysms showed intimal and medial disruption but no old or recent extravasation of blood outside of the aorta. This reported experience with "aneurysms" has dampened the enthusiasm for this procedure in many centers. The incidence of these lesions was small initially and does not seem to be increasing. Those "aneurysms" which are seen usually are small outpouchings in the area of dilation; they usually do not seem to enlarge and there have been only rare reports of long-term adverse consequences.[19] With these data, many centers still perform dilation of native coarctation, with the stipulation that these patients are to be followed closely and indefinitely.[4,12,20-22]

The criteria for choice of balloon and the technique for dilation of native coarctation are identical to those for recoarctation. In the VACA data,[4] a slightly better overall result was obtained when a balloon slightly larger than the adjacent aorta was used. In the registry there was no statistical correlation between balloon to coarctation size and complications; at that time the "aneurysms" had been neither recognized nor reported as a potential problem.

In the VACA registry and in subsequent series, dilation of native coarctation in the newborn or young infant was usually acutely successful and relieved the symptoms of heart failure and acidosis. Most of these lesions recurred over the course of 1 to 6 months. However, when they did recur it was without signs of heart failure or decompensation so that further treatment could be totally elective. Many of these infants have had redilation or elective surgery of the coarctation. In this group of newborns and young, sick infants where the surgery is of higher risk[23,24] and more likely to result in recoarctation, there is a greater interest in the dilation of native coarctation where the benefits appear to outweigh the risks.

PULMONARY ARTERY BRANCH STENOSIS

Pulmonary artery branch stenosis, sometimes referred to as coarctation of the branch pulmonary arteries, occurs congenitally ("native"),[25] as a result of previous surgery[26] on or near the involved pulmonary artery, or as a combination of both mechanisms. Congenital branch pulmonary stenosis occurs in multiple forms, most frequently occurring with tetralogy of Fallot and then with involvement of the proximal branches of the pulmonary arteries.[27] These patients are also the most common type to have both congenital stenosis and acquired postoperative stenosis as a result of a previous shunt. Congenital branch pulmonary artery stenosis may occur as the only cardiac abnormality, or as part of a syndrome such as Williams' or rubella syndrome.[28] In the syndromic congenital cases and those without other cardiac anomalies, the stenosis appears more diffuse and more distal, and it often involves many segments of the lung vasculature. The vessels appear diffusely narrowed, often having one or more very discrete areas of stenosis within the diffuse segments. Pure postsurgical branch stenosis can occur in any patient who has had surgery on the pulmonary arteries, but particularly following systemic to pulmonary shunts. Although all types of systemic to pulmonary anastomoses have led to stenosis, the direct ascending aorta to right pulmonary artery (Cooley or Waterston) anastomosis was the most notorious for producing branch pulmonary artery stenosis and one of the more difficult or impossible for the surgeons to correct.[29] The combination of the location of the stenosis behind the aorta and the compression by the high-pressure adjacent ascending aorta adversely affects corrective surgical reconstructions.

All types of pulmonary branch stenoses have undergone dilation procedures, all with varying degrees of success. The degree of success with branch pulmonary artery dilation seems to have more to do with the criteria for success than the type of lesion, the technique, or the institution performing the dilation.[6,30] When any improvement in stenotic area diameter or any decrease in pressure gradient across the stenosis is the criterion of success, the procedure is quite successful. When enlargement of the diameter of the adjacent normal vessels and persistence of this dilated diameter over time are the determinants of success, then most of these lesions, when reevaluated angiographically and hemodynamically, will be considered failures!

The technique for dilation of these lesions is similar regardless of the etiology of the stenosis. A single-balloon technique is used because of the expected "round" configuration of the adjacent normal vessel and the generally smaller size of the pulmonary branch vessels. Since repeated pressure measurements and angiocardiograms will be necessary during the balloon dilations, it is recommended that a second venous catheter be introduced and advanced to the proximal main (or right or left) pulmonary artery before the dilation procedure is begun. Because of the total blood stasis and propensity to thrombosis created in vessels distal to inflated balloons, these patients should be systemically heparinized.

The area of stenosis and the adjacent vessels must be accurately measured. A selective pulmonary artery angiocardiogram using a calibrated catheter or calibration grid for reference is performed and the diameters of the stenotic area and the normal adjacent vessels are measured. A balloon 25 to 50% larger than the adjacent normal vessel diameter or, alternatively, three to four times the diameter of the narrowest segment of stenosis is chosen. An end-hole catheter is passed through the area of stenosis. It is replaced with an exchange length guidewire of as large a diameter as the balloon catheter to be used will accommodate. The balloon dilation catheter is passed over the wire and centered in the area of the most severe or discrete stenosis, care being taken not to let the distal end of the balloon extend too far into the more distal and usually much smaller peripheral vessel.

While the wire and the balloon are carefully controlled so that the balloon does not "squirt" forward off of the wire into the more distal vessel, the balloon is inflated to its maximum pressure limit or until the waist on the balloon disappears. If the balloon begins to move during inflation, inflation should be stopped immediately and the balloon, the wire, or both repositioned to a more fixed position. Unless the contralateral pulmonary artery is absent or severely stenosed, the balloon can be left inflated for 15 to 60 seconds without compromise of overall hemodynamics. If the area does not respond to dilation by means of a standard balloon, a high pressure balloon can be tried. These high pressure balloons can be inflated with as much as 16 atmospheres of pressure but, of course, at these pressures may have a greater likelihood of vessel rupture. Although they are thinner walled, they do not "form" over the catheters as well as the polyethylene balloons.

After the waist on the balloon has successfully been abolished, the balloon is carefully withdrawn over the wire from the area of stenosis and an angiocardiogram is recorded before the wire is removed. This sequence is to make sure that there is no immediate recoil of the stenosis that may require further dilation and that there are no vessel tears that might need "tamponading" with a reinserted balloon.

Most branch pulmonary arteries can be dilated and the balloon can be expanded to its full diameter, eliminating the "waist." The diameter of the stenotic area that remains is usually more than doubled compared to the original lesion and the transstenotic gradient reduced significantly in the majority of these vessels. However, this seldom represents an enlargement of the stenotic area to the full diameter of the adjacent vessel, and few of these vessels will remain at the diameter achieved initially. Many of them will have an immediate recoil from the diameter achieved by the fully inflated balloon as soon as the balloon is withdrawn. Even more of these dilated areas will restenose further with time, leaving the net long-term results of branch pulmonary artery stenosis dilation less than ideal.

The procedure is not without complications. In the VACA registry of 182 dilations in 156 patients there were five deaths directly related to the procedure (with 2 fatal vessel ruptures, 1 cerebrovascular accident, one sinus arrest, and one low cardiac output) and at least eight other life-threatening complications.[6,31] However, because of the very poor success of any surgical approaches to these lesions, and in spite of the marginal success rate and significant complication rate, this procedure is still definitely indicated for the patient with significant branch stenosis.

One hopes that a more definitive and predictable means of opening the branch pulmonary artery stenoses will soon be clinically available. After 4 years of very promising animal work on intravascular stents in pulmonary arteries[32] and now almost 2 years of very successful immediate-term results in clinical trials of these stents in 30 patients[32] with various forms of branch pulmonary artery stenosis, it has been demonstrated that balloon expandable intravascular stents of sufficient size for even the large pulmonary arteries can be delivered to the previously dilated site and will hold these vessels open to their maximum degree of dilation both acutely and for at least 1 year. Despite dramatic early success and minimal complications with stents in this area, however, longer followup is necessary before they can be recommended routinely.

SYSTEMIC VENOUS STENOSIS

After the major lesions of coarctation of the aorta and branch pulmonary stenosis, the most frequent nonvalvular miscellaneous lesion in the VACA registry for which dilation was attempted was systemic venous stenosis. More favorable, yet still not universally successful, results are obtained with dilation of the acquired form. These stenoses are usually a result of previous surgery on, or in the vicinity of, these areas. The most commonly encountered and dilated in this category is the baffle stenosis at the superior or inferior vena cava following a venous switch (Mustard, Senning) repair of transposition of the great arteries.

The original report of attempts at dilating these areas[33] was disappointing, but the collaborative results from the VACA registry,[7] including the patients in the series from Texas Children's Hospital, generally showed good hemodynamic relief of obstruction and correspondingly good relief of symptoms. Dilation was successful in 15 patients out of 16 for whom results were recorded in the registry.[7] The obstruction in these cases is frequently at a postsurgical juncture of the baffle and the involved cava. As a consequence, it is deeply involved with, and encased in, scar tissue and is frequently resistant to dilation. At the same time the normal vessels and tissues in the area are very compliant and distensible. With these features, to disrupt the scar tissue and to obtain an opening that will persist, significant overdilation of the area to as much as 2.5 times the diameter of the adjacent normal structures is recommended.[34]

To accomplish this large dilating diameter without destroying the venous entry channels, a double-balloon technique is recommended.[35] Two exchange wires are positioned through the area of narrowing and two balloons with combined diameters of at least twice the diameter of the nearest normal structure are passed into the area and inflated. If the stenosis is extremely tight, one may have to begin the dilation with a single balloon or two much smaller balloons to gain access for the larger balloons. If the stenosis does not give way to the initial dilation, and so long as there is no angiographic evidence of vessel disruption, then higher pressure balloons should be used.

Immediate success may be followed by restenosis. Experience has shown that redilation to an even larger diameter may achieve a more permanent result and without significant risk to the patient. This is particularly pertinent when one considers the risks and morbidity of surgical revision of these complex lesions.

Again, the intravascular stents may offer a more promising method of permanently fixing these stenotic lesions in the dilated configuration. There also has been extensive and very favorable animal work on the use of intravascular stents in systemic venous channels.[36] These particular areas of restenosis are approved for clinical trials of the intravascular stents in two centers. The accumulated clinical material is insufficient for even a speculation concerning the clinical applicability of stents in this area.

SURGICALLY CREATED ANASTOMOSIS

Another nonvalvular area in which dilation has proved successful is in surgically created anastamoses.[37-40] The dilation of such an area, particularly in a patient who is a poor candidate for surgery or for whom more definitive surgery is not available, can spare the patient a premature or unnecessary surgical procedure. Only the "natural" or direct tissue to tissue anastomoses, ie, those without prosthetic tube grafts interposed, are considered potentials for this technique for two reasons. First, the balloon will not dilate the tubular prosthetic material. Second, and of equal importance, the tubular grafts develop a neointimal lining that is quite readily dislodged from the inner surface of the graft. When this occurs, the dislodged "peel" can totally occlude an already compromised lumen.

The greatest experience with the dilation of surgical anastamoses has been with the dilation of true Blalock-Taussig (direct end of subclavian artery to side of pulmonary artery) shunts. The vessels of these shunts tend to grow with the patients while the actual anastomotic site may remain fixed in diameter or actually constrict with tissue scarring. The native shunt vessel and the attached pulmonary artery remain very compliant. As a consequence, the stenotic area must be dilated to at least two and possibly even three times the narrowest diameter to achieve a lasting effect. The scarring around the anastomosis causes significant resistance to the dilation but, at the same time, also presumably provides some built-in safety with "tissue reinforcement" around the area being dilated.

The general technique is similar to other single-balloon dilations. The diameters of the stenosis and the adjacent vessels are determined from a selective angiocardiogram with injection just proximal to the stenosis and with the x-ray tubes angled to cut the narrowing precisely on edge. An end-hole catheter is passed through the anastomosis, preferably from a prograde venous catheter advanced out through the ascending aorta to the area of the shunt, or if that is not possible, then retrograde from a femoral artery. When the catheter passing through the shunt is well out into a distal pulmonary artery, it is replaced with a Teflon-coated exchange wire. If there were many curves or if the catheter's course through the shunt to the pulmonary artery is very tortuous, an extra-stiff exchange wire should be used.

The appropriate dilating balloon catheter is advanced over the wire and centered on the anastomosis site. To facilitate rapid inflation and deflation, the balloon is inflated with very dilute contrast material. Because the shunt being dilated may be the predominant, or the only, source of blood flow to the lungs and prolonged occlusion will lead to severe hypoxemia, the balloon inflation/deflation should be accomplished as rapidly as possible. The balloon diameter should be two or three times the diameter of the obstruction even if the adjacent vessel is smaller than that size. The vessel will overdilate to accommodate the balloon, whereas the stenosis will not be relieved unless the stenosis is markedly overdilated. The experience in the VACA registry[7] and the additional experience at Texas Children's Hospital suggest that this procedure will be successful in more than 50% of cases. When successful, it prevents or greatly delays subsequent surgery.

DISCRETE SUBAORTIC STENOSIS

Discrete subaortic stenoses have been dilated with variable acute success.[41-43] The subvalvular area is approached through the aortic valve retrograde from the femoral artery. Accurate measurements of the aortic valve annulus and left ventricular outflow tract are made from a left ventricular and/or an aortic root angiocardiogram using a calibrated marker catheter or calibration grid as a reference. A single-balloon technique is described here, but it is necessary to have two arterial lines, one for the balloon delivery and the other for arterial pressure monitoring during the balloon inflation. It is helpful to have a third line in the left ventricle during the dilation so that immediate results of the dilation are available without the necessity of removing the balloon from the vessel or the exchange wire from the left ventricle. The patients are given heparin at this point. An end-hole catheter is passed retrograde into the left ventricle. This is replaced with an exchange length Teflon wire which should be looped within the ventricle.

The balloon diameter is chosen to correspond to the diameter of the left ventricular outflow tract in the area of the membrane, but not to exceed the diameter of the aortic valve annulus. As with aortic valve dilations, a longer balloon provides more stability in the left ventricular outflow tract. Since the entire systemic output is obstructed by the balloon inflation, inflation and deflation must be accomplished as quickly as possible whether or not a waist appears and then disappears on the balloon. Repeat dilation, particularly using a larger balloon when the initial balloon appears smaller than the measured annulus, may improve less than satisfactory results.

The potential complications for dilation of subaortic stenosis are similar to those for aortic valve dilation. The likelihood of developing significant aortic regurgitation with subaortic membrane dilation is probably less than with aortic valve dilation, however.

The immediate results of dilation of subaortic membranes seem to be determined by exactly how discrete and thin the membrane is. It appears that a very thin membrane, close to the aortic valve and not associated with *any* tubular or tunnel stenosis, can be consistently opened with a balloon dilation. What becomes of the dilated tissue around the wall and what effect any remaining subvalvular tissue or stenosis will have on the aortic valve and particularly the development of aortic regurgitation is unknown. Additionally, the history of this lesion even after surgical excision is frequent recurrence of the membrane and stenosis. Dilation of this lesion has only been performed for a few years. With the many unanswered questions about the procedure and even the immediate results, it cannot be recommended routinely. (See also Chapter 13).

OTHER NONVALVULAR STENOSES

Many other vessels and surgical anastamoses have been dilated; however, these have been in very small numbers, using diverse techniques and with mixed reported success, so that no significant data are available for success or complication rates. The areas that have been attempted include pulmonary veins, Fontan anastomoses, Glenn anastomoses, subpulmonic membrane, prior pulmonary artery band sites, collateral vessels to pulmonary arteries, ascending aorta anastomosis in a postoperative arterial switch for transposition patient, and small atrial septal defects.[7] Of this group, probably the pulmonary vein dilation has had the least success, but the most unsatisfactory of these pulmonary vein procedures were performed before any of the vast experience with valvuloplasty or angioplasty of any other congenital lesions and before the availability of much more satisfactory equipment.[44] With the current wide experience with angioplasty in congenital lesions and the marked improvement in the dilation equipment, the effectiveness and safety of the procedures has dramatically improved over the past decade. Given the frequent high risks and unfavorable results of surgery for this last group of scattered lesions, attempted dilation of these stenoses is recommended as a first approach to therapy. As with the branch pulmonary artery stenosis and systemic venous stenosis, intravascular stenting of many of these vessels and structures may be possible in the future and afford a more permanent relief of the obstructions.

REFERENCES

1. Allen HD, Mullins CE: Results of the Valvuloplasty and Angioplasty of Congenital Anomalies Registry. *Am J Cardiol.* 65:772–774, 1990.

2. Stanger P, Cassidy SC, Girod DA, et al: Balloon pulmonary valvuloplasty: results of the Valvuloplasty and Angioplasty of Congenital Anomalies Registry. *Am J Cardiol.* 65:775–783, 1990.

3. Rocchini AP, Beekman RH, Shachar GB, et al: Balloon aortic valvuloplasty: results of the Valvuloplasty and Angioplasty of Congenital Anomalies Registry. *Am J Cardiol.* 65:784–789, 1990.

4. Tynan M, Finley JP, Fontes V, et al: Balloon angioplasty for the treatment of native coarctation: results of the Valvuloplasty and Angioplasty of Congenital Anomalies Registry. *Am J Cardiol.* 65:790–792, 1990.

5. Hellenbrand WE, Allen HD, Golinko RJ, et al: Balloon angioplasty for aortic recoarctation: results of the Valvuloplasty and Angioplasty of Congenital Anomalies Registry. *Am J Cardiol.* 65:793–797, 1990.

6. Kan JS, Marvin WJ Jr, Bass JL, et al: Balloon angioplasty—branch pulmonary artery stenosis: results of the Valvuloplasty and Angioplasty of Congenital Anomalies Registry. *Am J Cardiol.* 65:798–801, 1990.

7. Mullins CE, Latson LA, Neches WH, et al: Balloon dilation of miscellaneous lesions: results of the Valvuloplasty and Angioplasty of Congenital Anomalies Registry. *Am J Cardiol.* 65:802–803, 1990.

8. Kan JS, White RI Jr, Mitchell SE, et al: Treatment of restenosis of coarctation by percutaneous transluminal angioplasty. *Circulation.* 68:1087–1094, 1983.

9. Suarez de Lezo J, Fernandez R, Sancho M, et al: Percutaneous transluminal angioplasty for aortic isthmic coarctation in infancy. *Am J Cardiol.* 54:1147–1149, 1984.

10. Finley JP, Beaulieu RG, Nanton MA, et al: Balloon catheter dilatation of coarctation of the aorta in young infants. *Br Heart J.* 50:411–415, 1983.

11. Lock JE, Bass JL, Amplatz K, et al: Balloon dilation angioplasty of coarctations in infants and children. *Circulation.* 68:109–116, 1983.

12. Morrow WR, Vick GW III, Nihill MR, et al: Balloon dilation of unoperated coarctation of the aorta. Short- and intermediate-term results. *J Am Coll Cardiol.* 11:133–138, 1988.

13. Lababidi Z, Daskalopoulos DA, Stoeckle H Jr, et al: Transluminal balloon coarctation angioplasty. Experience with 27 patients. *Am J Cardiol.* 54:1288–1291, 1984.

14. Cerilli J, Lauridsen P: Reoperation for coarctation of the aorta. *Acta Chir Scand.* 129:391–394, 1965.

15. Cooper SG, Sullivan ID, Wren C: Treatment of recoarctation: balloon dilation angioplasty. *J Am Coll Cardiol.* 14:413–419, 1989.

16. Lorber A, Ettedgui JA, Baker EJ, et al: Balloon aortoplasty for recoarctation following the subclavian flap operation. *Int J Cardiol.* 10:57–63, 1986.

17. Burrows PE, Benson LN, Williams WG, et al: Iliofemoral arterial complications of balloon angioplasty for systemic obstructions in infants and children. *Circulation.* 82:1697–1704, 1990.

18. Marvin WJ, Mahoney LT, Rose EF: Pathologic sequelae of balloon dilation angioplasty for unoperated coarctation of the aorta in children (abstr.). *J Am Coll Cardiol.* 7:117A, 1986. Abstract.

19. Krabill KA, Bass JL, Lucas RV Jr, et al: Dissecting transverse aortic arch aneurysm after percutaneous transluminal balloon dilation angioplasty of an aortic coarctation. *Pediatr Cardiol.* 8:39–42, 1987.

20. Beekman RH, Rocchini AP, Dick M II, et al: Percutaneous balloon angioplasty for native coarctation of the aorta. *J Am Coll Cardiol.* 10:1078–1084, 1987.

21. Kaemmerer H, Ehrenheim C, Wilken W, et al: Clinical findings and magnetic resonance imaging in the follow-up of children after angioplasty of coarctation of the aorta (COA). *Z Kardiol.* 79:766–773, 1990.

22. Fontes VF, Esteves CA, Braga SLM, et al: It is valid to dilate native aortic coarctation with a balloon catheter. *Int J Cardiol.* 27:311–316, 1990.

23. John CN, Cartmill TB, Johnson DC, et al: Report of four cases of aneurysm complicating patch aortoplasty for repair of coarctation of the aorta. *Aust N Z J Surg.* 59:748–750, 1989.

24. DeSanto A, Bills RG, King H, et al: Pathogenesis of aneurysm formation opposite prosthetic patches used for coarctation repair. An experimental study. *J Thorac Cardiovasc Surg.* 94:720–723, 1987.

25. Adams FH, Emmanouilides, GC: *Heart Disease in Infants, Children and Adolescents.* Baltimore: Williams & Wilkins, 1983, p 253.

26. Edwards BS, Lucas RV Jr, Lock JE, et al: Morphologic changes in the pulmonary arteries after percutaneous balloon angioplasty for pulmonary arterial stenosis. *Circulation.* 71:195–201, 1985.

27. Baum D, Khoury GH, Ongley PA, et al: Congenital stenosis of the pulmonary artery branches. *Circulation.* 29:680–687, 1964.

28. Emmanouilides GC, Linde LM, Crittenden IH: Pulmonary artery stenosis associated with ductus arteriosus following maternal rubella. *Circulation.* 29:514–522, 1964.

29. Gill CC, Moodie DS, McGoon DC: Staged surgical management of pulmonary atresia with diminutive pulmonary arteries. *J Thorac Cardiovasc Surg.* 73:436–442, 1977.

30. Lock JE, Castaneda-Zuniga WR, Fuhrman BP, et al: Balloon dilation angioplasty of hypoplastic and stenotic pulmonary arteries. *Circulation.* 67:962–967, 1983.

31. Fellows KE, Radtke W, Keane JF, et al: Acute complications of catheter therapy for congenital heart disease. *Am J Cardiol.* 60:679–683, 1987

32. O'Laughlin MP, Perry SB, Lock JE, et al: Use of endovascular stents in congenital heart disease. *Circulation.* 83:1923–1939, 1991.

33. Waldman JD, Waldman J, Jones MC: Failure of balloon dilatation in mid-cavity obstruction of the systemic venous atrium after Mustard operation. *Pediatr Cardiol.* 4:151–154, 1983.

34. Lock JE, Bass JL, Castaneda-Zuniga W, et al: Dilation angioplasty of congenital or operative narrowings of venous channels. *Circulation.* 70:457–464, 1984.

35. Mullins CE, Nihill MR, Vick GW III, et al: Double balloon technique for dilation of valvular or vessel stenosis in congenital and acquired heart disease. *J Am Coll Cardiol.* 10:107–114, 1987.

36. Mullins CE, O'Laughlin MP, Vick GW III, et al: Implantation of balloon-expandable intravascular grafts by catheterization in pulmonary arteries and systemic veins. *Circulation.* 77:188–199, 1988.

37. Rao PS, Levy JM, Chopra PS: Balloon angioplasty of stenosed Blalock-Taussig anastomosis: role of balloon-on-a-wire in dilating occluded shunts. *Am Heart J.* 120:1173–1178, 1990.

38. Ishii K, Koga Y, Onitsuka T, et al: Balloon dilatation angioplasty of stenotic pulmonary artery simultaneously with a Blalock-Taussig shunt for extremely severe tetralogy of Fallot. *Kyobu Geka.* 41:971–975, 1988.

39. Scheel JN, Gardner TJ, Kan JS: Balloon dilatation of a stenotic Waterston shunt with long-term follow-up. *Am J Cardiol.* 68:821–822, 1991.

40. Snyder MS, Sos T, Levin AR, et al: Transluminal angioplasty of a stenotic Potts shunt and pulmonary arterial branch stenosis. *Am Heart J.* 113:198–200, 1987.

41. Suárez de Lezo J, Pan M, Sancho M, et al: Percutaneous transluminal balloon dilatation for discrete subaortic stenosis. *Am J Cardiol.* 58:619–621, 1986.

42. Lababidi Z, Weinhaus L, Stoeckle H Jr, et al: Transluminal balloon dilatation for discrete subaortic stenosis. *Am J Cardiol.* 59:423–425, 1987.

43. Alyousef S, Khan A, Lababidi Z, et al: Perkutane transluminale Ballondilatation der rein membranösen subvalvulären Aortenstenose (DMSS). *Herz.* 13:32–35, 1988.

44. Driscoll DJ, Hesslein PS, Mullins CE: Congenital stenosis of individual pulmonary veins: clinical spectrum and unsuccessful treatment by transvenous balloon dilation. *Am J Cardiol.* 49:1767–1772, 1982.

CHAPTER 22

A SURGEON'S POINT OF VIEW

ROBERT G. JOHNSON
RONALD M. WEINTRAUB

What may appear to be new technology today often has its roots in some previous, seemingly unrelated, technological developments. Percutaneous balloon valvuloplasty is an example of this phenomenon. Although the immediate origins of percutaneous balloon valvuloplasty are detailed elsewhere in this text, it is a procedure that has been made possible not only through a variety of recent improvements in catheterization technology, but also by prior surgical experience.

DEVELOPMENT OF THE BALLOON VALVULOPLASTY TECHNIQUE

Percutaneous balloon valve dilatation is currently employed to achieve, without operation, results that had been achieved through operative techniques many years before.[1] In 1902 Sir Lauder Brunton wrote[2]:

> Mitral stenosis is not only one of the most distressing forms of cardiac disease, but in its severe forms it resists all treatment by medicine. On looking at the contracted mitral orifice in a severe case of this disease one is impressed by the hopelessness of ever finding a remedy which will enable the auricle to drive the blood in a sufficient stream through the small mitral orifice, and the wish unconsciously arises that one could divide the constriction as easily during life as one can after death. The risk which such an operation would entail naturally makes one shrink from it.

This concept of direct relief of valvular stenosis was followed by an unsuccessful operation on the pulmonary valve by Doyen in 1913, digital dilatation of the aortic valve by Tuffier in 1914, and transcardiac incision of the mitral valve in 1923 by Cutler and associates. By 1929 twelve operations for chronic valve disease had been accomplished with a mortality of 83%. These discouraging outcomes led to more than a decade's passing before similarly bold attempts were undertaken in the midst of other technological improvements. In the late 1940s successful pulmonary valvotomy was accomplished by Brock in London, and the first successful mitral commisurotomy was performed by Bailey in Philadelphia. Days after Bailey's successful mitral operation Harken performed a similar procedure in Boston. It was the early 1950s before Bailey's group successfully performed the first aortic valve commissurotomy.[3] Indirect opening of stenotic valve commissures was accomplished by palpation without direct vision and was the mainstay of treatment until the advent of cardiopulmonary bypass technology (open commissurotomy) and the development of artificial valves (valve replacement).

The desire to avoid operation, cardiopulmonary bypass, and prosthetic valve replacement in patients with valvular stenosis provided the impetus for a resurgence of interest in balloon valvuloplasty techniques, which can now be accomplished percutaneously. Even while surgeons are increasingly avoiding valve replacement by using open valvuloplasty techniques whenever feasible, any successful treatment that can avoid operative and cardiopulmonary bypass risks has obvious appeal. Balloon dilatation of stenotic valves provides such an option. As alternative treatment options become available, it is the responsibility of those involved with the care of such patients to consider the risks and benefits of these options in an effort to treat patients individually.

In this chapter we review the surgical considerations regarding percutaneous balloon valvuloplasty. Recent surgical literature regarding the mortality and long-term followup of primary operative treatment for valve stenosis is cited, as it is necessary to have some knowledge of the operations that are alternatives to percutaneous balloon valvuloplasty. The operative experience in patients who have had previous percutaneous balloon valvuloplasty is specifically examined.

THE SURGEON'S ROLE

From 1985 through 1990, approximately 225 aortic and 200 mitral balloon valve dilatations were performed at Boston's Beth Israel Hospital. Cardiothoracic surgical support of this experience included involvement in four distinct areas. *Preprocedure consultation*, which early in the experience was required in all cases, provided the patient and responsible physicians with a specific assessment of the risks of operation, so that the appropriate procedure could be selected. *Emergency operations* for complications of percutaneous balloon valvuloplasty were required in a few cases. In those rare cases when the dilatation was unsuccessful or, more commonly, when late restenosis has occurred, *elective cardiac surgical consultation* was obtained. As cardiac surgeons our involvement with balloon valvuloplasty patients generally occurs at the request of a referring cardiologist, but on occasion it is *we who request the consultation for possible percutaneous balloon valvuloplasty.* There have been occasions when we have been asked to operate on patients in whom we thought the operative risks exceeded the benefits, or in selected patients whose condition we believed might be improved by an initial percutaneous reduction in valve gradient prior to an operative procedure.

PREPROCEDURE CONSULTATION

Prior to valvuloplasty a cardiac surgeon may be consulted to evaluate an individual patient with respect to his or her operative candidacy. The published short-term and long-term results of operative treatment of valvular stenosis must be considered. More important, each institution has a slightly different experience, and each patient may have characteristics that alter his or her chance of a satisfactory result with either operation. In this regard local surgical consultation can be critical in the selection of appropriate treatment.

Balloon Aortic Valvuloplasty

Balloon aortic valvuloplasty for adult aortic stenosis is currently performed at our institution only after surgical consultation has determined the patient to be an inappropriate candidate for operative valve replacement. The characterization of a patient as "a high risk surgical candidate" is always relative to the individual patient's current condition and the experience of the consulting surgeon. At least two thirds of the first 179 patients who were referred to this center for percutaneous balloon aortic valvuloplasty as "poor operative candidates" would not have been considered to have an excessive operative risk at our institution. Our review of these referred patients, however, failed to reveal whether each patient had been evaluated by a cardiac surgeon. Only through a collaborative interdisciplinary effort can the appropriate procedure be selected for these patients. Examples of some characteristics that we consider relative contraindications to operation include a life expectancy of less than 6 months, a porcelain aorta, and a history of hospitalizations that is not likely to be corrected by operation. Advanced age and poor left ventricular function are not independent contraindications to operation for aortic stenosis.

Aortic stenosis in children differs from the adult analog in its anatomic and pathologic features. Currently, operative valvulotomy offers a finite term of palliation until valve replacement can be performed. When valvulotomy is the anticipated treatment, percutaneous balloon dilatation may be considered as initial therapy. Balloon dilatation has also been successful in children who have previously undergone operative valvulotomy.[4] Accurate decisions regarding the use of percutaneous balloon valvuloplasty in lieu of operation will be difficult until more long-term data regarding the percutaneous procedure are available.

In adults, operations for aortic valve stenosis are quite successful, and this must be considered in the determination of an individual's therapeutic risk:benefit ratio. The reported operative mortality following isolated aortic valve replacement is as low as 2.1%.[5] Other recently published results reflect the results of combined procedures in an older, sicker population. In a large series of aortic valve replacements reported in 1990, inclusive of those patients requiring revascularization, the reported 30-day mortality has ranged from 4%[6] to 5.2%.[7] Octogenarians have been reported as having a greater risk of postoperative death. In 1989 Levinson and his colleagues at the Massachusetts General Hospital noted an in-hospital mortality of only 3% in isolated aortic valve replacement procedures for aortic stenosis in octogenarians, and a mortality of 9.4% for those who required associated procedures.[8] Long-term survival rates following aortic valve replacement are greatly affected by the preoperative condition and associated operations or cardiac disease but range from 69% to 86% at 5 years.[6,7] In evaluating these figures from surgical series it is appropriate to recognize that all operative experiences represent some selection bias. It is impossible to glean from the surgical literature data regarding patients who were not operated upon because of an assessment of high risk. If percutaneous balloon aortic valvuloplasty is performed only in high risk patients, then the results of the two treatments are impossible to compare. We note, however, that patients in whom percutaneous balloon aortic valvuloplasty fails may be reconsidered for operation. At that time, given the lack of therapeutic alternatives, valve replacement may be accepted despite the significant risk of death or complications.

Occasionally cardiac surgical consultation will be sought for patients who have aortic stenosis but who have a variety of severe co-morbidities. These may include pulmonary impairment, mitral regurgitation possibly secondary to the valve stenosis, or both. Co-morbidities such as neoplastic disease or "brittle" dialysis-dependent renal failure would have no direct relationship to the presence of a stenotic valve. In patients with stenosis-related co-morbidities percutaneous balloon valvuloplasty may be recommended as a diagnostic and therapeutic trial prior to a possible valve operation, and in the patient with non-stenosis-related co-morbidities the cardiac surgeon may suggest that the patient have percutaneous balloon aortic valvuloplasty in lieu of a valve operation.[9] In patients with stenotic aortic bioprosthetic valves, percutaneous balloon valvuloplasty may offer the hope of avoiding a reoperation, but the reported results of this have been poor, with resulting acute tears in the calcified, degenerated leaflets.[10] Reoperation should be considered the primary option in such situations. (See also Chapter 17).

Balloon Mitral Valvuloplasty

Patients who have isolated mitral stenosis rarely require any surgical evaluation prior to percutaneous balloon valvuloplasty. The results in these patients are good and mirror the earlier experience with mitral commissurotomies[1] without the trauma of an operation.[11]

Although balloon aortic valvuloplasty for aortic stenosis may be recommended only when operation is not an option, mitral valve operations for mitral stenosis may be appropriate only when balloon valvuloplasty is not recommended[11] or after it fails. The characteristics that may assist in the appropriate initial, therapeutic choice in patients with predominant mitral stenosis have been defined[12,13] and are discussed elsewhere in this volume. Obviously the most important contraindication to balloon valvuloplasty of the stenotic mitral valve is severe associated incompetence. Relative contraindications to percutaneous balloon mitral valvuloplasty include left atrial thrombus not isolated to the appendage, extensive subvalvular pathology identified by echocardiogram, heavy leaflet and annular calcification, and a clear indication for other cardiac operative procedures. On rare occasions transseptal catheterization will not be possible owing to a thickened atrial septum, and these patients will require operative intervention.

In general, operations for relief of aortic stenosis are associated with better clinical outcomes than operations for mitral stenosis. This difference has a number of explanations, including the chronic effect of stenosis of either valve on the left ventricle and the pulmonary vasculature. At operation the mitral valve offers the additional challenge of a subvalvular apparatus that may have significant functional importance and which may be destroyed by the disease process or by the valve operation. It is therefore important to the success of a mitral valve operation that the stenosis be relieved with conservative, reparative techniques whenever feasible, and that consideration be given to the salvage of the subvalvular apparatus even when the leaflets cannot be saved.

The hospital mortality associated with mitral valve operations varies according to preoperative clinical status, valvular pathology, and prior mitral valve operations. The risk for primary, isolated mitral valve operation is in the realm of 3%. Czer's recent series notes no operative deaths in a small group of patients having mitral commissurotomy and a 4% mortality in a similar group of patients having valve replacement.[7] In a large, retrospective series of over 20 years' experience with mitral valve operations from New York University (inclusive of reoperations and combined procedures), the operative mortality was reported as 5% with reconstruction, 16.6% with mechanical valve replacement, and 10.6% with porcine bioprosthesis insertion.[14] Obviously selection played a major role in determining the different results of these procedures, but the numbers reflect the significant operative mortality associated with operations for mitral valve disease in over 1200 patients. The 5-year survival — free from cardiac related deaths — was similar among the groups, ranging from 81% for those repaired to approximately 73% for those with valve replacement of either type.

In patients who have undergone prior mitral valve operations percutaneous balloon mitral valvuloplasty is an option. Patients who experience late restenosis after operative mitral commissurotomies, either open or closed, have had results similar to those seen in patients who have not been operated upon previously.[15] In addition, in contrast to aortic bioprosthetic valves, there has been at least one report of successful palliation of a patient with stenosis of a mitral bioprosthesis.[16]

EMERGENCY OPERATIONS

The need for emergency operation associated with percutaneous balloon valvuloplasty is rare. Over 420 adult balloon valvuloplasty procedures were performed by our cardiologic colleagues from 1986 to 1991, and we have operated emergently on only 7 patients. Six of the patients had emergency cardiac operations for complications related to the percutaneous balloon valvuloplasty technique. One of these 7 patients had a percutaneous balloon aortic valvuloplasty as a means of palliation/salvage when she experienced a cardiac arrest during a diagnostic catheterization for unstable angina in the presence of known aortic stenosis. An additional patient required an emergency vascular procedure to repair an iliac artery injury early in the experience. No emergency operations have been required in patients following percutaneous balloon valvuloplasty from September 1989 to the present (February 1991). The experience from our institution yields an incidence of emergency operation in 3 of 220 percutaneous balloon aortic valvuloplasty procedures and 4 of 200 mitral dilatations. These numbers are similar to those from Ferguson and colleagues at the Texas Heart Institute with 2 emergency operations after 73 percutaneous balloon aortic valvuloplasty procedures,[17] and the experience of Vahanian and associates with 2 emergency operations among 200 mitral dilatations.[18] Emergency operations in pediatric percutaneous balloon aortic or pulmonary valvuloplasty have not been reported. Many important considerations arise from the admittedly limited experience with emergency cardiac operations in adult balloon valvuloplasty patients. These include indications for operative treatment, the management of the patient until operation, and the operative management (repair of injury with or without valve treatment).

Mechanism of Injury, Presentation, and Indications for Emergency Operation

The most common complication of percutaneous balloon valvuloplasty necessitating· operation has been **cardiac perforation**[19,20,21,22] with a balloon catheter or guidewire. These injuries present with a complaint of sudden severe chest pain and associated hypotension, resulting from the pericardial tamponade physiology associated with an acute hemopericardium. Our experience and the case reports in the literature suggest that an emergency operation is more likely after balloon mitral dilatation than after percutaneous balloon aortic valvuloplasty. The location of the perforation depends somewhat on the targeted valve and the technique used. The right or left atrium may be punctured if the transseptal approach is used, but left ventricular perforation has occurred with both transatrial and retrograde-aortic techniques. There have been isolated reports of aortic annular disruption[23] and aortic rupture[24] associated with severe hypotension. The diagnosis of a cardiac perforation may, by itself, be considered an indication for operation. As noted below, however, there may be exceptions to this (for example when the perforation clearly involves only the atrium).

Acute severe valve regurgitation may also necessitate urgent operation.[19,25,26] This appears to be more common with balloon mitral dilatations, and it presents with refractory, severe pulmonary edema. Regurgitation may result from leaflet disruption[19,25] or subvalvar papillary damage.[19] In these cases the decision to operate is based on the severity of the regurgitation and, specifically in mitral pathology, the ability to control the regurgitation medically. Acute mitral insufficiency requiring emergency operation has been reported,[19,27,28] as have technical and anatomic subvalvular characteristics which may be associated with such injuries. We have never had to perform an emergency operation for acute mitral regurgitation, but one of our patients underwent operation 7 days after percutaneous balloon mitral valvuloplasty for increased mitral regurgitation poorly responsive to medical therapy. Our experience is mirrored in a report by Vahanian and colleagues,[18] who noted that no emergency operations were performed for mitral insufficiency but that 8 of 200 mitral dilatation patients did require mitral operations for regurgitation 2 to 8 weeks after percutaneous balloon mitral valvuloplasty. In contrast to the experience with mitral regurgitation, severe aortic valve regurgitation after percutaneous balloon aortic valvuloplasty is likely to be the result of a significant annular or wall injury[29] and is unlikely to improve without operation.

Although perforation and regurgitation are the primary reasons for emergency cardiac operations following percutaneous balloon valvuloplasty, there are acute situations that might require operations. **Transatrial shunts** are frequently present following transseptal catheterization. There are, however, no reported cases in which this lesion, in isolation, has required emergency operation. **Major vascular injuries** have also been reported, particularly in very young and elderly patients,[30-33] and may require emergency operation. Emergency operations may also be required following implementation of percutaneous balloon valvuloplasty **during a diagnostic catheterization** in a patient with critical aortic stenosis.[34,35] We have successfully operated on one such patient. These cases represent complications of diagnostic catheterization and not of percutaneous balloon valvuloplasty. Indeed, the percutaneous balloon valvuloplasty provided lifesaving palliation prior to a high risk emergency operation.

Preoperative Management

Cardiac perforation can be fatal[21] and requires immediate attention. Fluid infusion can be used to correct the hypotension rapidly, sedation is administered, and intubation is accomplished as required. Echocardiography should be immediately used to assess the degree of hemopericardium and to guide the placement of a pericardial catheter for aspiration. The temptation to reinfuse the aspirated blood should be resisted unless the patient is given anticoagulants or the blood is treated. This sequence of events has achieved hemodynamic stability in all six cases of perforation that we have taken to the operating room. Two had undergone percutaneous balloon aortic valvuloplasty and four had percutaneous balloon mitral valvuloplasty. Although nonoperative hemodynamic stabilization has been possible in each case at our institution, fatal ventricular perforation has been reported.[21] Percutaneous cardiopulmonary bypass has been successfully employed[22] to resuscitate and support a patient with aortic injury and tamponade until operation could be performed.

When **valve disruption** occurs it generally results in a manageable increase in preexisting regurgitation, and the definitive operative treatment can take place hours or days later. Afterload reduction, balloon counterpulsation, or both may help stabilize these patients with mitral insufficiency, and inotropic support may be helpful in managing either aortic or mitral regurgitation.

Once the operating room staff has been notified of the probability of an emergency operation, and after the initial effort to stabilize the patient, the timing of operation can be determined. In two of our patients with mitral stenosis, who had presumed atrial perforation, we found no bleeding from the site of injury at the time of operation. An absence of bleeding has also been observed by others.[18] If a patient is stabilized by pericardiocentesis, and if the perforation is certain to have been atrial, consideration may be given to correction of anticoagulation and a period of observation. After a period of an hour, if the patient remains stable, if echocardiographic evaluation shows no accumulation of pericardial fluid, and if there is no drainage from the pericardial catheter, then operation need not be performed as an emergency. If all the foregoing conditions are not met and the patient either remains hemodynamically unstable or shows an increasing hemopericardium or continued pericardial catheter drainage, then emergency operation is required. Pericardiocentesis must be continued to maintain stability, and in this regard, it may be appropriate to avoid any reversal of systemic anticoagulation because pericardial thrombosis may result in an unmanageable tamponade. Obviously, mitral regurgitation resulting in pulmonary edema refractory to medical therapy necessitates emergency operation as well.

Operative Management

There are reports of emergency operations with correction of the perforation without valve repair or replacement,[19] deferring definitive valve treatment until a subsequent operation. We have not found this approach necessary and have found it possible to perform definitive treatment of the valve, the vessels, and the injury. This has been true even for patients, referred from other institutions, who were having their percutaneous balloon aortic valvuloplasty in lieu of an operation that was considered to have excessive risk. One patient with mitral stenosis had commissurotomy and an annuloplasty, three had aortic valve replacement, one had mitral valve replacement, and two had mitral valve replacement with coronary revascularization.

Among our seven patients there was one hospital death. This 79-year-old patient had his percutaneous balloon aortic valvuloplasty very early in the experience of our institution, and experienced a left ventricular perforation. He had to await the availability of an operating room and surgeon, during which time he was hemodynamically stable, but blood was continuously drained from his pericardium and reinfused without sufficient anticoagulation or filtration. Intraoperatively a severe coagulopathy was evident, which was never corrected. The other six patients were discharged. One patient with percutaneous balloon mitral valvuloplasty who had mitral valve replacement, aortic valve replacement and aortic root replacement died 3 months later of persistent cardiac failure. The patient who had mitral valve repair required a valve replacement 6 months later for insufficiency. The five surviving patients were well at a mean of 36 months postoperatively.

Summary

On the basis of the literature and our experience with emergency cardiac operations associated with percutaneous balloon valvuloplasty we conclude the following:

1. Complications requiring emergency operation are rare (1–3% after percutaneous balloon aortic valvuloplasty and 1–2% after percutaneous balloon mitral valvuloplasty).
2. The most common cardiac injury is perforation, which is slightly more likely to occur with percutaneous balloon mitral valvuloplasty and is probably related to the transseptal technique.
3. Although it occurs more commonly with percutaneous balloon mitral valvuloplasty, valve disruption or insufficiency is more likely to require an emergency operation when it occurs after percutaneous balloon aortic valvuloplasty.
4. Surgical support for percutaneous balloon valvuloplasty should include the anticipated availability of an operating room and surgeon within two hours of the valve dilatation.
5. Immediate echocardiography and pericardiocentesis are critical to the preoperative management of these patients.
6. If an operative repair is required, definitive treatment of valvular and coronary pathology can generally be carried out.

ELECTIVE CONSULTATION FOLLOWING BALLOON VALVULOPLASTY

Aortic Stenosis

As compared with operation, percutaneous balloon aortic valvuloplasty offers two distinct advantages: It is a slightly less invasive procedure and it avoids valve replacement. The long-term, late risks associated with a prosthetic or bioprosthetic valve are real, and an alternative to aortic valve replacement would be desirable. Unfortunately, operative alternatives to valve replacement for aortic stenosis have not yielded promising results. Open valvulotomy in children has been used for years with some long-term successes, but mostly as a palliative measure.[36] Open valve debridement in adults, who often have a greater degree of valvular calcification, has been accomplished by a variety of techniques, and most recently with an ultrasonic aspiration device.[37-39] Restenosis, valvular insufficiency, or both have precluded this technique's widespread adoption. It is hoped that replacement with cryopreserved homografts will eliminate some of the long-term risks of prosthetic valve replacement by reducing the risk of leaflet degeneration, thromboembolism, and early endocarditis while potentially eliminating the need for anticoagulation.[40] Because valve replacement is the mainstay in the treatment of aortic stenosis, research efforts will continue to identify a biologic valve that will not degenerate or a mechanical valve that will resist thrombosis.

Because of the disappointing early and midterm restenosis rates in patients treated by percutaneous balloon aortic valvuloplasty, it is used only in adult patients who are not considered candidates for operation.[20,32,41] If this rule were applied in its strictest sense, there would be no experience with valve replacement in patients following percutaneous balloon aortic valvuloplasty. Indeed, as the percutaneous procedure is less liberally applied, the number of patients who will subsequently be offered an operation will surely diminish. Until absolute, unanimously accepted criteria can be established for operative candidacy, there will be patients who have percutaneous balloon aortic valvuloplasty as "noncandidates" but who deteriorate clinically and subsequently undergo valve operation at "high risk." Such clinical deterioration is most commonly the result of restenosis, but may occasionally be caused by aortic regurgitation.[42]

An experience with late operations in patients who have undergone percutaneous balloon aortic valvuloplasty was reported in a series from our institution in 1990.[20] Of 179 patients, 42 required late elective operation for symptomatic restenosis at a mean interval of 7.8 months following percutaneous balloon valvuloplasty. During the early experience 15 patients were accepted on the basis of their desire to avoid an operation, but the remaining 27 patients had originally been considered poor candidates for operative valve replacement. At operation 22 patients had isolated aortic valve replacement; 13 had aortic valve replacement and coronary artery bypass graft, 1 had aortic valve replacement, coronary artery bypass graft, and mitral valve replacement; 1 had an open aortic valvuloplasty, 3 had repeat coronary artery bypass graft and aortic valve replacement; and 2 had repeat sternotomy and aortic valve replacement (having had aborted operations at other institutions due to calcified aortas). There were 3 in-hospital deaths (8.9% operative mortality) following elective operation. All 16 patients over the age of 80 survived operation. Two of the deaths occurred in patients among the 30 considered poor candidates for operation prior to their percutaneous balloon valvuloplasty. Both of these patients experienced significant cerebrovascular accidents and the third death occurred in a 37-year-old patient who experienced a ventricular fibrillatory arrest in the postoperative period. The late followup studies revealed persistent clinical improvement in all discharged patients at a mean of 11 ± 7.5 months after elective operation.

Prior to elective operation the presence of a left-to-right shunt at the atrial level should be considered. If the previous percutaneous balloon aortic valvuloplasty has been performed in an "antegrade" fashion, requiring a transseptal approach, there may be a hemodynamically significant shunt which should be closed[43] at operation. At operation the use of retrograde coronary sinus cardioplegia has made administration of cardioplegia in these patients much simpler, obviating direct coronary cannulation. We routinely monitor the myocardial temperature in all such patients to avoid inadequate volume administration and unequal distribution. As noted previously many of these patients have other cardiac problems that were considered less critical than the aortic stenosis that was palliated with the percutaneous balloon valvuloplasty. In these cases the surgeon applies his or her usual criteria for the addition of coronary revascularization and mitral valve replacement.

The experience with percutaneous balloon aortic valvuloplasty points out the difficulty of accurately assessing the risk of operation in patients with aortic stenosis. Reliable risk determinations would predict that patients who undergo percutaneous balloon valvuloplasty (in lieu of operation, because of an elevated probability of an adverse outcome) would indeed have an increase in morbidity and mortality with any subsequent operation. No such increase has been demonstrated, however, suggesting that the risk criteria in current use need to be reevaluated, or that percutaneous balloon aortic valvuloplasty improved these patients, altering their assigned risks. Regarding this later probability, it seems clear that percutaneous balloon aortic valvuloplasty does provide a predictable period of valve area improvement, but the measurable improvement often disappears before the operations is performed.[20]

As surgeons, we conclude that patients should have careful surgical evaluation before balloon aortic valvuloplasty. We also recognize the possibility that percutaneous balloon aortic valvuloplasty might provide both diagnostic and therapeutic benefit for occasional patients who appear to be at high risk for operation. Such patients would include those with significant mitral regurgitation in whom the risk of double valve replacement might be considered prohibitive, but who might have a significant decrease in their mitral problem if their aortic valve gradient could be relieved. Another example would be a patient with significant pulmonary disease and pulmonary hypertension who might be considered to have an excessive operative risk if the pulmonary component is irreversible or unrelated to aortic stenosis. In each of these examples percutaneous balloon valvuloplasty may be used to achieve a temporary improvement in the aortic valve gradient, and if clinical and echocardiographic improvement ensues then operation for aortic valve replacement may be undertaken with less fear and a greater anticipation of a satisfactory clinical result. In view of the known palliative nature of percutaneous balloon aortic valvuloplasty, patients who have successful procedures should be considered for operative valve replacement during the interval of their improvement.

Mitral Stenosis

Operative alternatives to mitral valve replacement for mitral stenosis were noted in the introduction of this chapter. These surgical attempts to relieve mitral stenosis provide both a sound basis for the implementation of percutaneous balloon mitral valvuloplasty, as well providing some information regarding the limitations of the technique.[44-46] Open commissurotomy and, less frequently, closed commissurotomy have remained a part of the surgical armamentarium to the present day. In appropriately selected cases the option of open commissurotomy may actually offer a longer reoperation-free survival than valve replacement.[47] Enthusiasm for repair is limited only by the long-term results, which must be obtained at the risk of a procedure that is also capable of replacing the valve. Considering these facts, it was appropriate that the first report detailing clinical balloon mitral commissurotomy, by Inoue and colleagues, was published in a surgical journal in 1984.[48] They presented results with both transvenous and open (intraoperative) balloon dilatation. It remains to be determined whether percutaneous balloon mitral valvuloplasty has made operative commissurotomy obsolete. As previously cited, it is known that percutaneous balloon mitral valvuloplasty can be successfully performed in patients in whom restenosis occurs after operative commissurotomy.[15]

Only the development of an operative procedure that would avoid valve replacement while providing long-term results equal to or better than those obtainable with valve replacement could alter the current role of percutaneous balloon mitral valvuloplasty as treatment for isolated mitral stenosis. A recent report regarding the use of ultrasonic debridement for mitral stenosis[49] provides an example of the type of operative solutions that might be applied to improve current commissurotomy results.

The experience was limited to 8 patients with heavy valve calcification. Each had a satisfactory immediate postoperative result, but 2 required valve replacement for increasing insufficiency within 2 years of the debridement. The other 6 patients have not been followed long enough to assess the potential benefits of this procedure, but the results of aortic debridement[37-39] may make hesitation more appropriate than adoption of this technique.

There are no large published series of patients who have undergone mitral valve operations following percutaneous balloon mitral valvuloplasty. Carpentier's group[19] reported 10 patients, 7 of whom required operation in the first 12 hours postoperatively. The indications for operation were hemopericardium (3 patients), acute mitral insufficiency (5 patients), and left to right shunting (2 patients). Only those with an atrial septal defect and one with mitral regurgitation could be clearly classified as electively operated on. It is possible that the others with increased mitral regurgitation might have been managed medically for a longer time. As the authors noted in their report the incidence of operation after percutaneous balloon mitral valvuloplasty could not be established by them because they did not see all of the operative patients from their institution who required valve procedures.

Our unpublished experience with elective operation in these patients has also been modest, but we can attempt to quantify the incidence of operation relative to mitral dilatation procedures. Implementation of this technique at our institution was begun in November of 1985, when we saw an elderly, institutionalized gentleman with severe noncardiac pulmonary disease who was not considered to be a candidate for operation. From that time until January 1991 nearly 200 balloon mitral valvuloplasties have been performed at Boston's Beth Israel Hospital (Kuntz R, personal communication, Jan. 1991), and only 15 patients have required subsequent operation. Many patients who underwent balloon mitral valvuloplasty here were referred from other facilities, and five elected to have their operations nearer their homes. Ten of the fifteen subsequent operations have been performed here at a mean interval of 9.5 months (7 days–24 mo) after percutaneous balloon valvuloplasty. In that same time interval we performed 73 other mitral valve replacement procedures for mitral stenosis (with or without other operative procedures). Eight of these post–percutaneous balloon valvuloplasty patients presented with recurrent mitral stenosis, and only two had increasing mitral insufficiency as a major feature of their disease.

In reviewing the records of these patients it is clear that many of them could have had a second percutaneous balloon mitral valvuloplasty, but other cardiac problems led to the decision to perform a comprehensive operation. This is reflected by noting the procedures performed in these patients:

Two had isolated mitral valve replacement.

Two had mitral valve replacement plus closure of an atrial septal defect.

Two had mitral and aortic valve replacement.

Two had all three of the foregoing procedures.

One had mitral and aortic valve replacement plus coronary artery bypass graft.

One had mitral valve replacement and tricuspid annuloplasty.

There were no hospital deaths following these operations. Although four patients had closure of atrial septal defects at operation, only one of these was hemodynamically significant (Q_p:Q_s = 2.3).

When operation is required, the presence of a significant atrial septal defect must be considered. Recently transesophageal echocardiographic studies have demonstrated atrial shunts in 87% of patients one day after the transseptal balloon mitral valvuloplasty.[50] It should be noted that transthoracic evaluation was much less discerning. The incidence of shunts decreased with time so that at 6 months only 20% had significant shunts noted on transesophageal echocardiography.[50] In patients who have had balloon valvuloplasty we routinely perform transthoracic echocardiographic "microbubble" studies to search for a shunt. Right heart catheterizations and oxygen saturation sampling are also routine. If the pulmonary: systemic flow ratio is less than 1.5:1 then the decision to repair the defect may be made in the operating room. These small defects can generally be closed by one or two pledgeted horizontal mattress sutures. Only one of our four patients required the more traditional right atrial approach.

Other aspects of the operation in these patients are unchanged by the prior percutaneous balloon valvuloplasty. We have not performed valve repair in any of our patients, particularly noting that half of them required aortic valve replacement as well. Valve repair is certainly an option when insufficiency is the primary pathologic condition, as is commisurotomy when restenosis occurs,[19] but we have wished to avoid an additional palliative procedure (although some would consider valve replacement a form of palliation as well).

CONCLUSIONS

Emergency cardiac operations should be rare and their outcome good if patients are appropriately selected prior to dilatation and appropriately diagnosed and managed after injury. Operative support is absolutely necessary for these procedures, but the availability need not be instantaneous. Nearly all patients can have their definitive valve replacement at the time of their emergency operation.

Percutaneous balloon aortic valvuloplasty is indicated only for truly inoperable patients, and this decision requires serious consideration by a cardiac surgeon. Selected patients may benefit from percutaneous balloon aortic valvuloplasty as palliation prior to operation, but again this decision is a collaborative one.

Percutaneous balloon mitral valvuloplasty has become a primary modality in the treatment of patients with severe mitral stenosis. Certain anatomic considerations may be evaluated by echocardiography which will predict a more satisfactory long-term outlook (longer operation-free period). In patients who later require mitral valve replacement, if a significant atrial shunt exists, the associated atrial septostomy should be closed.

Surgeons should clearly be involved in decision making (procedure selection) for patients, and both the cardiologist and surgeon need a familiarity with the most recent results of percutaneous balloon valvuloplasty and operations at their institution.

REFERENCES

1. Hickey MSJ, Blackstone EH, Kirklin JW, et al: Outcome probabilities and life history after surgical mitral commissurotomy: implications for balloon commissurotomy. *J Am Coll Cardiol.* 17:29–42, 1991.

2. Brunton L: Preliminary note on the possibility of treating mitral stenosis by surgical methods. *Lancet.* 1:352, 1902.

3. Johnson SL: *The History of Cardiac Surgery 1896–1955.* Baltimore:Johns Hopkins Press, 1970, pp 87–107.

4. Meliones JN, Beekman RH, Rocchini AP, et al: Balloon valvuloplasty for recurrent aortic stenosis after surgical valvotomy in childhood: immediate and follow-up studies. *J Am Coll Cardiol.* 13:1106–1110, 1989.

5. Myers ML, Lawrie GM, Crawford ES, et al: The St. Jude valve prosthesis: analysis of the clinical results in 815 implants and the need for systemic anticoagulation. *J Am Coll Cardiol.* 13:57–62, 1989.

6. Lund O, Nielsen TT, Pilegaard HK, et al: The influence of coronary artery disease and bypass grafting on early and late survival after valve replacement for aortic stenosis. *J Thorac Cardiovasc Surg.* 100:327–337, 1990.

7. Czer LSC, Chaux A, Matloff JM, et al: Ten-year experience with the St. Jude Medical valve for primary valve replacement. *J Thorac Cardiovasc Surg.* 100:44–55, 1990.

8. Levinson JR, Akins CW, Buckley MJ, et al: Octogenarians with aortic stenosis: outcome after aortic valve replacement. *Circulation.* 80(suppl I):I-49–I-56, 1989.

9. Cheitlin MD: Severe aortic stenosis in the sick octogenarian. A clear indicator for balloon valvuloplasty as the initial procedure. *Circulation.* 80:1906–1908, 1989.

10. McKay CR, Waller BF, Hong R, et al: Problems encountered with catheter balloon valvuloplasty of bioprosthetic aortic valves. *Am Heart J.* 115:463–465, 1988.

11. McKay CR: Should patients with mitral stenosis who are acceptable surgical commissurotomy candidates now have balloon valvuloplasty treatment? *Cardiovasc Clin.* 21(1):175–195, 1990.

12. Reid CL, Chandraratna PAN, Kawanishi DT, et al: Influence of mitral valve morphology on double-balloon catheter balloon valvuloplasty in patients with mitral stenosis. Analysis of factors predicting immediate and 3-month results. *Circulation.* 80:515–524, 1989.

13. Abascal VM, Wilkins GT, O'Shea JP, et al: Predication of successful outcome in 130 patients undergoing percutaneous balloon mitral valvotomy. *Circulation.* 82:448–456, 1990.

14. Galloway AC, Colvin SB, Baumann FG, et al: A comparison of mitral valve reconstruction with mitral valve replacement: intermediate-term results. *Ann Thorac Surg.* 47:655–662, 1989.

15. Medina A, Suarez De Lezo J, Hernandez E, et al: Balloon valvuloplasty for mitral restenosis after previous surgery: a comparative study. *Am Heart J.* 120:568–571, 1990.

16. Cox DA, Friedman PL, Selwyn AP, et al: Improved quality of life after successful balloon valvuloplasty of a stenosed mitral bioprosthesis. *Am Heart J.* 118:839–841, 1989.

17. Ferguson JJ III, Riuli EP, Massumi A, et al: Balloon aortic valvuloplasty: the Texas Heart Institute experience. *Tex Heart Ins J.* 17:23–30, 1990.

18. Vahanian A, Michel PL, Cormier B, et al: Results of percutaneous mitral commissurotomy in 200 patients. *Am J Cardiol.* 63:847–852, 1989.

19. Acar C, Deloche A, Tibi PR, et al: Operative findings after percutaneous mitral dilation. *Ann Thorac Surg.* 49:959–963, 1990.

20. Johnson RG, Dhillon JS, Thurer RL, et al: Aortic valve operation after percutaneous aortic balloon valvuloplasty. *Ann Thorac Surg.* 49:740–745, 1990.

21. Robertson JM, de Virgilio C, French W, et al: Fatal left ventricular perforation during mitral balloon valvoplasty. *Ann Thorac Surg.* 49:819–821, 1990.

22. Aaron BL, Alyono D: Ventricular perforation with valvoplasty. *Ann Thorac Surg.* 50:1022, 1990.

23. Seifert, PE, Auer JE: Surgical repair of annular disruption following percutaneous balloon aortic valvuloplasty. *Ann Thorac Surg.* 46:242–243, 1988.

24. Lembro NJ, King SB III, Roubin GS, et al: Fatal aortic rupture during percutaneous balloon valvuloplasty for valvular aortic stenosis. *Am J Cardiol.* 60:733–736, 1987.

25. Cequier A, Bonan R, Crepeau J, et al: Massive mitral regurgitation caused by tearing of the anterior leaflet during percutaneous mitral balloon valvuloplasty. *Am J Med.* 85:100–103, 1988.

26. Lewin RF, Dorros G, King JF, et al: Percutaneous transluminal aortic valvuloplasty: acute outcome and follow-up of 125 patients. *J Am Coll Cardiol.* 14:1210–1217, 1989.

27. Ramondo A, Chirillo F, Dan M, et al: Mitral valve disruption following percutaneous balloon valvuloplasty. *Cathet Cardiovasc Diagn.* 21:239–244, 1990.

28. de Ubago JLM, Vasquez de Prada JA, Moujir F, et al: Mitral valve rupture during percutaneous dilation of aortic valve stenosis. *Cathet Cardiovasc Diagn. 16:115–118, 1989.*

29. Phillips RR, Gerlis LM, Wilson N, et al: Aortic valve damage caused by operative balloon dilatation of critical aortic valve stenosis. *Br Heart J.* 57:168–170, 1987.

30. Skillman JJ, Kim D, Baim DS: Vascular complications of percutaneous femoral cardiac interventions. *Arch Surg.* 123:1207–1212, 1988.

31. Letac B, Cribier A, Koning R, et al: Aortic stenosis in elderly patients aged 80 or older. Treatment by percutaneous balloon valvuloplasty in a series of 92 cases. *Circulation.* 80:1514–1520, 1989.

32. Berland J, Cribier A, Savin T, et al: Percutaneous balloon valvuloplasty in patients with severe aortic stenosis and low ejection fraction. Immediate results and 1-year follow-up. *Circulation.* 79:1189–1196, 1989.

33. Vogel M, Benson LN, Burrows P, et al: Balloon dilatation of congenital aortic valve stenosis in infants and children: short term and intermediate results. *Br Heart J.* 62:148–153, 1989.

34. Losordo DW, Ramaswamy K, Rosenfield K, et al: Use of emergency balloon dilation to reverse acute hemodynamic decompensation developing during diagnostic catheterization for aortic stenosis (bailout valvuloplasty). *Am J Cardiol.* 63:388–389, 1989.

35. Friedman HZ, Cragg DR, O'Neill WW: Cardiac resuscitation using emergency aortic balloon valvuloplasty. *Am J Cardiol.* 63:387–388, 1989.

36. Johnson RG, Williams GR, Razook JD, et al: Reoperation in congenital aortic stenosis. *Ann Thorac Surg.* 40:156–162, 1985.

37. Craver JM. Aortic valve debridement by ultrasonic surgical aspirator: a word of caution. *Ann Thorac Surg.* 49:746–753, 1990.

38. McBride LR, Naunheim KS, Fiore AC, et al: Aortic valve decalcification. *J Thorac Cardiovasc Surg.* 100:36–43, 1990.

39. Freeman WK, Schaff HV, Orszulak TA, et al: Ultrasonic aortic valve decalcification: serial Doppler echocardiographic follow-up. *J Am Coll Cardiol.* 16:623–630, 1990.

40. O'Brien MF, Stafford EG, Gardner MAH, et al: A comparison of aortic valve replacement with viable cryopreserved and fresh allograft valves, with a note on chromosomal studies. *J Thorac Cardiovasc Surg.* 94:812–823, 1987.

41. Sherman W, Hershman R, Lazzam C, et al: Balloon valvuloplasty in adult aortic stenosis: determinants of clinical outcome. *Ann Intern Med.* 110:421–425, 1989.

42. Brdlik O, Laub GW, Fernandez J, et al: Aortic valve disruption after percutaneous aortic balloon valvoplasty. *Ann Thorac Surg.* 49:822–823, 1990.

43. Lemmer JH Jr, Winniford MD, Ferguson DW: Surgical implications of atrial septal defect complicating aortic balloon valvuloplasty. *Ann Thorac Surg.* 48:295–297, 1989.

44. Grantham RN, Daggett WM, Cosimi AB, et al: Transventricular mitral valvulotomy.

Analysis of factors influencing operative and late results. *Circulation*. 50 (suppl II): II-200–II-211, 1974.

45. Ellis LB, Singh JB, Morales DD, et al: Fifteen- to twenty-year study of one thousand patients undergoing closed mitral valvuloplasty. *Circulation*. 48:357–364, 1973.

46. Housman LB, Bonchek L, Lambert L, et al: Prognosis of patients after open mitral commissurotomy. Acturial analysis of late results in 100 patients. *J Thorac Cardiovasc Surg*. 73:742–745, 1977.

47. Eguaras MG, Luque I, Montero A, et al: A comparison of repair and replacement for mitral stenosis with partially calcified valves. *J Thorac Cardiovasc Surg*. 100:161–166, 1990.

48. Inoue K, Owaki T, Nakamura T, et al: Clinical application of transvenous mitral commissurotomy by a new balloon catheter. *J Thorac Cardiovasc Surg*. 87:394–402, 1984.

49. Nakano S, Mitsuno M, Taniguchi K, et al: Ultrasonic debridement during mitral valve reconstruction for calcified mitral stenosis. *Ann Thorac Surg*. 50:923–926, 1990.

50. Yoshida K, Yoshikawa J, Akasaka T, et al: Assessment of left-to-right atrial shunting after percutaneous mitral valvuloplasty by transesophageal color Doppler flow-mapping. *Circulation*. 80:1521–1526, 1989.

CHAPTER 23

Future Prospects

TSUNG O. CHENG

It was only barely a decade ago that balloon dilatation was first introduced to treat stenotic lesions in both congenital[1] and acquired heart diseases.[2] Now percutaneous balloon valvuloplasty has become an accepted alternative to surgical treatment of many of these lesions. This successful outcome can be attributed in part to the establishment in the early course of its development of several data registries and cooperative studies: the Valvuloplasty and Angioplasty of Congenital Anomalies (VACA) Registry[3] in 1983; the French Cooperative Study of Percutaneous Mitral Valvotomy[4] and the Mansfield Balloon Aortic Valvuloplasty Registry[5] in 1986; and the National Heart, Lung, and Blood Institute (NHLBI) Aortic[6] and Mitral[7] Valvuloplasty Registries in 1987. These registries ensure proper, expedient, and safe development of the various procedures through coordination and open communication regarding techniques, success and complication rates, and long-term followup results among the different investigators and institutions engaged in these procedures. Although a registry is not a replacement for a well-designed clinical trial, it successfully achieves these expectations.[8]

BALLOON PULMONIC VALVULOPLASTY

Percutaneous balloon pulmonic valvuloplasty is now a well-established technique for the treatment of congenital pulmonic stenosis in all age groups.[9,10] The procedure has proved safe, with a lower mortality than surgery and probably a lower morbidity as well.[9,11] The immediate and late results of percutaneous balloon pulmonic valvuloplasty are comparable to those after surgery.[9,11,12] As a result the U.S. Food and Drug Administration (FDA) has approved percutaneous balloon pulmonic valvuloplasty for use in both children and adults.

Balloon pulmonary valvuloplasty is also a useful alternative to aortopulmonary shunts for the relief of cyanosis in children with tetralogy of Fallot.[13] It has the added advantage of promoting growth of the pulmonary valve annulus and pulmonary arteries.[13]

523

BALLOON MITRAL VALVULOPLASTY

Because percutaneous balloon mitral valvuloplasty can achieve hemodynamic results similar to those of surgery and may delay or postpone indefinitely the trauma and expense of surgery, it is an attractive and acceptable alternative to surgical mitral commissurotomy.[14] This is equally true for both young[15,16] and old[17,18] as well as surgical high risk patients.[19] The results, both immediate and late, are certainly comparable to those of closed surgical mitral commissurotomy[20,21] and perhaps also to those of open surgical mitral commissurotomy.[22] It is expected that the long-term results will be similar too.[23-25] Echocardiography rather than cardiac catheterization is the best way to follow these patients.[26] Moreover, percutaneous balloon mitral valvuloplasty improves not only the ventilatory function but also the exercise performance of these patients.[27]

Whether the single-balloon catheter or the double-balloon catheter technique is the procedure of choice remains to be seen. However, with the excellent results following the use of the Inoue balloon catheter on the largest series of patients in the world reported from China and Japan (see Chapter 10), as well as from Korea,[28,29] India,[30] France,[31] Belgium,[32] Spain,[33] South Africa,[34] Saudi Arabia,[35] and also the United States,[36,37] the single-balloon technique of Inoue may prevail eventually over the double-balloon technique. The only limiting factor is the cost and availability of the Inoue balloon catheter.[37] The catheter industry thus has the responsibility of making these catheters more readily available and affordable, especially in the developing countries where rheumatic mitral stenosis is still prevalent.

Besides the single- and double-balloon techniques of valvuloplasty, bifoil and trefoil balloon catheters have also been introduced recently.[38] Bifoil and trefoil balloon catheters have the theoretical advantage of avoiding complete obstruction of the valve orifice during inflation. In the presence of a bicuspid or tricuspid valve configuration, however, they could be potentially more occlusive than monofoil balloons because each of the two and three individual components of bifoil and trefoil balloons, respectively, may occupy the intercommissural spaces while inflated.[39]

BALLOON AORTIC VALVULOPLASTY

For congenital valvular aortic stenosis the VACA Registry data[40] suggest that percutaneous balloon aortic valvuloplasty provides effective acute relief in both infants and children. Serious complications are uncommon if balloon valvuloplasty is performed on children older than 1 month of age. Percutaneous balloon aortic valvuloplasty is equally effective for recurrent aortic stenosis after surgical valvuloplasty in childhood.[41] However, long-term followup data are necessary before balloon valvuloplasty can be established as a treatment of choice for congenital valvular aortic stenosis.

Although the Mansfield and NHLBI Registry data were not designed to compare balloon valvuloplasty directly with surgical treatment of acquired aortic stenosis, they have been useful in evaluating the efficacy and safety of the procedure on a large group of symptomatic patients with severe aortic stenosis, especially the elderly. The registries also provide data on the feasibility of a randomized trial to compare this new method of treating aortic stenosis with the more established surgical procedures.

The recently published results of the Mansfield Scientific Aortic Valvuloplasty Registry suggest that balloon aortic valvuloplasty can bring about immediate hemodynamic improvement in patients with aortic stenosis, with only a minimal risk of increasing aortic insufficiency.[42] Older patients have as good results in terms of objective measures of valve area and gradient reduction as do younger patients.[43] Followup of the patients in the Mansfield Registry suggests that modest clinical benefit was achieved by balloon valvuloplasty.[44] Palliation of symptoms occurred in two thirds of patients who survived to 6-month followup. Improvement as defined by doubling in valve area did impart a survival advantage, especially in patients with extremely severe aortic stenosis. Percutaneous balloon aortic valvuloplasty can be performed in patients with low gradient, low output states with an in-hospital mortality less than that of a comparable group undergoing aortic valve replacement.[45] Identifying which patients are associated with increased complications may improve patient selection and allow more accurate assessment of the risk:benefit ratio for this specific patient subset.

Future directions for clinical research are apparent. Procedural and catheter modifications must occur to lessen in-hospital morbidity. More effective methods of nonoperative improvement in valve orifice area must be sought (see below). Methods to limit restenosis must be developed. In the interim, guarded optimism for the use of balloon aortic valvuloplasty in elderly, nonoperable patients with aortic stenosis is warranted, because in many of them it may provide the only reasonable possibility for improving their condition.[46]

BALLOON TRICUSPID VALVULOPLASTY

To date, only a few isolated reports on the successful use of balloon valvuloplasty to treat tricuspid stenosis have appeared. Despite the scarcity of data on balloon tricuspid valvuloplasty, it is expected that balloon dilatation will offer a feasible and effective percutaneous method for treating this condition. Such long-term results as have been published have been very encouraging.[47] Given that the most common etiology of the disease is rheumatic, separation of fused commissures appears to be the underlying mechanism of success. A double-balloon technique will presumably be needed to achieve effective dilatation, given the size of the tricuspid anulus in most adults. In addition, given the proximity of the atrioventricular conduction system to the tricuspid valve, one may also expect complete heart block to be a possible complication of the procedure.[48]

Pure tricuspid stenosis is uncommon. The etiology is usually rheumatic and rarely congenital.[49,50] Carcinoid heart disease may manifest as tricuspid stenosis, although it is usually associated with tricuspid regurgitation.[51,52] Patients with severe tricuspid stenosis and mild to moderate tricuspid regurgitation are still potential candidates for balloon tricuspid valvuloplasty.[47,52] The decision to perform such a procedure in patients with significant tricuspid regurgitation accompanying moderate to severe tricuspid stenosis is a difficult one, because balloon tricuspid valvuloplasty may worsen tricuspid regurgitation. Only long-term followup of these patients will help resolve this dilemma.

PROSTHETIC AND CONDUIT VALVULOPLASTY

Balloon dilatation of prosthetic and conduit valves represents another potential application of percutaneous balloon valvuloplasty. Experience in the pediatric population suggests that such a procedure may be successfully performed without complications such as embolic phenomena or acute valvular insufficiency.[53,54] Published experience in adults is more limited. Although successful uncomplicated dilatation of calcified stenotic mitral prosthetic valves has been reported,[55,56] the possibility of peripheral embolism during balloon bioprosthetic valvuloplasty in adults poses a real risk.[57] The recent introduction of an embolization-preventing device[58] may be a solution. Further study is needed in this area.

Conduit obstruction may be amenable to balloon dilatation, depending on the level of the stenosis, and may allow a delay in reoperation.[59-61] On the other hand, the success rate may be limited,[62] and it is thus unclear how long conduit replacement may be postponed and whether the short-term palliation significantly decreases the risk of reoperation. More work needs to be done in this field.

MULTIVALVE BALLOON VALVULOPLASTY

The feasibility of using a balloon to dilate several cardiac valves in the same patient concurrently has already been demonstrated.[63] Because multivalvular stenoses, either congenital or acquired, are common, and in view of the recent demonstration that balloon aortic valvuloplasty can be done as successfully in antegrade fashion as retrogradely,[64] percutaneous balloon valvuloplasty can be readily performed transvenously to treat combined valvular stenoses of all four valves of the heart.

With increased operators' expertise and technical improvement of the balloon catheters, the amount of radiation exposure for multivalve balloon valvuloplasty would be comparable to multivessel percutaneous transluminal coronary angioplasty (PTCA) and therefore acceptable. Just as PTCA evolved from a single-vessel to a multivessel procedure, it would not be long before percutaneous balloon valvuloplasty of two, three, or even four cardiac valves will become a common practice. In developing countries where rheumatic heart disease is still prevalent, this nonoperative treatment of multivalve stenoses will have a major impact on the cost of health care.

BALLOON DILATATION OF NONVALVULAR CARDIOVASCULAR LESIONS

Besides the stenotic lesions of the four heart valves, either native or prosthetic, other stenotic lesions involving the parietal pericardium,[65] aorta,[66,67] pulmonary veins,[68] superior vena cava,[68,69] inferior vena cava,[70,71] aortopulmonary shunts,[68] supra- and subvalvular obstructions[68] (see also Chapter 21) have all been successfully dilated with balloon catheters. In fact, balloon dilatation is at present the treatment of choice in most patients with recoarctation because the results are good and the morbidity and mortality are insignificant when compared to reoperation.[72] Balloon angioplasty is equally successful in nonoperative treatment of native coarctation.[73] Furthermore, in contrast to surgical repair of coarctation, which is complicated by aneurysm formation in 30% of patients,[74] aneurysms seldom develop after balloon angioplasty.[75] Percutaneous balloon dilatation is also an effective and safe alternative to surgical treatment of Budd-Chiari syndrome due to membranous obstruction of the inferior vena cava[70,71] (Figs. 23.1 and 23.2).

Patent ductus arteriosus now can not only be closed by transcatheter delivery of occluding devices but also dilated with a balloon catheter. Corwin and associates[76]

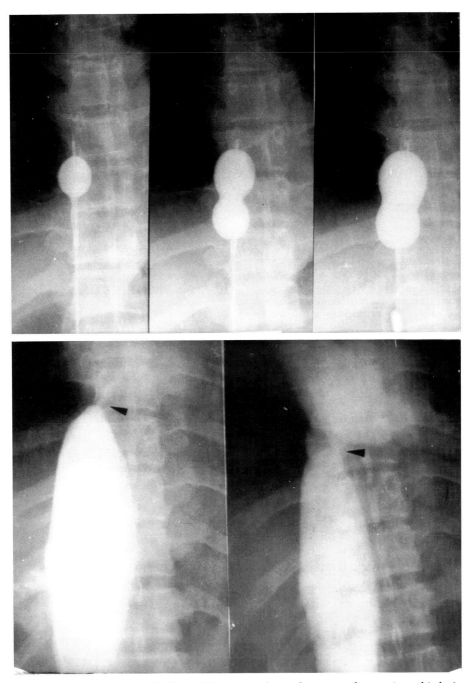

Figure 23.1 Percutaneous balloon dilatation of membranous obstruction of inferior vena cava in a 30-year-old Chinese man. *Top left,* Inoue balloon being inflated just above the obstruction. *Top center,* Further inflation showing "waisting" at the site of obstruction. *Top right,* Near disappearance of the waist after full balloon inflation. *Bottom left,* Inferior vena cavogram before balloon dilatation showing near-complete occlusion of the inferior vena cava as it enters the right atrium (*arrowhead*). *Bottom right,* Inferior vena cavogram after successful dilatation showing that the luminal diameter has increased from 2 to 20 mm (*arrowhead*) with prompt right atrial filling. The caval pressure decreased from 32 to 20 mmHg. (Courtesy of Chuan-Rong Chen, M.D. and Xue-Liang Yang, M.D.)

527

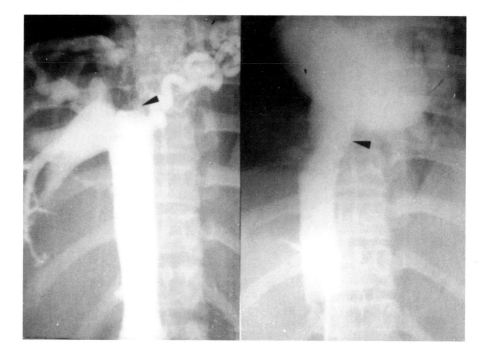

Figure 23.2 Percutaneous balloon dilatation of complete membranous obstruction of inferior vena cava in a 27-year-old Chinese woman. *Left,* Predilatation inferior vena cavogram showing complete caval obstruction (*arrowhead*) 2 mm below its entrance into right atrium with profuse collaterals visualized below the obstruction. *Right,* Postdilatation inferior vena cavogram showing luminal enlargement to near normal (*arrowhead*) with prompt filling of right atrium and disappearance of all the collaterals and less distention of the inferior vena cava. (Courtesy of Chuan-Rong Chen, M.D. and Xue-Liang Yang, M.D.)

used a 5F Berman angiographic catheter advanced prograde with the balloon inflated with air in an infant with an interrupted aortic arch and ventricular septal defect. They tried this approach as palliation just prior to taking the infant to surgery. Suarez de Lezo and associates[77] used a static, fluid-filled balloon catheter advanced from the main pulmonary artery and successfully dilated a patent ductus arteriosus in an infant with the hypoplastic left heart syndrome. More experimental work needs to be done in this area, because dilatation of stenotic ductus arteriosus could represent an alternative for palliative treatment of ductus-dependent congenital heart diseases. Furthermore, if permanent dilatation of the ductus arteriosus could be performed, fewer infants would require shunting operations.

When surgery is available for the above miscellaneous lesions, it is very complex, marginally successful, or both. Catheter dilatation of these lesions has demonstrated some acute success in each type of lesion and carries a low incidence of significant complications. Dilatation of most of these miscellaneous lesions, however, should still be undertaken as an investigational procedure under a protocol both for the technique and for the detailed followup of each patient. These procedures probably should be performed in institutions routinely performing other catheter dilatation procedures where both the experience and the often extensive inventory of special equipment are available.

PERCUTANEOUS CARDIOPULMONARY
BYPASS SUPPORT

Percutaneous balloon valvuloplasty for the management of aortic valvular stenosis is generally performed in patients who are high operative risks or in whom open heart surgery is contraindicated. Unfortunately, these patients also are at high risk during balloon valvuloplasty and the risk is even higher if concurrent PTCA is required. These patients will have a period of no forward flow when the balloon is inflated within the aortic orifice, leading to ischemia, hypotension, and ventricular arrhythmias.

In an effort to limit myocardial or cerebral ischemia during balloon inflation and to prevent cardiovascular collapse, these patients currently are being prophylactically placed on percutaneous cardiopulmonary bypass support.[78-80] This simple concept involves cardiopulmonary bypass using relatively new technology, and it is accomplished in the cardiac catheterization laboratory on awake patients. The cardiopulmonary bypass support system (CPS, Bard, Inc., Billerica, MA), instituted by means of femoral venous–right atrial and femoral arterial cannulas inserted percutaneously, can achieve a flow rate of up to 5 L/min.[80]

As interventional cardiology advances into the treatment of more complex and advanced valvular and coronary artery diseases, circulatory-supported procedures are likely to bridge the gap between standard transcatheter interventions and open heart surgery. The technique has also been used effectively to treat patients with such catastrophic complications as ventricular perforation during percutaneous balloon mitral valvuloplasty.[81,82] A 51-year-old woman at the author's institution in the United States suffered a left ventricular perforation during percutaneous balloon mitral valvuloplasty.[83] Rather than attempting to take a dying patient to the operating room, the surgeons immediately instituted the Bard CPS system in the cardiac catheterization laboratory. During the interval between ventricular perforation and open heart surgical repair, the pressures, perfusion, and oxygenation were well preserved. The patient arrived in the operating room in a relatively stable state, her ventricular perforation was closed and her mitral valve replaced, and she made an uneventful recovery.

LASER MYOPLASTY, TRANSCATHETER
MYECTOMY, AND ANGIOSCOPIC MYOTOMY

Isner and associates[84] reported successful laser myoplasty performed intraoperatively in a patient with hypertrophic cardiomyopathy, using a 200-micron fiber interfaced with an argon laser. They established the feasibility of using laser therapy to create a myoplasty trough that is similar in appearance to that typically achieved by the conventional blade technique. They further pointed out two principal advantages of laser myoplasty: constant illumination of the intraventricular operative field and precise modeling of the myoplasty trough. The feasibility of a nonoperative approach for percutaneous laser therapy is currently being investigated for treatment of medically refractory hypertrophic cardiomyopathic patients (Isner JM, personal communication, March 19, 1991).

Qureshi and associates[85] recently reported the successful use of an atherectomy catheter for percutaneous transcatheter myectomy of the infundibulum in a 2-year-old child with tetralogy of Fallot with severe subvalvular pulmonic stenosis. The right

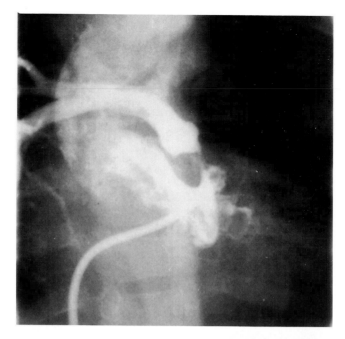

A

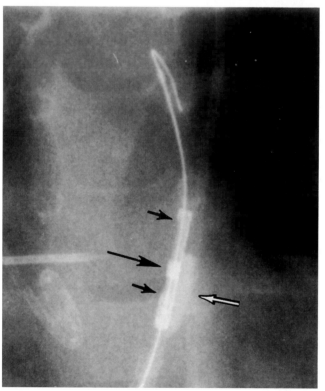

B

Figure 23.3 *A,* Selective angiogram in the infundibulum (AP projection) taken at start of procedure showing gross hypertrophy of the infundibulum. *B,* Atherectomy catheter (AP projection) in position during myectomy. The balloon was inflated (*hollow arrow*), the cutting window (*small arrows*) was in contact with the infundibulum, and the drill, which was being advanced, can be seen (*large arrow*).
C, Selective angiogram in the infundibulum (AP projection) after myectomy. The outflow tract was wider and the surface of the infundibulum (*arrow*) was irregular.

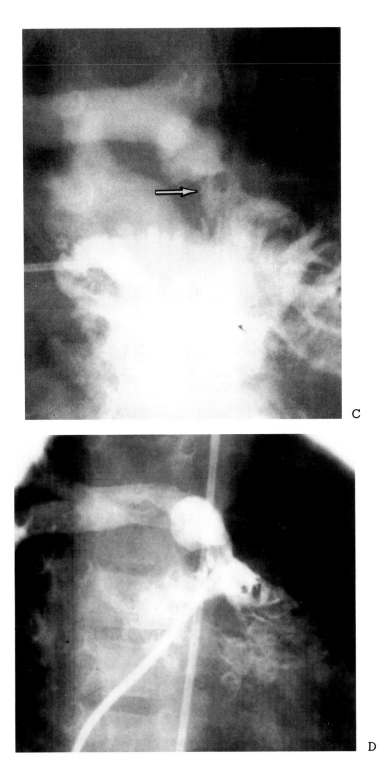

C

D

(*A, B,* and *C* from: Qureshi SA et al: Percutaneous transcatheter myectomy of subvalvar pulmonary stenosis in tetralogy of Fallot: a new palliative technique with an
atherectomy catheter. *Br Heart J.* 64:163–165, 1990. With permission.) *D,* Followup
angiogram 1 year later showed persistence of the irregularities and widening of the
outflow tract with some remodeling. (Courtesy of Shakeel A. Qureshi, M.D.)

531

ventricular outflow tract had been balloon-dilated when the patient was 14 months old. Seven months later angiography showed severe infundibular stenosis (Fig. 23.3A). He underwent further balloon dilatation of the right ventricular outflow tract followed by transcatheter myectomy of the infundibulum with an atherectomy catheter (Fig. 23, 3B). Although there was no change in the pressures across the right ventricular outflow tract, repeat angiography showed a wider outflow tract (Fig. 23.3C). A followup angiogram 1 year later showed maintenance of the widened outflow tract (Fig. 23.3D) (Qureshi SA, personal communication, April 15, 1991). Transcatheter resection of the infundibulum may be an important adjunct in the palliation of tetralogy of Fallot and possibly other conditions characterized by fibromuscular stenosis. However, further modifications of the atherectomy catheter are needed for this technique to become widely accepted.

The recent introduction of an angioscope-guided catheter-scissor system[86] may have clinical potential. When performed with angioscopic guidance, percutaneous cardiac myotomy or myectomy may be more accurate and safe (Fig. 23.4). The preliminary results in dogs have been encouraging.[86]

LASER BALLOON ANGIOPLASTY AND STENT IMPLANTATION

Laser balloon angioplasty is being used to alleviate the common causes (dissection, recoil, thrombosis) of suboptimal luminal results of conventional balloon coronary angioplasty, and has been found to be safe and effective.[87,88] Although laser treatment of valvular stenosis,[89] pulmonary atresia,[89] and coarctation of the aorta[89] was attempted experimentally almost a decade ago, the clinical application of this technique has only been reported recently.[90]

Various intravascular stents have been developed to avoid restenosis after PTCA.[91] An animal study aimed at stent implantation in pulmonary artery stenosis (Fig. 23.5) and venous obstructions[92] demonstrated a patency rate of 93% on followup. Twenty-seven stents were placed in 13 mongrel dogs through long sheaths (12 to 14 Fr.) and expanded up to 18-mm diameter. Stent embolization occurred in 11% without hemodynamic consequences. Intimal proliferation was mild and side branches along the stent remained patent.

Another animal study was reported recently on balloons to examine the feasibility of stent deployment in stenotic right heart valved conduits (Fig. 23.6).[93] The technique was successful in all (Fig. 23.7), resulting in significant hemodynamic improvement. Insertion of a valve conduit between the right ventricular outflow tract and the pulmonary artery during repair of certain types of complex congenital heart disease

Figure 23.4 Percutaneous angioscope–guided cardiomyotomy. *Top*, The system composed of a 9F guiding balloon catheter (*a*), scissors (*b*), 1.6F fiberscope (*c*), and a guidewire (*d*) fixed to the scissors. *Middle*, Schematic representation of the method of cardiomyotomy. *Bottom left*, Angioscopic view during cardiomyotomy of the left ventricle. The edges of the scissors (*a*) were opened and pushed against a trabecula. *Bottom right*, Angioscopic view showing the edges of the scissors (*a*) closed to excise the trabecula (*arrowheads*). (From: Uchida et al: Percutaneous cardiomyotomy and valvulotomy with angioscopic guidance. *Am Heart J.* 121:1221–1224, 1991. With permission.)

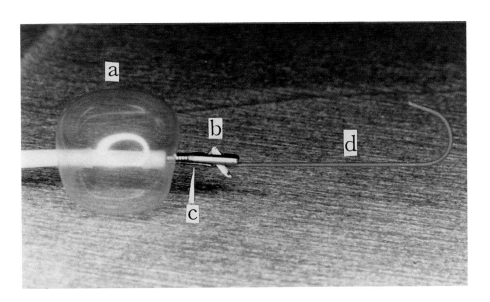

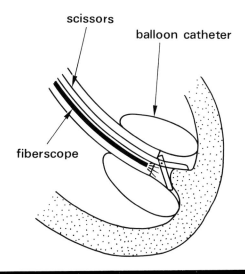

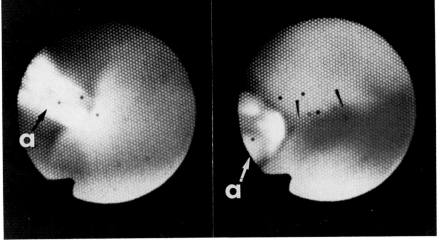

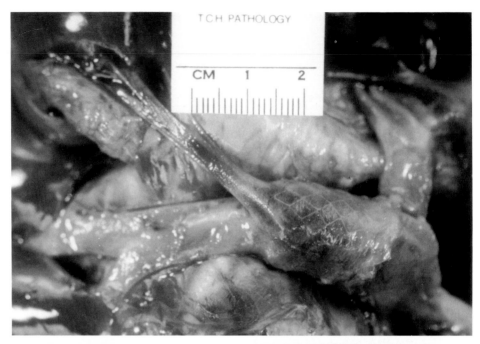

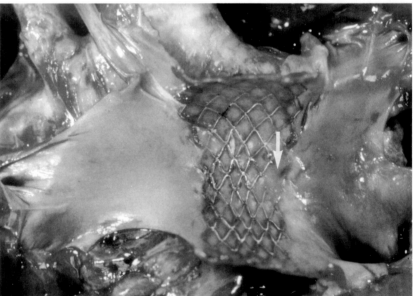

Figure 23.5 *Top*, Exterior of the right pulmonary artery from a dog (2-month follow-up). The expandable intravascular stent may be seen through the thin pulmonary arterial wall. The configuration of the struts is seen clearly. The artery has been dilated to greater than its native diameter, as seen by comparison with the left pulmonary artery in the background. *Bottom*, The stent was patent without thrombosis. The process of covering with neointima was progressing (*arrow*). (From: Mullins CE et al: Implantation of balloon-expandable intravascular grafts by catheterization in pulmonary arteries and systemic veins. *Circulation.* 77:188–199, 1988. With permission of the American Heart Association Inc.)

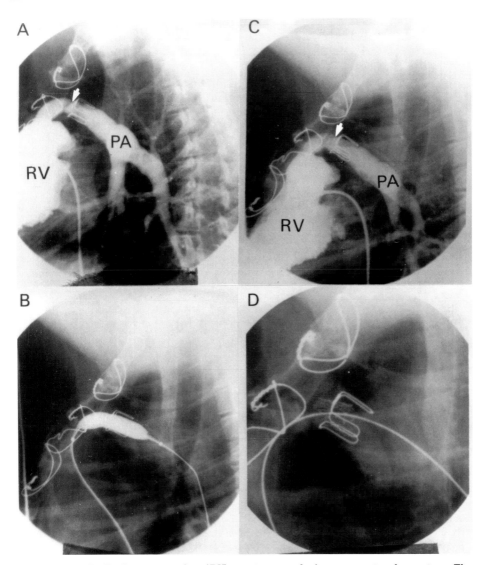

Figure 23.6 *A,* Right ventricular (*RV*) angiogram before stent implantation. The arrow is pointing toward the stenotic area in the right ventricular–pulmonary artery (*PA*) conduit. *B,* A fully expanded 15-mm balloon catheter across the stenosis during stent deployment. *C,* Right ventricular angiogram after stent implanation. The stenosis was resolved (*arrow*). *D,* Fully expanded stent across the valved conduit. (From: Almagor Y et al: Balloon expandable stent implantation in stenotic right heart valved conduits. *J Am Coll Cardiol.* 16:1310–1314, 1990. With permission.)

has been recommended. Applications include D-transposition of the great arteries with ventricular septal defect and pulmonic stenosis, pulmonary atresia, tetralogy of Fallot, and truncus arteriosus type 1; a biologic valve is generally used to avoid anticoagulation. This technique may be a useful alternative transcatheter procedure, especially in light of recent reports[54,61,62] indicating mixed results from percutaneous balloon dilatation in relieving valved-conduit stenosis. Stent implantation may help

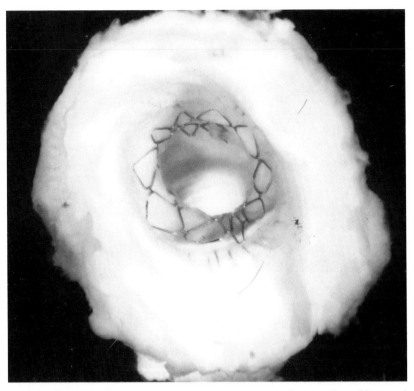

Figure 23.7 Gross pathologic section of the stent in the conduit. Notice the full expansion of the stent which is embedded in the fibrous peel. (From: Almagor Y et al: Balloon expandable stent implantation in stenotic right heart valved conduits. *J Am Coll Cardiol.* 16:1310–1314, 1990. With permission.)

defer conduit replacement in young children until a later age when a larger, definitive conduit can be inserted.

These experimental investigations suggest that stents hold promise for definitive dilatation of congenital or postoperative vessel stenosis. Early clinical application has confirmed their feasibility and safety.[94] Future study directions should include (1) thrombogenicity of stents in a low venous pressure circulation, (2) endothelialization and neointima formation over the stent surface, (3) assessment of long-term effects of stent implantation that may result in conduit restenosis, and (4) development of new equipment to improve the success of stent deployment. More flexible stents permitting expansion of longer conduit segments and stronger balloons with higher burst pressures will be necessary to improve clinical results.

LASER OR ULTRASONIC DECALCIFICATION AND SHOCK WAVE LITHOTRIPSY

Balloon aortic valvuloplasty offers immediate and dramatic relief of symptoms in most patients with severe aortic stenosis, but the results have been less satisfactory in adults with heavily calcified valves. Recently there has been a resurgence of interest and enthusiasm for mechanical decalcification by either laser or ultrasound.

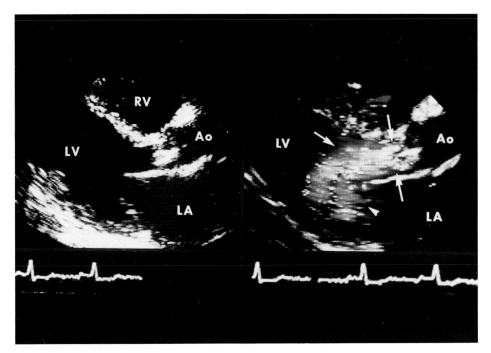

Figure 23.8 Composite two-dimensional Doppler echocardiographic findings in a patient with severe aortic regurgitation after ultrasonic aortic valve decalcification. *Left panel*, Parasternal long-axis image in diastole: the left ventricle is moderately dilated and residual calcific aortic valve disease is present. *Right panel*, Doppler color flow imaging reveals a broad aortic regurgitant jet (arrows) nearly filling the entire left ventricular outflow tract during diastole; mitral diastolic inflow is also visualized (*arrowhead*). *Ao*—aorta. *LA*—left atrium. *RV*—right ventricle. (From: Freeman WK et al: Ultrasonic aortic valve decalcification: serial Doppler echocardiographic follow-up. *J Am Coll Cardiol.* 16:623–630, 1990. With permission.)

Continuous-wave lasers, such as the argon and neodymium:yttrium-aluminum-garnet, (Nd:YAG), are ineffective in decalcifying valves.[95] Pulsed lasers, such as erbium:YAG and excimer, can achieve valve decalcification. However, perforation occurred with the erbium:YAG. Excimer, the other pulsed laser, at appropriate pulse energy and repetition rates may lead to selective ablation of calcified valve tissue.[95]

Ultrasonic aortic valve decalcification was associated with favorable early results.[96,97] However, a high restenosis rate and an unacceptably high rate of significant aortic insufficiency at followup evaluation (Fig. 23.8 and 23.9) prompted many early enthusiasts to abandon this technique.[98,99] More recently ultrasonic debridement during mitral valve reconstruction for calcific mitral stenosis with favorable short-term results was reported from Japan.[100] However, one has to await the long-term results to see if they will be similar to those of aortic valve decalcification.

Shock waves have been successfully used for nephrolith and gallstone fragmentation. Thus, one may presume that valvular calcific deposits also can be fragmented using shock wave treatment. The morphology of the calcified valves, however, is different from that in nephrolith. In the valves, even extensive calcifications do not consist of compact slabs but are embedded in fibrous tissue as a diffuse granulate. With fibroid conglutination of the commissures, the further fragmentation of these

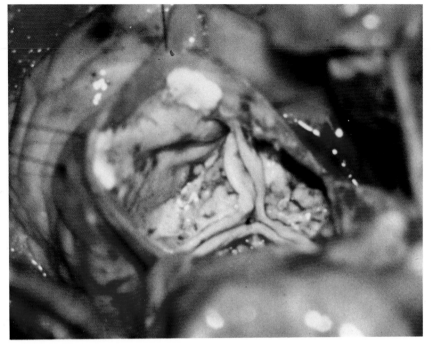

A

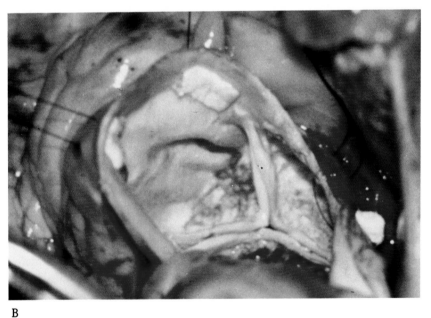

B

Figure 23.9 Intraoperative photography of the aortic valve as viewed from aortotomy. *A,* Severe senescent aortic stenosis before ultrasonic decalcification. *B,* Immediately after ultrasonic decalcification; most calcific excresences have been debrided and cusp coaptation is intact.

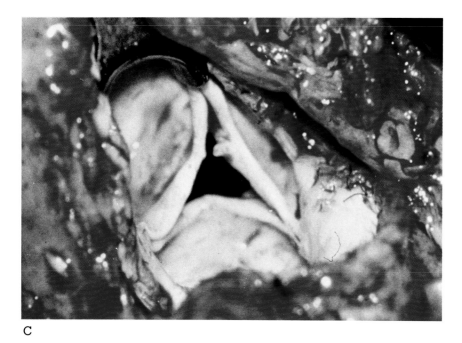

C

Figure 23.9 (continued) *C,* The same patient at reoperation 7.5 months later for severe aortic regurgitation. The previously decalcified aortic cusps are thickened and severely retracted with marked deficiency in central coaptation. (From: Freeman WK et al: Ultrasonic aortic valve decalcification: serial Doppler echocardiographic follow-up. *J Am Coll Cardiol.* 16:623–630, 1990. With permission.)

granulates does not lead to any significant increase in mitral valve opening area. Contrary to expectation, the mobility of the cusps was not improved.

Furthermore, shock wave treatment can cause calcium particles to be torn off. Serious danger of calcium embolism[101] makes this method unsuitable either as a pretreatment in or an alternative treatment to balloon valvuloplasty.

CONCLUSIONS

When Rashkind[102] a quarter of a century ago created an atrial septal defect in an infant by means of a balloon mounted at the tip of a catheter as a palliative approach to complete transposition of the great arteries, little did he know how many thousands more therapeutic procedures would be accomplished with a balloon (Fig. 23.10). Since that time balloon catheters have been used to dilate stenotic valves and stenotic blood vessels, to embolize congenital or surgically created systemic–pulmonary collateral blood vessels and pulmonary arteriovenous malformations, and finally to close congenital defects such as patent ductus arteriosus or atrial septal defect. Although this book deals only with their use for dilatation of stenotic valves and blood vessels, the sky is the limit to how far balloons will fly.

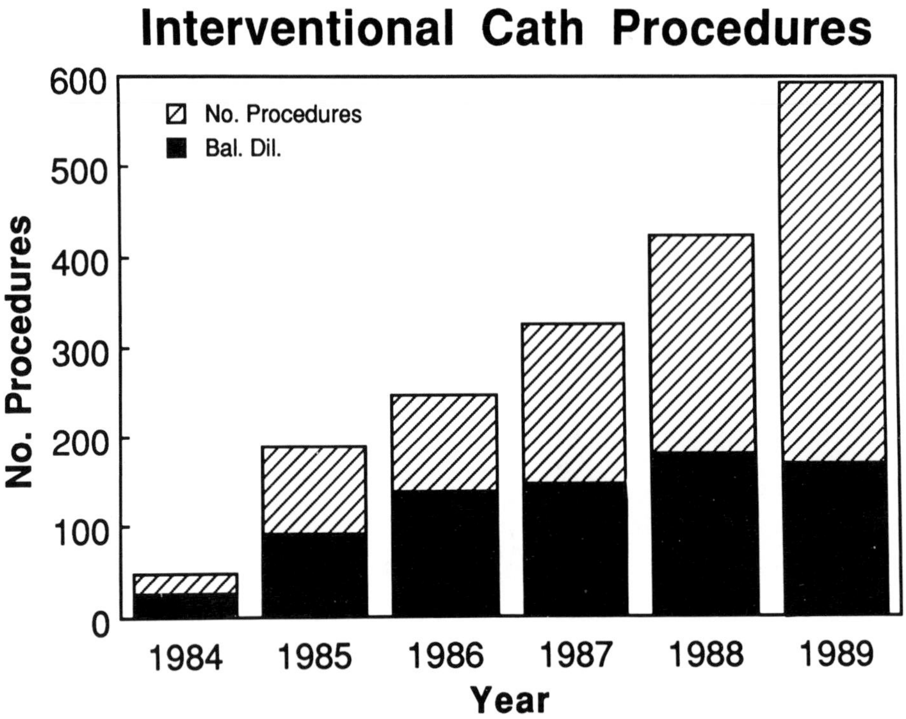

Interventional Cath Procedures

Figure 23.10 Therapeutic cardiac catheterizations at the Children's Hospital, Boston. Note the rapid increase in both total numbers of interventional catheterization procedures and balloon dilatation procedures from 1984 to 1989. (Courtesy of James E. Lock, M.D.)

Cardiologists in the catheterization laboratory cannot view the movie *Around the World in 80 Days* without thinking, "Where else can balloons take us?" They cannot listen to the radio without beaming at the lyrics, "up, up and away in my beautiful balloon." As Zeevi and associates[62] conclude: "We, hoping to defer surgical interventions, continue to attempt balloon dilation . . . with care, concern, caution and judicious, meticulous adherence to protocol, the balloon does not burst (figure of speech)."[103] As Mark Twain once said, "To a man with a hammer a lot of things look like a nail that needs pounding."

Over the past decade cardiologists, both pediatric and adult, have made remarkable progress in developing nonsurgical methods for treating many forms of congenital and acquired heart disease. With further modification of existing procedures, the validation of interventional procedures that are currently experimental — such as transcatheter closure of septal defects, transcatheter occlusion of patent ductus arteriosus, laser balloon angioplasty, laser myoplasty, transcatheter myectomy, angioscopic myotomy, balloon-expandable intravascular stents, and the advent of intravascular guided echocardiography[104] — and the development of even newer and innovative procedures, such as the recent application of valvuloplasty techniques to the fetus,[105,106] therapeutic catheterization alone in lieu of, or in combination with, a surgical procedure will become the standard of cardiologic care of the majority of patients with valvular heart disease. I predict that before the end of this century even transcatheter valve replacement will be feasible. It is ironic to note that, although Rashkind's balloon atrial septosomy for transposition is now seldom used, being replaced in many major medical centers by an arterial switch operation,[107,108] its impact on the therapeutic application of a balloon catheter in the practice of pediatric and adult cardiology will continue to be felt for many years to come.

REFERENCES

1. Kan JS, White RI, Mitchell SE, et al: Percutaneous balloon valvuloplasty: a new method for treating congenital pulmonary-valve stenosis. *N Engl J Med*. 307:540–542, 1982.

2. Inoue K, Owaki T, Nakamura T, et al: Clinical application of transvenous mitral commissurotomy by a new balloon catheter. *J Thorac Cardiovasc Surg*. 87:394–402, 1984.

3. Allen HD, Mullins CE: Results of the Valvuloplasty and Angioplasty of Congenital Anomalies Registry. *Am J Cardiol*. 65:772–774, 1990.

4. Petit J, Vahanian A, Michel P-L, et al: Percutaneous mitral valvotomy: French Cooperative Study: 114 patients. *Circulation*. 76:IV-496, 1987.

5. O'Neill WW for the Mansfield Registry Investigators: Long-term survival after percutaneous aortic balloon valvuloplasty: preliminary report of the Mansfield Scientific Registry. *Circulation*. 78:II-594, 1988.

6. McKay RG for the NHLBI Balloon Valvuloplasty Registry Coordinating Center: Clinical outcome following balloon valvuloplasty for severe aortic stenosis. *J Am Coll Cardiol*. 13:1218, 1989.

7. Block PC for the NHLBI Balloon Valvuloplasty Registry (BVR): Early results of mitral balloon valvuloplasty (MBV) for mitral stenosis: report from the NHLBI Registry. *Circulation*. 78:II-489, 1988.

8. O'Neill WW: Seminar on balloon aortic valvuloplasty, I: introduction. *J Am Coll Cardiol*. 17:187–188, 1991.

9. Stanger P, Cassidy SC, Girod DA, et al: Balloon pulmonary valvuloplasty: results of the Valvuloplasty and Angioplasty of Congenital Anomalies Registry. *Am J Cardiol*. 65:775–783, 1990.

10. Barraud P, de Guise P, Kratz K, et al: Adult balloon pulmonary valvuloplasty: immediate and long term results. *J Am Coll Cardiol*. 17:298A, 1991.

11. O'Connor BK, Beekman RH, Snider AR, et al: Late outcome after pulmonary balloon valvuloplasty: comparison to a matched surgical control group. *J Am Coll Cardiol*. 17:154A, 1991.

12. McCrindle BW, Kan JS: Long-term results after balloon pulmonary valvuloplasty. *Circulation*. 83:1915–1922, 1991.

13. Sreeram N, Saleem M, Jackson M, et al: Results of balloon pulmonary valvuloplasty as a palliative procedure in tetralogy of Fallot. *J Am Coll Cardiol*. 18:159–165, 1991.

14. Kirklin JW: Percutaneous balloon versus surgical closed commissurotomy for mitral stenosis. *Circulation*. 83:1450–1451, 1991.

15. Arora R, Nair M, Rajagopal S, et al: Percutaneous balloon mitral valvuloplasty in children and young adults with rheumatic mitral stenosis. *Am Heart J*. 118:883–887, 1989.

16. Cheng TO: Percutaneous balloon mitral valvoplasty for young patients with rheumatic mitral stenosis. *Int J Cardiol*. 33:339, 1991.

17. Berland J, Rath PC, Rocha P, et al: Balloon mitral valvotomy in patients above 40 years of age: immediate results and 2 years' follow up. *J Am Coll Cardiol*. 17:339A, 1991.

18. Shaw TRD, Elder AT, Flapan AD, et al: Mitral balloon valvuloplasty for patients aged over 70 years: an alternative to surgical treatment. *Age and Aging* 20:299–303, 1991.

19. Lefevre T, Bonan R, Serra A, et al: Percutaneous mitral valvuloplasty in surgical high risk patients. *J Am Coll Cardiol.* 17:348–354, 1991.

20. McKay CR: Should patients with mitral stenosis who are acceptable surgical commissurotomy candidates now have balloon valvuloplasty treatment? *Cardiovasc Clin.* 21(1):175–195,1990.

21. Turi ZG, Reyes VP, Raju S, et al: Percutaneous balloon versus surgical closed commissurotomy for mitral stenosis. A prospective, randomized trial. *Circulation.* 83:1179–1185, 1991.

22. Hickey MSJ, Blackstone EH, Kirklin JW, et al: Outcome probabilities and life history after surgical mitral commissurotomy: implications for balloon commissurotomy. *J Am Coll Cardiol.* 17:29–42, 1991.

23. Chen CR, Hu SW, Chen JY, et al: Percutaneous mitral valvuloplasty with a single rubber-nylon balloon (Inoue balloon): long-term results in 71 patients. *Am Heart J.* 120:561–568, 1990.

24. Chen CR, Chen JY, Zhou YL, et al; Long term results of percutaneous balloon mitral valvuloplasty by Inoue Balloon catheter technique, *J Am Coll Cardiol.* in press for March, 1992.

25. Hung JS, Chern MS, Wu JJ, et al: Short- and long-term results of catheter balloon percutaneous transvenous mitral commissurotomy. *Am J Cardiol.* 67:854–862, 1991.

26. Block PC, Tuzcu EM, Palacios IF: Two-year follow-up of percutaneous mitral valvotomy (PMV): cardiac catheterization; echocardiography; and clinical status. *J Am Coll Cardiol.* 17:340A, 1991.

27. Cheng TO: Improvement in cardiopulmonary function in mitral stenosis after percutaneous balloon mitral valvuloplasty. *Chest.* 100:295, 1991.

28. Shim WH, Jang YS, Cho SY, et al: Comparison of outcome between double and Inoue balloon techniques for percutaneous mitral valvuloplasty – single blind randomized prospective study. *J Am Coll Cardiol.* 17:83A, 1991.

29. Park S-J, Lee SJK, Kim JJ, et al: Percutaneous mitral balloon valvotomy using Inoue and double balloon technique (randomized trial): mechanism of dilation, immediate results and follow-up. *J Am Coll Cardiol.* 27:340A, 1991.

30. Natarajan D, Sharma VP, Sharma SC: Percutaneous mitral valvotomy with Inoue catheter in young patients of mitral stenosis. *Am Heart J.* (in press)123: (February), 1992.

31. Bassand J-P, Schiele F, Bernard Y, et al: The double-balloon and Inoue techniques in percutaneous mitral valvuloplasty: comparative results in a series of 232 cases. *J Am Coll Cardiol.* 18:982–989, 1991.

32. Benit E, Glazier JJ: Percutaneous balloon mitral valvuloplasty: Inoue balloon vs double balloon technique-Answer. Acta Cardiol 46:494, 1991.

33. Macaya C, Colman T, F-Ortiz A, et al: Percutaneous mitral valvotomy with the Inoue balloon catheter in a Western population. *Eur Heart J* 12 (Abstract Supplement): 47, 1991.

34. Patel JJ, Mitha AS, Hassen F, et al: Balloon mitral valvuloplasty: single catheter technique comparing bifoil/trefoil and Inoue balloons. *J Am Coll Cardiol.* 17:82A, 1991.

35. Ribeiro PA, Fawzy ME, Arafat MA, et al: Comparison of mitral valve area results of balloon mitral valvotomy using the Inoue and double balloon techniques. *Am J Cardiol.* 68:687–688, 1991.

36. Nishimura RA, Holmes DR Jr, Reeder GS: Efficacy of percutaneous mitral balloon valvuloplasty with the Inoue balloon. *Mayo Clin Proc.* 66:276–282, 1991.

37. Cheng TO: Single Inoue balloon catheter vs double Mansfield balloon catheter techniques in percutaneous balloon mitral valvuloplasty. *Am J Cardiol.* in press for 1992.

38. Vahanian A, Michel PL, Cormier B, et al: Mitral valvuloplasty: the French experience. In:

Topol EJ. *Textbook of Interventional Cardiology*. Philadelphia: WB Saunders Co, 1990, 868–886.

39. Plante S, van den Brand M, van Veen LCP, et al: Aortic valvuloplasty of calcific aortic stenosis with monofoil and trefoil balloon catheters: practical considerations. An evaluation of balloon design and valvular morphology relationship, derived from experimental and clinicopathological observations. *Int J Cardiac Imaging*. 5:249–260, 1990.

40. Rocchini AP, Beekman RH, Shachar GB, et al: Balloon aortic valvuloplasty: results of the Valvuloplasty and Angioplasty of Congenital Anomalies Registry. *Am J Cardiol*. 65:784–789, 1990.

41. Meliones JN, Beekman RH, Rocchini AP, et al: Balloon valvuloplasty for recurrent aortic stenosis after surgical valvotomy in childhood: immediate and follow-up studies. *J Am Coll Cardiol*. 13:1106–1110, 1989.

42. McKay RG for the Mansfield Scientific Aortic Valvuloplasty Registry Investigators: The Mansfield Scientific Aortic Valvuloplasty Registry: overview of acute hemodynamic results and procedural complications. *J Am Coll Cardiol*. 17:485–491, 1991.

43. Reeder GS, Nishimura RA, Holmes DR Jr, et al: Patient age and results of balloon aortic valvuloplasty: the Mansfield Scientific Registry experience. *J Am Coll Cardiol*. 17:909–913, 1991.

44 O'Neill WW for the Mansfield Scientific Aortic Valvuloplasty Registry Investigators: Predictors of long-term survival after percutaneous aortic valvuloplasty: report of the Mansfield Scientific Balloon Aortic Valvuloplasty Registry. *J Am Coll Cardiol*. 17:193–198, 1991.

45. Nishimura RA, Holmes DR Jr, Michela MA, et al: Follow-up of patients with low output, low gradient hemodynamics after percutaneous balloon aortic valvuloplasty: the Mansfield Scientific Aortic Valvuloplasty Registry. *J Am Coll Cardiol*. 17:828–833, 1991.

46. Cribier A, Letac B: Percutaneous balloon aortic valvuloplasty in adults with calcific aortic stenosis. *Curr Opin Cardiol*. 6:212–218, 1991.

47. Ribeiro PA, Al Zaibag M, Idris MT: Percutaneous double balloon tricuspid valvotomy for severe tricuspid stenosis: 3-year follow-up study. *Eur Heart J*. 11:1109–1112, 1990.

48. McKay RG, Grossman W: Balloon valvuloplasty. In: Grossman W, Baim DS. *Cardiac Catheterization, Angiography and Intervention*. 4th ed, Philadelphia:Lea & Febiger, 1991, pp 511–533.

49. Chen CR, Lo ZX, Huang ZD, et al: Concurrent percutaneous balloon valvuloplasty for combined tricuspid and pulmonic stenoses. *Cathet Cardiovasc Diagn*. 15:55–60, 1988.

50. Lokhandwala YY, Rajani RM, Dalvi BV, et al: Successful balloon valvotomy in isolated congenital tricuspid stenosis. *Cardiovasc Intervent Radiol*. 13:354–356, 1990.

51. Mullins PA, Hall JA, Shapiro LM: Balloon dilatation of tricuspid stenosis caused by carcinoid heart disease. *Br Heart J*. 63:249–250, 1990.

52. Cheng TO: Nonsurgical treatment of carcinoid heart disease. *Ann Thorac Surg*. 51:1046, 1991.

53. Fellows KE, Radtke W, Keane JF, et al: Acute complications of catheter therapy for congenital heart disease. *Am J Cardiol*. 60:679–683, 1987.

54. Waldman JD, Schoen FJ, Kirkpatrick SE, et al: Balloon dilatation of porcine bioprosthetic valves in the pulmonary position. *Circulation*. 76:109–114, 1987.

55. Calvo OL, Sobrino N, Gamallo C, et al: Balloon percutaneous valvuloplasty for stenotic bioprosthetic valves in the mitral position. *Am J Cardiol*. 60:736–737, 1987.

56. Fields CD, Isner JM: Balloon valvuloplasty in adults. *Cardiol Clin*. 6:383–419, 1988.

57. McKay CR, Waller BF, Hong R, et al: Problems encountered with catheter balloon valvuloplasty of bioprosthetic aortic valves. *Am Heart J*. 115:463–465, 1988.

58. Babic UU, Grujicic S, Vucinic M: Balloon valvoplasty of mitral bioprosthesis. *Int J Cardiol*. 30:230–232, 1991.

59. Greenberg MA, Menegus MA, Issenberg H, et al: Advances in interventional cardiology: endomyocardial biopsy, valvuloplasty, and pediatric interventional cardiology. *Curr Opin Radiol*. 2:616–627, 1990.

60. Waldmann JD, Lamberti JJ, Schoen FJ, et al: Balloon dilatation of stenotic right ventricle-to-pulmonary artery conduits. *J Cardiac Surg*. 3:539–546, 1988.

61. Ensing GJ, Hagler DJ, Seward JB, et al: Caveats of balloon dilation of conduits and conduit valves. *J Am Coll Cardiol*. 14:397–400, 1989.

62. Zeevi B, Keane JF, Perry SB, et al: Balloon dilation of postoperative right ventricular outflow obstructions. *J Am Coll Cardiol*. 14:401–408, 1989.

63. Cheng TO: Multivalve percutaneous balloon valvuloplasty. *Cathet Cardiovasc Diagn*. 16:109–112, 1989.

64. Block PC, Palacios IF: Aortic and mitral balloon valvuloplasty: the United States experience. In: Topol EJ. *Textbook of Interventional Cardiology*. Philadelphia: WB Saunders Co, 1990, pp 831–832.

65. Palacios IF, Tuzcu M, Ziskind AA, et al: Percutaneous balloon pericardial window for patients with malignant pericardial effusion and tamponade. *Cathet Cardiovasc Diagn*. 22:244–249, 1991.

66. Tynan M, Finley JP, Fontes V, et al: Balloon angioplasty for the treatment of native coarctation: results of Valvuloplasty and Angioplasty of Congential Anomalies Registry. *Am J Cardiol*. 65:790–792, 1990.

67. Cheng TO: Balloon angioplasty of aortic coarctation. *Ann Thorac Surg*. 52:581, 1991.

68. Mullins CE, Latson LA, Neches WH, et al: Balloon dilation of miscellaneous lesions: results of Valvuloplasty and Angioplasty of Congenital Anomalies Registry. *Am J Cardiol*. 65:802–803, 1990.

69. Grace AA, Sutters M, Schofield PM: Balloon dilatation of pacemaker induced stenosis of the superior vena cava. *Br Heart J*. 65:225–226, 1991.

70. Cheng TO: Membranotomy for Budd-Chiari syndrome. *Ann Thorac Surg*. 51:522–523, 1991.

71. Yang XL, Chen CR, Cheng TO: Nonoperative treatment of membranous obstruction of inferior vena cava by percutaneous balloon transluminal angioplasty. *Circulation*. 82 (supp II): II–27, 1991.

72. Perloff JK, Child JS: *Congenital Heart Disease in Adults*. Philadelphia: WB Saunders Co, 1991, p 227.

73. Rao PS, Chopra PS: Role of balloon angioplasty in the treatment of aortic coarctation. *Ann Thorac Surg*. 52:621–631, 1991.

74. Pinzon JL, Burrows PE, Benson LN, et al: Repair of coarctation of the aorta in children: postoperative morphology. *Radiology*. 180:199–203, 1991.

75. Cheng TO: Aneurysm formation following surgical repair of coarctation of aorta. *Radiology*. 181:905, 1991.

76. Corwin RD, Singh AK, Karlson KE: Balloon dilatation of ductus arteriosus in a newborn with interrupted aortic arch and ventricular septal defect. *Am Heart J*. 102:446–447, 1981.

77. Suarez de Lezo J, Lopez-Rubio F, Guzman J, et al: Percutaneous transluminal angioplasty of stenotic ductus arteriosus. *Cathet Cardiovasc Diagn*. 11:493–500, 1985.

78. Gundry SR, Brinkley J, Wolk M, et al: Percutaneous cardiopulmonary bypass to support angioplasty and valvuloplasty. *Trans Am Soc Artif Intern Organs*. 35:725–727, 1989.

79. Tommaso CL: Use of percutaneously inserted cardiopulmonary bypass in the cardiac catheterization laboratory. *Cathet Cardiovasc Diagn*. 20:32–38, 1990.

80. Shawl FA, Domanski MJ, Wish MH, et al: Percutaneous cardiopulmonary bypass support

in the catheterization laboratory: technique and complications. *Am Heart J.* 120:195–203, 1990.

81. Shawl FA, Domanski MJ, Yackee JM, et al: Left ventricular rupture complicating percutaneous mitral commissurotomy: salvage using percutaneous cardiopulmonary bypass support. *Cathet Cardiovasc Diagn.* 21:26–27, 1990.

82. Cheng TO: Left ventricular perforation following percutaneous balloon mitral valvuloplasty. *Can J Cardiol.* 7(4):XI, 1991.

83. Aaron BL, Alyono D: Ventricular perforation with valvoplasty. *Ann Thorac Surg.* 50:1022, 1990.

84. Isner JM, Clark RH, Pandian NG, et al: Laser myoplasty for hypertrophic cardiomyopathy. In vitro experience in human postmortem hearts and in vivo experience in a canine model (transarterial) and human patient (intraoperative). *Am J Cardiol.* 53:1620–1625, 1984.

85. Qureshi SA, Parsons JM, Tynan M: Percutaneous transcatheter myectomy of subvalvar pulmonary stenosis in tetralogy of Fallot: a new palliative technique with an atherectomy catheter. *Br Heart J.* 64:163–165, 1990.

86. Uchida Y, Nakamura F, Kido H, et al: Percutaneous cardiomyotomy and valvulotomy with angioscopic guidance. *Am Heart J.* 121:1221–1224, 1991.

87. Spears JR, Reyes VP, Wynne J, et al: Percutaneous coronary laser balloon angioplasty: initial results of a multicenter experience. *J Am Coll Cardiol.* 16:293–303, 1990.

88. Spears JR, Reyes VP, McMath LP, et al: Laser balloon angioplasty: current results and future directions. *Lasers Surg Med.* 3(suppl):17, 1991.

89. Riemenschneider TA, Lee G, Ikeda RM, et al: Laser irradiation of congenital heart disease: potential for palliation and correction of intracardiac and intravascular defects. *Am Heart J.* 106:1389–1393, 1983.

90. Parsons JM, Rees MR, Gibbs JL: Percutaneous laser valvotomy with balloon dilatation of the pulmonary valve as primary treatment for pulmonary atresia. *Br Heart J.* 66:36–38, 1991.

91. Baim DS: Intracoronary stenting – hope or hype? *Mayo Clin Proc.* 66:332–335, 1991.

92. Mullins CE, O'Laughlin MP, Vick GW III, et al: Implantation of balloon-expandable intravascular grafts by catheterization in pulmonary arteries and systemic veins. *Circulation.* 77:188–199, 1988.

93. Almagor Y, Prevosti LG, Bartorelli AL, et al: Balloon expandable stent implantation in stenotic right heart valved conduits. *J Am Coll Cardiol.* 16:1310–1314, 1990.

94. O'Laughlin MP, Perry SB, Lock JE, et al: Use of endovascular stents in congenital heart disease. *Circulation.* 83:1923–1939, 1991.

95. Wilson BH, Splinter R, Marroum M-C, et al: Laser valvuloplasty of calcified aortic valves: a comparison of continuous wave and pulsed lasers. *Circulation.* 82:III-79, 1990.

96. Mindich BP, Guarino T, Krenz H, et al: Aortic valve salvage utilizing high frequency vibrating debridement. *J Am Coll Cardiol.* 11:3A, 1988.

97. Freeman WK, Schaff HV, King M, et al: Ultrasonic aortic valve decalcification: Doppler echocardiographic evaluation. *J Am Coll Cardiol.* 11:229A, 1988.

98. Freeman WK, Schaff HV, Orszulak TA, et al: Ultrasonic aortic valve decalcification: serial Doppler echocardiographic follow-up. *J Am Coll Cardiol.* 16:623–630, 1990.

99. Schwinger ME, Colvin S, Harty S, et al: Clinical evaluation of high-frequency (ultrasonic) mechanical debridement in the surgical treatment of calcific aortic stenosis. *Am Heart J.* 120:1320–1325, 1990.

100. Nakano S, Mitsuno M, Taniguchi K, et al: Ultrasonic debridement during mitral valve reconstruction for calcified mitral stenosis. *Ann Thorac Surg.* 50:923–926, 1990.

101. Nowak B, Baykut D, Kaltenbach M, et al: Usefulness of shock wave lithotripsy as

pretreatment for balloon valvuloplasty in calcific mitral stenosis. *Am J Cardiol.* 63:996–997, 1989.

102. Rashkind WJ, Miller WW: Creation of an atrial septal defect without thoracotomy. A palliative approach to complete transposition of the great arteries. *JAMA.* 196:991–992, 1966.

103. Ritter SB: Balloon dilation: recession or inflation. *J Am Coll Cardiol.* 14:409–412, 1989.

104. Harrison JK, Sheikh KH, Davidson CJ, et al: Balloon angioplasty of coarctation of the aorta evaluated with intravascular ultrasound imaging. *J Am Coll Cardiol.* 15:906–909, 1990.

105. Bashore TM, Davidson CJ: *Percutaneous Balloon Valvuloplasty And Related Techniques.* Baltimore: Williams & Wilkins, 1991, p 332.

106. Maxwell D, Allan L, Tynan MJ: Balloon dilatation of the aortic valve in the fetus: a report of two cases. *Br Heart J.* 65:256–258, 1991.

107. Beitzke A, Stein JI, Suppan C: Balloon atrial septostomy under two-dimensional echocardiographic control. *Int J Cardiol.* 30:33–42, 1991.

108. Idriss FS, Paul MH: Arterial switch repair for transposition of the great arteries: historical overview. *Cardiac Surg.* 5:1–5, 1991.

Index

Page numbers followed by (f) indicate figure; page numbers followed by (t) indicate table.